Public Health Behind Bars

From Prisons to Communities

Public Health Behind Bars

From Prisons to Communities

Edited by

Robert B. Greifinger

John Jay College of Criminal Justice CUNY
New York, New York, USA

Deputy Editors

Joseph Bick

University of California,
Davis, California, USA

Joe Goldenson

Department of Public Health,
San Francisco, California, USA

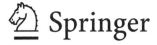 Springer

Robert B. Greifinger
John Jay College of Criminal Justice
32 Parkway Drive
Dobbs Ferry, New York 10522
USA
robert.greifinger@verizon.net

Library of Congress Control Number: 2007925690

ISBN 978-0-387-71694-7 (Hardbound)
ISBN 978-0-387-71695-4 (eBook)

Printed on acid-free paper.

9 8 7 6 5 4 3 2 1

springer.com

Foreword

America's health care system is failing those who are incarcerated. As Assistant Secretary for Health and the United States Surgeon General from 1998 to 2002, I had the opportunity to lead in the development of Healthy People 2010, a comprehensive, nationwide health promotion and disease prevention agenda to improve the health of all people in the United States during the first decade of the 21st century. Healthy People 2010's overarching goals are to increase the quality and years of healthy life and eliminate racial and ethnic health disparities. In America, we have gained over 30 years in life expectancy in the last century, from 47 years in 1900 to 77.6 years in 2003. Yet as we move closer to the year 2010, major disparities in health status and health outcomes still exist between African Americans and other racial and ethnic minorities when compared to whites.

There are factors called determinants of health that affect whether people are healthy or not. They include the social and economic environment, the physical environment, individual behavior and genetics, gender, policies and interventions, and access to quality health care. Health conditions, both mental and physical, are exacerbated by lifestyle. Many people (more men than women, more blacks than whites) who are poor, uneducated, and unemployed find themselves caught up in the criminal justice system and incarcerated. African-American men and other men of color have been incarcerated at rates disproportionate to their representation in the general population.

During my tenure as director of the Centers for Disease Control and Prevention (1993-1998), there was a concerted and major focus on correctional health care. This resulted in corrections-specific studies and recommendations for a variety of conditions prevalent among inmates. Correctional health care is now recognized as an important part of public health care. There are standards for correctional facilities and facilities can become accredited for meeting these standards. Correctional health care standards represent basic minimum standards. Correctional health professionals can become certified on these standards. However, there are still too many jails, prisons, and juvenile confinement facilities that do not meet these standards. They operate under their own set of rules.

Indeed, the current system is not serving people very well when they are in jails and prisons. The current system does far too little to ensure that people return to mainstream society in good health. Too often, health problems that remain unaddressed during confinement lead people back to jail after release. We all know that America's prison health system is in need of correction!

This book, *Improving Public Health through Correctional Health Care* takes a comprehensive look at factors that impact correctional health care and the related implications for public health and public health policy. It discusses the impact of public policy on correctional populations. Keeping in mind that the United States of America leads the world in the percentage of its population that is incarcerated, the book grapples with whether crime in our communities is diminished by incarcerating more and more people and whether health care behind bars could improve the health status of our communities. Special concerns arise when there are prisoners with physical or mental disabilities and others who are simply growing old. Basic oral health care has its own unique set of implications.

Inmates have a high prevalence of communicable and chronic diseases. Infection rates with hepatitis and HIV are more than 10 times those found in the general population. This book discusses the prevention and early detection of communicable and chronic diseases and how to reduce transmission in the communities to which these prisoners return.

Far too many people enter our criminal justice system due to an untreated or under-treated mental illness. Too often, we find our prison system substituting for the mental health care once provided in mental hospitals and other medical settings. It is estimated that one in six people in the correctional system lives with a serious mental illness. Compounding the problem is the co-occurrence of mental illness and substance abuse. *Improving Public Health through Correctional Health* Care leaves no stone unturned in its presentation and analysis of problems in correctional health.

Many of us have blinders on when it comes to the criminal justice system and those who "commit crimes." We just want these people out of our neighborhoods and communities. The belief is that once they are "put away" we will not have to worry about them anymore and our communities will be more secure, if not safe. Many people are not aware of, or have not thought about, incarceration in the context of what it means to their health and the health of their families.

The reality is that most inmates get out of jails and prisons and return to their communities. In fact, more than 95 percent of people living in prison will be released. Releasing people back into the community, without adequate identification and treatment of communicable diseases and mental disorders, and without a plan for follow-up and continued treatment, has a tremendous detrimental impact on communities, families, and individuals. So ensuring they are healthy upon release will benefit all of us.

In the section "Thinking Forward to Reentry—Reducing Barriers/Community Linkages," the authors discuss both the opportunities and challenges of making the transition from incarceration back to communities successful, for both the ex-inmate and the community to which the inmate returns.

Inmates and ex-inmates are part of the communities we live in. What happens to them is vital to the health of the community and to the public health. For all of these reasons and more, the public health implications of criminal justice policy is significant to our nation. We must never forget that regardless of reasons for incarceration, we are still dealing with fellow human beings.

For those of you who are unfamiliar or vaguely familiar with the challenges faced by the correctional health care system, *Improving Public Health through Correctional Health Care* provides an excellent introduction. It identifies problems; asks the hard questions; and offers viable solutions. The book puts a human face on people who are incarcerated and begs us to consider that they are still a part of us and our communities. Knowing this, we must persist in our efforts to improve the health of the incarcerated as we strive to improve the health of all Americans. *Improving Public Health through Correctional Health Care* is a must read for those who care and want to make a difference. It should educate, motivate, and mobilize every one who reads it.

David Satcher, MD, PhD
16th U.S. Surgeon General
Morehouse School of Medicine

Preface

This is a book of *what ifs*. What if we discovered a vast and untapped resource, a resource that could yield improved population health status and lower social costs? What if we could harness the energy in this mine toward public health benefit? What if this lode was right before our eyes and easier to tap than nutrition, exercise, air quality and global climate change? This book is a map to the mother lode of correctional health care.

Although it hasn't been kept as a secret, this mother lode has been hidden from public consciousness. What does it take to unlock the gates and find the rich veins of potential public health benefits? I have spent 20 years on this quest. Communication is an ongoing challenge in public health and medical care. To my knowledge, there has been no book written about the nexus of public health and criminal justice, until now.

Two years ago, in a fit of introspection, I began to think of how to leave a legacy. I asked myself how I could catalogue the public health opportunities that can be seized through medical care behind bars. "Would it make any difference?" I thought. "Of course it would make a difference," I said. All I had to do was to find the right prism through which others could see how to make this difference.

As a result of my internal dialogue, I took yet another turn in my professional direction. I enhanced my voice in public policy discussions, published more articles in journals, joined the faculty at John Jay College of Criminal Justice, and focused on trying to find a few novitiates in correctional medicine to mentor. Next, I got a call from Springer in the spring of 2006 asking me if I might be interested in editing a text at the nexus of criminal justice and public health. It took me about ten seconds to decide. I thought about the *what ifs* and was awestruck with the possibilities.

Who would be the audience for such a work? Public policy makers? Correctional administrators? Correctional health care practitioners? Inmate and patient advocates? Lawyers? Educators? Students? Public health scholars and practitioners? The answer was "yes" to each of these.

This text is the product of thinking about the *what ifs* and *for whom*. It is intended to be a guide to the mother lode of resources, resources that are untapped because of ignorance, attitudinal bias, and misallocated public resources. Through the prism of public health and public policy this book explores prevention opportunities in the criminal justice system and reentry process.

I hope the readers find answers to the following question: *as a rational society, what can we do for public benefit through attention to our captive population, a population that is disproportionately minority, under-educated, with a high burden of risk and illness?* Most of this burden of risk and illness is amenable to amelioration or remedy, if not cure. The book is about how we identify opportunities and how we can craft remedies that work toward improving the health of our free-world communities, the communities to which most prisoners return.

Alas (I might get away with using this word in the preface), this book is broad in scope, too broad for me to have written it myself. And why should I try, with so many experts who were eager to write a chapter within their expertise? We included the traditional categorical attention to communicable disease and we attend more broadly to prevention in a population at risk for, or with extant, dental, mental, addiction, age, and gender related illness. And this population is a captive one. The book addresses using the law to promote prisoner health care, information technology, international comparisons, innovative programs and research opportunities.

But the book is incomplete. We publish it without hubris. There is a paucity of research on efficacy with captive populations. Should we succeed with this venture, the next edition of this book should have sections on preventing transmission of skin infections, sanitation, performance measurement, outcome studies, cost-effectiveness, analyses of the effects of regulation, and more: How do we teach states and counties to specify intended outcomes for their correctional health programs? How do we measure and report health outcomes of interventions behind bars? How can we learn from our botches and mishaps? What are the pitfalls of various interventions? What do we need to know and how do we develop the resources to find out? Perhaps we will address these topics in the next edition or a Volume II.

As in other human work, there must be errors and omissions in ours. I apologize, in advance, and I invite constructive criticism to make subsequent editions more provocative and helpful.

So many people inspired me toward my work behind bars, some of them unknowingly. My mentors include some notables in public health and criminal justice; I am indebted to David Axelrod, Martin Cherkasky, Nancy Dubler, Richard Grossman, David Jones, Ross Kessel, Victor Sidel, Steve Spencer, Jeremy Travis and Harold Wise, among others. I am especially honored that David Satcher agreed to write the foreword. If I may borrow from the 2007 vernacular of youth, I *so appreciate* my editors at Springer, Khristine Queja and Bill Tucker for giving me opportunity, guidance and latitude. I thank the associate editors of this text, Joe Bick and Joe Goldenson, for turning their brains and hearts toward this work. Forty-nine authors contributed to this book, without tangible compensation. They did the most work and I applaud them foremost, although several of these authors managed to shake my equanimity with their tardiness, wreathing me with anxiety at times. Many of the academic authors are new colleagues for me. I appreciate their thoughtfulness, provocative analysis and responsiveness. The practitioners among the authors, those who work behind bars, labored the hardest. Although less experienced as writers, their voice is critical because of their exposure over time to the real world of medicine behind bars.

I've had substantial support from my wide-range of clients and colleagues in correctional medicine. While they go un-named, they are each appreciated, individually. You know who you are. Never wavering, my strongest support and inspiration comes from my nuclear family, Maura Bluestone, Rena Greifinger and Liza Greifinger.

Robert B. Greifinger
February 8, 2007

Contents

Section 2: Communicable Disease

Section 3: Primary and Secondary Prevention

Contributors

Rita Abraldes, MA
Independent Researcher, San Francisco, CA

Frederick L. Altice, MD
Yale University AIDS Program, New Haven, CT

Andrea F. Balis, PhD
John Jay College of Criminal Justice CUNY, New York, NY

Traci N. Bethea, MPA
Boston University School of Public Health, Boston, MA

Nicole M. Bekman, MA
Department of Mental Health Law and Policy, Louis de la Parte, Florida Mental Health Institute, University of South Florida, Tampa, FL

Joseph A. Bick, MD
California Department of Corrections and Rehabilitation, University of California, Davis, CA

Gail A. Bolan, MD
STD Control Branch, State of California Department of Health Services, Richmond, CA

R. Douglas Bruce, MD, MA
Yale University AIDS Program, New Haven, CT

Todd R. Clear, PhD
John Jay College of Criminal Justice, The City University of New York, New York, NY

Kaiyti Duffy, MPH
Physicians for Reproductive Choice and Health®, New York, NY

Nicholas Freudenberg, DrPH
Hunter College, City University of New York, New York, NY

Nicholas Freudenberg, DrPH
Distinguished Professor of Urban Public Health, Hunter College, City University of New York, New York, NY

Marshall W. Fordyce, MD
Department of Medicine, New York University, New York, NY

Richard L. Grant, MD
University of Illinois School of Medicine at Peoria, Peoria, IL

Robert B. Greifinger, MD
John Jay College of Criminal Justice, CUNY, NY, NY

Lindsay M. Hayes, MS
National Center on Institutions and Alternatives, Mansfield, MA

Mark Heath, MD
Department of Anesthesiology, Columbia University, New York, NY

Karen A. Hennessey, PhD, MSPH
Division of Viral Hepatitis, US Centers for Disease Control and Prevention, Atlanta, GA

Steven K. Hoge, MD
Bellevue Hospital Center, New York, NY

Charlotte K. Kent, PhD
STD Prevention and Control Services, San Francisco Department of Public Health, San Francisco, CA

Joshua D. Lee, MD, MS
Division of General Internal Medicine, New York University, New York, NY

Michael Levy, MD
School of Public Health, University of Sydney Victorian Institute of Forensic Medicine, Monash University, Australia

Thomas Lincoln, MD
Baystate Brightwood Health Center, Springfield, MA

Kamala Mallik-Kane, MPH
The Urban Institute, Washington, DC

Jeff Mellow, PhD
Department of Law, Police Science & CJ Administration, John Jay College of Criminal Justice, New York, NY 10019

John R. Miles, MPA
Baystate Brightwood Health Center, Springfield, MA

Mary E. Northridge, PhD, MPH
Mailman School of Public Health, New York, NY

Farah M. Parvez, MD
Division of Tuberculosis Elimination, Centers for Disease Control and Prevention, Atlanta, GA

Raymond F. Patterson, MD
Howard University School of Medicine, Washington, D.C.

R. Samuel Paz, JD
Loyola Law School, Culver City, CA

Roger H. Peters, PhD
Department of Mental Health Law and Policy, Louis de la Parte Florida Mental Health Institute, University of South Florida, Tampa, FL

Megha Ramaswamy, MPH
Urban Public Health at Hunter College, CUNY, New York, NY

Josiah D. Rich, MD, MPH
Brown University, The Miriam Hospital, Providence, RI

Michele Rorie, DrPH, MPA
Morehouse School of Medicine, Department of Community Health and Preventive Medicine, East Point, GA

David Satcher, MD, PhD
Morehouse School of Medicine Atlanta, GA

Steve Scheibel, MD
Community Oriented Correctional Health Services, Oakland,

Duncan Smith-Rohrberg, BA
Yale University AIDS Program, New Haven, CT

Sandra A. Springer, MD
Yale AIDS Program, Section of Infectious Diseases, Yale School of Medicine, New Haven, CT

Michelle Staples-Horne, MD, MS, MPH
Office of Health Services, Georgia Department of Juvenile Justice, Decatur, GA

Karen Terry, PhD
Criminal Justice Doctoral Program, CUNY, John Jay College of Criminal Justice, New York, NY

Henrie M. Treadwell, PhD
National Center for Primary Care, Morehouse School of Medicine, Atlanta, GA

Christy A. Visher, PhD
The Urban Institute, Washington, DC

Cindy Weinbaum, MD
Centers for Disease Control and Prevention, Atlanta, GA

Brie Williams, MD, MS
University of California School of Medicine, San Francisco, CA

Ralph P. Woodward, MD
New Jersey Department of Corrections, Blairstown, NJ

Jon Wool, JD
Vera Institute of Justice and Commission on Safety and Abuse in America's Prisons,
New York, NY (Organizations listed are solely for identification purposes)

Barry Zack, MPH
Community Health Systems at the University of California, San Francisco, CA

Chapter 1

Thirty Years Since *Estelle v. Gamble*: Looking Forward, Not Wayward

Robert B. Greifinger

How far have we come in the 31 years since the Supreme Court issued its landmark decision in *Estelle v. Gamble* (Estelle, 1976)? And how much will correctional health care develop in the next three decades? For all of these years, correctional health care has been isolated from public health and isolated further from community health care, two systems that are already remote from each other. How do we make the argument that medical care interventions behind bars have so much to do with the health of the communities to which the inmates return? How do we make the argument that public health is a piece of public safety? How easy is it to identify the barriers that prevent the application of public health and community health approaches to correctional medicine? How easy is it to break down these barriers and build bridges to enable timely access to reasonable and humane health care? Where exactly is the low-hanging fruit?

There are additional questions that need thought and analysis: how can we understand and empower correctional professionals? How can we link correctional health care with public health and community health providers? How can we increase the health literacy of public policy makers and correctional administrators?

The purpose of this book is to tackle these questions. The intent is to help develop a persuasive rationale to direct public policy toward seizing the public health opportunities that present themselves in a captive population beset by an extraordinary burden of illness. Much of this burden derives from poverty and drug abuse. This book is:

- an exploration of the next evolutionary steps in public health practice, from the perspective of the criminal justice system;
- about the implications on public health when prevention opportunities are seized behind bars;
- about reentry and the public health impact of the cycle of incarceration.

The chapters of this book are authored by some of the foremost experts in correctional health care, public health, criminal justice, and civil rights law. The objective is to outline the elements of an infrastructure for improving the health of the community through attention to prisoners' medical care. If we want to protect the public health, the time is ripe to develop public policy that takes advantage of the period of incarceration. In this introductory chapter, I will describe:

1. constitutional requirements to provide access to medical care;
2. the growing population behind bars;
3. the burden of illness in correctional populations;
4. the effects of *Estelle*;
5. eight conundrums of public policy, medical care, and public health behind bars; and
6. a preview of the later sections of the book.

Constitutional Standard: No Deliberate Indifference to Serious Medical Needs

In the United States, the legal foundation for reasonable medical care behind bars is the case of *Estelle v. Gamble*, decided by the Supreme Court in 1976. For the first time in almost 200 years, the Court codified what it called "the evolving standard of decency" for health care behind bars. The Eighth Amendment constitutional standard prohibiting cruel and unusual punishment was applied to the personal medical services provided to prisoners. Because they were deprived of their liberty, the Court ruled that it was unconstitutional to deny medically necessary care to a prisoner. The Court concluded that "deliberate indifference to serious medical needs" was the "unnecessary and wanton infliction of pain," and thereby a violation of the Eighth Amendment. In *Estelle*, the Court ruled that prisoners were entitled to:

1. access to care for diagnosis and treatment;
2. a professional medical judgment; and
3. administration of the treatment prescribed by the physician.

The same standards apply to pretrial detainees and juveniles in detention, through the due process clause in the Fourteenth Amendment (Bell, 1979).

In court, the plaintiff must first establish that a "serious medical need" was present. A good working definition for corrections should be consistent with the definition used by managed care organizations as part of their process to consider whether to approve diagnostic tests and treatments. In effect this is a community standard. A good working definition for this objective test is:

A serious medical need is defined as a valid health condition that, without timely intervention, will result in unnecessary pain, measurable deterioration in function (including organ function), death or substantial risk to the public health. (Greifinger, 2006)

"Deliberate indifference" is a trickier phrase. Nevertheless, it is a term we are stuck with. In 1994, the Supreme Court helped define the meaning of this oxymoron. The Court ruled that, although defendants did not necessarily have to show malicious intent to do harm, the plaintiff must demonstrate that the defendants knew of and disregarded the risk to the prisoner (Farmer, 1994). This is a subjective test that follows the objective test of establishing that there is a serious medical need.

Growing Inmate Population

By the end of 2004, more than 2.2 million people were behind bars in the United States, an increase of 1.9% from the previous year, but lower than the average growth during the last decade (3.2%) (Beck, 2005). This represents more than a sixfold increase compared to the incarcerated population of 325,400 in 1970 (Beck, 2000). The steady increase in the number of incarcerated individuals is attributed to harsh sentencing guidelines legislated during the 1990s (Butterfield, 2003), a time when states could afford to build more prisons. By 2003 more than half (55%) of all sentences in federal prisons were attributed to drug offenses, more than one-quarter (27%) to public-order offenses, and the rest to violent and property offenses. Among state prisons, violent crimes (51%), property (20%) and drug offenses (21%) constituted the majority of sentences in 2002 (Beck, 2005). As a result, the U.S. incarceration rate is at a historical zenith, straining corrections systems resources, particularly in health care (Federal Bureau of Prisons, 2006). The increasing size of the correctional population is compounded by the increasing costs of medical care in the United States, a more than sevenfold increase since 1980 (Kaiser, 2006). As a consequence of the increased population and rise in medical care costs, it is a difficult task to develop the resources for a socially responsible health care system for inmates, especially one that seizes public health opportunities.

Burden of Illness

As a result of poverty and drug abuse, prisoners have a uniquely high prevalence of communicable disease, including HIV/AIDS, tuberculosis, sexually transmitted diseases, and viral hepatitis B and C (NCCHC, 2002) owing in part to their drug abuse. As a result of their poverty, inmates have high rates of mental illness and chronic diseases, such as asthma, diabetes, and hypertension. Drug addiction, poor access to health care, poverty, substandard nutrition, poor housing conditions and homelessness contribute to increased morbidity from these and other debilitating conditions.

Close to 80% of chronically ill inmates have not received routine medical care prior to incarceration and are likely to have used hospital emergency rooms as their source of primary care (Davis & Pacchiana, 2004; Hammett, 1998; Conklin et al., 1998). As a group, inmates report more disabling conditions, have poorer perceptions of their health status, and have lower utilization of primary health care services than the general population. Twenty to twenty-six percent of all people living with HIV, 29 to 43% of all those infected with the hepatitis C virus, and 40% of those with active tuberculosis in the United States passed through correctional facilities during 1997 (NCCHC, 2002; Hammett et al., 1997). While the focus of correctional health care is often on the people behind bars, correctional health care interventions benefit custody staff, their families, prisoner families, and the communities to which inmates return. Correctional facilities are linked to our nation's communities through population dynamics. Virtually all return to their communities and families (Corrections, 2003; Roberts et al., 2004).

The Effects of *Estelle*

The consequence of *Estelle* and ensuing decisions on medical care for inmates has been considerable. In large part, driven by litigation based on *Estelle* and other related Court decisions, we have witnessed improvements in health care behind bars since 1976:

- Standards have evolved, such as those promulgated by the National Commission on Correctional Health Care, the Joint Commission on Accreditation of Healthcare Organizations, the American Correctional Association, and the American Public Health Association.
- Policies and practices have improved.
- There is more professionalism in correctional health care.
- Timely access to care is more the rule than the exception.
- Staff are better qualified and have better training and supervision.
- There is better continuity and coordination of care.
- Performance measurement and quality management programs have improved with increasing self-criticism.
- Oversight has increased somewhat.

In 1996, Congress passed the Prison Litigation Reform Act (PLRA, 1995), a law that restricted some of the legal remedies that had been available to prisoners through class-action litigation for injunctive relief and individual complaints for damages. But Congress opened another avenue for litigation to improve health care behind bars with the Americans with Disabilities Act (ADA, 1990), passed in 1990. In 1998, the U.S. Supreme Court ruled that the ADA applies in the prison context. Prisoners are entitled to reasonable accommodations for their disabilities under Title II of the ADA (Pennsylvania, 1998). The latter decision became a new avenue for prisoners to seek redress through the Courts.

Conundrums[1] Behind Bars

The list of improvements (above) in correctional health care is not to say that our correctional health care systems are uniformly excellent. Too often, correctional health care is compromised by strained resources, isolation, and pressures to conform to the punitive aspects of command-control environments. Too often, correctional health professionals begin to stereotype their patients and thereby distrust them. This stereotyping results in cynicism that is destructive to therapeutic relationships. And too often, there are inadequate linkages to community health care providers and public health authorities.

---

[1] In this section of the chapter, I use the term *conundrum* instead of *challenge, obstacle, barrier,* or *hurdle.* To me, these are puzzles that can be solved with rational analysis. Once the puzzles are solved, there is no detritus to bar the way.

Isolation of Correctional Health Professional from Mainstream Medicine

We have a triple system of medical care in the United States: care for the affluent in private offices and group practices; care for the poor in community health centers and hospital clinics; and care for prisoners behind bars. But at least 95% of these prisoners will return to their communities (Hughes & Wilson, 2003). The first conundrum for public policy makers to solve is how to coalesce these diverse medical care systems for better communication of medical information, access to specialty care and hospitals, and linkages for continuity of care on release.

Nexus of Correctional Medical Care with Public Health

A second conundrum is how to address the nexus of personal medical care and public health. We have learned lessons at the interface of public health and criminal justice. In the 1980s we learned about HIV and the disproportionate percentage of infected people who were behind bars. In the 1990s we learned about the prevalence and incidence of tuberculosis and the high risk of transmission in correctional facilities. And in the first decade of the twenty-first century, we are learning about viral hepatitis C and community-acquired methicillin-resistant *Staphylococcus aureus* (MRSA).

Every inmate who leaves a correctional facility with untreated sexually transmitted disease, viral hepatitis, HIV, or tuberculosis might be a source of transmission in the community. These are diseases typically addressed by public health authorities, agencies that because of their categorical funding may not have the resources to join efforts with correctional agencies. Every inmate who is treated for communicable disease behind bars reduces the risk to the public health. The community also benefits from treatment of chronic disease and mental illness behind bars, through the savings from early intervention (Freudenberg et al., 2005).

Episodic versus Primary Models of Care

A third conundrum is the archaic model of medical care in most prison and jail systems. Most facilities use what they call a "sick call" system. This episodic care is appropriate for acute illness, but it has no place in the care and treatment of patients with chronic disease and mental illness. There are nationally accepted guidelines, each with an evidence basis, for a wide variety of chronic conditions. If patients are treated according to these guidelines, including treatment plans for prisoners with special needs, there will be reduced morbidity and mortality. The reduction in morbidity is a substantial cost-saving for the communities to which inmates return because of their dependence on public resources for access to care in the community.

Integration of Care for Patients with Coexisting Illness

The fourth conundrum is the artificial walls between treatment for drug abuse and mental illness behind bars. For a variety of reasons, correctional systems typically provide medical care and drug treatment through parallel, but unrelated programs. And there is not enough drug treatment behind bars to help reduce recidivism. These are barriers to recovery for patients with coexisting illness.

Transfer of Medical Information

The fifth conundrum is the challenge of transfer of medical information between community and correctional providers. It is a cumbersome process. As a consequence, it happens infrequently. This interferes with continuity and coordination of care, putting incoming and outgoing prisoners at risk of harm.

Quality Management Systems

The sixth conundrum is the development of meaningful self-critical analysis, a process called quality management or quality improvement in community health care facilities. Very few correctional agencies have incorporated valid and reliable performance measurement into their medical care programs. As a consequence, they are unable to measure their problems and then reduce barriers to improved outcomes of care. Performance measurement with quantitative and qualitative analysis of data is an opportune way to improve care and reduce risk of harm and costly litigation. This has been amply demonstrated in the community. There is no reason why the same approach cannot be used behind bars.

Command-Control versus Collaboration

The seventh conundrum is the apparent contradiction of the command-control organizational model, so essential for safety, and the collaborative-autonomy model used in health care. For example, there are challenges to provide meaningful diagnosis and treatment for inmates who are confined in isolation for breaking facility rules, typically with disruptive behavior. Many inmates are disruptive because of mental illness. Segregation for 23 hours per day is not likely to be an effective treatment for mental illness. To the contrary, isolation is contraindicated for serious mental illness, yet correctional agencies often rely on deprivation as a way to reduce disruptive behavior. This is but one of the ongoing challenges between the command-control model of correctional facility operations and a public health model of care.

Command-control is critical to safety behind bars. It requires rigorous adherence to rules and does not easily tolerate uncertainty. Even in their most scientific modes, medicine and public health are filled with uncertainty, more uncertainty than is often tolerated in command-control environments. Physicians and other health professionals are used to managing with much more uncertainty than is often tolerated by custody staff. This creates a natural tension, even when the leadership of correctional facilities works hard both to keep a facility safe and to provide good medical care through autonomous health professionals.

Reentry—Seven Tasks

The eighth conundrum is reentry. Until recently, the responsibility of correctional agencies stopped at the gate. Recent public attention to reentry offers correctional and public health professionals the finest opportunity to make a difference, for the prisoners themselves and for the communities to which they return. But it requires a revised scope of responsibility for correctional agencies. A revised scope often means a revised budget. With increasing attention to reentry among public policy makers and correctional system leaders, social conditions are favorable for personal health care and public health practitioners to make a real difference here. This is a time and place where their advantage to our communities can shine. It is a place where correctional and public health practitioners can honor their moral duty to provide continuity of care for their patients (AMA, 2001).

Among many other risks, recently released inmates are at higher risk of death after release than people in the community, matched for age, sex, and race (Binswanger, 2007). The reentry process contributes to excess mortality relative to incarceration itself, which might have a small protective effect, especially among blacks (Mumola, 2007). In the Binswanger study, conducted in the State of Washington, the relative risk of death within 2 weeks of release was 12.7 times expected and the overall risk of death in the several years following release was 3.5 times expected, and higher among women. In the studied cohort, the most frequent causes of death were overdose, cardiovascular disease, homicide, suicide, cancer, motor vehicle accidents, and liver disease. Surely, some of this risk could be reduced by thoughtful reentry planning.

From a medical perspective, a successful reentry program has seven tasks (Mellow, 2006):

1. *Define the target population.* Of course this would include patients with incompletely treated communicable disease such as tuberculosis, HIV, skin infections, and sexually transmitted diseases. And it would include patients with acute medical conditions, such as alcohol withdrawal, organ failure (e.g., heart, kidney, or liver failure), fevers, trauma and those who are recovering from surgery, and patients with suicidal behavior and uncompensated psychosis. There are other questions that correctional programs should answer to help define the target population:
   - Will the program target patients at risk of serious illness, such as those with abnormal Pap smears, pregnancy, and abnormal laboratory tests?
   - Will the program target patients with well-compensated chronic mental illness (on medication), such as major depression, schizophrenia, bipolar disorder, posttraumatic stress syndrome, or any mental illness being treated with medication?
   - How about patients with severe chronic diseases, such as uncompensated cirrhosis, moderate or severe asthma, poorly controlled diabetes, and symptomatic coronary artery disease? Or all patients with chronic diseases, including hypertension, asthma, diabetes, stroke, arthritis, viral hepatitis and partially treated latent or active tuberculosis?
   - For a larger target, could facilities target patients with nonemergent dental or gum disease, or a history of drug and/or alcohol abuse?
   - How much medication will be supplied at release? Will the facility provide written prescriptions and an address of a pharmacy that might fill the prescriptions for impoverished patients, in addition to the medications dispensed?
   - What are the limitations on distributing certain medications at the time of release, for example, antipsychotic medication, narcotics, benzodiazepines, medication for tuberculosis?
2. *Develop formal linkages with commonly accessed community providers including public health departments, community health centers, and public or private hospitals.*

3. *Determine an individual patient's risk and eligibility for reentry services as early as the intake process.*
4. *Summarize essential information for the patient and the subsequent provider of care.*
5. *Provide medication or a combination of medication and written prescriptions.*
6. *Enable access to care on release with community providers, including an appointment and information for access to community-based organizations.*
7. *Designate staff with a clearly defined discharge planning function.*

Improving Public Health Through Correctional Health Care

With our high rates of incarceration and high burden of illness, there are social policy conundrums that go beyond the authority of correctional administrators and correctional health practitioners. Public policy makers will be dealing with increasing costs for medical care, not just because of health care inflation, but because the inmate population is aging. What is the effect of our current policies on communities? Inmates are returning to their home communities without treatment, education, skills, housing, jobs, and self-confidence. Each of these topics is covered in this book. How do we make the expense of incarceration into an investment in our communities? Who do we lock up and who can we safely divert, perhaps in a more constructive manner? How to think about the potential effect of reentry for healthier communities? And, how do we improve the health literacy of public policy makers so as to improve the public health?

Inmates are beacons of public health opportunity. It is my hope that this book will provide a sound basis for a public health perspective on criminal justice policy and operations. It should provide information for policy analysis and direction for correctional medical care programs. Beyond the introductory materials, the book is divided into five sections. Within a section, each chapter is intended to provide both scholarly analysis and practical advice for public health interventions through the criminal justice system. Although I did distinguish communicable disease prevention with its own section, readers may note that I did not separate the psychiatric chapters in their own sectional cocoon. I did this to make the point that we need to reduce the barriers created by mind–body distinctions. Illness is illness. Illness can cause functional disabilities, whether it is somatic or psychiatric.

Section One of the book is about the impact of law and public policy on correctional populations, addressing the following questions: What is the impact of criminal justice policies on communities? What are inmates' constitutional rights to timely and appropriate medical care and how has litigation driven the standard of care? What are the rights of disabled inmates and which ones are disabled? How do we compare to other countries, especially with programs to minimize harm? What are the special needs of aging inmates and has anyone considered the cost of reasonable accommodation for a rapidly aging prison population? And, how does the medicalization of lethal injection contribute to a moral dilemma for physicians and pain and suffering for the condemned inmates?

Section Two is about categorical public health. From a prevention point of view, we address how to reduce morbidity, mortality, and transmission of diseases that are highly prevalent in inmate populations: tuberculosis, viral hepatitis, HIV, and sexually transmitted disease.

Section Three is about primary and secondary prevention. What can we do to prevent disease in the first place and how can we devise programs for early detection (screening) and treatment, using evidence-based protocols? How do we prevent suicides? How can we improve the diagnosis of mental illness? Why is oral health care important? How are women's health issues different from men's health issues? How are youth different from adults behind bars?

Section Four is about tertiary prevention. For patients with established diagnoses, how do we treat them for rehabilitation and prevention of mortality and end-organ damage? In this section, because of the high prevalence among prisoners, we focus on mental illness, addictive disorders, and coexisting disease. How can we do a better job at diagnosis, treatment planning, coordinating care and managing co-occurring disorders?

Finally, Section Five is about developing a better infrastructure for reentry. How can we improve communication, especially with electronic information systems? What research needs to be done? How do we manage sexual predators? And, how can we manage reentering patients with HIV and mental illness?

Public Health Behind Bars should be a provocative guide to developing the next evolutionary steps in public policy for a better future for our communities.

References

ADA Americans with Disabilities Act, 42 U.S.C. § 12101 (1990).

AMA (American Medical Association) Code of Ethics 2001. Accessed October 20, 2006, at http://www.ama-assn.org/apps/pf_new/pf_online?f_n=resultLink&doc=policyfile s/HnE/E-8.115.HTM&s_t=continuity+of+care&catg=AMA/HnE&&nth=1&&st_ p=0&nth=12&

Beck, A.J. (2000). *Prisoners in 1999.* Washington, DC: U.S. Department of Justice, Office of Justice Programs, Bureau of Justice Statistics.

Beck, A.J. (2005). *Prisoners in 2004.* Washington, DC: U.S. Department of Justice, Office of Justice Programs, Bureau of Justice Statistics.

Bell v. Wolfish, 441 U.S. 520 (1979).

Binswanger, I.A., Stern, M.F., Deyo, R.A., et al. (2007). Return from prison—A high risk of death for former inmates. *N Engl J Med, 356*, 157–165.

Butterfield, F. (2003). Study finds 2.6% increase in U.S. prison population. *New York Times*, July 28.

Conklin, T.J., Lincoln, T., & Flanigan, T.P. (1998). A public health model to connect correctional health care with communities. *Am J Public Health, 88*, 1249–1250.

Corrections Agency Collaborations with Public Health: Special Issue in Corrections. (2003). Longmont, Co: National Institute of Corrections Information Center, U.S. Department of Justice.

Davis, L.M., & Pacchiana, S. (2004). Health profile of the state prison population and returning offenders: Public health challenges. *Journal of Correctional Health Care, 10*, 325–326.

Estelle v. Gamble, 429 U.S. 97 (1976).

Farmer v. Brennan (92–7247), 511 U.S. 825 (1994).

Federal Bureau of Prisons quick facts. (2006, September 18). Available at http://www. bop.gov/news/quick.jsp (updated monthly).

Freudenberg, N., Daniels, J., et al. (2005). Coming home from jail: The social and health consequences of community reentry for women, male adolescents, and their families and communities. *Am J Public Health*, *95*, 1725–1736.

Greifinger, R.B. (2006). Health care quality through care management. In M. Puisis (Ed.), *Clinical practice in correctional medicine*. Amsterdam: Elsevier.

Hammett, T.M. (1998). *Public health/corrections collaborations: Prevention and treatment of HIV/AIDS, STDs and TB*. National Institute of Justice and Centers for Disease Control and Prevention Research in Brief. Washington, DC: U.S. Department of Justice, Office of Justice Programs, National Institute of Justice.

Hammett, T.M., Harmon, M.P., & Rhodes, W. (2002). The burden of infectious disease among inmates of and releasees from US correctional facilities, 1997. *Am J Public Health*, *92*, 1789–1794.

Hughes, T., & Wilson, D.J. (2003). Bureau of Justice Statistics. Washington, DC: U.S. Department of Justice. Accessed October 20, 2003, at http://www.ojp.usdoj. gov/bjs/reentry/growth.htm

Kaiser Family Foundation. (2006). Trends and indicators in the changing health care marketplace. Accessed October 20, 2006, at http://www.kff.org/insurance/7031/print-sec1.cfm

Klein, S.J., et al. (2002). Building an HIV continuum for inmates: New York State's criminal justice initiative. *AIDS Educ Prev*, *14*(5 Suppl. B), 114–123.

Mellow, J., & Greifinger, R.B. (2006). Successful reentry: The perspective of private correctional health care providers. *Journal of Urban Health*, *84*, 85–98.

Mumola, C.J. (2007). *Medical causes of death in state prisons, 2001–2004*. Washington, DC: Bureau of Justice Statistics, U.S. Department of Justice (NCJ 216340).

National Commission on Correctional Health Care. (2002). *The health status of soon-to-be-released inmates: A report to Congress*. Accessed October 20, 2006, at http://www.ncchc.org/pubs/pubs_stbr.html

Pennsylvania Department of Corrections v. Yeskey, 524 U.S. 206, 212 (1998).

PLRA Prison Litigation Reform Act of 1995, 18 U.S.C. § 3626.

Roberts, C.A., Kennedy, S., & Hammett, T.M. (2004). Linkages between in-prison and community-based health services. *Journal of Correctional Health Care*, *10*, 333–368.

Section 1

Impact of Law and Public Policy on Correctional Populations

The purpose of this section of *Public Health Behind Bars* is to provide a backdrop for later chapters. This section is about the effect of law and public policy on correctional health care and public health. The chapters offer new and different public policy options to consider, focusing on the health of our communities and what the legal bases are for inmates' rights to medical care. The chapters help us ask and answer questions about what can be done through laws themselves, for example laws about sentencing, and what can be done to improve health care through litigation. This section provides a basis for dealing with the puzzles of prevention and reentry.

During the past few decades, the growth in imprisonment in the United States has been startling, both for its volume and for its concentration of poor, young men, disproportionately African-American. Todd Clear is a social scientist who looks at communities and the impact of incarceration on the people who live in them. His chapter on the impact of incarceration on community public safety and public health describes the characteristics of the home communities of prisoners and the impact of incarceration on the families and communities to which prisoners return. Professor Clear makes a compelling argument that the high incarceration rate is a direct impediment to public health and public safety. In effect, he makes a compelling argument that the imprisonment of a high proportion of community residents is a punishment for the home community as well as for the individuals.

Jon Wool, an attorney working in public policy, explains the current status of litigation as a driving force for improving health and health care for inmates. He describes the vehicles for this litigation including constitutional entitlements through the Eighth and Fourteenth Amendments, the Americans with Disabilities Act, and the Constitutional Rights of Institutionalized Persons Act. Mr. Wool also describes the barriers to legal enforcement created by the Prisoner Litigation Reform Act. Behind bars, litigation has driven constructive change for more than 30 years, yet it has been frustrating for correctional administrators and policy makers when they are the objects of these lawsuits. The author posits the value of litigation for improving medical care in prisoners.

Likewise, Sam Paz, a civil rights attorney, writes about accommodating disabilities behind bars and the legal protections that Congress awarded the disabled, including prisoners, with the passage of the Americans with Disabilities Act

(ADA). The ADA is being used increasingly in inmate litigation, for patients with either physical or mental disabilities. Mr. Paz clearly describes the rights of disabled people and the responsibilities of correctional administrators to accommodate these people.

And there will be more disabled people behind bars unless public policy changes. Brie Williams, a geriatrician, researcher, and correctional health practitioner, elucidates the elements of managing disabled inmates. Because of high incarceration rates and long sentences, the proportion of elderly inmates is increasing. Dr. Williams addresses the numbers and the potential costs for care for a larger elderly population. The cost implications for public policy makers are mind-boggling. These data scream for some sound economic analysis of the implications of the aging inmate population.

In his chapter on international public health models, Michael Levy, a public health physician who works with correctional systems, provides us with a view that we often miss, i.e., there are other ways to do things. With descriptions of harm minimization programs in jails and prisons around the world, Dr. Levy offers us a lot of ideas on how we might craft improved prevention programs behind bars and for reentry.

Mark Heath, a professor of anesthesiology, writes about the implications of the medicalization of lethal injection, currently the dominant mode of capital punishment in the United States. He explains the horror of the pain and suffering of the condemned that is caused by botched executions. Dr. Heath describes the spectacle of lethal injection and asks the reader why we are "witnessing the foreseeable and gratuitous suffering of condemned prisoners?" This is both a practical question and a moral one, so long as the execution process is medicalized with pharmaceuticals and intravenous delivery methods.

Chapter 2

Impact of Incarceration on Community Public Safety and Public Health

Todd R. Clear

The purpose of the paper is to provide data and theory to support three propositions:

- Incarceration rates have grown in concentrated ways, especially effecting poor minority males who come from impoverished neighborhoods.
- High levels of incarceration, concentrated in impoverished neighborhoods, damage the social capital of those who live there, destabilizing the capacity for informal social control.
- Reductions in informal social control have devastating consequences for public safety and public health.

The implications of this argument are that incarceration policy in the United States is an obstruction to the well-being of poor, especially minority, communities. With crime rates that have fallen nationally for about a decade, the source of growth in imprisonment is not new felons having committed dangerous crimes, but a largely inexhaustible supply of potential drug felons combined with a system that provokes high rates of failure among those who get caught up in it. This situation suggests that any chance for real reform requires changes in drug law enforcement policy.

The Growth in Incarceration Rates

In 1971, there were about 200,000 prisoners in the daily U.S. head-count. In the generation since then, we have added about 1 million people to the daily population of those in prison; counting all forms of incarceration, more than 2 million Americans are behind bars on any given day in the United States. That means that about 1.6% of all U.S. adults aged 18–50 are incarcerated. In the quarter century between 1974 and 2001, the likelihood that a U.S. citizen would go to prison sometime in his or her lifetime increased from 1.9% to 6.6% (Bonczar, 2003).

Counting probationers and parolees as people *at risk* of incarceration, there are over 6 million people for whom jail or prison time is a reality or a direct threat—an astonishing 5% of the adult population. As contrast, 7% of adults are diagnosed with serous diabetes, and 3.5% will experience potentially lethal forms of cancer.

The U.S. prison population in 1971 was high compared to other countries, but not as extreme as is the case by today's standards. Our current incarceration rate of 724 per 100,000 is the highest in the world, approached only by Russia (564), St. Kitts (539), Belarus (532), and Bermuda (532). Among Western democracies, we are an order of magnitude higher in the use of confinement: England (145), Australia (120), Canada (116), Germany (97) and France (88) all use prison at a rate that is a fraction of ours. Compared to third-world countries, we are at the top of a list that, among those making the most use of imprisonment, might not make us feel so progressive: compare our rate to the totalitarian states of Cuba (487) and China (118). Even with regard to some of the world's more despotic governments, we still lead the pack.[1] Knowing nothing else about the United States than our rate of imprisonment, an unbiased observer would be more likely to think we are an economically underdeveloped dictatorship rather that the self-proclaimed "leading voice for freedom in the world."

The United States has achieved its distinctive incarceration rate through a range of policies that have grown the penal system with little relationship to crime. The general picture is as follows: In the 1970s, the growing prison population closely mirrored increases in rates of felony crime; contrary to many predictions, the increase in imprisonment did not drive down the rate of crime. In the 1980s, however, crime first fell precipitously, then rose at a roughly equivalent rate, ending the decade about where it started. Prison populations grew annually during these shifts in crime, largely as a consequence of a reduction in the use of probation as a sentence for felony crime. In 1990, probation was the most common sentence for felony offenses. By the end of the decade, sentences to confinement outnumbered sentences to probation by a ratio of 2:1. In the early 1990s, crime rates began to fall, and did so for more than a decade. That trend appears to be ending, though it is too early to be certain. Because of declining crime, the annual number of new felony commitments to prison *also* declined. Prison populations grew nonetheless, because the amount of time served by those going to prison increased as much as 50%. [For a discussion of these three time periods, see Blumstein & Beck (2005).] Today, we have a prison population about six times larger than it was in 1971, an incarceration rate five times larger, and about the same crime rate.

It is important to emphasize how unique this prison growth is to the United States, and to accept how ingrained the prison system is in our socio-political psyche. Prisons grew in all areas of the country, under Democrat and Republican leadership, during good economic times and bad, while we were at war and during peacetime, before welfare reform and after, during the baby-boom years and after they had ended. The current stock of prisoners serving very long sentences will guarantee that prison populations will continue to grow regardless of any realistic changes in crime patterns. No other nation has this pattern of prison use. It is a peculiarly American idea to use the prison as the first-choice reaction to crime.

---

[1] Incarceration rate comparisons taken from Mauer (2005).

Impact on Human and Social Capital in Poor Communities

The growth in imprisonment is not a random social phenomenon. Rather, it concentrates itself within society in four important ways: age, gender, race, and place.[2]

Age. Confinement is disproportionately a young person's experience. Americans aged 18–44 are about two-fifths of the U.S. population, but they are more than three-quarters of the people behind bars. Young people end up in prison largely because crime is more prominent among the young. The peak age of arrest is the late teens. People rarely go to prison as a consequence of their first arrest, so it is a few years later when subsequent arrest leads to prison. The median prison stay is about 30 months (Irwin & Austin, 2006). Thus, the typical person who ends up behind bars went to prison for the first time at the age of 25 and will, by the end of his sentence, have spent a major portion of his young adulthood behind bars.

Gender. Adult men are slightly less than half of the general population, but they are more than nine-tenths of the prison population and are more than nine times more likely to end up in prison than women. Males are more prevalent in all aspects of the criminal justice system. They represent 68% of juvenile arrests, 76% of adult arrests, and 95% of prison commitments. Men end up in prison in part for the same reason young people do: they are more likely than others to be criminally active. Today 80% of men aged 18–44 are behind bars.

Race. African Americans are five times more likely to go to prison than whites, and almost twice as likely as Hispanics. Unlike age and gender data, the prominence of blacks among those who break the law is less clear. For example, blacks in high school are slightly *less* likely to report illicit drug use than whites, and victims of violent crime report that their assailants were black at a differential far less than 5:1 (Walker et al., 2004). Nonetheless, almost one-fifth of African Americans will go to prison during their lifetimes.

Place. Poor people go to prison at rates much greater than the nonpoor. In his epic study of the role of prisons in inequality, Princeton sociologist Bruce Western (2006) shows how those who enter prison are predominantly those with low human capital: undereducated, underemployed, and underskilled. Due to racial and economic segregation, those who are incarcerated tend to come in concentrated numbers from impoverished neighborhoods. Thus, some deeply poor neighborhoods in major cities have as many as one-fifth or more of their adult male residents behind bars on any given day. Of course, they cycle in and out at fairly high rates, so that over time, almost every family in some locations currently has or recently had a member in prison. In Brooklyn, high incarceration neighborhoods see one person go to prison or jail for every 8 adult males aged 18–44; in contrast, low incarceration neighborhoods send people to prison at less than one-tenth that rate. [For a detailed description of concentration by place, see Clear et al. (2005).]

The collective effect of these four types of concentration is that certain sub-groups of Americans bear the brunt of U.S. prison growth. Young black males who come from impoverished places and develop limited human capital are more

---

[2] Unless otherwise cited, data for this section are taken from various federal reports of prison population demographics (especially Bonczar, 2003), justice processing statistics, and the U.S. census.

likely to go to prison in their lifetimes (see Western, 2006). This has substantial impact on social networks, social capital, and informal social control.

Social Networks. The array of personal relationships people find themselves involved in comprises their "social network." It is upon one's social network that one relies for social support: when a problem arises, this is the set of relationships upon which a person can call for help; when opportunities are sought, the network is the cast of people whose real-world relationships are the foundation for those opportunities. Volumes have been written on social networks, much more than can be adequately reviewed here. But a few points are important to make concerning incarceration and social networks.

First, poor people—people who are likely to go to prison—tend to have social networks that are diminished in several respects. Their networks are dominated by what is called "strong ties," that is, ties that are reciprocal, to people whose networks include roughly the same array of relationships. Family members, for example, are often strong ties. They have fewer "weak ties," or relationships with people whose networks include a far different cast of relationships. We develop weak ties with many of those at our workplaces. This is important (Granovetter, 1974) because strong ties do not provide access to a new set of potential relationships, whereas weak ties do (through an important weak tie to someone in a person's network, access is given to many people in the contact's network but not in that person's network). Second, poor people's social networks tend not to span outside of their local residential area, except for family ties, which are often good examples of strong ties. Thus, when a poor person is in need of some form of social support (help with a problem, intervention with some external set of forces), poor people tend to be limited to relationships in physical proximity to where they live. Thus, poor people tend to have "thin" networks comprised dominantly of "strong" ties. Third, young men play crucial relationship-building roles in social networks—they are referred to as "entrepreneurs." They take jobs that open up employment-related social ties, they leave their local neighborhood to work and socialize, bringing outsiders into their networks and, by contact to others, into the weak ties of their families and close friends.

When young, poor black men go to prison, those who are in their social networks, especially family members, are affected in important—but largely invisible—ways. First, many family members maintain contact with a young male who has gone to prison, especially when he goes for the first time and especially if the sentence is expected to be short. This means that the energy of those who remain behind which could have been devoted to expanding and strengthening a social network is instead spent maintaining the network with the person behind bars. Since these networks were thin to begin with, the effect of the imprisonment is to further weaken them. Studies of networks find that incarceration has a small destabilizing effect, reducing the size of already depleted networks [for a discussion, see Rengifo & Waring (2006)]. The size of the network may be only part of the problem. Because young men should be contributing dynamically to the networks of those associated with them, men who are in prison constitute missing "entrepreneurs" whose absence invisibly diminishes the networks of others, not because of what they do but because of what missing men *cannot* do.

Social Capital. Social capital is the capacity a person has to obtain "goods" (support, resources, assistance, materials) through relationships with others.

Classic examples are the way parents can deal with the problems of sick children and college entrance applications. Adults with good social capital rely on friends to identify the best available medical care, or they use friendships to bring their children's applications into a positive light. Thus, social networks are the foundation for social capital. That is why weak ties are so much more valuable than strong ties—weak ties add new layers of relationships to a network that can serve as potential sources of social capital when inevitable problems come along. One way of looking at the intersection of social networks and social capital is that when a person's human capital—his or her own personal skills and abilities—and wealth are insufficient to deal with a problem in life, the resources available to one's social networks are activated though the mechanism of interpersonal relationships, and the dormant capacity of those networks is a person's social capital.

By definition, social capital is lacking in poor neighborhoods. People who live in poor places do not have many personal resources to call upon for social support, other than their immediate family and their personal capabilities. They tend to go to state supported services for help when they are in need, making use of public welfare, free counseling, and drop-in health clinics. If these services are not adequate, they often do without help.

The weakening of social networks that results from incarceration of young adults, especially men, has profound implications for social capital. This begins as social networks are affected in the way described above. This small deterioration in social networks adds up, when there is an entire community of people who are similarly affected. Each small diminishment in capacity is multiplied across family units and related networks. Most people whose social networks took a temporary "hit" would compensate by turning to others, but this is not possible in communities where networks were weak to begin with, on top of which virtually *every* network is damaged by incarceration in much the same way. The impact of incarceration becomes multiplied when it becomes ubiquitous, because the usual compensations are unavailable. The result is that state-sponsored and volunteer services grow in importance for places with limited social capital, simply as a result of the ever diminishing set of options [see Rose & Clear (1998)].

Informal Social Control. Hunter (1985) has defined three levels of social control. Public controls are operated by the state: police, courts, and prisons on the one hand; schools, welfare, and social services on the other. Parochial social controls are community-level groups that stabilize a place's community life; for example, the barbershop has historically played this role in black communities and religious institutions do the same. Private social control includes intimate interpersonal relations, most characteristically the family [for an expanded discussion, see Bursik & Grasmick (1993)]. Two important points can be made from this classification. First, these levels of social control can operate independently, but they typically are in interplay with each other to provide public safety. Second, of the three, the public safety importance of public social control pales in comparison to private and parochial levels of social control.

These can also be seen as (at least potentially) compensatory forms of social control. If private social controls are effective, there is little pressure on parochial or public social controls. When private controls fail, parochial controls can be strained, and public controls attempt to enter the breach. Without the benefit of viable private and parochial controls, public social control is challenged to provide safety for communities.

Incarceration of large numbers of adults in concentration affects both parochial and private controls. Parochial controls require enough adults to be around to participate in them. Participation is made more difficult when the adult population has limited long-term commitment to a residential area: places with high levels of outward mobility do not sustain the long term relationships that are the foundation for parochial control (Shaw & McKay, 1943) and in these places a degree of isolation develops that keeps people from interacting with one another (Skogan, 1990). Places with large numbers of adults going to prison are also places that have many single-parent families (Sabol & Lynch, 2003). The rate of adult incarceration is an indicator of the rate of deterioration in informal social control.

In this regard, the incarceration of women, although occurring in smaller numbers than men, may have impact exceeding the sheer question of numbers. Women play crucial roles in poor, especially black, communities. They provide the stability that makes parochial social control possible (in particular, churches and religious institutions) and they are the main providers of child socialization and childcare. Their ability to perform functions of informal social control is impeded when men are absent, because they have to concentrate their energies on filling in the missing functions men might have performed. They provide none of this social control when they themselves are behind bars.

Public Safety and Public Health Outcomes

There are good reasons, then, to believe that high rates of incarceration, concentrated in impoverished residential areas, will have negative impact on the health and safety of those areas. Studies of this question are mixed, but tend to bear this out.

Health Outcomes. Several studies have investigated the relationship between incarceration and health. The most direct impact has been documented for STDs. Johnson and Raphael (2005) have shown that the disparity in HIV rates between black and white *women* closely parallels the disparity in incarceration rates between black and white *men*. They speculate that the cause is the higher rate of HIV infection transmission that occurs in prison, and the resulting community-based transmission of the disease after men are released from prison. But epidemiologist James Thomas, of the University of North Carolina, has a different explanation. He has argued that the *removal* of large numbers of men provides the explanation for higher rates of STDs in these neighborhoods, not their *return*. His position is, essentially, that the way incarceration destabilizes social networks and private social control leads to unsafe sex that increases the transmission of sexual diseases in poor communities. His study (2005) of Durham, North Carolina, finds that incarceration rates in counties and smaller geographical units at one time predict STD rates at a later time. In the same way that incarceration weakens interpersonal bonds that promote informal social control, it weakens the bonds of commitment that promote sexual fidelity and responsible sex practices. His argument is bolstered by the fact that teenage births follow the same pattern (and it is more logical to believe teenage birth rates rise because of irresponsible sex practices that increase when men are in short supply, rather than the mere presence of many men who have been released from prison). In addition, ethnographic work in Durham confirms that the distorted ratio of young women to sexually desirable male partners has distorted the patterns of sexuality in these places.

A larger body of work has been published regarding the health of families and children. Divorce (and breakup) rates are high for families where the male goes to prison. Studies show that men who have been to prison are less likely to marry after incarceration, than men of the same background who have never gone to prison. They cohabit, even in long-term relationships, but they tend not to marry (Western et al., 2004). It is no surprise, then, that places with high rates of incarceration have high rates of single-parent families (Sabol & Lynch, 2003). Because men who go to prison earn less money for the rest of their lives, perhaps as much as 40% less (Western, 2006), they provide less economic support to the families with whom they cohabit. There is a pattern of mutually reinforcing problems here: places that produce lots of people going to prison are always places with very low economic resources; the people who leave prison to return to these places will themselves face diminished earning capacity. The result is a cycle of diminished family health and well-being.

Children of incarcerated fathers have been found to suffer a range of problems in adjustment. The quality of studies on this topic varies, as do the findings. But parental incarceration has been identified as a risk factor for a range of child age maladies, including: truancy, academic underperformance, depression, anxiety, and violent acting out. In general, the effects when the incarcerated parent is a man are moderate compared to when the incarcerated parent is a woman. Here again, the damaging effects for women are larger than those for men, suggesting that even though fewer women are behind bars, the impact of their incarceration is greater. Studies have consistently shown that having a parent who was incarcerated is a major risk factor for a child to end up in prison, and the reasons cited above suggest why.

Research carried out in Australia (Weatherburn & Lind, 2004) sheds light on the way that the destabilization of families can lead to delinquency. Their study found that economic deprivation led to dysfunctional parenting practices (faulty disciplinary methods and risk of abuse). These practices weakened the bonds between parent and children, and the latter substituted an enhanced attachment to peers for the unsatisfactory attachment to parents. Because those suffering from economic deprivation tend to live in neighborhoods with a greater supply of delinquents as peers, the youth who become alienated from their parents become attached to delinquent colleagues. Thus, delinquency becomes amplified.

Safety Outcomes. Several studies have investigated the impact of concentrated incarceration on crime rates.[3] The original argument that very high rates of imprisonment would lead to higher rates of crime was first

---

[3] There is a body of literature assessing the impact of incarceration, generally, on crime. This literature covers a range of studies reaching a broad range of conclusions. For a review of these studies, see Chapter 2 of Clear (forthcoming).

made by Rose and Clear (1998) who said that there would likely be a "tipping point" after which the deterrence and incapacitation benefits of imprisonment would be outweighed by the way it has destabilized the neighborhood's capacity for informal (parochial and private) social control. In a later paper (Clear et al., 2002), they found strong evidence in support of the tipping point thesis, analyzing crime and incarceration data in Tallahassee, Florida. They show that neighborhoods with low levels of incarceration in one year experience less crime in the following year, but neighborhoods with the highest levels of incarceration experience increases in crime rather than decreases in the following year. Similar effects have been found in Portland, Oregon, Columbus, Ohio, and Chicago [see Chapter 7 of Clear (forthcoming)].

The "tipping point" thesis and the evidence in support of it are controversial, because the exact relationship is difficult to model. Crime and incarceration are reciprocally related; that is, incarceration is undoubtedly a result of crime, because with only the rarest of exceptions, people do not get locked up unless crimes have been committed. Yet the model also posits a complicated relationship in the opposite direction: up to a point, incarceration will reduce crime; after a point, it will increase it. The available data and math to statistically model this sort of effect are not very satisfactory.

For example, Lynch and Sabol (2004) analyzing data in Baltimore and Cleveland found a similar kind of pattern to incarceration and crime as Clear and his colleagues when they replicated that modeling method. When they used a different statistical technique (instrumental variables), not only did the nature of the impact change, it reversed itself, suggesting that higher rates of incarceration *decrease* crime (though it also increased fear of crime and had other problematic effects). They conclude that the tipping point models of crime and incarceration are inconclusive, at best, and potentially wrong.

Taylor et al. (2006) entered this debate by investigating the impact of adult incarceration on serious *juvenile* crime. They argue that using juvenile crime is a solution to this problem, because it breaks the reciprocality of the crime–incarceration relationship: it is irrational to argue that juvenile crime "causes" adult incarceration. When they investigate incarceration and juvenile crime (arrest) rates in Philadelphia neighborhoods, they find support for the tipping point thesis: high adult incarceration rates in one year lead to increasing juvenile crime rates in the years that follow.

In a review of this and other work on the topic, Clear (forthcoming) argues that the weight of the evidence supports the tipping point thesis. The argument is simple. To argue in favor of the tipping point thesis is to argue that incarceration, at high rates of concentration, clearly destabilizes families, weakens bonds between parents and children, decreases economic well-being, diminishes the capacity of social networks, reduces long-term job market viability, increases serious juvenile delinquency, *and increases crime*. The opposite argument is that concentrated incarceration has all of these same negative effects, each of which might be expected to increase crime, *yet it does not increase crime*. On balance, it seems more logical to accept the idea that although the assertion that incarceration at the highest levels tends to increase crime has not been definitively proven, the evidence to support that conclusion is strong.

Incarceration, Public Health, and Public Safety

If the arguments of this paper are correct, then one of the impediments to health and safety in poor communities is, paradoxically, the high incarceration rate its residents must endure. What is to be done?

It goes without saying that to stop locking people up from certain communities, just because that neighborhood has reached a "tipping point," is untenable. There are all kinds of people convicted of crimes in these places, some of whom would seem dangerous to any eye. Likewise, it seems implausible to segment a certain stratum of crime, say drug sales, and treat residents of this location differently than others when convicted of this crime, merely because of where they live. There is no obvious way to treat residents here differently, in terms of punishment, and not raise basic objections of equity and justice.

There are at least two possible routes, however: sentencing reform and justice reinvestment.

Sentencing Reform. The prison population is fully determined by two numbers: how many people go in and how long they stay. To reduce the prison population, either number (or both) must be changed.

It is possible to reduce the prison population proportionately by reducing (average) length of stay. It is difficult to see how public safety will be affected much, if at all, by releasing people a few months earlier than we do now. Almost everyone who goes into prison comes out. The length of stay in prison has little or no effect on recidivism (if there is an effect, it is that longer stays lead to higher rates of failure). If the general population experienced a 3-month, across-the-board reduction in stay, it would make people's return to the streets more rapid in the marginal sense, and would have potentially significant impact on the number of people behind bars. One group of criminologists has estimated that a 3-month reduction in length of stay for felony offenders, and a 6-month reduction for arrested parole violators, would result in a reduction in the average daily prison population by over 200,000 prisoners (Irwin & Austin, 2006).

Reducing length of stay will not reduce the rate at which men of color enter prison, and will therefore have little ameliorative impact on the negative consequences described above. For maximum effect, the number of prisoners who enter prison on new felonies and probation and parole revocations must be reduced. The obvious target for the former figure is to reduce or eliminate imprisonment for drug felony convictions. The obvious strategy for the latter is to prevent return to prison for pure technical violations (rules violations without new arrests) of probation or parole. Jacobson (2005) has shown that strategic changes in drug sentencing and broad changes in enforcement practices for probation and parole can reduce prison populations by 20–40%.

Justice Reinvestment. There are two "good news" items in this story. First, the number of areas in our major cities that are negatively affected by high incarceration rates is not large; usually, it is but a handful of places, less than three or four neighborhoods in most large cities. That means that the target of change is not jurisdictionwide, but much more targeted than that. The small number of affected places opens the possibility for targeted strategies that focus their efforts in those places.

Second, there is already a great deal of money being spent on the public safety problem. In 2003, about $140 billion (Hughes, 2006) was spent on the formal criminal justice system. This money is concentrated, just as incarceration is concentrated. Cadora et al. (2002) showed that there are single blocks in Brooklyn, New York, in which over $2 million was spent locking up its residents *in a single year*. Some of that money, say 10%, could be diverted to the places that are now negatively affected by criminal justice in order to change the pattern.

Recently, a few scholars have called attention to the potential benefits of community justice models that are focused on heavily affected communities and divert existing resources in a strategy called "justice reinvestment" (Tucker & Cadora, 2003). These strategies entail a variety of programs that integrate community residents and formerly convicted felons in projects that promote community well-being. Working on these projects operates as a substitute for some portion of the incarceration a person might experience as a result of a felony conviction. The intended result is win-win: the community is improved through targeted efforts, and the effects of incarceration are ameliorated because the projects both replace incarceration and target the negative consequences of incarceration, such as substandard housing, school failure, and economic decay.

Conclusion

This paper has linked the growing rates of incarceration to the health and safety problems of certain subgroups of the U.S. population, and it has shown how concentrated incarceration within those subgroups has had deleterious effects on the neighborhoods within which they live. Research demonstrating the negative impact of high rates of incarceration on public health and public safety has been summarized, with attention to both settled matters of empirical fact and controversial matters currently under debate. The paper concluded with some suggested ways of addressing this problem.

There is a moral imperative that has not yet been stressed. The penal apparatus in the United States is meant to be an instrument of public safety and institutional justice. To the degree that people who break the law should not be allowed to do so without consequences that symbolize the wrongfulness of that conduct, the criminal justice system is an essential instrument of social order. Yet in the United States, the system has grown to the point that it no longer can claim the high moral ground that derives form a careful and deliberative concern for a social order grounded in basic social justice. In some places, the punitive apparatus of the penal system is now one of the proximate causes of declining public safety. For the children who grow up in those areas, the criminal justice system is now a source of social injustice that robs them of life chances and places a low ceiling on their lifelong prospects. We must change this.

References

Blumstein, A., & Beck, A. (2005). Reentry as a transient state between liberty and recommitment. In J. Travis & C. Visher (Eds.), *Prisoner reentry and crime in America*. New York: Cambridge University Press.

Bonczar, T. P. (2003). *The prevalence of imprisonment in the U.S. population, 1974–2001*. Washington, DC: U.S. Bureau of Justice Statistics.

Bursik, R. J., Jr., & Grasmick, H. G. (1993). *Neighborhoods and crime: The dimensions of effective community control*. New York: Lexington Books.

Cadora, E., Swartz, C., & Gordon, M. (2002). Criminal justice and human services: An exploration of overlapping needs, resources and interests in Brooklyn neighborhoods. In J. Travis & M. Waul (Eds.), *Prisoners once removed: The impact of incarceration and reentry on children, families, and communities*. Washington, DC: Urban Institute Press.

Clear, T. R. (Forthcoming). *Incarcerating and communities: How mass incarceration damages poor communities*. New York: Oxford University Press.

Clear, T. R., Rose D. R., Waring, E., Scully, K. (2003). Coercive mobility and crime: A preliminary examination of concentrated incarceration and social disorganization. *Justice Quarterly, 20*, 33–64.

Clear, T. R., Waring, E., Scully, K. (2005). Communities and reentry: Concentrated reentry cycling. In J. Travis & C. Visher (Eds.), *Prisoner reentry and crime in America* (pp. 179–208). New York: Cambridge University Press.

Granovetter, M. S. (1973). The strength of weak ties. *American Journal of Sociology, 78*, 1360–1380.

Hughes, K. A. (2006). *Justice expenditure and employment in the United States, 2003*. Washington, DC: U.S. Bureau of Justice Statistics.

Hunter, A. J. (1985). Private, parochial and public social orders: The problem of crime and incivility in urban communities. In G. D. Suttles & M. N. Zald (Eds.), *The challenge of social control: Citizenship and institution building in modern society* (pp. 230–242). Norwood, NJ: Aldex.

Irwin, J., & Austin, J. (2006). *A blueprint for reducing crime and incarceration in the United States*. Report of the Open Society Institute by JRA Associates.

Jacobson, M. (2005). *Downsizing prisons: How to reduce crime and end mass incarceration*. New York: New York University Press.

Johnson, R. C., & Raphael, S. (2005). *The effects of male incarceration dynamics on AIDS infection rates among African-American women and men*. Unpublished paper: www.popcenter.umd.edu/events/Raphael.pdf (July).

Lynch, J.P., & Sabol, W. J. (2004). Effects of incarceration on informal social control in communities. In M. Patillo, D. Weiman, & B. Western (Eds.), *Imprisoning America: The social consequences of mass incarceration*. New York: Russell-Sage.

Mauer, M. (2005). Thinking about prison and its impact in the twenty-first century. Walter C. Reckless Memorial Lecture, *Ohio State Journal of Criminal Law*, *2*, 607.

Rengifo, A., and Waring E. 2005, November 17. *A Network Perspective on the Impact of Incarceration on Communities*. Paper presented to the-annual meetings of the American Society of Criminology, Toronto.

Rose, D. R., & Clear, T. R. (1998). Incarceration, social capital and crime: Examining the unintended consequences of incarceration. *Criminology, 36*, 441–479.

Sabol, W. J., & Lynch, J. P. (2003). Assessing the longer-run consequences of incarceration: Effects on families and employment. In D. Hawkins, S. L. Myers, Jr., & R. Sone (Eds.), *Crime control and social justice: The delicate balance*. Westport, CT: Greenwood Press.

Shaw, C. R., & McKay, H. D. (1942). *Juvenile delinquency and urban areas*. Chicago: University of Chicago Press.

Skogan, W. (1990). *Disorder and decline: Crime and the spiral of decay in American neighborhoods*. New York: Free Press.

Taylor, R., Goldkamp, J., Harris, P., Jones, P., Garcia, M., McCord, E. (2006). *Community justice impacts over time: Adult arrests rates, male serious delinquency prevalence, rates within and between Philadelphia communities*. Presentation to the Eastern Sociological Society Meetings, Boston.

Thomas, J. (2005). *STDs, prisons and communities*. Paper presented to the 2005 meetings of the American Society of Criminology, Toronto.

Tucker, S. B., & Cadora, E. (2003). Justice reinvestment: To invest in public safety by reallocating justice dollars to refinance education, housing, healthcare, and jobs. *Ideas for an Open Society. Occasional Papers Series, 3*(3). New York: Open Society Institute.

Walker, S., Spohn, C., & DeLone, M. (2004). *The color of justice: Race, ethnicity, and crime in America*. Belmont, CA: Wadsworth.

Weatherburn, D., Lind, B. (2001). *Delinquency-prone communities*. New York: Cambridge University Press.

Western, B. (2006). *Punishment and inequality*. New York: Russell-Sage.

Western, B., Lopoo, L. M., & McLanahan, S. (2004). Incarceration and the bonds between parents in fragile families. In M. Pattillo, D. Weiman, & B. Western (Eds.), *Imprisoning America: The social effects of mass incarceration*. New York: Russell-Sage.

Chapter 3

Litigating for Better Medical Care

Jon Wool

Litigation to improve correctional health care has been—and, indeed, continues to be—a critical catalyst to better medical care for prisoners, and therefore to better public health. We no longer openly accept, as we once did, that prisoners are entitled to bare scraps of medical care, the leavings of a facility's lean resources. We now recognize and enforce the right of incarcerated persons to receive adequate professional care for their serious medical and mental health needs. It was the coercive power of litigation, rather than an enlightened public policy, that made this right meaningful.

However, much of the early promise of litigation has been quashed by the courts and Congress. As with so much else in the formation of criminal justice policy, political opportunism and retribution have led to policies (in practice, statute, and decisional law) that endanger the public health and safety. Just as our sentencing policies overly rely on thoughtless, punitive, and long-lasting confinement at the expense of rehabilitative and reintegrative opportunities, so policymakers and judges seek to curtail opportunities for prisoners to improve the conditions of confinement. Among the most important of those conditions is accessible and adequate physical and mental health care.

In this chapter, I first examine the peculiar nature of and context for lawsuits that seek to improve prison medical care. I next discuss the present state of the legal right to that care and the obstacles to realizing that right. I then suggest some promising ways in which litigation can successfully be used—despite those obstacles—to drive medical care forward. I hope to show that restricting prison medical care litigation is bad correctional policy and bad public health policy. Because the political process disfavors prisoners and the litigation that protects their rights (even when the public health is at stake), it is critical to have access to the courts to achieve what the majoritarian branches neglect. The protection, even support, of litigation to help ensure good quality care is necessary to improve the prognosis for prisoners and for the public as well.

Prisoners' Medical Litigation in Context

The principal source of prisoners' right to medical care is found in the Eighth Amendment's prohibition against cruel and unusual punishments. The Amendment applies to sentenced federal and state prisoners, while the due process clauses of the Fifth and Fourteenth Amendments offer an analogous, perhaps somewhat broader protection to federal and state detainees prior to adjudication. Federal statutes also provide the basis for broader rights to the provision of care. The Americans with Disabilities Act, which is fully discussed in a separate chapter, provides state and local prisoners the right to have one's disability fully accommodated in correctional settings (Americans with Disabilities Act of 1990). The Federal Tort Claims Act offers federal prisoners the right to sue for medical negligence in prison. (Federal Tort Claims Act). Yet, judicial decisions and federal and state statutes have limited prisoners' rights to medical care and have raised significant obstacles to ensuring that those rights are realized. The value of litigation to improve medical care turns as much on the ability to overcome these barriers to a judicial hearing and judicially enforced remedies as it does on the scope of the right in question.

In general, there are two different but often closely linked ways in which litigation, especially class action litigation, drives improvement in correctional health care. The first involves a degree of tacit cooperation between the parties. The second uses the lawsuit as part of a broader strategy for change.

Litigating medical care issues can be the rare key that unlocks the resources—principally money, but also expertise—required to ensure the facilities, staff, and institutional commitment to adequate care. The problems of prison medical care may seem intractable to legislators because the cost of providing even minimally adequate care is enormous. Even in its present state, health care accounts for a large and growing portion of correctional budgets. Health care in prisons often is dismal because of the reluctance of political actors to invest the enormous sums necessary to provide critical services to so many medically needy people. Courts can do what legislators and executive officials feel they cannot; they have the power to supersede the political obstacles to gaining sufficient resources for prisoners' health.

Indeed, corrections officials often welcome and may actively, although always quietly, support litigation to free up resources needed to improve the medical care delivery systems for which they are responsible (Schlanger, 2006). Many middle- and upper-level administrators are deeply concerned about their ability to provide adequate health care to prisoners, for the prisoners' sake as well as that of staff and the greater community. And given enormous and steadily increasing prison and jail populations (in almost all jurisdictions), they are often unable to secure the necessary resources to provide even minimally satisfactory care. Or to do so they must sacrifice other important programs such as education or job training or even security staffing. Prisoners' rights cases that provide an opportunity for corrections administrators to gain resources have the best chance of success. Medical care cases often present such a circumstance.

In cases in which there are not sufficiently cooperative corrections administrators, or the administrators see insufficient opportunities presented, correctional health litigation nonetheless can influence policy well beyond the claims raised in the legal action and regardless of the ultimate resolution of the suit. Sometimes, sympathetic administrators may accede to a two-pronged approach of not resisting the litigation too forcefully while also accepting a broader public policy strategy. They may quietly participate in the use of discovery and other avenues for public information to pressure the legislature or the executive to more quickly achieve the litigation demands or to seek greater change than can be achieved through litigation.

A class action can shake loose documentary evidence of the need for change that is not available to the public from any other source (litigation often provides the only form of independent outside oversight of correctional systems). Class actions are the lawsuits that seek to change a facility's policies and practices, often through long-term court intervention, rather than simply to recover for damages in an individual case. The evidence disclosed, bolstered by the analyses of independent expert consultants, can be put to effective use in advocacy efforts directed to the press and ultimately to executive and legislative leaders. Importantly, the change that results from such political processes is not limited by the minimal dictates of the Constitution and sparse relevant statutes, a fact not lost on litigators and other advocates.

Regardless of how the litigation proceeds, medical care cases present opportunities that other prisoner suits do not. Unlike cases involving allegations of staff violence, or officials' failure to protect prisoners from other prisoners, or serious effects of overcrowded conditions, or restrictions on First Amendment rights, medical care cases are less threatening to corrections administrators and their lawyers, and to some extent to other government decision makers. Allegations of failures of medical care in prisons and jails may seem less personally accusatory; these cases tend to address the deficiencies of an entire system rather than the culpability of individual actors. A prisoner's medical suffering might garner sympathy with corrections officials and lawyers and ultimately with a judge or jury. Everyone has experienced the fear of illness and pain and can envision being unable to access care or being offered only substandard care. Moreover, there is some awareness that the care prisoners receive directly affects the entire correctional community, and even those beyond the walls.

Suits alleging constitutionally deficient medical care also may be more sympathetically received by the judges who control their fate than other claims made by prisoners. Judges may be less likely to defer to the judgment of corrections professionals in medical matters. Prison officials generally are not physicians or public health experts and, in class-action litigation at least, judges will hear from plaintiffs' correctional medicine experts who are. Moreover, judges, like administrators or legislators, are more apt to see adequate medical care as a matter of human dignity that should not and need not be sacrificed as an incidence of incarceration, as part of a prisoner's sentence. Security concerns are only tangentially implicated if at all and so the often-used argument that "the court must not intrude" rings hollow.

Federal court litigation about conditions of confinement focuses heavily on claims of constitutionally deficient medical care. An analysis of prior studies of prisoners' federal civil rights litigation found that medical care was among the top four bases for constitutional claims, ranging from 10.8 to 25% of the docket and "is consistently one of the most prominent topics in inmate litigation" (Schlanger, 2003). The proportion of civil rights class actions that focus on medical issues is likely even greater. By one rough measure, medical care ranks second only to overcrowding as the basis for ongoing court intervention. In 2000, among the 320 state or private prisons that were under the supervision of a court order or consent decree for a specific condition of confinement, 166 related to the prisons' medical facilities or mental health treatment. Another 95 related to "accommodation of the disabled" (U.S. Department of Justice, 2000).

It is not only prisoners who think their constitutional rights are violated by deliberate indifference to their medical care; the United States Department of Justice thinks so as well. Virtually all of the Department's recent investigations of adult prisons and jails that led to formal demands for change included findings of constitutionally deficient medical or mental health care. The Department's website lists 12 letters providing the results of investigations of constitutional violations from 2001 through 2006. All 12 included findings of unconstitutional conditions in the provision of medical or mental health care, and usually both (U.S. Department of Justice, 2007). For example, the most recent findings letter required changes in:

intake; medication administration and management; nursing sick call; provider sick call; scheduling, tracking, and follow-up on outside consultations; monitoring and treatment of communicable diseases; monitoring and treatment of chronic diseases; medical records documentation; scheduling; infirmary care; continuity of care following hospitalizations; grievances; and patient confidentiality. [And] care for patients with acute medical urgencies was also constitutionally inadequate (U.S. Department of Justice, 2006 Letter)

There are several reasons for the prevalence of medical care claims among prisoners' federal civil rights actions. First, there is a federal constitutional right to some level of medical care among those who are detained or imprisoned and there is the availability of federal court review. Second, these lawsuits have a significant, if small, chance of success. And when they succeed, they can bring compensatory and punitive monetary damages in individual cases and broad institutional reform in class-action cases. Third, a fair number of jurisdictions are doing a poor job of providing adequate care. This is because of the immensity of the task and because of a failure of political will and wisdom.

Our representatives too seldom recognize that good correctional health care is essential to good public health policy and that their constituents can be made to understand that, if they do not already. Litigation, therefore, is a critical tool to achieving what the political process fails to deliver. But, litigation to advance the rights of prisoners also is under attack.

Prisoners' Right to Medical Care and Enforcing that Right

Prisoners (and other involuntarily institutionalized people) are the only persons in this country with a federal constitutional right to medical care. This often repeated claim—sometimes raised as an exhortation and sometimes trotted out to deride—is true enough in theory. But there are powerful forces that keep it from being fully realized in practice.

Prior to the late 1960s, prisoners had no recognized constitutional right to health care and few avenues of judicial review of the conditions in which they were made to live. The federal courts, in what has been labeled the "hands-off doctrine," broadly declined to interfere with the practices of correctional administrators. The courts' abstention was not absolute, but nearly so.

As one sympathetic federal judge put it in dismissing a prisoner's claim, "the treatment as alleged was not so far below the standards of ordinary humanity as to permit or require judicial interference" (*United States* ex rel. *Yaris v. Shaughnessy*, 1953). Judges very rarely encountered facts sufficiently far below humane standards to merit their intervention.

As demands for civil rights moved from the streets to the courthouses, prisoners too insisted on relief from oppressive conditions. Disturbances and full-scale uprisings such as at Attica and in the New York City jails in part were responses to inhumane medical care (McDonald, 1999). Presented with evidence of the most egregious conditions, a small number of federal trial judges declined to look the other way. In 1972, for example, in one of the earliest decisions holding a state prison system's medical care constitutionally deficient, Chief Judge Frank Johnson described intentional denials of needed care, unconscionable waits for emergency care, and such woefully insufficient and unqualified staff as to lead prisoners to diagnose and treat other prisoners. The judge concluded that Alabama's prison medical care was characterized by "a degree of neglect of basic medical needs of prisoners that could justly be called 'barbarous' and 'shocking to the conscience'" (*Newman v. State*, 1972).

In a brief period of expansiveness, the U.S. Supreme Court began to embrace the lower courts' less constricted view of the judiciary's role in prison conditions cases generally, and in medical cases specifically. In 1974, the Court put an end to the hands-off doctrine: "But though his rights may be diminished by the needs and exigencies of the institutional environment, a prisoner is not wholly stripped of constitutional protections when he is imprisoned for crime. There is no iron curtain drawn between the Constitution and the prisons of this country" (*Wolff v. McDonnell*, 1974). Two years later, in *Estelle v. Gamble*, the Court explicitly found in the Eighth Amendment's prohibition against cruel and unusual punishment a right to medical care, a conclusion that many federal courts of appeals had already reached (*Estelle v. Gamble*, 1976; *Westlake v. Lucas*, 1976).

In response to Mr. Gamble's handwritten *pro se* complaint alleging the indifference of Texas prison officials to his serious back injury, the Court set out the right. "In order to state a cognizable claim, a prisoner must allege acts or omissions sufficiently harmful to evidence deliberate indifference to serious medical needs. It is only such indifference that can offend 'evolving standards of decency' in violation of the Eighth Amendment" (*Estelle v. Gamble*). A constitutional right to the provision of medical care to prisoners had at last been formally unveiled. Yet, from its inception, the Court's formulation of that right—the extremely high and difficult-to-prove "deliberate indifference" standard—paved the way for considerable future retrenchment.

Justice Stevens, perhaps the Court's most liberal member, recognized the hidden danger of this formulation. He decried the Court's eagerness to limit the scope of the right to care before the lower courts had fully fleshed it out, as they were in the process of doing. And he specifically objected to conditioning a viable claim on terms that "incorrectly relate to the subjective motivation of persons violating the Eighth Amendment rather than to the standard of care required by the Constitution" (*Estelle v. Gamble*, Stevens, J., dissenting). Justice Stevens's hope that the constitutional standard "should turn on the character of the punishment rather than the motivation of the individual who inflicted it," was not to be (*Estelle v. Gamble*, Stevens, J., dissenting).

A tug of war between rights-sensitive trial court judges and an increasingly parsimonious Supreme Court ensued. Over time, the Court made clear that an Eighth Amendment medical claim turns on the mental culpability of individual actors, regardless of the seriousness of the harm inflicted. In other words, a prisoner must show that a prison official acted or failed to act with the subjective mental state of deliberate indifference (something akin to recklessness, requiring disregard of a known risk) to a serious medical need of the prisoner (an objectively determined standard, posing a significant threshold) (*Wilson v. Seiter*, 1991; *Farmer v. Brennan*, 1994).

As a matter of legal theory, the Court reached its standard by concluding that the Eighth Amendment only controls "punishments" and that the conditions under which a prisoner is confined do not constitute part of the punishment. "If the pain inflicted is not formally meted out *as punishment* by the statute or the sentencing judge, some mental element must be attributed to the inflicting officer before it can qualify" (*Wilson v. Seiter*). Whether accurate as a gloss on the cruel and unusual punishment clause or not, the standard is woefully inadequate to protect against serious threats to public health that arise from often deplorable conditions of medical care in correctional institutions. As Justice Blackmun warned in 1994: "Where a legislature refuses to fund a prison adequately, the resulting barbaric conditions should not be immune from constitutional scrutiny simply because no prison official acted culpably" (*Farmer v. Brennan*, Blackmun, J., concurring). That is precisely the threat we now face.

As it scaled back the scope of a prisoner's right to medical care, the Court—its own constitution changing dramatically—began to narrow the avenues by which prisoners might exercise the newly established right. In 1979, returning to the language of great deference to prison administrators, the Court announced that "the operation of our correctional facilities is peculiarly the province of the Legislative and Executive Branches of our Government, not the Judicial." The Court's jurisprudence has leaned ever more toward looking the other way than actively and meaningfully ensuring that "barbaric prison conditions [are not] beyond the reach of the Eighth Amendment" (*Farmer v. Brennan*, Blackmun, J., concurring). The hands-off doctrine has not fully returned, but the Supreme Court has made it clear that prisoners should not rely too heavily on judicial intervention and trial judges should not be too eager to remedy alleged constitutional violations behind bars.

There are other legal obstacles that prisoners face in their efforts to vindicate constitutional rights, including the right to adequate medical care. If the facts underlying the claim fall within the narrow constitutional window, there still are restrictions on what or whom the prisoner can sue. A state or local prisoner (or detainee) brings a suit challenging a constitutional violation in federal court by way of the Civil Rights Act of 1871 (42 U.S.C. §1983). Known as "section 1983" actions, these suits provide court access when alleging violations of law by persons acting on behalf of a state or local government. [Federal prisoners cannot resort to section 1983, but the courts have created a corollary route, known as a "*Bivens* action" (*Bivens v. Six Unknown Named Agents of Federal Bureau of Narcotics*, 1971).] The Eleventh Amendment, however, bars federal courts from entertaining a claim against a state (although not against a county or municipality). Thus, a state prisoner may only sue individual government officials or staff.

Yet, an individual government actor enjoys a qualified immunity to suit. In order to proceed with a lawsuit against the individual, the courts have held that the prisoner must show that the individual violated a specific "clearly established" legal right or was objectively unreasonable in believing that he was not violating such a right. Designed to give individuals sufficient latitude to carry out their discretionary functions, qualified immunity can dramatically restrict the availability of remedies for constitutional violations. Here is one example, taken from a recent case: A jail mental health caseworker who allegedly failed to secure adequate mental health treatment for an 18-year-old detainee in her care—who subsequently hanged himself—was granted immunity from suit because no clearly established right guided her conduct. The judge made this determination despite allegations that the caseworker took the detainee off suicide watch soon after he had attempted suicide, that she determined that he was acting manipulatively and was not suicidal, and that she moved him to a single cell without observation (*Perez v. Oakland County*, 2006).

If prisoners, individually or as a class, are able to overcome these and other legal hurdles, they nonetheless remain vulnerable to the skepticism and animosity of the fact finder, whether judge or jury, toward a convicted criminal's claims regarding the conditions he or she faces in prison. Prisoners prevail at trial infrequently, at the rate of roughly 10% (Schlanger, 2003). Although claims of deliberate indifference to serious medical needs may be more positively received than other claims arising in custody, prisoners still face a very steep climb. And most prisoners must litigate their cases without the assistance of a lawyer.

While the Supreme Court was solidifying its constricted view of prisoners' legal right to medical care and restricting access to judicial determination of that right, Congress entered the action by dramatically narrowing access to the federal courts and limiting the ability of the courts to provide relief when they find a constitutional violation. It was the mid-1990s and it was a particularly bad time to be a criminal defendant or a prisoner. Crime and the public concern it engendered were disconcertingly high and the politicization of criminal justice flourished. State legislatures reacted by increasing the harshness of sentencing statutes, including dramatic uses of mandatory minimum sentences. And they joined with Congress in eliminating discretionary parole release for violent offenders—leading to longer terms of incarceration. These so-called "truth-in-sentencing" provisions were a condition of federal funding for the building of new state prisons, a "self-filling" prophecy (Violent Offender Incarceration and Truth-in-Sentencing Incentive Grants). Congress increased the range of federal crimes and ratcheted up the lengths of federal sentences (Violent Crime Control and Law Enforcement Act of 1994), leading to a still continuing expansion of the federal prison system. Congress drastically curtailed access to federal habeas corpus relief to challenge the lawfulness of one's detention (Antiterrorism and Effective Death Penalty Act of 1996). And federally funded legal services offices were barred from representing prisoners in civil rights cases (Omnibus Consolidated Rescissions and Appropriations Act of 1996).

With similar enthusiasm, Congress turned directly to the "reform" of prison litigation by enacting the Prison Litigation Reform Act of 1995 (PLRA) (Prison Litigation Reform Act of 1995). Consistent with the looseness of its title—it was enacted in 1996—this sweeping limitation on the availability of federal judicial remedies for constitutional violations suffered by incarcerated persons was passed with virtually no deliberation; it was attached to an appropriations bill. The PLRA, the principal aim of which was claimed to be the elimination of unnecessary federal court litigation, has spawned so much litigation that one outraged federal appellate court was moved to write: "When Congress penned the Prison Litigation Reform Act … the watchdog must have been dead" (*McGore v. Wrigglesworth,* 1997).

There is no question that the PLRA has succeeded in reducing prisoners' individual civil rights lawsuits and, perhaps to a small extent, class actions. The courts were burdened with a large and increasing number of prisoner lawsuits, roughly 41,000 in 1995, the year before the Act was passed (that number represented a 47% increase from 1990) (Administrative Office of the U.S. Courts, 2007). By 2005, the number of suits had decreased to roughly 23,000, despite a 45% increase in the prisoner population over that period. What remains in question is whether, as the proponents of the PLRA claimed, much of that litigation was frivolous and whether the PLRA has had a net positive effect on the quality, and not just the quantity, of prisoner suits.

The claims of frivolousness are hard to judge but it appears that the Act's proponents did not distinguish between truly frivolous and legally insufficient claims. A medical care claim that fails to fully allege that an individual actor was deliberately indifferent to a clearly established right regarding the prisoner's serious medical need, although acting with gross negligence causing serious injury or death, would be dismissed, just as would a truly frivolous claim. But, the former does not suggest a burden on the federal courts that warrants wholesale diminution in the rights of access. In retrospect, the claims of frivolousness seem grossly exaggerated. Many of the claims that were advanced as demonstrating frivolousness appear to be the product of mental illness, rather than intent to maliciously or recreationally litigate. Indeed, these claims may further suggest the need for improved correctional mental health care, and perhaps the need to litigate for better care. Nonetheless, in its massive chilling of prisoner suits in federal court, it is likely that a fair portion of truly frivolous claims have been eliminated.

In any event, the PLRA's assault on prisoners' civil rights litigation was not solely a response to the burdens of frivolous lawsuits. It was in large part a product of the contemporaneous politics of greater punishment and fewer rights for those arrested, charged with a crime, or imprisoned. It set upon an easy target to score points with the public. But, as with so much of good politics, the Act makes bad public policy. A large number of meritorious claims are, as a consequence of the PLRA, either now not brought or are dismissed in their early stages, and the ability of the federal courts to monitor court-ordered relief from unconstitutional conditions has therefore been weakened. With regard to claims of inadequate medical or mental health care, a critical tool in the public health toolbox has been rendered less effective.

The PLRA takes two broad approaches to inhibiting prisoner civil rights litigation, each with distinct deleterious effects. It takes aim at prisoners directly and it targets those who would help prisoners, their attorneys and the judges who oversee their cases.

The statute precludes a federal court from granting damages to a prisoner or detainee (the PLRA applies equally to both) for mental or emotional injury alone [42 U.S.C. §1997e(e); 28 U.S.C. §1346(b)(2)]. In many contexts this physical injury requirement has pernicious effects, such as precluding relief from the emotional effects of sexual coercion or assault. Yet, it may have limited impact in the context of correctional health care, where the Eighth Amendment already restricts relief to acts or omissions relating to one's serious medical needs. Nonetheless, in some instances, such as the failure to treat mental illness or the willful disclosure of HIV status, the PLRA may bar a remedy for a significant constitutional wrong. Importantly, the courts have construed this provision's twisted language to allow a prisoner with no physical injury to obtain a nonmonetary remedy, such as an injunction ordering the correctional facility to change its practices to preclude future mental or emotional injury.

Taking an economic approach to suppressing prisoners' individual lawsuits, the PLRA requires prisoners who seek and qualify for indigent status, as virtually all do, to pay the regular filing fee (presently $350 and $450 for an appeal) over time from their prison accounts, including a partial payment up front [28 U.S.C. §1915(b)(1-2)]. This provision, which singles out poor prisoners over all other poor civil rights claimants, is likely one of the biggest reasons for the dramatic decline in the number of suits filed. Prisoners have very little earning power—jobs, to the extent they are available, generally pay less than $1 per hour—and they may rationally forego a medical care claim that has only a small chance of delivering a relatively small recovery. In addition, the statute requires full, up-front payment of the filing fee (which is often simply not possible) when a prisoner has three times previously filed a claim that was deemed frivolous, malicious, or legally insufficient [28 U.S.C. §1915(g)]. The filing fee provisions may even affect medical care class actions. Class actions may begin as individual *pro se* filings and thus the pool of meritorious claims that reach the light of day may be diminished.

The PLRA requires that prisoners, as a right of entry to the federal courts, first pursue all available administrative grievances, including each level of administrative appeal [42 U.S.C. §1997e(a)]. This "exhaustion rule" poses the highest hurdle for aggrieved prisoners seeking to remedy violations of their constitutional right to medical care while incarcerated. The PLRA substituted an inflexible rule for a system in which judges had the discretion to allow a non-exhausted claim to go forward. The exhaustion rule does not turn on whether the administrative process is a meaningful one, which it too often is not, or whether the remedies available are in any way equivalent to those available in federal court, which they never are, or, indeed, the merits of the prisoner's claims.

In a series of decisions, the Supreme Court has dramatically expanded the scope of the PLRA's exhaustion rule. Most important, it recently held that the rule includes a further requirement that prisoners meet all administrative time-lines, which are often extremely short, 2 to 4 weeks or less (*Woodford v. Ngo*, 2006). The failure to meet any deadline forever bars an Eighth Amendment or statutory claim. For the unschooled prisoner, the highly technical and some-times inconsistently applied administrative rules and timelines pose a series of Catch-22s. The PLRA has created a paradoxical system in which prison officials both control the administrative process and are arbiters of whether the prisoner has properly exhausted by completing the process within the allotted time. In effect, the statute takes away the authority of federal judges to declare whether a lawsuit can proceed and gives it to prison officials, the putative defendants in the lawsuit at issue.

In a heartening reversal 7 months after *Woodford v. Ngo*, the Supreme Court unanimously blocked a lower court's efforts to further expand the reach of the exhaustion requirement (*Jones v. Bock*, 2007). This was the Court's first decision that did not expand its scope.

The breadth of the exhaustion rule as it has been interpreted by the Supreme Court allows for an almost unlimited opportunity for an unsympathetic judge to dismiss a prisoner's constitutional medical claim. For the sympathetic judge, it demands creativity to allow meritorious claims to go forward. A typical case looks something like this: An officer slammed the door to the segregated prisoner's food slot on the prisoner's hand. Medical staff then refused any but the most cursory care. He filed a timely grievance alleging that one officer used unjustifiable force in slamming the door on his hand and followed up with the necessary appeals. Later, after learning that his hand had been fractured and improperly healed, the prisoner filed a second, untimely grievance regarding the failure to treat his broken hand. In the ensuing lawsuit claiming both excessive use of force and deliberate indifference to a serious medical need, the court held that the prisoner had adequately stated an Eighth Amendment medical claim but dismissed that claim for his failure to allege it with specificity in his initial prison grievance (*Murray v. Artz*, 2002).

Congress was not content to suppress frivolous prisoner lawsuits. In a further sign that it had the vitality of the Eighth Amendment in its sights, it also took aim at the persons who would ensure the vindication and ongoing protection of those rights, lawyers and judges. In two sets of provisions, the PLRA threatens litigation that seeks to permanently improve the conditions of confinement, often centering on the provision of medical care.

First, it sets out a series of limitations on the fees that attorneys for prisoners can recover. If Congress had intended to improve the quality of prisoners' suits, as the Supreme Court has opined (*Porter v. Nussle*, 2002), the last thing one would have expected it to do would be to make it more difficult for prisoners to be represented by attorneys. Yet, it did so by imposing three restrictions on prisoners' attorney fees. It bars any fees that are not "directly and reasonably incurred in proving an actual violation of the plaintiff's rights" [42 U.S.C. §1997e(d)(1)(a)]; it caps those fees at 1.5 times the rate paid to federal appointed counsel in criminal cases [42 U.S.C. §1997e(d)(3)]; and it limits fees to 1.5 times the amount awarded in damages [42 U.S.C. §1997e(d)(2)]. The first provision is a disincentive to attorneys in that fees are not recoverable when a case is settled favorably to the prisoner because there has been no proof of a violation of the plaintiff's rights. Settlements are favored in part because they avoid the admission or proof of liability. The latter two provisions strongly discourage representation. One-and-one-half the appointed counsel rate would be warmly received among appointed attorneys in criminal cases, who are paid for every hour they work regardless of the outcome. But for a prisoner's constitutional claim, attorneys are awarded fees only in those cases in which the prisoner prevails. And when one prevails the damages are often not large. The rate and total fee caps mean attorneys who choose to represent prisoners cannot expect to cover their overhead.

The PLRA's second assault on efforts to use the federal courts to remedy prisoners' constitutional violations comes through a series of restrictions on judges' authority to oversee court-ordered or consensual remedies. These restrictions impact litigation seeking systemic reform. Unlike the range of a federal court's authority in all other civil rights cases, the Act limits the duration of an injunction—an order requiring the prison take steps to cure a constitutional violation—to 2 years, unless the court finds anew an ongoing constitutional violation [18 U.S.C. §§3626(b)(1)(A)(i) and (b)(3)]. It also requires the suspension of the injunction when a prison official defendant moves to terminate it after the 2-year limit [18 U.S.C. §3626(e)(2)]. This allows any ongoing violation to go unchecked while the matter is adjudicated. And it limits preliminary injunctions to 90 days [18 U.S.C. §3626(a)(2)]. More generally, the PLRA restricts the nature of a court's ongoing relief to that which is "narrowly drawn," "extends no further than necessary," and is "the least intrusive means to correct the violation" [18 U.S.C. §3626(a)(1)(A)]. In practice, the power of these provisions to limit a federal court's critical oversight role depends significantly on the degree to which the defendants contest the court's role. But it is precisely in the most contested cases that a court's oversight may be most critical.

While Congress has been particularly active in quashing prisoners' ability to achieve judicial redress from federal constitutional and statutory violations, the states have not sat idly by. A great number of state legislatures have enacted provisions similar to the PLRA that operate to limit access to state courts for a broader range of claims involving prison conditions, including claims of inadequate medical care that do not reach the level of Eighth Amendment constitutional violations, as the Supreme Court has interpreted it. Taken together, these limitations on the federal right to correctional health care and the barriers to accessing judicial remedies have restricted the force of correctional health care litigation, especially prisoners' individual lawsuits.

Meaningful access to justice for the individual prisoner is extremely important and its diminution is not a healthy development. It is at the core of the guarantee of adequate care. But, it also has a more direct effect on prisoners' health. For an incarcerated person, the ability to have one's legitimate grievances relating to serious mental or physical illness or suffering be heard by a federal court is a source of self-respect. And self-respect is both a necessary ingredient in the rehabilitative process and one that is hard to come by in the crowded, unhealthy, and often degrading conditions in which prisoners live. As two keen observers of prison life have pointed out, the right to file a lawsuit "tells the guards and the warden and the whole world that prisoners have rights that must be respected," which is critical because "[i]n order for a man to feel good about himself, he has to be able to affect his situation" (Specter & Kupers, 2001). Feeling good about oneself is an aspect of personal health and the entire prison culture benefits when prisoners can expand their sense of dignity. Moreover, the free community benefits when prisoners are given opportunities to grow healthier, psychologically as well as physically, and otherwise better prepare for reintegration. The judicial and legislative suppression of individual prisoner lawsuits has ignored these collateral benefits.

The Continuing Vitality of Prisoners' Medical Litigation

Notwithstanding the restrictions imposed by the courts and legislatures, litigation—especially class action litigation—remains one of the most important tools in forcing or encouraging better care, and better public health outcomes. The judicial and legislative restrictions seem to affect class action litigation less severely than they do individual cases. These are the lawsuits—brought to remedy a range of constitutional deficiencies in a facility or even an entire state or local correctional system—that most believe are responsible for the bulk of the change in prison conditions, including the provision of medical care, in the past 40 years. Other than those individual lawsuits that develop into larger, counseled actions seeking broad change through injunctive relief, individual suits rarely affect the operational practices of the correctional facilities involved. Corrections officials and their attorneys more often respond to the facts presented in each case rather than the systemic deficiencies underlying the facts. They have no institutional reason to do otherwise. Class-action litigation, however, can impose such a reason, or present an opportunity to develop one. In the absence of the political will or courage to adopt policies that embrace prisoners as members of the public, or prison medical care as a core factor in public health, class action litigation remains essential.

The developing legal restrictions may have changed somewhat the character of class-action prison cases. These lawsuits are less often wholesale interventions into the operation of a prison or prison system. More often class-action prison cases are now intensive attacks on one or a few particular aspects of prison medical conditions, such as inadequate screening and treatment for infectious diseases, the use of isolation for persons with serious mental illness, or deficiencies in prenatal care. But, there remain situations in which the courts and the parties face circumstances so completely dire that wholesale oversight is required.

Ongoing litigation involving California's prison medical system provides such an example. *Plata v. Schwarzenegger*, filed in 2001, alleged constitutionally deficient medical care throughout the largest prison system in the country (*Plata v. Schwarzenegger*, 2001; Civil Rights Litigation Clearinghouse). *Plata* is the latest in a series of class actions (*Madrid v. Gomez*, 1990; *Shumate v. Wilson*, 1995) to challenge one or another element of California's provision of medical care to its 170,000 prisoners. In 2005, following lengthy discovery, a series of specific court orders, a stipulated agreement, regular reports of court-appointed experts, and a period of intensive negotiations, the judge took drastic action. Concluding that "[t]he problem of a highly dysfunctional, largely decrepit, overly bureaucratic, and politically driven prison system, which these defendants have inherited from past administrations, is too far gone to be corrected by conventional methods," he subsequently ordered that all aspects of correctional medical services be taken over by a court-appointed receiver (*Plata v. Schwarzenegger*, May 2005). The conditions of care, which generally were not disputed by the defendants, were found to be so poor that "on average, an inmate in one of California's prisons needlessly dies every six to seven days due to constitutional deficiencies in the CDCR's medical delivery system" (*Plata v. Schwarzenegger*, October 2005).

The desperation of corrections officials seems nearly to have matched that of the judge and they clearly welcomed the order shifting responsibility and authority to a receiver. The judge noted that the second-ranking official in the system had testified "that medical care simply is not a priority within the CDCR, is not considered a 'core competency' of the Department, and is 'not the business of the CDC, and it never will be the business of the Department of Corrections to provide medical care,'" and that the official "could not even estimate when significant improvements to the system might be made if the State were left to its own devises" (*Plata v. Schwarzenegger*, October 2005).

The judge recognized that the political process had continually failed to ensure that California's experiment in mass incarceration would be accompanied by even minimally constitutionally sufficient medical care. "To a significant extent, this case presents a textbook example of how majoritarian political institutions sometimes fail to muster the will to protect a disenfranchised, stigmatized, and unpopular subgroup of the population. This failure of political will, combined with a massive escalation in the rate of incarceration over the past few decades, has led to a serious and chronic abnegation of State responsibility for the basic medical needs of prisoners" (*Plata v. Schwarzenegger*, October 2005). Even with such litigation, reforming California's prison medical system still poses unimaginable obstacles. But without the broad and forceful intervention of the court, and the cooperation of the defendants, there would be little hope for even modest reform.

While California corrections officials cooperated with the appointment of a receiver and other aspects of the litigation, another presently vital model of litigation was at work on the other coast. This can be seen in three lawsuits directed at medical care in New York, one challenging the care provided to persons with HIV in New York prisons, and the other two to persons with mental illness who are incarcerated in prisons and jails. In each case, the litigation has functioned as part of a broader advocacy effort, designed to propel change through the political as well as the judicial process.

In the first case, a class of HIV-positive prisoners filed suit in federal court in 1990, alleging multiple constitutional deficiencies in the provision of care (*Inmates of New York State with Human Immune Deficiency Virus v. Cuomo*, 1990). The litigation proceeded slowly through discovery battles and other adversarial steps. All the while, in large part because of the pressure of litigation and the information that was revealed through discovery, the state began to improve care in a number of ways. Screening improved. Regional medical centers within the prison system were organized to accommodate greater access to specialty care for people with HIV. And more resources were committed to give prisoners access to new, life-saving medications. Although there are reportedly still delays in care and additional infectious disease specialists are needed, the medical conditions for prisoners infected with HIV have, reportedly, greatly improved.

In the second case, the advocacy bent of the litigation was evident from the outset. The plaintiff was not a prisoner but an organization statutorily authorized to advocate for persons with mental illness. The organization filed suit in 2003 alleging wholesale deficiencies in correctional mental health care (*Disability Advocates, Inc. v. New York State Office of Mental Health*, 2003). In 2004, another group, statutorily authorized to monitor conditions in the New York prisons, prepared and published a detailed report on the state of that care (Correctional Association of New York, 2004). The Department of Correctional Services began to adjust its policies, particularly with regard to the isolation of persons with serious mental illness, and the Department of Mental Health began to focus more attention and resources on prisoners' care, supported by substantial new funding from the governor and legislature. In both cases, the gains in improved mental health care and protection were not all the plaintiffs sought, but they were in some respects deeper and perhaps more long-lasting than what they might have achieved from litigation alone.

The third case also involves the care of persons with mental illness and focuses on discharge planning, an area that seems particularly ripe for an advocacy-based approach to litigation. Although the case was filed in state rather than federal court, at least in part because it relied on favorable New York statutes ensuring care for the mentally ill, it is another helpful example of the advocacy reach of correctional medical litigation. There is a fast-expanding understanding of the importance of adequately preparing prisoners for release and a greater appreciation generally of the community effects of prisoners' health. Even if purely based on self-interest, the public as well as correctional staff and officials will support investment in identifying and treating prisoners' infectious diseases and mental illnesses. Jails are even more porous than prisons when it comes to disease, as prisoners come and go so quickly. In 1999, recognizing the serious medical needs of prisoners as well as the public health and public relations opportunities, a coalition of advocates filed a class action lawsuit on behalf of all persons with mental illness released from New York City's jails, estimated at 25,000 persons each year (*Brad H. v. City of New York*, 1999).

For a few years, the litigation proceeded in typical adversarial fashion. The city appealed the issuance of a temporary injunction. After the injunction was upheld, the litigation turned to whether the city was to be held in contempt for failing to abide by its demands. Press coverage was favorable to the plaintiffs, public pressure was mounting, and the city had a new mayor. In early 2003, the parties agreed to settle the case and to provide for independent monitoring, which continues today. The monitors report a slow and unsteady process that nonetheless collectively brought about a vast improvement in the planning and follow-up care available for persons with mental illness leaving prison (Urban Justice Center). And the settlement is a model that a number of jurisdictions are using voluntarily to improve their discharge planning systems—another way that litigation can more broadly spur positive change.

There is one other type of litigation to address prison conditions that could be a far greater force for improved correctional health care. The Civil Rights of Institutionalized Persons Act (CRIPA), enacted in 1980, authorizes the Civil Rights Division of the U.S. Department of Justice to investigate and, as necessary, litigate allegations of violations of the constitutional or statutory rights of prisoners in state and local facilities (42 U.S.C. §1997a). A lawsuit under CRIPA functions like a class action. Although the plaintiff is the federal government, it is brought to vindicate the rights of prisoners as a class. And unlike civil rights actions brought by individual or classes of prisoners, such suits are not subject to the Prison Litigation Reform Act's restrictions on court-ordered relief and there is no Eleventh Amendment prohibition to directly suing the state or its corrections department. CRIPA suits follow a cooperative approach to investigation and litigation, with ample opportunities for the target institutions to voluntarily come into compliance prior to the formal filing of the lawsuit. The statute also has the benefit of authorizing investigators to visit facilities and review documents, allowing for much more efficient and expeditious development of the factual record. Most of its investigations lead to a settlement prior to the filing of a court action.

Whether this approach achieves all it might, CRIPA can be an effective tool in driving improvements in prison and jail medical care. For example, in March 2006, the Department of Justice notified the State of Delaware that it would investigate medical care conditions in its prisons. It visited the facilities with its experts and reviewed documents in the summer and fall. The state hired its own experts to conduct an investigation. By December, the state stipulated to the findings of unconstitutional conditions and the parties signed an agreement outlining a 3-year comprehensive remedial plan to be overseen by a jointly selected monitor (U.S. Department of Justice, 2006 Memorandum). The Memorandum of Agreement was published the same day as the Department's letter detailing its findings of constitutional violations.

CRIPA agreements such as these have their limitations. They are not enforceable in court, and indeed require the Department to mediate any dispute regarding compliance before it files suit. CRIPA settlements do not seek or achieve the same breadth and depth of remedy as successful private class action settlements or court-ordered relief. Moreover, CRIPA has never been widely used, perhaps because of the political obstacles to adequately funding and pursuing federal government lawsuits to protect prisoners against state and local governments. And in recent years the Department of Justice has been extremely sluggish in bringing new investigations and particularly new lawsuits against prisons and jails.

Is What Remains Enough?

William Collins, who as coeditor of the *Correctional Law Reporter* is as familiar as anyone with the present state of correctional litigation, recently asked: "Is what remains [of litigation] enough to hold correctional institutions and agencies accountable for the care and treatment they provide inmates?" (Collins, 2004). It is a national failure that we have to ask and that the answer is uncertain. We should not have to rely on litigation brought by private citizens to serve a de facto oversight role for institutions that have such enormous impact on millions of individuals and on our society as a whole. But we do. Unlike in most European countries, there are virtually no systems of independent oversight in America's prisons and jails. At the very least, public health departments must have the authority and responsibility to oversee the care prisoners receive, just as they do throughout the rest of the public health system.

So long as the political process continues to fail to provide a sensible and far-seeing public health policy that fully embraces the needs of prisoners, litigation will remain essential. Indeed, litigation can move the political process along to a better, public health-centered approach to medical and mental health care for incarcerated people. And there are allies to be found from within the institutions. Corrections officials can be, and often are, among the most enlightened government officials. They know what life is like behind bars and are witnesses to the suffering prisoners face. And they often are deeply committed to improving the care and treatment their facilities and staff provide. They may be jaded—as everyone gets in a thankless job with largely unattainable goals—but they know an opportunity when it comes along. Litigating for better medical care can provide that opportunity.

References

Administrative Office of the U.S. Courts. (2007). *Judicial Facts and Figures, U.S. District Courts, Prisoner Petitions Filed by Nature of Suit*. Retrieved January 14, 2007, from http://www.uscourts.gov/judicialfactsfigures/Table406.pdf (1995 figures).

Americans with Disabilities Act of 1990, Pub. L. No. 101–336, 104 Stat. 327 (1990).

Antiterrorism and Effective Death Penalty Act of 1996, Pub. L. No. 104–132, 110 Stat. 1214 (1996).

Bell v. Wolfish, 441 U.S. 520, 548 (1979).

Bivens v. Six Unknown Named Agents of Federal Bureau of Narcotics, 403 U.S. 388 (1971).

Brad H. v. City of New York, No. 11782/99 (Sup. Ct. N.Y. County, filed 1999).

Civil Rights Litigation Clearinghouse (2007). St. Louis; http://www.clearinghouse.wustl.edu/

Collins, W. (2004). Bumps in the road to the courthouse: The Supreme Court and the Prison Litigation Reform Act. *Pace Law Review*, *24*, 651, 674.

Correctional Association of New York. (2004). *Mental health in the house of corrections*. Retrieved January 17, 2007, from http://www.correctionalassociation.org/PVP/publications/Mental-Health.pdf

Disability Advocates, Inc. v. New York State Office of Mental Health, No. 03-CV-3309 (S.D. N.Y., filed 2003).

Estelle v. Gamble, 429 U.S. 97, 106, 109, 116 (1976).

Farmer v. Brennan, 511 U.S. 825, 835–38, 851, 855 (1994).

Federal Tort Claims Act, 28 U.S.C. §1346.

Inmates of New York State with Human Immune Deficiency Virus v. Cuomo, No. 90-CV-2052 (N.D.N.Y., filed 1990).

Jones v. Bock, 2007 WL 135890 (January 22, 2007).

Madrid v. Gomez, No. 90–3094 (N.D. Cal., filed 1990).

McDonald, D. (1999). Medical care in prisons. In M. Tonry & J. Petersilia (Eds.), *Crime and justice: A review of research* (Vol. 26, p. 427). Chicago: University of Chicago Press.

McGore v. Wrigglesworth, 114 F.3d 601, 603 (6th Cir. 1997).

Murray v. Artz, 2002 WL 31906464 (N.D. Il. 2002).

Newman v. State, 349 F. Supp. 278, 281 (M.D. Ala. 1972).

Omnibus Consolidated Rescissions and Appropriations Act of 1996, Pub. L. No. 104–134, 110 Stat. 1321, Title V (1996).

Perez V. Oakland County, 466 F.3rd 416 (6th Cir. 2006)

Plata v. Schwarzenegger, No. C-01-1351 (N.D. Cal., filed 2001).

Plata v. Schwarzenegger, 2005 WL 2932243, p. 1 (N.D. Cal. May 10, 2005).

Plata v. Schwarzenegger, 2005 WL 2932253, pp. 1, 4, 24 (N.D. Cal. October 3, 2005).

Porter v. Nussle, 534 U.S. 516, 525 (2002).

Prison Litigation Reform Act of 1995, Title VIII of the Omnibus Consolidated Rescissions and Appropriations Act of 1996, Pub. L. No. 104–134, 110 Stat. 1321 (1996).

Schlanger, M. (2003). Inmate litigation, *Harvard Law Review*, *116*, 1555, 1570–1572, 1659, 1676, fn. 390.

Schlanger, M. (2006). Civil rights injunctions over time: A case study of jail and prison court orders. *New York University Law Review*, *81*, 550, 562–563.

Shumate v. Wilson, No. 2:95-CV-00619 (E.D. Cal., filed 1995).

Specter, D., & Kupers, T. (2001). Litigation, advocacy, and self-respect. In D. Sabo, T. Kupers, I. & W. London, (Eds.), *Prison masculinities* (pp. 239–241). Philadelphia: Temple University Press.

United States ex rel. *Yaris v. Shaughnessy*, 112 F. Supp. 143, 145 (S.D. N.Y. 1953).

Urban Justice Center. Quarterly Reports of the Compliance Monitors. Retrieved January 27, 2007, from http://www.urbanjustice.org/ujc/litigation/mental.html

U.S. Department of Justice, Office of Justice Programs, Bureau of Justice Statistics. (2000). Census of State and Federal Correctional Facilities (p. 9). Retrieved January 13, 2007, from http://www.ojp.usdoj.gov/bjs/pub/pdf/csfcf00.pdf

U.S. Department of Justice, Civil Rights Division, Special Litigation Section. (2006). Letter to Governor Ruth Ann Minner, RE: Investigation of Delaware Correctional Center, Smyrna, Delaware; Howard R. Young Correctional Institution, Wilmington, Delaware; Sussex Correctional Institution, Georgetown, Delaware; John L. Webb Correctional Facility, Wilmington, Delaware; and Delores J. Baylor Women's Correctional Institution, New Castle, Delaware. December 29, 2006 (p. 4). Retrieved January 13, 2007, from http://www.usdoj.gov/crt/split/documents/delaware_prisons_findlet_12-29-06.pdf

U.S. Department of Justice, Civil Rights Division, Special Litigation Section. (2006). Memorandum of Agreement Between the United States Department of Justice and the State of Delaware Regarding the Delores J. Baylor Women's Correctional Institution, the Delaware Correctional Center, the Howard R. Young Correctional Institution, and the Sussex Correctional Institution. December 29, 2006. Retrieved January 16, 2007, from http://www.usdoj.gov/crt/split/documents/delaware_prisons_moa_12-29-06.pdf

U.S. Department of Justice, Civil Rights Division, Special Litigation Section. (2007). Investigative Findings. Retrieved January 13, 2007, from http://www.usdoj.gov/crt/split/findsettle.htm#FindingsLetters.

Violent Crime Control and Law Enforcement Act of 1994, Pub. L. No. 103–322, 108 Stat. 1796 (1994).

Violent Offender Incarceration and Truth-in-Sentencing Incentive Grants, 42 U.S.C. ch. 136, subch. 1, §13701 et. seq. (1996).

Westlake v. Lucas, 537 F.2d 857, 859 fn. 2 (6th Cir. 1976) (listing Court of Appeals decisions prior to *Estelle v. Gamble*).

Wilson v. Seiter, 501 U.S. 294, 300 (1991) (emphasis in original).

Wolff v. McDonnell, 418 U.S. 539, 555–556 (1974).

Woodford v. Ngo, 126 S.Ct. 2378 (2006).

18 U.S.C. §3626(a)(1)(A).
18 U.S.C. §3626(a)(2).
18 U.S.C. §§3626(b)(1)(A)(i) and (b)(3).
18 U.S.C. §3626(e)(2).
28 U.S.C. §1346(b)(2).
28 U.S.C. §1915(b)(1–2).
28 U.S.C. §1915(g).
42 U.S.C. §1997a.
42 U.S.C. §1997e(a).
42 U.S.C. §1997e(d)(1)(a).
42 U.S.C. §1997e(d)(2).
42 U.S.C. §1997e(d)(3).
42 U.S.C. §1997e(e).

Chapter 4

Accommodating Disabilities in Jails and Prisons

R. Samuel Paz

Introduction

In 1990, Congress passed the Americans with Disabilities Act[1] (ADA), an optimistic and comprehensive civil rights law intended to provide equal opportunity in employment and public life to individuals living with physical and mental disabilities. Title I addresses discrimination in employment[2]; Title II guarantees disabled persons equal access to state services and programs, an assurance that the rights these programs fulfill will be protected[3]; and Title III mandates "reasonable accommodation" to the needs of the disabled in public facilities.[4] The federal statute includes both a prohibition against discrimination against disabled persons and a provision for redress. Legislators recognized that without the prospect of "effective enforcement provisions," the states would be unlikely to move into compliance with the new legislation.

The ADA began with the principle that its purpose is enforcement of the Fourteenth Amendment's command that "all persons similarly situated should be treated alike."[5] The Supreme Court observed that classifications based on disability violate that constitutional command if they lack a rational relationship to a legitimate governmental purpose.[6] If an entity's policies and practices discriminate against a plaintiff because he or she was mentally or physically disabled and in need of services and programs which are available, then the policies of the entity treat the plaintiff differently.

The traditional remedies for unconstitutional treatment of prisoners in our nation's courts generally have been found in case law decided under 42 U.S.C. 1983, the "civil rights" statute enacted in 1871.[7] However, over the years, the Supreme Court and many circuit courts have made prosecution of civil rights cases more difficult, and there are numerous examples of plaintiffs being successful at the trial level but verdicts having been overturned on appeal.[8] One hurdle is that proving a case under Section 1983 is not just proving the traditional breach of a duty causing harm, the requirement to prove most claims under state law negligence theory. Section 1983 requires a high degree of proof described as "deliberate indifference" requiring that the evidence prove that a prison official acted with a "sufficiently culpable state of mind," which entails more than mere negligence, but less than conduct undertaken for the very purpose of causing harm.[9] Over the years the courts have interpreted the concept of "deliberate indifference" in many ever increasingly higher degrees of proof of the subjective mental state of the individual custodial officer under the factual circumstances presented by the case.[10] When combined with a number of judicial doctrines which allow an individual officer to escape liability and deprive a plaintiff of a remedy for even an admitted violation of constitutional rights, the road to justice for many persons who suffer a multitude of unconstitutional harms, intentional abuse, and even death, is a difficult one indeed.[11] The case law interpreting the ADA over the last decade appears to offer an alternative concept for vindicating the rights of incarcerated people with physical and mental disabilities and in many instances the ADA fills a void left by the federal courts interpreting prisoners' rights under Section 1983. In some situations, ADA claims by disabled prisoners are well paired with the rights protected under Section 1983 and constitute a more comprehensive range of options for correcting repetitive violations of constitutional rights and inhumane conditions.[12]

As will be seen by many of the cases discussed below, the prisoner litigants whose cases proceed in federal court are often those with compelling facts: paraplegic, incontinent, or severely disabled individuals. But the ADA definition of a "disability" is defined more broadly: "(A) a physical or mental impairment that substantially limits one or more of the life activities of such individual; (B) a record of such an impairment; or (C) being regarded as having such an impairment."[13]

Of the general population in the United States, the Census Bureau has found that 18%, or 51.2 million people, have a disability and 12%, or 32.5 million, have a severe disability.[14] People with severe disabilities are poorer, with a median annual income of $12,800. Prisoners and detainees are poorer and sicker than those responding to the Census surveys.[15] Estimates of mental illness among those in prison range from 16%[16] upward to a majority—the finding of a current study released by the Bureau of Justice Statistics in September 2006.[17] These are people who are at risk either physically or mentally. They are vulnerable to substandard care because of erroneous assumptions about them.[18] In practice, those disabled persons are simply not chosen to participate in educational or training programs. Whether or not the prison officials engage in conscious discrimination, the impact on disabled prisoners is to limit their opportunities for employment and reintegration on release.

Consequences of failing to make provision for those who live in prison with disabilities can be grave for the individuals concerned. Mentally ill prisoners are much more likely to suffer physical abuse, earn disciplinary sanctions for breaking prison rules or failing to respond promptly to orders, and to accrue further criminal punishment that extends the length of their confinement.[19] Although some prison administrators do recognize mental illness as a mitigating factor as they assess infractions, those prisoners whose disabilities make it hard for them to comply with prison rules often end up with long periods of isolation. Isolation can deepen and exacerbate mental illness, and can prompt acts of self-harm.[20]

It would not be unrealistic to expect that a third of prisoners would qualify for reasonable accommodation if we were to take seriously a rehabilitative purpose for imprisonment. For the growing percentage of life-sentenced prisoners who are now aging into their 60s and 70s in state and federal prisons, and for the increasing proportion of middle-aged and elderly in the prison population,[21] the questions are: what accommodations should be considered and what are the core activities (of a life in prison) that should be protected? The fledgling, but growing, body of case law interpreting the claims of the incarcerated under the protections provided by the ADA gives some indication of some of the answers to these questions.

Basic Concepts of Title II of the ADA in Jails and Prisons

Title II of the ADA provides that "[n]o qualified individual with a disability shall, by reason of such disability, be excluded from participation in or be denied the benefits of the services, programs, or activities of a public entity, or be subjected to discrimination by any such entity" (42 U.S.C. §12132). Thus, the ADA not only prohibits public entities from discriminating against the disabled, it also prohibits public entities from excluding the disabled from participating in or benefiting from a public program, activity, or service "solely by reason of disability."[22] If a public entity denies an otherwise "qualified individual" "meaningful access" to its "services, programs, or activities" "solely by reason of" his or her disability, that individual may have an ADA claim against the public entity.[23]

One judge explained that the "ADA was cast in terms not of subsidizing an interest group but of eliminating a form of discrimination that Congress considered unfair and even odious"[24] and the ADA essentially assimilates the disabled into those groups that by reason of sex, age, race, religion, nationality, or ethnic origin are believed to be victims of discrimination. "Rights against discrimination are among the few rights that prisoners do not park at the prison gates" even if the special conditions of incarceration allow for deprivation of liberty that would not be tolerated in a free environment, nonetheless, there is no general right of prison officials to discriminate against prisoners on grounds of race, sex, religion, and so forth. Succinctly, the court explained the basic concept of the ADA:

If a prison may not exclude blacks from the prison dining hall and force them to eat in their cells, and if Congress thinks that discriminating against a blind person is like discriminating against a black person, it is not obvious that the prison may not exclude the blind person from the dining hall, unless allowing the person to use the dining hall would place an undue burden on prison management. *Id.*

The ADA defines a "qualified individual with a disability" to include any disabled person "who, with or without reasonable modifications to rules, policies, or practices, ... or transportation barriers, or the provision of auxiliary aids and services, meets the essential eligibility requirements for the receipt of services or the participation in programs or activities provided by a public entity" [42 U.S.C. §12131(2)].[25] However, simply because the person is disabled and excluded from a program is not sufficient, they must also prove that without their handicap, i.e., the medical or mental disability, they would have been eligible for treatment in the program.[26]

A plaintiff need not show intentional discrimination in order to make out a violation of the ADA.[27] The ADA broadly defines "public entity"[28] to include[29] state prisons[30] and local law enforcement agencies. However, there is at least one district court case which has held that the ADA does not apply to a federal immigration detention facility.[31] The implications for the ADA as a vehicle for protection of human rights for disabled persons among the population of those in prisons and jails become evident given that this population is now more than 2 million.[32]

Application of the ADA by the Courts

In the prison context the Supreme Court has provided some guidance on whether a modification in programs would be reasonable to accommodate a disability. In *Turner v. Safley*,[33] the court identified factors the lower courts should consider: (1) whether there is a valid, rational connection between the prison policy and the legitimate governmental interest that the prison officials put forward to justify the policy; (2) whether there are any alternative means for the prisoner to be able to exercise the right; (3) the impact that accommodating the constitutional right will have on guards, other inmates, or the allocation of prison resources; and (4) whether the policy is an exaggerated response to prison concerns. Finally, the court said that the burden is on the inmate to show that the challenged regulation or policy is unreasonable. One example of the application of the *Turner v. Safley* factors is *Bullock v. Gomez*,[34] where an HIV-positive inmate and his wife, also HIV-positive, sued the prison alleging that the prison's refusal to allow them to participate in a conjugal visits program violated the ADA. The court rejected the prison's claim of summary judgment and held the plaintiffs' claim could go to trial because a genuine issue of material fact existed that the plaintiffs were qualified for purposes of the ADA. The court noted that the wife was not able to bear children, minimizing any chance of her being a direct threat to others, such as a newborn (she was not able to bear children) or herself (she was already HIV-positive). Successful ADA claims were also found where an HIV-positive pretrial detainee in a county jail alleged inappropriate medical care and segregation by the jail officials.[35]

There are some good examples of reform in prisons and jails by use of the ADA in combination with Section 1983 and state laws in response to the efforts of litigators who have pursued the rights of those least able to assert them.[36].

ADA Applies to Nondisabled "Otherwise Qualified" Persons

The scope of the ADA has been extended to nondisabled persons who are associated with disabled persons who are denied "services, programs, or activities of a public entity." In *Niece v. Fitzner*,[37] both plaintiffs, a nondisabled inmate and his girlfriend, a person with numerous disabilities, were found to be "otherwise qualified" under the ADA.[38] They alleged that the girlfriend was discriminated against on the basis of her disabilities and that the inmate was discriminated against in the range of options available to him in the prison because he associated with a person with a disability. *Id.*

Equal Access to Facilities

Equal use of a state prison dining hall or a prison library has been held as an "activity" under the ADA that a public entity may be required to provide to a disabled person who is denied access to services, programs, or activities of public entity.[39] An educational program provided by a state prison may be a program that a public entity is required to provide to a disabled individual under the ADA.

Accommodation Within the Facility

The area of jail conditions which discriminate against a disabled person requiring accommodation under the ADA have been extended to jails as well as prisons. In one case, a bilateral amputee parole violator confined in county jail while awaiting trial successfully raised claims against a sheriff and county jail nurses as to whether the design of the cell's shower causes it to be inaccessible to him and whether he should be provided with a shower chair and a portable commode.[40] A similar result in the prison context involved a double amputee who, although he was actually able to use most of the jail services, did not preclude his claims against jail officials under the ADA because he was able to do so only by exceptional and painful exertion that was contraindicated to his physician's instructions.[41] Another successful extension of accommodations required by the ADA to city jails required a city to make the jail shower accessible to and usable by an inmate who wore an artificial leg and had suffered burns on his body that required him to take medication and shower on a regular basis.[42]

Equal Participation in Custody Programs and Proceedings

A deaf and visually impaired prisoner was held to be entitled to interpreters for meaningful participation in prison counseling sessions, administrative or disciplinary hearings, and medical treatment and diagnosis.[43] Hearing-impaired inmates successfully raised claims that the prison had violated their rights under the ADA by failing to provide qualified interpreters for various aspects of reception and classification; failing to provide timely access to telephone communication devices; closed-caption decoders for televisions; special alarms to alert in the event of fire; failing to establish an effective grievance procedure for deaf and hearing-impaired inmates regarding accommodations for services; and by conducting disciplinary, grievance, and parole hearings without affording them interpretive services or assistive devices necessary to render their opportunity to be heard meaningful.[44]

A visually disabled inmate prevailed on an ADA claim that prison officials were required to provide him with a recorder and tapes. It was reasonable to interpret the phrase "service, program, or activity" to include whatever reading and educational opportunities were provided to fully sighted inmates.[45]

Inmate Rights to Medical and Mental Health Under the ADA

Medical and mental health to the incarcerated are "services, programs, or activities of a public entity" within the meaning of the ADA section prohibiting discrimination of qualified individuals with disabilities.[46] For example, regarding a detainee denied medication required for his HIV condition while he was incarcerated in a detention center for 3 days, the court found that the prescription services offered by the detention center were programs or services of a public entity for purposes of the ADA prohibition on discrimination against qualified persons with disabilities.[47]

Diabetic inmates successfully raised claims under the ADA that they were denied the benefits of the services, programs, or activities of a prison treatment and diagnostic center by presenting evidence of failure to adequately treat the inmates' diabetes and the complications of diabetes.[48] An inmate who needed crutches to assist his mobility, but was denied the use of them, successfully alleged a claim for violation of the rights protected by the ADA that required the prison to make the crutches available to him when appropriate.[49]

Mental Health Under Civil Rights Law

In the area of mental health, more and more mentally ill persons are incarcerated because of conduct arising from their mental illness, often exacerbated by homelessness, drug addiction, and alcoholism. The frequency of jail suicide and failure to train staff on issues of mental health have been revealed in civil rights cases.[50] However, it bears discussing the increasingly high burdens which the courts have placed on plaintiffs under the civil rights statute to understand how the ADA has changed the landscape.

The issues of denial of access to mental health causing a suicide in a jail are areas of the law under 42 U.S.C. §1983 are not firmly established. In one of the earlier cases defining the applicable law in cases involving a suicide as a denial of medical treatment in the area of mental health, the circuit extended the principles developed in the medical cases to establish liability in situations involving the denial and interference with mental health treatment.[51] It was essentially a recognition that mental health treatment was the same as treatment required under constitutional principles discussed above for medical conditions.[52] The circuit upheld liability after a trial rejecting the jail defendants' argument that there was no showing of a policy of deliberate indifference to the decedent's medical and psychiatric needs because he was not denied *access* to medical and psychiatric help (emphasis in the original). They point to the uncontested evidence in the record that the decedent was evaluated on several occasions by various medical personnel. However, the Circuit pointed out that "access to medical staff is meaningless unless that staff is competent and can render competent care."[53]

The Supreme Court vacated the *Cabrales*[54] circuit opinion and remanded for consideration in light of *City of Canton v. Harris,*[55] and the Ninth Circuit reinstated its opinion.[56] The standard for liability under 42 U.S.C. §1983 involving a suicide was made more onerous in the Seventh Circuit under the Eighth Amendment by requiring the plaintiff to prove both an objective and a subjective element: (1) the harm that befell the prisoner must be objectively, sufficiently serious and a substantial risk to his or her health or safety, and (2) the individual defendants were deliberately indifferent to the substantial risk to the prisoner's health and safety.[57] In prison suicide cases, the objective element is met by virtue of the suicide itself, as "[i]t goes without saying that 'suicide is a serious harm.'"[58] Where the harm at issue is a suicide or attempted suicide, the second, subjective component of an *Eighth Amendment* claim requires a dual showing that the defendant: (1) subjectively knew the prisoner was at substantial risk of committing suicide and (2) intentionally disregarded the risk.[59] With respect to the first showing, "it is not enough that there was a danger of which a prison official *should have been* aware," rather, "the official must *both* be aware of facts from which the inference could be drawn that a substantial risk of serious harm exists, and he must also draw the inference."[60] In other words, the defendant must be cognizant of the significant likelihood that an inmate may imminently seek to take his own life.[61]

The impact of the Seventh Circuit inserting a subjective component into the level of proof the plaintiff must prove is to imbalance the law to favor the jail or prison officer. The "subjective" element means the officer can simply say "I don't remember, I did not see, hear or know anything" and the plaintiff loses, even where the officer has an affirmative duty to observe the prisoner, protect the prisoner, provide access to the prisoner. In essence, the individual officer who may be responsible for ignoring his or her duties is able to admit to negligence, dereliction of duty, abandonment of responsibilities, violations of policy, and still not be held responsible under the civil rights law. Over the years, the Supreme Court has continually moved to an "objective standard" as to what the reasonable officer should have done in the situation presented by the facts of the case.[62]

Mental Health Under the ADA

Given the increasingly high levels of proof the circuit courts have required to prove that a jail or prison is responsible for denial of access to medical or mental health treatment under the evolving standards discussed above, the ADA provides an alternative remedy having a different burden to prove a case. The ADA creates the affirmative duty on the institution to accommodate persons with mental disabilities and, of course, suicidal ideation or with a history of suicide attempts. Accommodation under the ADA may include training of jail staff on observation handling of such inmates, housing alternatives, access to focused medical care and increased programs of observation and reporting to specialists. It is well established that persons incarcerated may not be discriminated against because of their mental illness.[63]

Mental health services undertaken by law enforcement and provided by correctional facilities to those incarcerated are "services, programs, or activities of a public entity" within the meaning of the ADA.[64] The result of reducing the threshold to prove liability is an increased likelihood of improving training, programs, and services to address the increasing frequency of suicides of mentally disabled in jails and prisons across the nation.

Limitations to the Reach of the ADA

There are many cases where the plaintiff cannot meet the elements of the ADA because they fail to present facts that they are a "qualified individual with a disability" or that "by reason of such disability" they are "excluded from participation in or be denied the benefits of the services, programs, or activities of a public entity" or "subjected to discrimination" by the public entity as required by 42 U.S.C. §12132. The preceding cases provide concrete examples of the reach of the ADA so that a proper assessment can be made before launching litigation.

There are more subtle limits to the reach of ADA. One area is that claims that "[t]he treatment, or lack of treatment, concerning plaintiff's medical condition does not provide a basis upon which to impose liability under the [Rehabilitation Act] or the ADA."[65] However, there is a major distinction between those claims that limit the plaintiff from making a claim for denial of medical care and those where the plaintiff has successful presented a claim under the ADA for denial of medical services or programs because she is disabled.[66] For example, where a prisoner with an amputated left leg alleged that he was provided old wheelchairs that later broke, causing him to fall or cut himself, and that he received inadequate medical care following such incidents, this was determined by the court to merely challenge the prisoner's medical care, not his lack of access to prison programs or other benefits.[67]

The ADA does not create a right for an inmate to demand that a prison system or a specific prison facility implement a specific type of rehabilitation or educational program that is not already available or create any right for an inmate to be housed at a specific prison.[68]

Implications for the Future

As federal courts continue to consider the scope and limitations of the ADA, three general questions are relevant: (1) What percentage of prisoners will qualify as disabled? (2) What counts as "reasonable accommodation" to the needs of physically challenged and mentally ill prisoners? (3) Does it not make sense to consider alternatives to incarceration for many disabled prisoners, thereby reducing the potential cost of providing reasonable accommodations behind bars?

These are practical and achievable objectives:

- Medical care and physical plant accommodations for patients with multiple chronic medical illnesses such as chronic respiratory disease, diabetes, arthritis, and heart disease, diseases that are highly prevalent among the poor, who are overrepresented in prisons and jails.[69] In addition, there are conditions whose prevalence is uniquely high behind bars, including paraplegia secondary to gunshot wounds, advanced liver disease from alcohol abuse and/or viral hepatitis C, and end-stage kidney disease from injection drug use and/or HIV infection. Geriatric patients are at special risk for acute infections, such as influenza and pneumonia.[70]
- Mental health care and physical plant accommodations for patients with serious mental illness, such as schizophrenia, bipolar disorder, major depression, and posttraumatic stress disorder. The prevalence of each of these is higher behind bars than in the community.[71]
- Medication for patients with chronic medical problems and mental illness.
- Protection from heat injury for those especially susceptible, including those with chronic illnesses such as diabetes and those who are on medications that increase the likelihood of heat injury, for example, medications for psychosis and heart disease.[72]
- Skilled nursing care for patients with functional disabilities that interfere with their activities of daily living: bathing, dressing, eating, transferring, and toileting. Some patients with physical disabilities need mobility aids that can be hard to come by behind bars. In prison, there are activities that are unique to daily life, called "prison activities of daily living." These necessary

actions include dropping to the floor for alarms, standing for head count, moving to dining areas, climbing on top bunks, and hearing orders. Rates of functional impairment are higher when these activities are measured.[73]

- Programming for patients with physical or functional disabilities, including those with chronic disease, mental illness, and developmental disabilities. Patients with vision and hearing problems are common among older people.[74] These conditions can result in falls, social isolation, depression, and functional physical disability. Patients with cognitive impairments, such as dementia, from aging or medical conditions such as HIV or viral hepatitis C are physically vulnerable.
- Training for correctional staff to recognize that failure to cooperate with prison rules can be caused by impairments of sense (hearing or vision), dementia, or mental illness. These patients are too often disciplined with segregation status instead of being referred for evaluation, treatment, and protective housing. Likewise, patients with physical disabilities that cause problems such as vomiting or incontinence too often get disciplined for soiling instead of being evaluated by medical care staff.
- Personal safety protection for those with physical or mental disabilities, especially the elderly.

The modifications that would be warranted by a scrupulous application of the ADA to prisons and jails—increasing physical access within a facility, increasing timely contacts between prisoners and social service and medical staff, increasing congregate time for education and training—run immediately up against the security provisions, some of which are policy-driven and others of which result from the design of a particular facility. As was expressed by lawyers for the group of states arguing for sovereign immunity in the case of *Goodman v. Georgia*:

Like most Americans, amici applaud the ADA's goal of ensuring that disabled citizens are protected from invidious discrimination and have every opportunity to participate fully in the benefits our society provides to other citizens. Prisons, however, are dangerous places for all who work or live there. ... Recognition of private ADA claims has the potential to disrupt sound prison administration which, as this Court has often noted, is peculiarly within the province and professional expertise of corrections officials.[75]

It should be more of a concern to the states and the federal government that there is widespread failure on the part of states, and state departments of correction, to enact the provisions of the ADA.[76] It is not acceptable that the ADA mandate should simply be waived—or considered a principle less significant than that of punishment. If it is not feasible to treat disabled prisoners fairly and without discrimination in prison settings, then alternative settings should be considered.

Imprisonment is the default punishment in the United States, but whether incarceration achieves the purposes of punishment is much less certain. That the ADA is yet to be fully implemented should not mean a retreat from its principles: the opportunity and challenge is for criminal justice professionals to envision less restrictive settings in which disabled prisoners can live without constant suffering, and those who are eligible can prepare for life after imprisonment. It is, after all, generally not they who pose the greatest threat to society.

Endnotes

1 Americans with Disabilities Act, ch. 126, 42 U.S.C. §12101.

2 42 U.S.C. §§12111–12117.

3 42 U.S.C. §12131 et seq.

4 42 U.S.C. §12181 et seq.

5 *Board of Trustees v. Garrett,* 531 U.S. 356, 365 (2001).

6 *Id.,* 366.

7 42 United States Code Section 1983, which applies to state and local government and officials, includes claims alleged against the federal government and its officials through what is known as a "Bivens action." See *Bivens v. Six Unknown Agents,* 403 U.S. 388 (1971) (federal government may be sued for actions of its agents conducted under governmental authority for violations of constitutional protections found in the Bill of Rights). Federal courts have consistently extended rulings under section 1983 to Bivens actions.

8 See James C. Harrington, *The ADA and Section 1983: Walking Hand in Hand,* 19 Rev. Litig. 43, U. Texas, 2000 and James C. Harrington, *Section 1983: Civil Rights Litigation 2007* (April 9, 2007), Georgetown U. Law Center.

9 *Estelle v. Gamble,* 429 U.S. 97, 50 L. Ed. 2d 251 (1976) (denial of medical care).

10 See Justice Scalia's discussion in *County of Sacramento v. Lewis,* 523 U.S. 833, 849 (1998), describing the range of "deliberate indifference" standards to evaluate an officer's culpability under the Fourteenth Amendment "shock the conscious" test.

11 See Michael Avery, David Rodovsky, & Karen Blum, *Police Misconduct: Law and Litigation,* 3d ed. 2004, for a comprehensive discussion of the myriad areas of federal law under Section 1983 that have developed to address individual and repetitive violations of the rights of persons in custody and at liberty, discussing the doctrines of qualified ("good faith") immunity, interlocutory appeals from the denial of qualified immunity, municipal immunity, and sovereign immunity.

12 James C. Harrington, *The ADA and Section 1983: Walking Hand in Hand,* 19 Rev. Litig. 43, U. Texas, 2000, discussing the increasing difficulties in protecting rights under Section 1983 and contrasting the ADA as an alternative vehicle for vindicating the rights of people with physical, developmental, and mental disabilities.

13 42 U.S.C. §12102 (2).

14 "More Than 50 Million Americans Report Some Level of Disability," Census Bureau News Release, May 12, 2006 <http://www.census.gov/Press-Release/www/releases/archives/aging population/006809.html>.

15 Doris L. James, *Profile of Jail Inmates, 2002* (Washington, DC: Bureau of Justice Statistics, U.S. Department of Justice, 2005) <http://www.ojp.usdoj.gov/bjs/pub/pdf/pji02.pdf>.

16 Paula M. Dixon, *Mental Health and Treatment of Inmates and Probationers* (Washington, DC: Bureau of Justice Statistics Special Report, 1999) <http://www.ojp.usdoj.gov/bjs/pub/pdf/mhtip.pdf>.

17 D.L. James & L.E. Glaze, *Mental Health Problems of Prison and Jail Inmates* (Washington, DC: Bureau of Justice Statistics, 2006).

18 Department of Health and Human Services, *The Surgeon General's Call to Action to Improve the Health and Wellness of Persons with Disabilities* (Rockville, MD: Public Health Service, 2005) <http://www.Surgeongeneral.gov/library/disabilities/calltoaction/calltoaction.pdf>.

19 See, e.g., U.S. Department of Justice, Civil Rights Division, 1997 CRIPA investigation into the conditions at Los Angeles County Jail established that mental health care at the jail violated the inmates' constitutional rights. It found "unconstitutional conditions exist at the Los Angeles County Jail, including *deliberate indifference to inmates' serious mental health needs.*" They found "abuse of mentally ill inmates

by sheriff's deputies working in the jail; some have their illnesses misdiagnosed and their medications improperly administered. … they have been abused by correctional staff; the jail does not adequately prevent abuse of mentally ill inmates and does not adequately investigate allegations of such abuse when it occurs."

20 *Madrid v. Gomez,* 190 F.3d 990 (9th Cir.1999).

21 Harrison & Beck, *Prisoners in 2003,* Bureau of Justice Statistics, U.S. Department of Justice 2004: NCJ 205335.

22 *Weinreich v. Los Angeles County Metro. Transp. Auth.,* 114 F.3d 976, 978-79 (9th Cir. 1997).

23 *Id.* (cites omitted).

24 *Crawford v. Indiana Dept. of Corrections,* 115 F.3d 481, 22 A.D.D. 22, 6 A.D. Cas. (BNA) 1416 (7th Cir. 1997) (rev'd on other grounds by *Erickson v. Board of Governors of State Colleges and Universities for Northeastern Illinois University,* 2000 WL 307121 (7th Cir. 2000)).

25 See, e.g., *Peacock v. Terhune,* 2002 U.S. Dist. LEXIS 1136, *2 (E.D. Cal. 2002) (holding plaintiff's claim valid where he alleged that the state defendants discriminated against him and other disabled inmates by "requiring them to go on a daily basis to health care providers for medical supplies based on the allegation that "the prison changed its policy on providing medical care and supplies so that paralyzed inmates were required to go on a daily basis to another location to get their supplies," and this policy change "treated non-disabled inmates differently from disabled persons." *Id.* at *7–8.

26 See *Harris v. Oregon Health Sciences University,* 1999 U.S. Dist. LEXIS 16231, *10 (D.C. Oreg. 1999) (plaintiff was mentally ill. She was expelled from a mental services program because her medical needs were too complex for a resident to handle. However, she could not show that without her handicap—her mental disability—she would have been eligible for treatment in the program. *Id.* In fact, without her disability the plaintiff clearly would *not* have been eligible for treatment since the entire reason for entering the program was her mental disability. *Id.* "Without a showing that the non-handicapped received the treatment denied to the 'otherwise qualified' handicapped, the appellants cannot assert that a violation of section 504 [and the ADA] has occurred." *Id.* at *13.

27 *See Martin v. PGA Tour, Inc.,* 994 F. Supp. 1242, 1247–48 (D. Oreg. 1998) (aff'd *Martin,* 204 F.3d 994 (9th Cir. 1999)) ("Congress intended to protect disabled persons not just from intentional discrimination but also from 'thoughtlessness,' 'indifference,' and 'benign neglect.'"). See also *Tyler v. City of Manhattan,* 857 F. Supp. 800, 818–819 (D. Kan. 1994) (finding discrimination based on disability despite defendant's good faith effort to remove particular barriers).

28 42 U.S.C. §12131(1).

29 ADA's broad language brings within its scope "'anything a public entity does.'" *Pennsylvania Dep't of Corr. v. Yeskey,* 118 F.3d 168, 171 & n.5 (3d Cir. 1997), aff'd 524 U.S. 206 (1998) This includes programs or services provided at jails, prisons, and any other "'custodial or correctional institution.'" *Id.* "Although 'incarceration itself is hardly a "program" or "activity" to which a disabled person might wish access,'" mental health services and other activities or services undertaken by law enforcement and provided by correctional facilities to those incarcerated are "services, programs, or activities of a public entity" within the meaning of the ADA.

30 *Pennsylvania Dep't of Corr. v. Yeskey,* 524 U.S. 206, 209 (1998); *Bogovich v. Sandoval,* 189 F.3d 999, 1002 (9th Cir. 1999).

31 *Hurtado v. Reno,* 34 F. Supp. 2d 1261 (D. Colo. 1999) (deaf alien awaiting deportation as an aggravated felon at an INS detention facility).

32 P. M. Harrison & A. J. Beck, *Prisoners in 2003* (Washington, DC: Bureau of Justice Statistics, U.S. Department of Justice, 2004).

33 482 U.S. 78, 107 S. Ct. 2254, 96 L. Ed. 2d 64 (1987).

34 929 F. Supp. 1299, 18 A.D.D. 542, 6 A.D. Cas. (BNA) 1275 (C.D. Cal. 1996).

35 *Roop v. Squadrito,* 70 F. Supp. 2d 868 (N.D. Ind. 1999).

36 See, e.g., *Coleman v. Wilson,* 912 F. Supp. 1282 (E.D. Cal. 1995) (requiring reforms in conditions for mentally ill prisoners in California prisons); *Plata v. Schwarzenegger,* 01-1351 (N.D. Cal., filed April 5, 2001) (massive restructuring of California's prison health care system); *Armstrong v. Wilson,* 942 F.Supp. 1252 (N.D. Cal. 1996) aff'd, 124 F.3d 1019 (9th Cir. 1997) (finding that the Cal. Department of Corrections was violating the Americans with Disabilities Act and the Rehabilitation Act and issuing an injunction to improve access to prison programs for prisoners with physical disabilities at all of California's prisons and parole facilities); and *VonColln v. County of Ventura,* 189 F.R.D. 583 (C.D. Cal.) 1999 U.S. Dist. LEXIS 20956 (preventing torture by use of a restraint chair in pretrial booking).

37 922 F. Supp. 1208, 6 A.D. Cas. (BNA) 335 (E.D. Mich. 1996).

38 *Id.* In holding that, the court noted that "otherwise qualified" means a person who meets the eligibility requirements for the receipt of services provided by a public entity, with or without the provision of auxiliary aids. Observing that most courts have construed the term "service" very broadly, the court concluded that prisons supply a service to persons, not inmates, by allowing them to be called by inmates and allowing them to visit inmates in prison.

39 *Crawford v. Indiana Dept. of Corrections,* 115 F.3d 481, 22 A.D.D. 22, 6 A.D. Cas. (BNA) 1416 (7th Cir. 1997) (rev'd on other grounds, *Erickson v. Board of Governors of State Colleges and Universities for Northeastern Illinois University,* 2000 WL 307121 (7th Cir. 2000)).

40 *Kaufman v. Carter,* 952 F. Supp. 520 (W.D. Mich. 1996).

41 *Schmidt v. Odell,* 64 F. Supp. 2d 1014 (D. Kan. 1999).

42 *Outlaw v. City of Dothan, Ala.,* 8 A.D.D. 560, 3 A.D. Cas. (BNA) 939 (M.D. Ala. 1993).

43 *Bonner v. Arizona Dept. of Corrections,* 714 F. Supp. 420 (D. Ariz. 1989) (decided under §504 of the Rehabilitation Act, 29 U.S.C.A. §794).

44 *Clarkson v. Coughlin,* 898 F. Supp. 1019, 10 A.D.D. 642, 4 A.D. Cas. (BNA) 1056 (S.D. N.Y. 1995).

45 *Walker v. Washington,* 13 Nat'l Disability Law Rep. P 60, 1998 WL 30701 (N.D. Ill. 1998).

46 *Lee v. City of Los Angeles,* 250 F.3d 668 (9th Cir. 2001).

47 *McNally v. Prison Health Services,* 46 F. Supp. 2nd 49 (D. Me. 1999), reconsideration denied, 52 F. Supp. 2d 147 (D. Me. 1999).

48 *Rouse v. Plantier,* 997 F. Supp. 575 (N.J. 1998), vacated on other grounds, 182 F.3d 192 (3rd Cir. 1999).

49 *Owens v. Chester County,* 2000 WL 116069 (E.D. Pa. 2000).

50 See, e.g., *Hare v. City of Corinth,* 135 F.3d 320, 327 (5th Cir.1998) discussing a series of suicide cases and *Flores v. County of Hardeman,* 124 F.3d 736, 736–739 (5th Cir. 1997).

51 *Cabrales v. County of Los Angeles,* 864 F.2d 1454 (9th Cir.1988) (duty to provide medical care encompasses detainees' psychiatric needs). *Cabrales* 864 F.2d 1461 (9th Cir. 1988), vac'd, 490 U.S. 1087, 104 L. Ed. 2d 982, 109 S. Ct. 2425 (1989), opinion reinstated, 886 F.2d 235 (9th Cir. 1989), cert. denied, 494 U.S. 1091, 108 L. Ed. 2d 966, 110 S. Ct. 1838 (1990); see also *Wellman v. Faulkner,* 715 F.2d 269, 272 (7th Cir. 1983) and *Ramos v. Lamm,* 639 F.2d 559, 574 (10th Cir. 1980).

52 The 7th Circuit also applies the medical deliberate indifference standard for pretrial detainee suicide cases. See *Brandich v. City of Chicago,* 413 F.3d 688, 690 (7th Cir. 2005) citing *Bell v. Wolfish,* 441 U.S. 520, 535 n.16, 60 L. Ed. 2d 447, 99 S. Ct. 1861 (1979) and *Matos v. O'Sullivan,* 335 F.3d 553, 556–57 (7th Cir. 2003).

53 *Cabrales* established that the affidavits relied on by the district court adequately demonstrated that the medical understaffing at the jail directly contributed to the

decedent's suicide. The psychiatric staff could only spend minutes per month with disturbed inmates. The district court could conclude that lack of time and resources meant, in the decedent's case, that any psychological illness he had would go undiagnosed and untreated. The omission by the County and its policymakers in providing adequate medical care at the Men's Central Jail was the policy or custom that was the "moving force" behind the deprivation of the decedent's constitutional rights without due process. *Id.*, 1461.

54 *Cabrales v. County of Los Angeles,* 864 F.2d 1454 (9th Cir.1988) vacated 490 U.S. 1087, 109 S. Ct. 2425, 104 L. Ed. 2d 982 (1989).

55 489 U.S. 378 (1989).

56 *Cabrales v. County of Los Angeles,* 886 F.2d 235, 236 (9th Cir. 1989) ("We conclude that *Harris* does not alter our previous opinion on either of these points. In *Harris,* the Supreme Court determined that a municipality can be held liable for a constitutional policy if it is culpable for an unconstitutional application of its policy. Because the policy of understaffing was considered unconstitutional, there was no need for us to determine separately whether the County could be held culpable for an unconstitutional application of its policy.")

57 *Collins v. Seeman,* 2006 U.S. App. LEXIS 23092, *7–8 (7th Cir. 2006) (citing *Farmer v. Brennan,* 511 U.S. 825, 832, 128 L. Ed. 2d 811 (1994)).

58 *Sanville v. McCaughtry,* 266 F.3d 724, 733 (7th Cir. 2001).

59 *Matos ex. rel. Matos v. O'Sullivan,* 335 F.3d 553, 557 (7th Cir. 2003). See also *Estate of Novack ex rel. Turbin v. County of Wood,* 226 F.3d 525, 529 (7th Cir. 2000) (defendant must be aware of the significant likelihood that an inmate may imminently seek to take his own life and must fail to take reasonable steps to prevent the inmate from performing the act).

60 *Estate of Novack,* 226 F.3d at 529 (emphasis added).

61 See also *Sanville, supra,* 266 F.3d at 737 (the issue is whether the defendant was subjectively "aware of the substantial risk that [the deceased prisoner] might take his own life"). Liability cannot attach where "the defendants simply were not alerted to the likelihood that [the prisoner] was a genuine suicide risk." *Boncher ex rel. Boncher v. Brown County,* 272 F.3d 484, 488 (7th Cir. 2001).

62 See, e.g., *Saucier v. Katz,* 533 U.S. 194 (2001) (sets forth a two-prong inquiry to resolve all qualified immunity claims. First, "taken in the light most favorable to the party asserting the injury, do the facts alleged show the officers' conduct violated a constitutional right?" *Id.*, 201. Second, if so, was that right clearly established? *Id.* "The relevant, dispositive inquiry in determining whether a right is clearly established is *whether it would be clear to a reasonable officer that his conduct was unlawful in the situation he confronted." Id.*, 202. This inquiry is wholly objective and is undertaken in light of the specific factual circumstances of the case. *Id.*, 201 emphasis added.

63 *Sites v. McKenzie,* 423 F. Supp.1190 (N.D W.Va. 1976) (denial of access to vocational rehabilitation programs violated Section 504 of the Rehabilitation Act), and *D.M v. Terhune,* 67 F. Supp.2d 402, 412 (D.C. N.J. 1999) (class action settlement of claims by inmates with mental disorders alleging denial of appropriate treatment and medications).

64 42 U.S.C.A. §12132. *Lee v. City of Los Angeles,* 250 F.3d 668 (9th Cir. 2001).

65 *Wilson v. Woodford,* 2006 U.S. Dist. LEXIS 12330, *10 (E.D. Cal. 2006). See also *Burger v. Bloomberg,* 418 F.3d 882, 882 (8th Cir. 2005) (medical treatment decisions are not a basis for Rehabilitation Act or ADA claims); *Fitzgerald v. Corr. Corp. of America,* 403 F.3d 1134, 1144 (10th Cir. 2005), and *Schiavo ex rel. Schindler v. Schiavo,* 403 F.3d 1289, 1294 (11th Cir. 2005).

66 See *McNally v. Prison Health Services,* 46 F. Supp. 2d 49, 58 (D. Me. 1999), reconsideration denied, 52 F. Supp. 2d 147 (D. Me. 1999) (discussing the distinction between the claims).

67 *Moore v. Prison Health Services,* 201 F.3d 448 (10th Cir. 1999).

68 *Garrett v. Angelone,* 940 F. Supp. 933 (W.D. Va. 1996), aff'd, 107 F.3d 865 (4th Cir. 1997),

69 C.A. Hornung, R.B. Greifinger, & S.Gadre, *A Projection Model of the Prevalence of Selected Chronic Diseases in the Inmate Population.* National Commission on Correctional Healthcare, The Health Status of Soon-to-Be-Released Inmates, Report to Congress (August 2002) <http://www.ncchc.org/stbr/Volume2/ Report3_ Hornung.pdf>.

70 R.H. Aday, *Aging Prisoners: Crisis in American Corrections* (Westport, CT: Praeger, 2003).

71 National Commission on Correctional Healthcare, The Health Status of Soon-to-Be-Released Inmates, Report to Congress (August 2002) <http://www.ncchc.org/ pubs_stbr.html>.

72 Arthur L. Kellerman & Knox H. Todd, "Killing Heat," *New England Journal of Medicine* 335 (1996): 126–27; E.M. Kilburne, K. Choi, T.S. Jones, & S.B. Thacker, "Risk Factors for Heatstroke: A Case-Control Study," *Journal of the American Medical Association* 247 (1982): 3332–36; "Heat-Related Mortality—Chicago, July 1995," *Morbidity and Mortality Weekly Report* 44 (1995): 577–79.

73 Brie A. Williams, Karla Lindquist, Rebecca L. Sudore, Heidi M. Strupp, Donna J. Willmott, & Louise C. Walter, "Being Old and Doing Time: Functional Impairment and Adverse Experiences of Geriatric Female Prisoners," *Journal of the American Geriatric Society* 54, no. 4 (April 2006): 702–07.

74 C. Seth Landefeld, Robert Palmer, Mary Anne Johnson, & Catherine Bree Johnston, *Current Geriatric Diagnosis and Treatment* (New York: McGraw–Hill, 2004); <http://www.ahrq.gov/clinic/uspstfix.htm> U.S. Preventive Services Task Force (USPSTF), Agency for Healthcare Research and Quality.

75 *United States v. Georgia, Goodman v. Georgia,* 126 S.Ct. 877, 163 L.Ed.2d 650 (2006). Brief of Amici Curiae Tennessee, Alabama, Colorado, Delaware, Idaho, Michigan, Nevada, New Hampshire, Oklahoma, Oregon, Puerto Rico, Washington, Wyoming in Support of Respondent, US v. Georgia.

76 Michael Waterstone, "The Untold Story of the Rest of the Americans with Disabilities Act," *Vanderbilt Law Review* 55 (2002):1807.

Chapter 5

Growing Older: Challenges of Prison and Reentry for the Aging Population

Brie Williams and Rita Abraldes

Introduction

The United States is experiencing an aging crisis in its prisons, with an exponential increase in the number of older inmates (Aday, 2003; Anno, Graham, Lawrence, & Shansky, 2004). In 2003, only 4.3% of incarcerated inmates were aged 55 years or older, but this percentage is increasing dramatically every year (Harrison & Beck, 2004). There are many consequences of this change in demographics, including surging costs associated with incarceration. Older prisoners cost approximately $70,000 per year—two to three times that of younger prisoners (Anno et al., 2004; Mitka, 2004).

In the community, geriatrics is the discipline of medicine specializing in care of the aged, defined as 65 years and older. In prison, the age at which an inmate is deemed "geriatric" varies from state to state (Lemieux, Dyeson, & Castiglione, 2002). In some states, inmates as young as 50 are defined as geriatric; in other states, inmates are not considered geriatric until they reach age 55 or 60 (Anno et al., 2004; Lemieux et al., 2002). Despite these differing definitions, there is consensus that inmates undergo a process of *accelerated aging* compared to their age-matched counterparts outside of prison (Aday, 2003).

The accelerated aging of inmates is reflected in their development of chronic illness and disability at a younger age than the general U.S. population (Aday, 2003; Baillargeon & Pulvino, 2000; Colsher, Wallace, Loeffelholz, & Sales, 1992; Fazel, Hope, O'Donnell, Piper, & Jacoby, 2001; Williams et al., 2006). This accelerated aging process is likely due to the high burden of disease common in people from poor backgrounds, who comprise the majority of the prison population, coupled with unhealthy lifestyles prior to and during incarceration (Aday, 2003; Hornung, Anno, Greifinger, & Gadre, 2002). These factors are often further exacerbated by substandard medical care either before or during incarceration (Aday, 2003). To account for accelerated aging, many state correctional departments now define prisoners aged 55 years and older as "geriatric" (Baillargeon & Pulvino, 2000; Fazel et al., 2001; Mitka, 2004; Voelker, 2004).

Outside of prison, people often encounter new physical, psychological, and social challenges as they age. In prison, an environment designed for younger inhabitants, aging introduces additional challenges in safety, functional ability, and health. As older ex-prisoners reenter their communities, they may face additional challenges such as being frail in an unsafe neighborhood, having multiple medical conditions with limited access to medical care, and leaving the familiarity of the place they have lived in for decades.

In this chapter, we describe some of the special challenges related to the aging of the population both inside prison and on reentry into the community. Despite the public health and economic implications of the surging geriatric prison population, little research has been conducted in these areas, particularly regarding reentry.

Demographics

In the United States, the rapid rise in the population of geriatric prisoners has been well documented (Aday, 2003; Anno et al., 2004). The states with the most older inmates are California, Texas, and Florida, reflecting the overall size of these state prison systems and their longer prison sentences (Lemieux et al., 2002). The aging of the prison population is not limited to the United States. An expansion in the aging inmate population is also described in England and Wales (Crawley & Sparks, 2006). The aging population affects the correctional system both within prison and throughout reentry.

Although the number of geriatric prisoners is still small relative to the overall prison population (4.3% of the overall U.S. prison population in 2003; Harrison & Beck, 2004), the growth rate for geriatric prisoners has been dramatic. The Bureau of Justice Statistics 2004 report states that the "US prison population is aging" (Harrison & Beck, 2004). For example, in California, the percentage of male inmates aged 50 and older increased from 4.7% of the census in 1995 to 10.2% in 2004; the percentage of female prisoners aged 50 and older increased from 3.7% of the census to 8.7% during the same period (*California Prisoners and Parolees 2004, 2005*). It is expected that by 2022, geriatric inmates will account for 16% of California's inmate population (Strupp & Willmott, 2005). In some states, the percentage of geriatric inmates already far exceeds the national average. In Florida, the population of geriatric prisoners (aged 50 and over) represented 11.7% of the inmate population in 2005 (http://www.dc.state. fl.us/pub/annual/0405/index.html, 2005).

According to the Department of Justice, the number of geriatric persons sentenced to state or federal jurisdiction increased from 32,600 in 1995 to 60,300 in 2003, an 85% increase (Harrison & Beck, 2004). This rate of growth is expected to continue in part because of a burgeoning middle-aged inmate population (40–54 years) that comprised 28% of the overall prison population at the end of 2003, a 22% increase from 1995 (Harrison & Beck, 2004). In fact, the middle-aged population alone accounted for 46% of the total growth in the prison population between 1995 and 2003 (Harrison & Beck, 2004).

Reasons for the dramatic aging of the inmate population are manifold. First, more older people are being sentenced to prison (Anno et al., 2004; Harrison & Beck, 2004; Linder, Enders, Craig, Richardson, & Meyers, 2002). Second, the balance of sentencing and release has been tipped. Due to steadily increasing mandatory minimum sentencing laws, second and third strike legislation, strict drug-related sentencing, deinstitutionalization of the mentally ill, and the discontinuation of discretionary parole, an increasing number of people are sentenced to prison while fewer qualify for release (Anno et al., 2004; Hill, Williams, Cobe, & Lindquist, 2006; Mitka, 2004).

Table 5.1 The mean age and average terms of inmates are rising (Harrison & Beck, 2004).

Year	Mean age of sentenced state inmates	Average term served among released inmates
1995	31 years	23 months
2003	33 years	30 months

The result is a rapidly increasing geriatric prison population marked by a "gradual rise in the average age of state inmates at the time of admission compounded by a sharp increase in time served in prison" (Table 5.1) (Harrison & Beck, 2004). Given these synergistic forces, current trends in the progressive aging of the prison population are not likely to be reversed without significant legislative changes.

Cost of Care

The increased burden of illness, disability, and special needs among geriatric prisoners make them expensive. Nationally, the average cost for incarcerating a geriatric prisoner is approximately $70,000 per year (Aday, 2003; Anno et al., 2004), two to three times that of younger prisoners. As it is in the community, older age is among the strongest predictors of morbidity and medical care utilization (Faiver, 1998; Lindquist & Lindquist, 1999). The high cost is due to higher health care expenses among geriatric prisoners including hospitalization, medications, diagnostic tests, and skilled nursing care. In addition, there are substantial custodial costs associated with off-site health care, primarily related to the cost of providing security (Hill et al., 2006). In California, inmates aged 55 and older represent approximately 5% of the inmate population, but account for 22% of the off-site hospital admission cost. California's off-site hospital costs are 35% higher for inmates 55 and older than for younger inmates (Hill et al., 2006). Given the surging geriatric population and the consequent escalating costs of older inmates, expenses for sustaining the prison system are likely to soar.

Special Challenges for Geriatric Prisoners

There are a number of special challenges faced by the incarcerated geriatric population. In prison, aging often introduces new medical and health care needs, geriatric syndromes, changes in functional ability, and personal safety and social considerations. Older inmates with health deterioration must also cope with loss of independence and recognition of the permanence of their medical conditions (Aday, 2003).

Medical and Health Care Needs

Multiple Chronic Medical Illnesses
On average, geriatric prisoners have more chronic diseases than adults of similar age living outside of prison (Anno et al., 2004; Baillargeon & Pulvino, 2000; Colsher et al., 1992; Fazel et al., 2001). Many of these chronic medical

conditions are similar to those also found in the older U.S. population such as chronic obstructive pulmonary disease, arthritis, diabetes, and heart disease. Geriatric inmates may also have conditions that have unusually high prevalence in prison, including: paraplegia secondary to gunshot wounds, advanced liver disease from alcohol use and/or viral hepatitis, and end stage renal disease from injection drug use and/or HIV. Geriatric inmates are also more vulnerable to acute infections in prison, such as influenza and pneumonia (Aday, 2003).

The likelihood of having more than one chronic medical condition is common among geriatric inmates. Having multiple chronic medical conditions, in turn, puts geriatric prisoners at special risk for "polypharmacy."

Polypharmacy

"Polypharmacy" means the inappropriate use of multiple medications. In the United States, it accounts for up to 27% of annual hospitalizations (Landefeld, Palmer, Johnson, Johnston, & Lyons, 2004). This is because the use of multiple medications increases the risk of adverse medication side effects (Landefeld et al., 2004). Older adults are at particular risk for adverse medication reactions due to age-related changes in the metabolism, clearance, and delivery of many medications (Landefeld et al., 2004). For this reason, medications that should be avoided or are contraindicated in older adults have been compiled into the "Beer's Criteria" list (Fick et al., 2003). Despite this list and others similar to it, the prevalence of inappropriate drug use outside of prison is as high as 40% (Landefeld et al., 2004).

An example of a Beer's list medication class that should be avoided in older adults is anticholinergic medication. Many medications have anticholinergic properties including antihistamines (diphenhydramine, hydroxyzine), some benzodiazepines (alprazolam, oxazepam), and some antibiotics (ampicillin, clindamycin). Anticholinergics' myriad side effects in the elderly include falls, delirium (acute confusion), and urinary retention (Landefeld et al., 2004). Given these side effects and their associated costs, it is imperative that prison health care providers know which medications to avoid giving older inmates.

One way to prevent polypharmacy is to treat geriatric patients as whole patients, rather than as a sum of their multiple medical conditions. For example, many older inmates have multiple concurrent medical conditions such as diabetes, hypertension, heart disease, and COPD. Since many diabetic patients are on multiple medications, a geriatric patient who has diabetes and any additional medical condition is at great risk for polypharmacy.

In an effort to treat chronic disease, many prisons have developed high-risk chronic disease management programs for common illnesses instead of relying on sick call for chronic disease management. Such programs help to ensure the up-to-date treatment of chronic diseases. For example, under the California Department of Corrections and Rehabilitation chronic care program, any inmate with hypertension, diabetes, or asthma is seen on a regular basis in a clinic visit for that particular medical condition (Hill et al., 2006). The goal of the visit is to address the medications and treatment of only that particular disease.

Since the majority of older inmates have more than one chronic disease (Baillargeon, J.,& Pulvino, 2000), they may be seen in more than one chronic care clinic. This compartmentalized health care approach runs the risk of increasing polypharmacy among geriatric inmates by focusing on the medications for only one disease at a time rather than the medication list as a whole. Instead, for geriatric inmates the best way to minimize polypharmacy is to review the entire medication list, to add new medications cautiously, and to regularly assess the need for each medication while considering the possibility of drug–drug interactions with other concurrent medications (Landefeld et al., 2004). One approach would be to create a geriatrics clinic to periodically assess older adults with multiple medical conditions and/or disability.

Preventive Services

Preventive health care can decrease the incidence of both disease and disability. Preventive interventions benefiting older people include screening for a risk of falls, depression, and hypertension, providing influenza, tetanus, and pneumococcal vaccines, and encouraging exercise. Preventive interventions also include cancer screening tests. Although screening and preventive services are covered elsewhere in this book, the approach to cancer screening for geriatric patients differs slightly from that for younger patients.

Selecting which cancer screening tests are appropriate for an individual older person requires consideration of his or her life expectancy (Landefeld et al., 2004). For example, a healthy older person with a favorable life expectancy should be offered cancer-screening tests such as colonoscopy or mammography. In contrast, an unhealthy older person with a limited life expectancy will be more likely to suffer the immediate harms of cancer screening, such as the workup of false negative test results, without having the time to accrue the benefits of screening (Walter & Covinsky, 2001).

The consideration of life expectancy and patient preferences is especially important when approaching the decision to screen for prostate cancer. There is currently no conclusive evidence that PSA screening reduces prostate cancer mortality at any age or life expectancy (Walter, Bertenthal, Lindquist, & Konety, 2006). When reviewing the evidence about PSA screening, the U.S. Preventive Service Task Force found "inconclusive evidence that early detection improves health outcomes" (http://www.ahrq.gov/clinic/uspstfix.htm). This is particularly true for people with limited life expectancies; the American Cancer Society and the American Urological Society only recommend annual screening for men 50 years if they have at least a 10-year life expectancy (Walter et al., 2006). Since it is not clear that PSA screening has any health benefit in younger men, the decision to perform PSA screening in older men with limited life expectancies exposes the patient more to the harms associated with screening rather than to the benefits (Walter et al., 2006). Thus, in geriatrics, preventive care follows a model of shared decision-making between patient and provider in which the focus is on discussing the risks and benefits of each test based on the patient's life expectancy and individual goals (Table 5.2) (Landefeld et al., 2004).

Table 5.2 Steps to individualize decision making for screening tests.

1. Estimate the individual's life expectancy
2. Estimate the risk of dying from the condition
3. Determine the potential benefit of screening
4. Weigh the direct and indirect harm of screening
5. Assess the patient's values and preferences

Mental Health Issues in Aging

Depression and depressive symptoms are common in the geriatric population. The prevalence of major depression in the United States is approximately 1–2% of community-dwelling older adults and is up to 27% for those who have significant depressive symptoms (Landefeld et al., 2004). The prevalence of depression rises among permanently institutionalized nursing home elders—43% have been found to have major depression (Landefeld et al., 2004). One study found that the prevalence of major depression was 50 times higher among incarcerated older men compared to community-dwelling men. The study also found that generalized anxiety disorders were prevalent and that, overall, 54% of the older inmates met criteria for psychiatric disorders (Koenig, Johnson, Bellard, Denker, & Fenlon, 1995). Another study showed that older female inmates more frequently experience social isolation than do older male inmates (Kratcoski & Babb, 1990). In prison, 15% of inmates of all ages have serious mental illness, such as schizophrenia (Aday, 2003; Lurigio, Rollins, & Fallon, 2004). In one report from a maximum-security hospital, 75% of elderly prisoners were admitted between age 20 and 30, and the majority were schizophrenic (Aday, 2003).

While not all older inmates have serious mental health diagnoses, many experience stress and psychological trauma related to incarceration (Crawley & Sparks, 2006). In the United Kingdom, a study of older male inmates investigated the psychological impact of incarceration. Elderly "first-timers" were frequently found to be anxious, depressed, and to experience incarceration as a form of psychological trauma (Crawley & Sparks, 2006). After a long incarceration, older prisoners may also lose contact with the outside world and become "institutionalized," leading to significant anxiety about the possibility of release (Aday, 2003; Crawley & Sparks, 2006).

Geriatric Syndromes and Functional Ability

Geriatric Syndromes

Complex problems that primarily affect older adults are referred to as "geriatric syndromes." These include vision and hearing loss, falls, cognitive impairment, and urinary incontinence. Geriatric syndromes are common among older inmates and put them at risk for adverse events while in prison (Aday, 2003; Colsher et al., 1992; Fazel et al., 2001; Hill et al., 2006; Williams et al., 2006).

Vision and Hearing Impairment

Vision and hearing problems are common among older people. Common causes of visual impairment include presbyopia, cataracts, macular degeneration, glaucoma, and diabetic retinopathy (http://www.ahrq.gov/clinic/uspstfix.htm; Landefeld et al., 2004). Vision impairment can greatly decrease independence and is associated with falls, social isolation, depression, and physical disability (http://www.ahrq.gov/clinic/uspstfix.htm; Landefeld et al., 2004).

In prison, visually impaired geriatric inmates should be considered at risk for falls, especially in cluttered areas where there are unseen obstacles or in areas with poor lighting (Hill et al., 2006). In the community, home safety evaluations and rehabilitation programs are designed to help older adults with decreased visual acuity improve and maintain their independence (Landefeld et al., 2004). Similar interventions could be offered in prisons.

Routine vision exams with an eye specialist are recommended for all older adults (http://www.ahrq.gov/clinic/uspstfix.htm; Landefeld et al., 2004). Regular eye exams are especially important for those older adults at high risk for glaucoma or diabetes-related vision problems (http://www.ahrq.gov/clinic/uspstfix.htm). A vision exam should be performed on any older inmate who falls.

The prevalence of significant hearing impairment increases rapidly after the age of 50; 25% of adults aged 51 to 65 have hearing loss, increasing to 33% of adults aged 65 and older, and to nearly 50% of adults aged 85 and older (http://www.ahrq.gov/clinic/uspstfix.htm; Mulrow & Lichtenstein, 1991). Adult hearing impairment is associated with social isolation, clinical depression, and limited activity (Bogardus, Yueh, & Shekelle, 2003). Development of adverse reactions to hearing loss increases markedly with age (Bess, Lichtenstein, Logan, Burger, & Nelson, 1989; Bogardus et al., 2003; http://www.ahrq.gov/clinic/uspstfix.htm). People with significant hearing loss who receive hearing aids have improved communication, social function, and emotional status (http://www.ahrq.gov/clinic/uspstfix.htm). Audiology screening tests include whispered voice, finger rub, and use of a portable audiometer. Although the portable audiometer is the most reliable and accurate method, another practical approach is to administer a self-assessment questionnaire to patients (Landefeld et al., 2004). These questionnaires, such as the "Hearing Handicap Inventory for the Elderly," are reliable and valid methods for identifying patients with hearing loss and also patients who are willing to accept further evaluation and treatment (Landefeld et al., 2004). Older inmates should be screened periodically for hearing loss and, when indicated, offered hearing aids.

Hearing loss in prison can also affect an older inmate's safety. For example, a hearing impaired inmate might fail to respond to the request of another inmate and this could result in a physical confrontation. In addition, rule violation charges could be filed when hearing–impaired inmates do not hear orders from staff (Hill et al., 2006; Lemieux et al., 2002). Loss of hearing can also lead to social isolation and falls (Hill et al., 2006).

Falls

Falls increase in frequency with advancing age and are associated with serious injury, loss of function, increased health care usage, nursing home placement, and mortality (Brown & Norris, 2006b). Approximately 30% of community-living U.S. adults aged 65 and older fall each year (Marshall et al., 2005). In contrast, a study in California found that 51% of geriatric women prisoners aged 55 and older reported a fall in the past year (Williams et al., 2006).

Falls are the most common cause of hip fracture and contribute to the high health-care costs of the elderly (Hill et al., 2006). In the United States in 2001, the cost of hip fracture repair was $8900 for the hospitalization and, with physician fees, follow-up care, and physical therapy, the total cost was $81,300 (Braithwaite, Col, & Wong, 2003).

In the community, 44% of falls are associated with environmental factors including poor lighting, loose rugs, and lack of handrails (Brown & Norris, 2006a). In prison, there are additional environmental stressors that might contribute to falls such as strenuous work assignments, quickly moving younger inmates, and top bunk assignments (Hill et al., 2006; Williams et al., 2006).

Cognitive Impairment

Cognitive impairment in the elderly includes a spectrum of neurologic changes from normal age-related changes to severe dementia. Normal age-related neurologic changes include slower reaction times and slower performance on timed tasks (Landefeld et al., 2004). Dementia, the most severe form of cognitive impairment, leads to significant morbidity and mortality. The diagnosis of dementia includes memory impairment and the presence of at least one other impairment including language deficits, apraxia (inability to perform previously learned tasks), visuospatial deficits, and/or decreased executive functioning such as poor abstraction, planning, or judgment (Landefeld et al., 2004).

Approximately 15% of men and 11% of women aged 65 and older in the United States have dementia (Federal Interagency Forum, 2004). The prevalence of dementia doubles every 5 years after age 60, and by age 85 the prevalence is 25–45% (Landefeld et al., 2004). In older persons, dementia is one of the most expensive illnesses, as nearly 90% of patients with dementia are eventually institutionalized in long-term care facilities (Landefeld et al., 2004). Average annual costs for dementia range from $4000 to $10,000 (Taylor, Schenkman, Zhou, & Sloan, 2001) and in the last year of life the average Medicare expenses exceed $25,000 (Newcomer, Clay, Yaffe, & Covinsky, 2005).

As the prison population ages, correctional officers and staff will encounter more inmates with memory impairment. Some older adults may enter prison already having cognitive impairment while others will develop it once incarcerated. One study of prisoners over age 60 found that nearly 15% had organic brain disorders(Aday, 2003), and court liaison referrals for older prisoners have found rates of dementia ranging from 19 to 30% (Aday, 2003).

With more cognitively impaired inmates, new approaches will have to be developed to discipline older adults with cognitive impairment. For example, if a demented, bed-bound inmate were to inappropriately grab a nurse, he might receive disciplinary action whereas in a community nursing home this occurrence would trigger a behavioral care plan (Hill et al., 2006). An accumulation of disciplinary actions could then delay release for cognitively impaired inmates (Hill et al., 2006).

Urinary Incontinence

Urinary incontinence is not a normal part of aging, but instead has numerous pathophysiologic causes including obstructive overflow incontinence due to prostatic hypertrophy, neurogenic bladder due to diabetes, medication side effects, and functional and cognitive impairment. In the U.S. community-dwelling population aged 65 and older, urinary incontinence affects 15–30% of women and 5–10% of men (Landefeld et al., 2004). After age 85, men and women are equally likely to be affected (Landefeld et al., 2004). Incontinence is also common in prison; one study found 13.9% of inmates aged 50–59 and 37.8% of inmates aged 60 and older reported urinary incontinence (Colsher et al., 1992).

In prison, urinary incontinence can pose special challenges for inmates. First, prisons do not always carry incontinence supplies such as incontinence briefs; when they do, inmates are sometimes charged a co-pay for them (Hill et al., 2006). Second, incontinence may lead to isolation among older inmates and could cause them to be ridiculed or even a target of violence. Since the majority of patients with urinary incontinence will improve with treatment (Landefeld et al., 2004), asking patients about it, identifying the etiology of urinary incontinence, and treating it are of great importance in the geriatric prisoner population.

Functional Ability

Central to geriatric care and assessment is functional ability. Functional ability reflects the extent to which an older person is independent and is measured by assessing a person's need for help with their Activities of Daily Living (ADL: bathing, dressing, eating, transferring, and toileting). The prevalence of ADL dependence increases with advancing age; 15–25% of persons aged 65 and 50% of persons aged 85 and older need help in performing one or more ADL (http://www.census.gov/hhes/www/disability/sipp/disab9495/ds94t1h.html; Landefeld et al., 2004).

Functional impairment is common among geriatric inmates and is associated with high health care costs, future functional decline, and mortality (Carey, Walter, Lindquist, & Covinsky, 2004; Reuben et al., 2004) . In Iowa, 11% of male prisoners aged 50 and older had limitations in self-care activities(Colsher et al., 1992) and in the United Kingdom, 10% of male prisoners aged 60 and older reported disability in one or more ADL (Fazel et al., 2001). In California, 16% of female prisoners aged 55 and older needed help in one or more ADL (Williams et al., 2006).

Independence is also affected by mobility. Mobility impairment is often defined as requiring aids such as canes, walkers, or wheelchairs or needing assistance during ambulation. Some inmates who would have no mobility difficulties outside of prison may face ambulation difficulties while in prison. For example, mobility aids may be difficult to acquire, or inmates may be reluctant to use such aids because they might appear weak and vulnerable. Even older inmates without mobility impairment might need protective housing and supervision or assistance in certain circumstances, such as walking while handcuffed since this is more difficult for older adults and can make them unsteady, putting them at increased risk for falls (Hill et al., 2006).

Environmental and Functional Mismatch

It is difficult to accurately assess an older person's functional ability without accounting for the environment in which they live and the daily activities they need to perform in order to remain living independently (Verbrugge & Jette, 1994). Incarceration introduces daily physical activities necessary to independent functioning that are unique to prison life. For this reason, functional ability in prison should take into account the unique daily activities faced by geriatric prisoners. One study termed such prison-specific activities "prison activities of daily living" (PADL) (Williams et al., 2006). PADL included dropping to the floor for alarms, standing for head count, getting to the dining hall for meals, hearing orders from staff, and climbing on and off the top bunk.

When PADL were measured, functional impairment was much more common than measures of ADL would indicate; 69% of older women reported an impairment in daily activities of prison life whereas only 16% of women would be identified as functionally impaired based on traditional measures of ADL (Williams et al., 2006). Thus, people who are independent in the community might be impaired in prison.

An older person's functional impairment and their environment's functional requirements are frequently mismatched (Gill, Robison, Williams, & Tinetti, 1999). The extent of this mismatch is intensified in prison. Prisons, which are designed for young, healthy inmates without functional limitations (Mara, 2003), raise the physical level at which older adults must function by requiring physically challenging activities such as climbing onto a top bunk and dropping to the floor for alarms. Adaptive devices that can help older adults maintain independence such as bathroom handrails, nonslip surfaces, and doorknobs that can easily be turned even with arthritic hands are frequently unavailable in prison. [Such devices should be considered accommodations for the disabled, and are required by the Americans with Disability Act (ADA, 1990).] The environmental demands of the prison setting can lead to decreased independence among older inmates.

Personal Safety and Social Considerations

The relationship between older and younger inmates is complex. Older inmates often report a fear of victimization by younger inmates (Aday, 2003; Williams et al., 2006). This fear is especially prevalent among older inmates who are new to prison (Aday, 2003). Chronic illness may also contribute to the sense of vulnerability among older inmates (Aday, 2003). Yet in prison there is also often an informal caregiving system in which younger inmates provide care to frail, older inmates (Crawley & Sparks, 2006; Mara, 2003; Williams et al., 2006). In addition, studies indicate that older inmates frequently attain prestige and respect from younger peers(Lemieux et al., 2002) and that older inmates can function as a stabilizing influence in the general prison population (Mara, 2003).

Geriatric Prisons

A common debate about aging prisoners is whether they should be placed in specialized, segregated housing units. Advocates point to the common fears that geriatric inmates have about victimization from younger inmates (Aday, 2003; Mara, 2003). In one study, 65% of older inmates stated that if their health declined, they would feel more comfortable in a segregated unit (Marquart, Merianos, & Doucet, 2000). Specialized housing units can also offer more adaptive aids such as ramps, grab bars, and nonslip surfaces to mitigate some of the functional demands of prison. However, those opposed to segregating geriatric inmates point to the stabilizing force of elders in the prison community, and that separate housing would eliminate this positive influence (Mara, 2003). Segregated units also may contribute to social isolation and boredom due to the lack of programming. Some older inmates perceive integration within the general population as enhancing independence (Aday, 2003). Finally, many older inmates have biological family members or friends in the general prison population and segregation could compromise these social ties.

Long-Term and Skilled Nursing Care

Long-term and skilled nursing care describes the care provided in assisted living facilities or nursing homes to adults with limitations in independence.

Such limitations are usually due to functional dependence or severe cognitive impairment such as dementia. Community-living older adults move into skilled nursing facilities when they cannot function independently and have no one to give them adequate assistance. In the United States, nearly 50% of adults reaching age 65 will spend some time in a nursing home (Landefeld et al., 2004). In prison, most inmates requiring long term care are geriatric, although some younger inmates, such as those paralyzed by a gunshot wound, may also require long term care (Mara, 2003).

In prison, informal or formal systems of inmate-provided care are used to help older inmates continue living in the general population (Mara, 2003; Williams et al., 2006). When an inmate is no longer independent, the options for long-term care depend on the prison. Some inmates stay in the general population despite multiple needs, others are moved to special housing, the infirmary, the prison hospital, or a long-term-care/skilled nursing prison (Mara, 2003). In recent years, more prisons are building nursing-home type environments in which to house older, functionally dependent inmates (Aday, 2003). In rare cases, an inmate is moved temporarily to a contracted community hospital for nursing-level care if no appropriate prison bed is available. This is a costly option.

Hospice

Much like older people in the community, "older inmates in poor health are more likely to think frequently about death" and the probability of dying in prison is a significant stressor (Aday, 2003; Crawley & Sparks, 2006). This fear is grounded in reality; with the aging of the prison population and strict release policies, more and more people are dying while incarcerated (Linder et al., 2002). At Angola State Prison in Louisiana, 97% of inmates die in prison (Fields, 2005). Increasing attention has thus been paid to prison hospice, or end of life care (Enders, Paterniti, & Meyers, 2005; Linder et al., 2002).

Although individual prisons have different rules governing who is hospice eligible, all hospice-eligible inmates must minimally have a physician certification that they have a life expectancy of 6 months or less, a do-not-resuscitate (DNR) order, and the inmate must consent to the transfer (Aday, 2003; Linder et al., 2002). The hospice-eligibility criteria can be problematic in prison (Aday, 2003; Linder et al., 2002). Inmates may feel conflicted about DNR orders because they fear dying in prison (Boyle, 2002). This is not so much a denial of impending death as it is a "struggle to come to terms with dying in prison. Many inmates cannot surrender the hope that, somehow, they can die free people" (Boyle, 2002). In addition, inmates might be reluctant to use prison hospice services since they often do not trust the health care staff.

Many variations are seen among prison hospice programs. All programs should adhere to the national hospice guidelines and standards. Correctional agencies have to consider various options to determine whether hospice patients should be integrated with hospital patients; how to best balance comfort care with security needs; and how to provide appropriate pain control in the setting of restrictive opioid medication dispensing policies (Aday, 2003; Linder et al., 2002). Also, prisons differ as to whether they allow other inmates to assist with activities of daily living. Most hospice programs utilize inmate volunteers (Aday, 2003).

Release and Parole of Older Inmates

Citing the very low recidivism rate of this population (Holman, 1998; Turley, 2003), and in order to relieve overcrowding in prison and the rising cost of incarcerating older inmates, some have called for the early release of non-violent geriatric inmates. Proposed alternatives to incarceration have included house arrest or community release with an electronic bracelet (Aday, 2003; Strupp & Willmott, 2005), expansion of the compassionate release programs to include people who are permanently disabled or mentally incapacitated (Strupp & Willmott, 2005), and early parole with more frequent intervals for parole review (Aday, 2003; Legislative Analyst's Office, Analysis for the 2003–2004 Budget Bill, 2003).

One parole program targeted specifically to the aging inmate is the Project for Older Prisoners (POPS), run by George Washington University law professor Jonathan Turley, which partners law schools and state departments of corrections to allow early release for nonviolent older inmates (http://www.gwu.edu/~ccommit/law.htm). According to Aday, "POPS is first and only organization in the country to work exclusively with the elderly and infirm to influence their early release" (Aday, 2003). As of 2003, the POPS program had organized the early release of more than 200 older prisoners without a single instance of recidivism (Aday, 2003).

Aging and Reentry Issues

As the prison population ages, so does the parole population. Between 1990 and 1999, the percentage of new parolees aged 55 and older increased from 1.5% to 2.1% of the total U.S. parolee population and the number of state prisoners aged 55 or older leaving custody on parole nearly doubled from approximately 5000 in 1990 to approximately 9000 in 1999 (http://www.ojp.usdoj.gov/bjs/pub/pdf/reentry.pdf, 2003). Despite these changing demographics, little research has been done on the care and well-being of older ex-prisoners.

On release, geriatric ex-prisoners may face unique challenges reentering the community. These challenges are social as well as medical, and include: frailty in an unsafe neighborhood; concerns about employability as an older person; multiple chronic illnesses with functional limitations; and/or lack of medical insurance or prescription drug benefits. In addition, serious mental illness and the psychological syndrome of institutionalization cannot be underestimated as challenges to long-term inmates when they are released to the community. With long-term incarcerations, older adults who are to be released may not have made up for opportunities missed in their life such as education, job advancement, and strengthening family relationships (Aday, 2003). Despite this, the Bureau of Justice reports that geriatric parolees have lower recidivism rates (54%) during their parole terms, and increasing age is one of the most reliable predictors of low recidivism as older ex-prisoners are the least likely to return to prison (Turley, 2003).

A series of interviews with elderly male prisoners aged 65 to 84 in England and Wales revealed that inmates commonly had concerns about release. These concerns were predominantly social and medical and centered on discharge planning. They included where they would live, how they would get there, and with whom they would be living. They were also fearful for their personal safety and about where they would get medical care (Crawley & Sparks, 2006).

Social Factors

Ex-prisoners usually reenter communities that are similar to those from which they came (Pogorzelski, Wolff, Pan, & Blitz, 2005). Many of these communities are unsafe. In contrast to when they were young, older ex-prisoners may now be less physically fit and less able to defend themselves. Some may have lost contact with family and friends. There may be no one to turn to for financial, physical, emotional, or economic support; for many older ex-prisoners, family and friends remain in prison (Aday, 2003; Crawley & Sparks, 2006).

When older adults reenter the community, finding employment can be difficult due to their age, especially if they used to work as hard laborers. The stigma of incarceration is a substantial barrier to a smooth reintegration into the community. In addition, job prospects may be further limited by educational attainment; studies show that fewer older probationers have completed high school or a GED than their younger counterparts (Aday, 2003). Also, after being in prison for many years and possibly for the majority of their lives, older adults many have acquired very few independent living skills such as cooking, shopping, and balancing a checkbook and would benefit from "community placement orientation" before release (Aday, 2003; Crawley & Sparks, 2006; Terhune et al., 1999).

Medical and Psychological Factors

Older ex-prisoners frequently have multiple medical conditions and may encounter several obstacles in optimizing their medical care. While older inmates are often on multiple medications at the time of release, many are discharged with little or no medication (Hornung et al., 2002). Insufficient health-related discharge planning may lead to release without a health care appointment. Reinstating Medicare and/or Medicaid can take many weeks to months, so the only health care option for many older parolees with chronic health care needs may be to use high cost emergency services for routine care or after medical decompensation (Hornung et al., 2002). In addition, some older parolees will require discharge to a nursing home or other long term care facility. This entails a special discharge coordination effort to find an accepting location and enrollment in Medicaid to obtain the funds necessary to pay for the care (Terhune et al., 1999).

Older inmates transitioning into the community may also have new health care providers who do not know of their incarceration history. This can pose a significant problem as ex-prisoners are at particularly high risk for certain diseases such as STDs, hepatitis, and HIV (Hornung et al., 2002; http://www.ojp.usdoj.gov/bjs/pub/pdf/reentry.pdf, 2003). Although all older adults should be screened for these diseases, they often are not because health care providers rarely consider older adults at risk (Skiest & Keiser, 1997). Thus, without knowledge of a history of incarceration, many health care providers might fail to screen older ex-prisoners for STDs or infectious disease.

Older parolees are also at higher risk for adverse psychological reactions to prison release. They display high rates of anxiety about release (Crawley & Sparks, 2006), and are also at increased risk for post-release suicide (Pratt, Piper, Appleby, Webb, & Shaw, 2006). Parole officers and health care providers should be familiar with these increased risks so that mental health crises can be avoided or identified early. In addition, older parolees with dementia could violate parole by missing their parole officer meetings, or might intentionally violate parole hoping to be returned to prison due to their inability to function on the outside (Terhune et al., 1999). For these reasons, some advocate changing the role of parole officers to serve as bridges and support systems for older parolees transitioning back into the community (Terhune et al., 1999).

Preventive Measures that Can Be Taken Before Release

Steps can be taken before prison release to smooth the transition back into the community. Prior to release, older adults who have been incarcerated for a long time may benefit greatly from training in independent living skills such as cooking, shopping, banking, and money management. It is imperative that older adults have a transition plan that includes health care and medication access. Ideally, a summary of the individual's medical problems would be provided to their post-release physician. In addition, classes in health care promotion and, for those who have a chronic disease, education about their illness and disease self-management can be valuable.

Intensive case management that links the older inmate to community resources can be a helpful step in promoting a smoother transition. Community-based organizations can also reach out to older adults who are being paroled or released. An example program is the Senior Ex-Offenders Program (SEOP) in San Francisco. SEOP helps the older ex-prisoner identify his or her needs, such as medical or mental health referrals or assistance with Medicare applications, and then mobilizes the necessary resources to meet these needs. Innovative organizations like SEOP also help ex-prisoners identify meaningful contributions that they can make to the community, such as being anger management counselors, HIV test counselors, or soup kitchen volunteers, and train them to develop these skills. In this way, such transition programs can provide purpose and a social network to older individuals as they reenter the community while also having a positive impact on the community to which they return.

Conclusion

The exponential growth of the aging inmate population has broad-reaching public policy, economic, and community health consequences both within prison and throughout the reentry process. The fundamental principle in caring for any older adult is to maintain independence and functional ability. In order to do so, attention must be paid to physical and mental health through chronic disease management, environmental modification, and social support. While this approach to geriatric care may be used to promote the health and safety of older prisoners, the special challenges facing older adults in the prison environment and during community reentry need to be addressed as well. These challenges must be met with innovative collaboration between many different disciplines including correctional staff, parole officers, community organizations, and health care providers. Improved coordination between these groups coupled with training in geriatric issues could lead to policies that will promote the health and safety of geriatric inmates and of the communities to which they return.

- Prisoners are often considered "geriatric" at age 55
- Consider the aging of the population when planning health and safety interventions
- Project physical plant and staffing needs for a population with increased illness and disability
- When projecting future medical care costs, consider that geriatric prisoners are more expensive than younger prisoners
- Monitor the use of potentially risky medications in older adults
- Design a geriatrics clinic for older prisoners with chronic disease and/or disability
- When using screening tests, discuss the risks and benefits and consider life expectancy and individual goals
- Assess physical and mental health status and risk by focusing on common geriatric syndromes
- Develop approaches to address behavior infractions among prisoners with cognitive impairment
- Adapt the environment to mitigate physically challenging tasks
- Remember that people who are independent in the community might be impaired in prison
- For reentry, provide bridge medications, postdischarge medical appointments, summarized health records, and community agency referrals

Acknowledgment

The authors appreciate the helpful advice of Michael Harper, M.D.

References

ADA. (1990). Americans with Disabilities Act of 1990.

Aday, R. H. (2003). *Aging prisoners: Crisis in American corrections.* Westport, CT: Praeger Publishers.

Anno, B. J., Graham, C., Lawrence, J. E., & Shansky, R. (2004). *Correctional health care: Addressing the needs of elderly, chronically ill, and terminally ill inmates.* Middletown, CT: Criminal Justice Institute.

Baillargeon, J. B. S., Pulvino, J., & Dunn, K. (2000). The disease profile of Texas prison inmates. *Ann Epidemiol, 10*, 74–80.

Bess, F. H., Lichtenstein, M. J., Logan, S. A., Burger, M. C., & Nelson, E. (1989). Hearing impairment as a determinant of function in the elderly. *J Am Geriatr Soc, 37*, 123–128.

Bogardus, S. T., Jr., Yueh, B., & Shekelle, P. G. (2003). Screening and management of adult hearing loss in primary care: Clinical applications. *JAMA, 289*, 1986–1990.

Boyle, B. A. (2002). The Maryland Division of Correction hospice program. *J Palliat Med, 5*, 671–675.

Braithwaite, R. S., Col, N. F., & Wong, J. B. (2003). Estimating hip fracture morbidity, mortality and costs. *J Am Geriatr Soc, 51*, 364–370.

Brown, C. J., & Norris, M. (2006a). Falls. In *PIER, Physicians' Information and Education Resource*. Philadelphia: American College of Physicians.

Brown, C. J., & Norris, M. (2006b). *PIER, Physicians' Information and Education Resource*. Philadelphia: American College of Physicians.

California Prisoners and Parolees 2004. (2005). California Department of Corrections and Rehabilitation, Offender Information Services, Estimates and Statistical Analysis Section, Data Analysis Unit. Sacramento.

Carey, E. C., Walter, L. C., Lindquist, K., & Covinsky, K. E. (2004). Development and validation of a functional morbidity index to predict mortality in community-dwelling elders. *J Gen Intern Med, 19*, 1027–1033.

Colsher, P. L., Wallace, R. B., Loeffelholz, P. L., & Sales, M. (1992). Health status of older male prisoners: A comprehensive survey. *Am J Public Health, 82*, 881–884.

Crawley, E., & Sparks, R. (2006). Is there life after imprisonment? How elderly men talk about imprisonment and release. *Criminology and Criminal Justice, 6*, 63–82.

Enders, S. R., Paterniti, D. A., & Meyers, F. J. (2005). An approach to develop effective health care decision making for women in prison. *J Palliat Med, 8*, 432–439.

Faiver, K. L. (ed.). (1998). *Health care management issues in corrections*. Lanham,MD: American Correctional Association.

Fazel, S., Hope, T., O'Donnell, I., Piper, M., & Jacoby, R. (2001). Health of elderly male prisoners: Worse than the general population, worse than younger prisoners. *Age Ageing, 30*, 403–407.

Federal Interagency Forum on Aging-Related Statistics. (2004). *Older Americans 2004: Key indicators of well-being*. Washington, DC: U.S. Government Printing Office.

Fick, D. M., Cooper, J. W., Wade, W. E., Waller, J. L., Maclean, J. R., & Beers, M. H. (2003). Updating the Beers criteria for potentially inappropriate medication use in older adults: Results of a US consensus panel of experts. *Arch Intern Med, 163*, 2716–2724.

Fields, G. (2005, May 18). Life and death: As inmates age, a prison carpenter builds more coffins. *Wall Street Journal*.

Gill, T. M., Robison, J. T., Williams, C. S., & Tinetti, M. E. (1999). Mismatches between the home environment and physical capabilities among community-living older persons. *J Am Geriatr Soc, 47*, 88–92.

Harrison, P. M., & Beck, A. J. (2004). *Prisoners in 2003* (Publication No. NCJ 205335). Washington, DC: U.S. Department of Justice.

Hill, T., Williams, B. A., Cobe, G., & Lindquist, K. J. (2006). *Aging inmates: Challenges for healthcare and custody. A report for the California Department of Corrections and Rehabilitation*. San Francisco.

Holman, B. (1998). Nursing homes behind bars: The elderly in prison. *Coalition for Federal Sentencing Reform, 2*(1), 1–2.

Hornung, C. A., Anno, B. J., Greifinger, R. B., & Gadre, S. (2002). Health care for soon-to-be-released inmates: A survey of state prison systems. In *The health status of soon-to-be-released inmates*. Vol. 2. National Commission on Correctional Health Care.

http://www.ahrq.gov/clinic/uspstfix.htm. U.S. Preventive Services Task Force (USPSTF), Agency for Healthcare Research and Quality. Retrieved August 15, 2006.

http://www.census.gov/hhes/www/disability/sipp/disab9495/ds94t1h.html.United States Census Bureau Website. Retrieved October 20, 2005.

http://www.dc.state.fl.us/pub/annual/0405/index.html. (2005). Florida Department of Corrections 2004–2005 Annual Report. Retrieved August 10, 2006.

http://www.gwu.edu/~ccommit/law.htm. George Washington Law School Website. Retrieved April 1, 2004.

http://www.ojp.usdoj.gov/bjs/pub/pdf/reentry.pdf. (2003). *Reentry Trends in the United States*. Retrieved August 1, 2006.

Koenig, H. G., Johnson, S., Bellard, J., Denker, M., & Fenlon, R. (1995). Depression and anxiety disorder among older male inmates at a federal correctional facility. *Psychiatr Serv, 46*, 399–401.

Kratcoski, P. C., & Babb, S. (1990). Adjustment of older inmates: An analysis of institutional structure and gender. *Journal of Contemporary Criminal Justice, 6*, 264–281.

Landefeld, C. S., Palmer, R. M., Johnson, M. A., Johnston, C. B., & Lyons, W. L. (2004). *Current geriatric diagnosis and treatment*. New York: McGraw–Hill.

Legislative Analyst's Office, Analysis for the 2003–2004 Budget Bill. (2003). Sacramento.

Lemieux, C. M., Dyeson, T. B., & Castiglione, B. (2002). Revisiting the literature on prisoners who are older: Are we wiser? *Prison Journal, 82*, 440–458.

Linder, J. F., Enders, S. R., Craig, E., Richardson, J., & Meyers, F. J. (2002). Hospice care for the incarcerated in the United States: An introduction. *J Palliat Med, 5*, 549–552.

Lindquist, C. H., & Lindquist, C. A. (1999). Health behind bars: Utilization and evaluation of medical care among jail inmates. *J Community Health, 24*, 285–303.

Lurigio, A. J., Rollins, A., & Fallon, J. (2004). The effects of serious mental illness on offender reentry. *Federal Probation, 68*(2), 45–52.

Mara, C. M. (2003). A comparison of LTC in prisons and in the free population. *Long-Term Care Interface,* November, 22–26.

Marquart, J. W., Merianos, D. E., & Doucet, G. (2000). The health-related concerns of older prisoners: Implications for policy. *Aging and Society, 20*, 79–96.

Marshall, S. W., Runyan, C. W., Yang, J., Coyne-Beasley, T., Waller, A. E., Johnson, R. M., et al. (2005). Prevalence of selected risk and protective factors for falls in the home. *Am J Prev Med, 28*, 95–101.

Mitka, M. (2004). Aging prisoners stressing health care system. *JAMA, 292*, 423–424.

Mulrow, C. D., & Lichtenstein, M. J. (1991). Screening for hearing impairment in the elderly: Rationale and strategy. *J Gen Intern Med, 6*, 249–258.

Newcomer, R. J., Clay, T. H., Yaffe, K., & Covinsky, K. E. (2005). Mortality risk and prospective Medicare expenditures for persons with dementia. *J Am Geriatr Soc, 53*, 2001–2006.

Pogorzelski, W., Wolff, N., Pan, K. Y., & Blitz, C. L. (2005). Behavioral health problems, ex-offender reentry policies, and the "Second Chance Act." *Am J Public Health, 95*, 1718–1724.

Pratt, D., Piper, M., Appleby, L., Webb, R., & Shaw, J. (2006). Suicide in recently released prisoners: A population-based cohort study. *Lancet, 368*, 119–123.

Reuben, D. B., Seeman, T. E., Keeler, E., Hayes, R. P., Bowman, L., Sewall, A., et al. (2004). The effect of self-reported and performance-based functional impairment on future hospital costs of community-dwelling older persons. *Gerontologist, 44*, 401–407.

Skiest, D. J., & Keiser, P. (1997). Human immunodeficiency virus infection in patients older than 50 years. A survey of primary care physicians' beliefs, practices, and knowledge. *Arch Fam Med, 6*, 289–294.

Strupp, H. M., & Willmott, D. J. (2005). *Dignity denied: The price of imprisoning older women in California*. San Francisco: Legal Services for Prisoners with Children.

Taylor, D. H., Jr., Schenkman, M., Zhou, J., & Sloan, F. A. (2001). The relative effect of Alzheimer's disease and related dementias, disability, and comorbidities on cost of care for elderly persons. *J Gerontol B Psychol Sci Soc Sci, 56*, S285–S293.

Terhune, C. A., Cambra, S., Steinberg, S. J., Duveneck, S., Baumgardner, E., & Cummings, C. (1999). *Older inmates: The impact of an aging population on the correctional system.* Unpublished manuscript.

Turley, J. (2003). *Statement of Professor Jonathan Turley: California's aging prison population*. Paper presented at the Joint Hearing of the Senate Subcommittee on Aging and Long Term Care, Senate Committee of Public Safety and the Senate Select Committee on the California Correctional System.

Verbrugge, L. M., & Jette, A. M. (1994). The disablement process. *Soc Sci Med, 38*, 1–14.

Voelker, R. (2004). New initiatives target inmates' health. *JAMA, 291*, 1549–1551.

Walter, L. C., Bertenthal, D., Lindquist, K., & Konety, B. R. (2006). PSA screening among elderly men with limited life expectancies. *JAMA, 296*, 2336–2342.

Walter, L. C., & Covinsky, K. E. (2001). Cancer screening in elderly patients: A framework for individualized decision making. *JAMA, 285*, 2750–2756.

Williams, B. A., Lindquist, K., Sudore, R. L., Strupp, H. M., Willmott, D. J., & Walter, L. C. (2006). Being old and doing time: Functional impairment and adverse experiences of geriatric female prisoners. *J Am Geriatr Soc, 54*, 702–707.

Chapter 6

International Public Health and Corrections: Models of Care and Harm Minimization

Michael Levy

John Howard has visited all Europe—not to survey the sumptuousness of palaces, or the stateliness of temples; or to make accurate measurements of the remains of ancient grandeur, to form a scale of the curiosity of modern art; not to collect medals or collate manuscripts—but to dive into the depths of dungeons and plunge to the infection of hospitals; to survey the mansions of sorrow and pain; to take the gauge and measure of misery, depression and contempt; to remember the forgotten, to attend to the neglected, to visit the forsaken, and compare and collate the miseries of all men in all countries. His plan is original; and it is full of genius as it is of humanity. (Edmund Burke, 1780)

Introduction

The development of the prison as the unchallenged institution of punishment is relatively recent compared to other social institutions, such as the asylum, the workhouse, and the hospital—being less than 250 years old (Morris & Rothman, 1995; Human Rights Watch). In contrast to these other social institutions, prisons have continued to grow. The International Centre for Prison Studies (Kings College, London) estimates that three in four jurisdictions throughout the world are currently expanding their prison systems (International Centre for Prison Studies).

In this situation, and with the downgrading of other institutions, the modern prison is taking on functions previously carried by others, such as the mental asylum (mental illness) (Rosen, 2006) and the poorhouse (welfare and accommodation).

Incarceration is an institution of "unequal power," between the dominant social structure and the individual who is contained within. Apart from the ethical and philosophical issues implicit in this "relationship," the health consequences are extreme on the individual, but also on the community from which the prisoner comes and will return. The modern prison, while posing health risks to the community (Freudenberg, 2001), also promises to deliver health gains to individuals engaged in it, albeit nonconsensually.

By its nature a coercive institution framed in a paramilitary mold, the modern prison is scrutinized by human rights and international law. There is a rich body of international human rights instruments which direct signatory states to implement minimum standards for the care of persons deprived of their liberty.

> Human rights frameworks demand of governments that minimum standards are adhered to consistently. The principle of "due diligence" requires that when states know, or ought to know, about abuses of human rights, and fail to take appropriate steps to prevent violations, then the State bears responsibility for the consequences. Exercising due diligence includes steps to prevent abuses, including to investigate them when they occur, prosecute the alleged perpetrators and bring them to justice in fair proceedings, and ensure adequate reparation for the victims, including rehabilitation and redress.
>
> Steps to prevent violence can be legal, educational, or practical (Amnesty International).

The medical profession, primarily through the World Medical Association, has enunciated further standards of professional conduct (World Medical Association). While primarily directed toward ethical conduct, the principles also have relevance for public health practice.

Loss of liberty carries with it diminished ability to control one's health. Prisons are crowded. Airborne, foodborne, and waterborne diseases have enhanced opportunities to be propagated; the prisoner (and to a lesser extent the prison worker) has little ability to control initial exposure, and subsequent propagations of a range of diseases of public health importance. In the seventeenth century, typhus (also called "gaol fever"), along with smallpox, posed dangers to prison inmates, jailers, and court officers. In more recent times, the spread of tuberculosis from within former Russian prisons and its spread into the general community have been well described (Spradling et al., 2002), as has been the transmission of multi-drug-resistant tuberculosis between prisoners and prison guards (Valway et al., 1994). The propagation of hepatitis C within prisons has been substantiated (Butler, Kariminia, Levy, & Kaldor, 2004), although the propagation into the community is yet to be elucidated.

Public Health and Corrections

Public health is the art and science of preventing disease and injury, prolonging life, and promoting health through the organized efforts of society. Public health practice informs and empowers individuals and communities, and creates healthy environments through the use of evidence-based strategies and accountability mechanisms. The balance of health risks and health gains is the essential issue in considering the public health impacts of prisons (Glaser & Greifinger, 1993).

The systematic management of risks in the correctional setting associated with air, food, and water, through the science of environmental health has been poorly developed. The California Department of Corrections and Rehabilitation has uniquely developed an audit tool for prisons (California Department of Corrections and Rehabilitation), but apart from this there is little accessible information or a strong evidence base.

Crowding within prisons is almost normative (Walmsley, 2005)—increased incarceration across the world brings with it increased occupancy levels. The normalization of physical violence and extreme lack of privacy, with the ever-present possibility of sexual abuse are almost inevitable consequences of this situation. Few countries limit the occupancy of their prisons to the actual bed capacity of their facilities. Norway and Iceland, notably, do not exceed their capacity; this is achieved through the delay of entry to prison once a person is sentenced, or explicit release of one prisoner to make room for a "more needy" occupant.

Some prison systems are underpinned by complex transport systems for moving prisoners between prisons and between prisons and courthouses; this provides further conduits for disease transmission and propagation (Levy et al., 2003).

Harm Minimization

Harm minimization is an approach to risks and hazards that takes into consideration the actual harms associated with the specific exposure. This approach weighs the range of potential harms of a particular risk and how these harms can be minimized or reduced. It recognizes that risk behaviors are, and will continue to be, a part of our society irrespective of the harms associated with their use (Hughes, 2003; World Health Organization, 2005).

Harm minimization, in the context of prisoner health, has led to improved cooperation between the health, social, justice, and law enforcement sectors and services. For example, needle syringe programs provide sterile equipment, information, and referral to other services, for people who use illegal drugs. Harm-reduction strategies such as needle syringe programs are effective in attracting drug users who may otherwise never have contact with other drug treatment services, medical, legal, or social services.

Extension of community injecting equipment exchange programs into prisons has been implemented in a number of countries (Dolan, Rutter, & Wodak, 2003): Switzerland, Germany, Luxembourg, Spain, Moldova, Belarus, and Scotland currently have such programs. While the number of countries implementing this strategy is increasing, the coverage on a world scale is minimal, and still considered controversial—or not considered at all!

Drug and Alcohol Misuse and Dependence

The convergence of drug and alcohol problems and the prisoner population is intense, because a crime may be commissioned while under the influence of a drug or alcohol, and because some forms of drug use are criminalized in most countries. Additionally, harmful use of alcohol is disproportionately associated with serious accidents, violent crimes, and driving-related crimes.

Coexistence of mental illness and drug and alcohol health problems is noted—either being a precipitator, or because of self-medication in otherwise poorly compliant mentally ill individuals (Abram, Teplin, & McClelland, 2003).

Much of the burgeoning in prison populations around the world is directly connected to this legal position. As an important aspect of public health practice is regulatory, the issues of drug laws and the criminalization of drug use have resonance in the areas of incarceration and public health.

Given that so many prisoners are directly or indirectly incarcerated because of drug-related crimes, legalization of personal drug use has the potential of drastically decreasing prisoner populations. Drug law reform has been pursued most aggressively in Portugal and Spain, where decriminalization of personal drug use is complete and absolute.

In the context of drug misuse and dependence, harm minimization encourages a change in attitudes toward people who use drugs, including those who are physically and psychologically dependent on drugs, such as heroin and cocaine. This approach moves away from stereotyping drug users as antisocial and directing them through the criminal justice system, rather than through treatment services. The more complex relationships between the individual, their community, the drug, and the environment and circumstances in which they are using it, are considered. Rather than seeking to "treat" or "cure," this approach considers other problems associated with the person's harmful drug use, such as the availability of the drug in the community, the prevalence of their use, and how much is known about the drug and its effects and harms in the community. Harm minimization highlights that a range of physical and chemical exposures has the potential to cause harm, not just the illegal drugs. This is especially important when we consider that legal drugs, such as tobacco and alcohol, are responsible for the greatest social and economic harms.

Using a variety of strategies in response to drug misuse and dependence, harm minimization works to reduce the harmful consequences of drug use, by reducing the demand for drugs, the supply of drugs, and the drug harms—assistance for people who choose to use drugs to do so in the safest possible way. Demand-reduction strategies work to discourage people from starting to use drugs, and encourage those who do use drugs to use less or to stop. Evidence supports a combination of information and education, along with regulatory controls and financial penalties, to help to make drug use less attractive (European Monitoring Centre for Drugs and Drug Addiction).

Health workers can offer clients a range of options for their desired treatment outcomes, which encourages more people to participate in treatment and prevention programs. The harms associated with a client's drug use can be reduced or minimized simply by their participation in targeted treatment programs. It is instructive to reflect on the lack of control that prisoners have over informed choices. As they relate to health risks, knowledge is far from sufficient—it has been said that prisoners are the most informed group in the population when it comes to risk assessment—but their capacity to respond appropriately is seriously impeded by the lack of options available to them.

Supply control strategies involve legislation, regulatory controls, and law enforcement. Supply reduction has received disproportionate support from custodial authorities, be it in boundary surveillance or interception of staff and visitors—generally with little proven effect (Australian National Council on Drugs, 2004).

Harm-reduction strategies have received little favor within the correctional environment—with some notable exceptions. Providing injecting drug users with access to clean equipment through needle syringe programs is a community standard in many countries. By reducing the risk of bloodborne infections such as hepatitis C, hepatitis B, and HIV being transmitted, the risks could be reduced for the individual prisoner, prison workers, and the community as a whole.

Bloodborne Viruses

The impact of bloodborne viruses on prisoner populations has been well documented in a number of countries (Estebanez et al., 2002; van Beek, Dwyer, Dore, Luo, & Kaldor, 1998; Zamani et al., 2006). Treatment opportunities benefit the individual prisoner, while public health concerns are focused on prevention, through education, and in isolated prison systems through the provision of the means of prevention—condoms for protected male sexual activity, dental dams for protected female sexual activity, liquid bleach for the cleaning of injecting equipment, or sanctioned tattooing.

HIV

The World Health Organization has provided a framework for the response to HIV in prisons (World Health Organization and UNAIDS, 2006). The framework stresses a human rights approach to the diagnosis, care, and management of HIV in the prison setting, identifying issues such as stigma, discrimination, intersectoral work (i.e., health services working both beyond health while in prison, and beyond the prison with the community), and workforce training (both health and custodial).

The prevalence of HIV among prisoners is typically four to five times that in the general community. Prison has a profound impact on the lived experience of too many persons living with HIV/AIDS: It has been reported that 25% of all HIV-positive individuals in the United States pass through a jail every year (Hammett, Harmon, & Rhodes, 2002).

The public health risks that prisons pose have been highlighted by a number of epidemiological studies of HIV transmission (Dolan & Wodak, 1999; Goldberg et al., 1998; Centers for Disease Control and Prevention, 2006). The single documented case of HIV transmission to a prison guard has attracted much attention as an issue of occupational safety, and consequent vehement, yet unsubstantiated, denial of harm minimization measures (Jones, 1991).

The responses of prison systems to HIV vary greatly (Resch, Altice, & Paltiel, 2005; Cotten-Oldenburg, Jordan, Martin, & Sadowski, 1999). Some systems have proven resistant to external pressures not to further discriminate against prisoners infected with HIV—western European and Scandinavian prisons operate under community standards of diagnosis, treatment, care, and respect for the confidentiality of inmates. Some countries have taken a different approach—including nonconsented compulsory testing, and linkage to community HIV registers (Estonia), and segregation of known HIV-positive prisoners (Singapore and Cuba).

Hepatitis C

The strong associations between illicit drug use, injecting with contaminated equipment, the criminalization of drug use in most jurisdictions throughout the world, and incarceration leads to a collision between the dual "epidemics" of incarceration and hepatitis C. In Western countries that have assessed the prevalence of hepatitis C virus among their prisoner populations, in excess of 50% are infected (Ogilvie, Veit, Crofts, & Thompson, 1999).

More disturbing, for the public health, is that the incidence of infection is also extremely high (Butler et al., 2004). Prisons have been referred to as the "powerhouses" of the hepatitis C epidemic.

Incarceration has proven an opportunity to address part of the hepatitis C problem—treatments have been successfully offered in a very limited number of prison systems, with success rates mirroring those achieved in the community (Skipper, Guy, Parkes, Roderick, & Rosenberg, 2003; Spaulding et al., 2006).

Evidence-Based Interventions

A range of initiatives aimed at minimizing the risks of transmission of bloodborne viruses have been introduced across the world, in response to the range of risk activities experienced in prisons:

Injecting drug use in prisons—there is a mounting body of evidence that injecting drug use continues within prisons (Griffin, 1994; Small et al., 2005; Seamark & Gaughwin, 1994; O'Sullivan et al., 2003). The response of different prison systems has been polarized to two relatively extreme positions—denial and acceptance, with introduction of injecting equipment exchange. The latter response has been implemented in Switzerland, Germany (Berlin), Spain, Moldova, Belarus, Luxembourg, and most recently in Scotland (Jacob & Stover, 2000; Lines, Jürgens, Betteridge, & Stöver, 2005).

Health education—to address knowledge deficits and misconceptions, and to provide skills for peer-education, of benefit during incarceration, and possibly once released into the community (Squires, 1996; Dolan, Bijl, & White, 2004). However, to advise/educate prisoners on the means to protect their health and the health of their fellow prisoners, and then not provide the means for protection could be considered "double jeopardy"!

Violence amelioration—to minimize the harms of incarceration; not merely the physical injury, but also the normalization of antisocial behaviors (Butler & Kariminia, 2006).

Pharmacotherapies—particularly useful for opiate dependence and addiction. Methadone has been utilized for more than 20 years in the prison environment; other pharmacotherapies include buprenorphine and naltrexone (Cropsey, Villalobos, & St Clair, 2005). Treatments for other drug dependencies are less well tested.

Conjugal visits—virtually no evidence supports intimate family visits as a measure to minimize harms associated with bllodborne viruses; however, a human rights focus would be strongly supportive (Carlson & Cervera, 1991). A similar approach may apply to the issue of children in prisons—in some jurisdictions, children are allowed to stay with their mother, providing the mother is compliant with regulations (e.g., "drug free"). This dispensation is variously for 12 months (e.g., Thailand) of school-entry age (Australia). Only one jurisdiction (Nepal) is known to allow male children to live with their fathers while imprisoned. In some South American prisons, entire families encamp within the prison perimeter. The intergenerational impacts of incarceration are intense, and of public health interest (Quilty, Levy, Howard, Barratt, & Butler, 2004).

Body piercing and tattooing—are highly prevalent, albeit risky activities in prisons (Hellard, Hocking, & Crofts, 2004; Babudieri et al., 2005). A tattoo parlor pilot was established in six federal Canadian prisons in 2005.

> ### Canada
>
> The Canadian federal prison system has trailed sanctioned tattooing over an 18-month period in 2005–2006. In six prisons prisoner-artists are taught in detail the infection control skills necessary for safe tattooing. Prison authorities register the artwork. There are restrictions on types of tattoos that can be applied (e.g., gang symbols, hate symbols are prohibited). The infection control standards set for the prison pilots exceed those currently in the community. At this time, there is no skin piercing done officially in any prisons, worldwide.

Mental Illness

The links between institutions of mass incarceration and those for the mentally ill are diverse (Fazel & Lubbe, 2005; Fazel, Bains, & Doll, 2006; Lamberti et al., 2001).

Persons incarcerated can manifest mental illness at any stage of the criminal proceedings.

- On entry, the first connect, reconnect, to health services may reveal emerging or established (but neglected) mental illness.
- The stress associated with arrest and detention may "unmask" mental illness.
- Mental illness may be provoked by the stresses associated with social isolation of incarceration.
- Mental illness may be considered the critical element in the commissioning of a crime, with the person considered "criminally insane."
- Regrettably, with the deinstitutionalization of mental asylums in the 1980s, secure accommodation for the mentally ill decreased, without a coincident increase in community-based housing. The prevalence of mental illness among prisoners exceeds that of the community (White, Chafetz, Collins-Bride, & Nickens, 2006). The links between prisoners, ex-prisoners, and persons in unstable accommodation have been convincingly made (Kushel, Hahn, Evans, Bangsberg, & Moss, 2005).

Many jurisdictions have mental health legislation that recognizes differing levels of accountability for people with mental illness committing crimes—to the extreme position of "criminal insanity" where the commission of the crime is not admissible to the court.

Women

Universally, male incarceration overwhelms that for females; in fact, incarceration is almost synonymous with male incarceration. Typically, women account for 4–8% of the prisoner estate; in Hong Kong, over 20% of prisoners are female. However, incarceration of women deserves particular attention (Rehman, Gahagan, DiCenso, & Dias, 2004). In most Western countries, the incarceration rate of females has exceeded that of males: In Australia, the number of incarcerated women has doubled in the last 10 years; from a low base, the proportion of elderly women (>45 years of age) has increased the highest; the crimes often relate to credit card fraud and gambling debts—they are rarely violent. Where violence is involved, too often it is an act of desperation within an abusive and violent relationship.

The public health issue beyond the disproportionate criminological issue, is that mothers and grandmothers are the long-term carers of children of prisoners; conversely, fathers isolated from their partner by incarceration, rarely act as long-term carers for affected children.

Female prisoners are consistently reported to be even more socially disadvantaged than their male counterparts. They have a shared experience of high rates of prior sexual abuse, physical violence (often in the domestic setting), and dangerous drug use (Arnold et al., 2003).

Women tend to receive shorter sentences, but have higher reincarceration rates than males. The consequences for health service delivery are profound. Treatments tend to be more opportunistic, and less successful when longer-term compliance is demanded.

Models of Care

All prison services would state that they provided some level of health care for their prisoners. The actual service delivery will depend on the legislative framework governing the correctional service, but rarely also the laws regulating the health service. Western European countries, additionally, apply a human rights framework to their prisons, and by extension, to the health services provided to prisoners.

Five models of prisoner health care are identifiable:

1. The prison health authority is directly related to the custodial authority. In this model, the custodial authority employs the health care staff. In some prison systems, the trade union affiliation of custodial and health staff may be the same; in some systems the same paramilitary structure applies to custodial and health staff. This is the most common model for the delivery of prisoner health services, worldwide.
2. A prison health authority is the primary health care provider. This service is either the community health service, or a dedicated health authority for prisoners.
3. The prison health authority is a public or private entity that has been tendered by a central custodial/health authority.
4. Custodial officers or prisoners themselves are the health service provider. In this circumstance, former health workers who have subsequently been incarcerated are utilized as auxiliary health workers [this is observed in Myanmar (Burma)].
5. No health entity [inmates have to seek their own care, or there simply is no health care for prisoners (this has been observed in some prisons in Papua New Guinea)]; when nongovernment or missionary organizations may temporarily fill a "void", but usually there is no sustained care.

Iceland

Prison health care is delivered from the neighboring community to the prison. Most workers are part-time. For example, the main 80-bed prison, near Stelfoss (Litla Hraun), has a nurse (32 hours per week), a doctor (10 hours per week), and a psychiatrist visiting 6 hours per week.

United Kingdom

The Primary Care Trusts of the National Health Service have become responsible for health care provision to prisoners in England and Wales. A central coordinating unit in the Ministry of Health provides guidance in policy and monitoring. The Inspectorate of Prisons for England and Wales has provided independent direction encouraging the transfer of services from the Home Office (Her Majesty's Inspectorate of Prisons for England and Wales, 1996; Hayton & Boyington, 2006).

How do Models of Care Impact on Public Health?

The competent prison health care service needs to do much more than simply provide health care to persons in custody. As a minimum, it is appropriate that it assume dual roles:

- as the independent advocate for the health of prisoners (and their families), and
- as the advocate for the public health—the health impacts of incarceration are to be minimized.

The models of care adopted by the health service need to consider the needs of different groups of detainees and the needs of the community.

Earlier in the incarceration process, the immediate health needs of prisoners will dominate. Newly received prisoners typically will have a burden of unmet health needs, as lack of compliance with treatment is a predictor of being arrested—particularly where drug misuse and mental illness are concerned. This is a time to offer resource-low and high-impact interventions, such as hepatitis B immunization, cervical screening, and vision testing.

As the stay in prisons extends, the health needs of a more chronic nature assume more importance, interspersed with prison-induced illness, and trauma.

Whether prisoner health services should be based on the principle of "equivalence" or "equity" (Levy, 1997) has been debated. Equivalence would require that inputs to the prisoner health service be on the same level of those provided in the community. The argument for "equity" states that the outputs, or health outcomes, of the service be the same. Noting that the health of prisoners is worse than a comparable group of free citizens, the inputs required for the same outcome to be achieved for prisoner, would be greater than those allocated for the community.

Utilization of Services

Access to services becomes a key issue in health service delivery to prisoners. Differing security classifications, and limitations placed by the physical environment, impose strict limits on accessing the clinic, and health staff. Given that many prisoners come from the community, having previously accessed services poorly, the physical proximity of the accommodation area to the clinic may provide opportunities for accessing services—until operational issues intervene, making access no easier than it had been in the community!

Few studies have looked at the nature of services provided to prisoners. An English study determined that prisoners consulted generalist medical practitioners 3 times more frequently than an equivalent community cohort, and primary health care providers 80 times more than community counterparts. That study did not consider the role that pharmacists play in the provision of health information in the community (and the absence of this service in the prison—by default provided by nurses) (Marshall, Simpson, & Stevens, 2001). In an Australian study, prisoners could reflect on the relative virtues of different service providers within the health care system (community and prison), and attribute different levels of satisfaction to each (Barling, Halpin, & Levy, 2005).

Clinical services for prisoners vary between jurisdictions, and where central coordination is weak or absent, it varies between prisons within the same system. In principle, custodial care is strongly based within primary care, where independent health practitioners work in relative isolation from their community-based professional colleagues. Standardized policies and procedures support "protocol-driven" care. This is efficient and addresses the majority of immediate health needs of the prisoner-patient.

Some prison health services maintain inpatient facilities, usually with low-level care. This provides an immediate level of care between ambulatory and (community standard) inpatient care. While providing a limited amount of clinical supervision and safety for the prisoner-patient, these facilities are too readily utilized as a disciplinary option for the custodial authority—particularly with prisoners having behavioral or "management" problems.

In some jurisdictions, the prisoner health care provider is called on to deliver health care to custodial officers. There is no evidence to support this model, and unpublished reports indicate that this distracts from health care for prisoners.

In principle, health services within prisons should only provide emergency care to non-prisoners.

Texas, USA

Dedicated funding for hepatitis B immunization for prisoners was also applied to a custodial officer immunization program. A funding shortfall for the expanded program required the program to cease prematurely—for both prisoners and custodial officers.

Thereafter, prison workers could complete their immunization through their community provider (but the prisoners could not).

Health benefits of incarceration are few, and relate primarily to opportunistic interventions, rather than treatments for chronic diseases, where longer-term compliance to complex treatments is demanded. The areas of interest in this context include pregnancy (specifically the infants of imprisoned mothers) (Martin, Kim, Kupper, Meyer, & Hays, 1997) and immunization (Day, White, Ross, & Dolan, 2003).

Reentry

Postrelease care poses the ultimate challenge to prisoner health care. The difficulties in reintegration to community living carry with it complex inter-actions between legal, housing, social welfare, and health care systems—to name only a few.

The burden of illness manifest by prisoners at the point of entry into the criminal justice system, gives some insight into the problems to be faced by these same people, on their reentry to the community. Resumption of chaotic lifestyles, decreased employment prospects, difficulty in accessing health services in an ordered manner, lead to overuse of emergency services, uncoordinated care of multiple symptom complexes, and poor management of multiple coexisting chronic health conditions (Leukefeld et al., 2006). Limited access to managed care, or exclusion from some government "safety net" schemes, exacerbates this disadvantage (Lee, Vlahov, & Freudenberg, 2006). Rarely, ex-prisoners are excluded from public funded health programs (Warren, Bellin, Zoloth, & Safyer, 1994). Such an anomaly establishes a system where individuals must decide to relinquish their physical freedom in order to maintain, sometimes life-saving, treatment.

Attention of many prison authorities is to the issue of deaths in custody. In Australia, in response to 99 deaths in custody, a Royal Commission into Aboriginal Deaths in Custody was conducted in the 1990s. The resultant report noted poignantly that Aborigines did not die disproportionately to non-Aborigines, merely "too many Aborigines go to prison too often" (Whimp). However, the magnitude of postrelease mortality (Pratt, Piper, Appleby, Webb, & Shaw, 2006; Christensen, Hammerby, Smith, & Bird, 2006) far exceeds that of deaths while in prison. Ex-prisoners with previous histories of mental illness or drug dependencies present particular risks of early death—either from drug overdose, suicide, or violence.

Diversion

In recent years, diversion programs for people with serious mental illness and co-occurring substance use disorders have received increasing attention (Greenberg & Nielsen, 2003; Draine, Blank, Kottsieper, & Solomon, 2005). Previous studies suggest that diversion programs have the potential to achieve positive outcomes—both in terms of successful referral (return) to treatment programs, and decreased rearrest rates. A study of six jail diversion programs (three prebooking and three postbooking) compared outcomes at 12 months following diversion with those of a comparison group. The findings suggested that jail diversion reduces time spent in jail without increasing the public safety risk, while linking participants to community-based services (Steadman & Naples, 2005).

A cooperative, community-oriented "public health model of correctional healthcare" was developed to address the needs of persons temporarily displaced into jail from the community, and to improve the health and safety of the community. It emphasizes five key elements: early detection, effective treatment, education, prevention, and continuity of care. In the program, physicians and case managers are "dually based"—they work both at the jail and at community healthcare centers, as a mechanism for promoting continuity of care for inmates with serious and chronic medical conditions (Lincoln et al., 2006).

The lack of success in reintegration programs has been noted. In one study in New York, interventions were judged to be too modest (Freudenberg, Daniels, Crum, Perkins, & Richie, 2005).

Numerous models have been developed, including planned release at the very point of entry to jail, to an acknowledgment of failure to connect with community health services by establishing a "community" clinic at the entrance to a prison, dedicated to ex-prisoners (The Modello in Barcelona, Spain).

Practical Guidance for Public Policy Makers and Health Practitioners

> The minimum principles for a prison health service are that it is an Independent Health Authority, with independent oversight (inspection) (Council of Europe, 2004)' and has links to academic health organizations, with avenues open to teaching and research (Raimer & Stobo, 2004).

Applying a stronger evidence-base to modern prisons could enhance the health of prisoners and the community through:

• Strengthening the independence of prisoner health services,
• Strengthening standards setting and independent review of the health service,

- Supporting diversion programs from the criminal justice system, using health-related criteria, and
- Strengthening both prisoner and community health service provision, on entry to prison, in anticipation of the return, and on returning to the community.

References

Abram, K. M., Teplin, L. A., & McClelland, G. M. (2003). Comorbidity of severe psychiatric disorders and substance use disorders among women in jail. *American Journal of Psychiatry, 160,* 1007–1010.

Amnesty International. Making rights a reality. How can states be held responsible for violence against women by private individuals? http://web.amnesty.org/wire/July2004/svaw (accessed November 2006).

Arnold, E. M., Kirk, R. S., Roberts, A. C., Griffith, D. P., Meadows, K., & Julian, J. (2003). Treatment of incarcerated, sexually-abused adolescent females: An outcome study. *Journal of Childhood Sexual Abuse, 12,* 123–139.

Australian National Council on Drugs. (2004). Research Paper No. 9—Supply, demand and harm reduction strategies in Australian prisons: Implementation, cost and evaluation. Canberra. http://www.ancd.org.au/publications/pdf/rp9_australian_prisons.pdf (accessed November 2006).

Babudieri, S., Longo, B., Sarmati, L., Starnini, G., Dori, L., Suligoi, B., Carbonara, S., Monarca, R., Quercia, G., Florenzano, G., Novati, S., Sardu, A., Iovinella, V., Casti, A., Romano, A., Uccella, I., Maida, I., Brunetti, B., Mura, M. S., Andreoni, M., & Rezza, G. (2005). Correlates of HIV, HBV, and HCV infections in a prison inmate population: Results from a multicentre study in Italy. *Journal of Medical Virology, 76,* 311–317.

Barling, J., Halpin, R., & Levy, M. (2005). Capturing perceptions: Prisoners assess their health services—Australia 2001 and 2004. *International Journal of Prisoner Health, 1,* 183–198.

Butler, T., & Kariminia, A. (2006). Prison violence: Perspectives and epidemiology. *New South Wales Public Health Bulletin, 17,* 17–20.

Butler, T., Kariminia, A., Levy, M., & Kaldor, J. (2004). Prisoners are at risk for hepatitis C transmission. *European Journal of Epidemiology, 19,* 1119–1122.

California Department of Corrections and Rehabilitation. Health Inspection Checklists. http://www.cya.ca.gov/divisionsboards/csa/health_inspection_checklists.htm (accessed November 2006).

Carlson, B. E., & Cervera, N. J. (1991). Incarceration, coping, and support. *Social Work, 36,* 279–285.

Centers for Disease Control and Prevention. (2006). HIV transmission among male inmates in a state prison system—Georgia, 1992–2005. *Morbidity and Mortality Weekly Report, 55,* 421–426.

Christensen, P. B., Hammerby, E., Smith, E., & Bird, S. M. (2006). Mortality among Danish drug users released from prison. *International Journal of Prisoner Health, 2,* 13–20.

Cotten-Oldenburg, N. U., Jordan, B. K., Martin, S. L., & Sadowski, L. S. (1999). Voluntary HIV testing in prison: Do women inmates at high risk for HIV accept HIV testing? *AIDS Education and Prevention, 11,* 28–37.

Council of Europe. (2004) European Committee for the Prevention of Torture and Inhuman or Degrading Treatment or Punishment. The CPT standards… CPT/Inf/E (2002). 1—Rev. 2004. http://www.cpt.coe.int/EN/documents/eng-standards-prn.pdf (accessed November 2006).

Cropsey, K. L., Villalobos, G. C., & St Clair, C. L. (2005). Pharmacotherapy treatment in substance-dependent correctional populations: A review. *Substance Use and Misuse, 40,* 1983–1999, 2043–2048.

Day, C., White, B., Ross, J., & Dolan, K. (2003). Poor knowledge and low coverage of hepatitis B vaccination among injecting drug users in Sydney. *Australian and New Zealand Journal of Public Health, 27*, 558.

Dolan, K. A., Bijl, M., & White, B. (2004). HIV education in a Siberian prison colony for drug dependent males. *International Journal of Equity and Health, 3*, 7.

Dolan, K., Rutter, S., & Wodak, A. D. (2003). Prison-based syringe exchange programmes: A review of international research and development. *Addiction, 98*, 153–158.

Dolan, K. A., & Wodak, A. (1999). HIV transmission in a prison system in an Australian State. *Medical Journal of Australia, 171*, 14–17.

Draine, J., Blank, A., Kottsieper, P., & Solomon, P. (2005). Contrasting jail diversion and in-jail services for mental illness and substance abuse: Do they serve the same clients? *Behavioral Science and Law*, 23, 171–181.

Estebanez, P., Zunzunegui, M. V., Aguilar, M. D., Russell, N., Cifuentes, I., & Hankins, C. (2002). The role of prisons in the HIV epidemic among female injecting drug users. *AIDS Care, 14*, 95–104.

European Monitoring Centre for Drugs and Drug Addiction . www.emcdda.europa.eu/ (accessed November 2006).

Fazel, S., Bains, P., & Doll, H. (2006). Substance abuse and dependence in prisoners: A systematic review. *Addiction, 101*, 181–191.

Fazel, S., & Lubbe, S. (2005). Prevalence and characteristics of mental disorders in jails and prisons. *Current Opinions in Psychiatry, 18*, 550–554.

Freudenberg, N. (2001). Jails, prisons, and the health of urban populations: A review of the impact of the correctional system on community health. *Journal of Urban Health, 78*, 214–235.

Freudenberg, N., Daniels, J., Crum, M., Perkins, T., & Richie, B. E. (2005). Coming home from jail: The social and health consequences of community reentry for women, male adolescents, and their families and communities. *American Journal of Public Health, 95*, 1725–1736.

Glaser, J. B., & Greifinger, R. B. (1993). Correctional health care: A public health opportunity. *Annals of Internal Medicine, 118*, 139–145.

Goldberg, D., Taylor, A., McGregor, J., Davis, B., Wrench, J., & Gruer, L. (1998). A lasting public health response to an outbreak of HIV infection in a Scottish prison? *International Journal of STD and AIDS, 9*, 25–30.

Greenberg, D., & Nielsen, B. (2003). Moving towards a statewide approach to court diversion in New South Wales. *New South Wales Public Health Bulletin, 14*, 227–229.

Griffin, S. (1994). The extent of injecting and syringe sharing in prison reported by Edinburgh drug clinic attenders. *Journal of Clinical Forensic Medicine, 1*, 83–85.

Hammett, T. M., Harmon, M. P., & Rhodes, W. (2002). The burden of infectious disease among inmates of and releasees from US correctional facilities, 1997. *American Journal of Public Health, 92*, 1789–1794.

Hayton, P., & Boyington, J. (2006). Prisons and health reforms in England and Wales. *American Journal of Public Health, 96*, 1730–1733.

Hellard, M. E., Hocking, J. S., & Crofts, N. (2004). The prevalence and the risk behaviours associated with the transmission of hepatitis C virus in Australian correctional facilities. *Epidemiology and Infection, 132*, 409–415.

Her Majesty's Inspectorate of Prisons for England and Wales. (1996). *Patient or prisoner? A new strategy for health care in prisons*. London: Home Office.

Hughes, R. (2003). Drugs, prisons, and harm reduction. *Journal of Health and Social Policy, 18*, 43–54.

Human Rights Watch. http://www.hrw.org/prisons/ (accessed November 2006).

International Centre for Prison Studies, Kings College London. http://www.kcl.ac.uk/ depsta/rel/icps/worldbrief/world_brief.html (accessed November 2006).

Jacob, J., & Stover, H. (2000). The transfer of harm-reduction strategies into prisons: Needle exchange programmes in two German prisons. *International Journal of Drug Policy, 11*, 325–335.

Jones, P. D. (1991). HIV transmission by stabbing despite zidovudine prophylaxis. *Lancet, 338*, 884.

Kushel, M. B., Hahn, J. A., Evans, J. L., Bangsberg, D. R., & Moss, A. R. (2005). Revolving doors: Imprisonment among the homeless and marginally housed population. *American Journal of Public Health, 95*, 1747–1752.

Lamberti, J. S., Weisman, R. L., Schwarzkopf, S. B., Price, N., Ashton, R. M., & Trompeter, J. (2001). The mentally ill in jails and prisons: Towards an integrated model of prevention. *Psychiatric Quarterly, 72*, 63–77.

Lee, J., Vlahov, D., & Freudenberg, N. (2006). Primary care and health insurance among women released from New York City jails. *Journal of Health Care for the Poor and Underserved, 17*, 200–217.

Leukefeld, C. G., Hiller, M. L., Webster, J. M., Tindall, M. S., Martin, S. S., Duvall, J., Tolbert, V. E., & Garrity, T. F. (2006). A prospective examination of high-cost health services utilization among drug using prisoners reentering the community. *Journal of Behavioral Health Service and Research, 33*, 73–85.

Levy, M. (1997). Prison health services. *British Medical Journal, 315*,1394–1395.

Levy, M. H., Quilty, S., Young, L. C., Hunt, W., Matthews, R., & Robertson, P. W. (2003). Pox in the docks: Varicella outbreak in an Australian prison system. *Public Health, 117*, 446–451.

Lincoln, T., Kennedy, S., Tuthill, R., Roberts, C., Conklin, T. J., & Hammett, T. M. (2006). Facilitators and barriers to continuing healthcare after jail: A community-integrated program. *Journal of Ambulatory Care and Management, 29*, 2–16.

Lines, R., Jürgens, R., Betteridge, G., & Stöver, H. (2005). Taking action to reduce injecting drug-related harms in prison: The evidence of effectiveness of prison needle exchange in six countries. *International Journal of Prisoner Health, 1*, 49–64.

Marshall, T., Simpson, S., & Stevens, S. (2001). Use of health services by prison inmates: Comparisons with the community. *Journal of Epidemiology and Community Health, 55*, 364–365.

Martin, S. L., Kim, H., Kupper, L. L., Meyer, R. E., & Hays, M. (1997). Is incarceration during pregnancy associated with infant birthweight? *American Journal of Public Health, 87*, 1526–1531.

Morris, N., & Rothman, D. J. (Eds.). (1995). *The Oxford history of the prison. The practice of punishment in Western society*. Oxford. Oxford University Press.

Ogilvie, E. L., Veit, F., Crofts, N., & Thompson, S. C. (1999). Hepatitis infection among adolescents resident in Melbourne Juvenile Justice Centre: Risk factors and challenges. *Journal of Adolescent Health, 25*, 46–51.

O'Sullivan, B. G., Levy, M. H., Dolan, K. A., Post, J. J., Barton, S. G., Dwyer, D. E., Kaldor, J. M., & Grulich, A. E. (2003). Hepatitis C transmission and HIV post-exposure prophylaxis after needle- and syringe-sharing in Australian prisons. *Medical Journal of Australia, 178*, 546–549.

Pratt, D., Piper, M., Appleby, L., Webb, R., & Shaw, J. (2006). Suicide in recently released prisoners: A population-based cohort study. *Lancet, 368*, 119–123.

Quilty, S., Levy, M. H., Howard, K., Barratt, A., & Butler, T. (2004). Children of prisoners: A growing public health problem. *Australian and New Zealand Journal of Public Health, 28*, 339–343.

Raimer, B. G., & Stobo, J. D. (2004). Health care delivery in the Texas prison system: The role of academic medicine. *The Journal of the American Medical Association, 292*, 485–489.

Rehman, L., Gahagan, J., DiCenso, A. M., & Dias, G. (2004). Harm reduction and women in the Canadian national prison system: Policy or practice? *Womens Health, 40*, 57–73.

Resch, S., Altice, F. L., & Paltiel, A. D. (2005). Cost-effectiveness of HIV screening for incarcerated pregnant women. *International Journal of STD and AIDS, 38*, 163–173.

Rosen, A. (2006). The Australian experience of deinstitutionalization: Interaction of Australian culture with the development and reform of its mental health services. *Acta Psychiatrica Scandinavica Supplement, 429*, 81–89.

Seamark, R., & Gaughwin, M. (1994). Jabs in the dark: Injecting equipment found in prisons, and the risks of viral transmission. *Australian Journal of Public Health, 18*, 113–116.

Skipper, C., Guy, J. M., Parkes, J., Roderick, P., & Rosenberg, W. M. (2003). Evaluation of a prison outreach clinic for the diagnosis and prevention of hepatitis C: Implications for the national strategy. *Gut, 52*, 1500–1504.

Small, W., Kain, S., Laliberte, N., Schechter, M. T., O'Shaughnessy, M. V., & Spittal, P. M. (2005). Incarceration, addiction and harm reduction: Inmates experience injecting drugs in prison. *Substance Use and Misuse, 40*, 831–843.

Spaulding, A. C., Weinbaum, C. M., Lau, D. T., Sterling, R., Seeff, L. B., Margolis, H. S., & Hoofnagle, J. H. (2006). A framework for management of hepatitis C in prisons. *Annals of Internal Medicine, 144*, 762–769.

Spradling, P., Nemtsova, E., Aptekar, T., Shulgina, M., Rybka, L., Wells, C., Aquino, G., Kluge, H., Jakubowiak, W., Binkin, N., & Kazeonny, B. (2002). Anti-tuberculosis drug resistance in community and prison patients, Orel Oblast, Russian Federation. *International Journal of Tuberculosis and Lung Disease, 6*, 757–762.

Squires N. (1996). Promoting health in prisons. *British Medical Journal, 313*, 1161.

Steadman, H. J., & Naples, M. (2005). Assessing the effectiveness of jail diversion programs for persons with serious mental illness and co-occurring substance use disorders. *Behavioral Science and Law, 23*, 163–170.

Valway, S. E., Richards, S. B., Kovacovich, J., Greifinger, R. B., Crawford, J. T., & Dooley, S. W. (1994) Outbreak of multi-drug-resistant tuberculosis in a New York State prison, 1991. *American Journal of Epidemiology, 140*, 113–122.

van Beek, I., Dwyer, R., Dore, G. J., Luo, K., & Kaldor, J. M. (1998). Infection with HIV and hepatitis C virus among injecting drug users in a prevention setting: Retrospective cohort study. *British Medical Journal, 317*, 433–437.

Walmsley, R. (2005). Prison health care and the extent of prison overcrowding. *International Journal of Prisoner Health, 1*, 9–12.

Warren, N., Bellin, E., Zoloth, S., & Safyer, S. (1994). Human immunodeficiency virus infection care is unavailable to inmates on release from jail. *Archives of Family Medicine, 3*, 894–898.

Whimp, K. Final Report of the Royal Commission into Aboriginal Deaths in Custody: A Summary. Reconciliation and Social Justice Library. http://www.austlii.edu.au/au/special/rsjproject/rsjlibrary/rciadic/rciadic_summary/ (accessed November 2006).

White, M. C., Chafetz, L., Collins-Bride, G., & Nickens, J. (2006). History of arrest, incarceration and victimization in community-based severely mentally ill. *Journal of Community Health, 31*, 123–135.

World Health Organization. (2005). *WHO status paper on prisons, drugs and harm reduction*. European Surveillance 10: E050714.5, Copenhagen.

World Health Organization and UNAIDS. (2006). *HIV/AIDS prevention, care, treatment and support in prison settings: A framework for an effective national response*. Geneva.

World Medical Association. Declaration of Tokyo. Guidelines for physicians concerning torture and other cruel, inhuman or degrading treatment or punishment in relation to detention and imprisonment. http://www.wma.net/e/policy/c18.htm (accessed November 2006).

Zamani, S., Kihara, M., Gouya, M. M., Vazirian, M., Nassirimanesh, B., Ono-Kihara, M., Ravari, S. M., Safaie, A., & Ichikawa, S. (2006). High prevalence of HIV infection associated with incarceration among community-based injecting drug users in Tehran, Iran. *Journal of Acquired Immune Deficiency Syndrome, 42*, 342–346.

Chapter 7

The Medicalization of Execution: Lethal Injection in the United States

Mark Heath

> If we could have been satisfied that executions could be carried out [by lethal injection] quickly, painlessly and decently in all cases, we should have recommended its adoption unanimously. But we are bound to conclude from our expert evidence that there is not at present a reasonable certainty of this.[1]

Since its introduction in the United States in 1977, lethal injection has supplanted other methods (firing squad, hanging, lethal gas, and electrocution) and has virtually become the sole method of execution.[2] The apparent clinical nature of the method seems to appeal to the public—to observers, it looks like putting down a dog, one injection and it's over, quickly and painlessly. The reality is far different. Over the past several years the method has received close scrutiny from the courts and the press. Consequently, as of early 2007, eleven states have temporarily suspended executions while medical, regulatory, and legal issues surrounding the method are thrashed out. During this recent period of challenges, volumes of data and documentation about the actual conduct of lethal injection have highlighted the medical nature of the procedure and the need for the participation of qualified medical personnel. Not previously available, this information has demonstrated significant inadequacies in the staffing and conduct of many executions by lethal injection. In many cases, the personnel so inadequately understand the medical underpinnings of the procedure that they fail to take important steps to ensure that executions reliably comply with the Eighth Amendment prohibition against cruel punishment or with contemporary standards of decency. Interestingly, despite the intense active public scrutiny, lethal injection procedures continue to be botched in foreseeable and visible ways and it has become increasingly clear that inmates can and do suffer consciously during execution.

This paper aims to provide a "nuts and bolts" explanation and depiction of the medical and scientific mechanics of lethal injection. Most of the source information derives from material produced during litigation in which the author served, or is serving, as an expert witness for plaintiffs who are litigating in civil court to remedy perceived deficiencies in the lethal injection procedures employed by various state departments of corrections. Of note, the author has in the past and will in the future receive compensation for many, but not all, of these legal cases. Further, it is important to recognize that some of the data and documentation that has been reviewed by the author and that contributes to the author's opinions has been placed under seal by court orders. Lastly, the author believes in the importance of disclosing that, as a result of his involvement in the legal challenges to lethal injection, he has developed a strong opposition to the imposition of the death penalty as it is presently administered in the United States.

Before delving into the mechanics of the procedure as currently implemented, it is worthwhile to review the process by which lethal injection was conceived, developed, and enacted in the United States. One might think that the official introduction of a new and complex method for causing human death would involve detailed consideration, contemplation, and review in order to ensure that it would properly serve its intended purpose. In particular, it might seem reasonable and appropriate to form a committee or panel of expert medical and correctional personnel to hold hearings and to review any proposed implementation of lethal injection procedures. In the United Kingdom, a Royal Commission on Capital Punishment was formed to investigate whether methods of execution were reliably humane. To the surprise of many, however, no such careful review or study was ever undertaken in the United States; instead, lethal injection was adopted without any guidance from qualified experts. The introduction of lethal injection was conceived by a state representative in Oklahoma, who hoped to devise a more humane death than that delivered by electrocution. Unable to obtain technical guidance from the Oklahoma Board of Medical Licensure, he ultimately contacted the state medical examiner, who dictated to him the following statutory language:

The punishment of death must be inflicted by continuous, intravenous administration of a lethal quantity of an ultrashort-acting barbiturate in combination with a chemical paralytic agent until death is pronounced by a licensed physician according to accepted standards of medical practice.[3]

Although clearly not expert in the administration of drugs, the medical examiner recommended using the anesthetic drug thiopental,[4] in combination with a neuromuscular blocking agent, pancuronium bromide, and a killing agent, potassium chloride. This proposal was cursorily reviewed by a prominent Oklahoma anesthesiologist who confirmed that the loss of consciousness produced by the administration of thiopental is a pleasant experience.[5] Little attention was paid to whether the actual implementation of the procedure would or could be constitutionally compliant. Other states soon followed Oklahoma's example and enacted laws using similar statutory language. The first execution by lethal injection was carried out in Texas in 1977.

Importantly, the precise recipe originally provided by Oklahoma's medical examiner (not detailed by the statutory language) appears to have been used in only one execution in Oklahoma, and the precise procedure that eventually spread across the United States failed to meet the expectations and intents of its designer, in both the manner of its implementation and the qualifications of the personnel performing it. In fact, the medical examiner has recently said that, when he provided the design of the procedure, he assumed that it would be supervised and conducted by qualified personnel: "The question [of the drugs] being administered properly, that never came up in my mind. I never knew we would have complete idiots injecting these drugs. Which we seem to have."[6]

Outline of the Generic Protocol

While there is a small amount of variation between states in the details (doses, timing, instructions) of lethal injection protocols, as of early 2007 all jurisdictions employ the same fundamental framework. Lethal injection, as presently conducted in the United States, is best thought of a four-step process. First, because the lethal injection drugs are to be administered intravenously, the prison must achieve adequate intravenous (IV) access to the condemned prisoner. Next, three drugs are administered in sequence: a general anesthetic (thiopental) to cause unconsciousness; a neuromuscular blocking agent (usually pancuronium bromide) to paralyze the prisoner so that body movements are masked; finally, potassium chloride to cause cardiac arrest and death. Because concentrated potassium chloride is unquestionably extremely painful on administration, and neuromuscular blocking agents will paralyze all voluntary muscles, including those which permit respiration, eventually causing asphyxiation, it is of utmost importance that a condemned prisoner be placed in a state of deep anesthesia before these drugs are administered.

Although there are variations across the country, the execution procedure from the State of California is a reasonably typical lethal injection protocol after IV access has been achieved:

f) When the Signal to Commence is Given By the Warden:

- The Luer Lock tip of Syringe #1 (Sodium Pentothal) shall be locked on to the stopcock, running to the right arm. After the stopcock is manipulated, the injection shall commence. A steady even flow of the injection shall be maintained with only a minimum amount of force applied to the syringe plunger. When the entire contents of the syringe have been injected;
- The stopcock is manipulated allowing the Normal Saline to continue to flow and syringe #1 is removed from the stopcock.
- The Luer Lock tip of Syringe #2 (Sodium Pentothal) shall be locked onto the stopcock, the stopcock manipulated, and the injection shall commence. A steady, even flow of the injection shall be maintained with only a minimum amount of force applied to the syringe plunger. After the entire contents of the syringe have been injected, the CAIR clamp to the 250 ml bag containing the 5 gm of Sodium Pentothal will be opened and an IV drip of a minimum of 75 drips per minute will be set allowing a continuous flow of Sodium Pentothal to the left IV. After the drip is set:

  (a) The syringe of normal saline marked "FLUSH" shall be locked on to the right stopcock, the stopcock manipulated, and the entire contents injected to flush the line. After the stopcock manipulation;
  (b) The "FLUSH" syringe shall be removed and syringe #3 containing the Pancuronium Bromide shall be locked on. After stopcock manipulation, the entire contents shall be injected with slow even pressure on the plunger.
  (c) After stopcock manipulation, syringe #4 containing Potassium Chloride shall be locked on, the stopcock manipulated, and the entire contents injected. After stopcock manipulation, syringe #5 containing Potassium Chloride shall be locked on, the stopcock manipulated, and the entire contents injected. After stopcock manipulation, syringe #6 containing Potassium Chloride, shall be locked on, the stopcock manipulated, and the entire contents injected.

- Upon completion of the injections, or at such earlier time as may be appropriate, the physician shall pronounce death. After the announcement of the completion of the execution, the witnesses will be escorted from the chamber.[7]

Intravenous Access

The first step in the execution process is achieving intravenous access. As the British Royal Commission on Capital Punishment presciently noted in 1949, reliably achieving venous access will be difficult for a variety of reasons: inattentiveness or lack of skill of the execution participants (which I discuss more fully below); the population to be cannulated has a higher than normal incidence of past IV drug use and associated venous damage and may be in poor health; and the circumstances of the execution render the subject fearful, stressed, or cold. As anticipated, the facts show that IV access has been, and continues to be, a tremendous problem in executions. Autopsy records often show multiple attempts at venous access on prisoners (with verified instances of up to 18 failed attempts to place a catheter in a peripheral vein—and when that was unsuccessful, followed by a surgical incision and retractors to reveal the vein to be cannulated).[8]

Some states have considered that peripheral IV access is so difficult to reliably achieve that they have elected to use femoral central line placement of catheters. However, a femoral central line placement is problematic, too, because of the difficulty in placement and the intrusiveness and painfulness of the placement of the catheters.[9] One example is an execution in Missouri where, during femoral IV placement, the femoral artery was nicked, causing bleeding and bruising around the IV site.

Qualifications of the Personnel

Even highly skilled persons may have difficulty in achieving IV access during executions, given the circumstances under which the access is to be performed. But what makes executions in the United States especially problematic are the patently unqualified persons who often participate in the process. For example, in California, there have been notable problems with execution personnel:

[O]ne former execution team leader, who was responsible for the custody of sodium thiopental (which in smaller doses is a pleasurable and addictive controlled substance), was disciplined for smuggling illegal drugs into San Quentin; another prison guard led the execution team despite the fact that he was diagnosed with and disabled by post-traumatic stress disorder as a result of his experiences in the prison system and he found working on the execution team to be the most stressful responsibility a prison employee ever could have.[10]

With respect to difficulties in achieving IV access reliably "team members had attitudes that allowed them to say 'shit happens,' after observing Witness #6 struggle for 15 minutes and fail to set the Williams IV."[11] In Maryland one of the executioners manning the injection apparatus had been convicted of poisoning dogs in his home neighborhood, and another had been disciplined for spitting in prisoners' food. The screening of personnel who volunteer to serve as executioners is often negligible and ineffective, and is typically performed by wardens who themselves lack the experience, training, and background to interview and evaluate medical qualifications and credentials.

The participation of poorly qualified and unconcerned personnel in the execution process heightens the risk of the process and creates an increased need for vigilant monitoring of the condemned prisoner by qualified persons.

The Drugs

If a foolproof protocol for lethal injection were devised and implanted, it might arguably be the case that less qualified personnel could perform the procedure. However, as currently designed, the drugs that have been selected are risky and complex and have a low tolerance to error. Thus, the inherent design of current lethal injection procedures greatly heightens the risk of an inhumane execution.

Thiopental

Thiopental is an ultrashort-acting barbiturate that is intended to be delivered intravenously to induce anesthesia. In typical clinical doses, the drug has both a quick onset and short duration, although its duration of action as an anesthetic is dose dependent.

When anesthesiologists use thiopental, we do so to temporarily anesthetize patients while we intubate the trachea and institute mechanical support of ventilation and respiration. Once this has been achieved, additional drugs are administered to maintain a "surgical depth" or "surgical plane" of anesthesia (i.e., a level of anesthesia deep enough to ensure that a patient feels no pain and is unconscious). The medical utility of thiopental derives from its ultrashort-acting properties: if unanticipated obstacles hinder or prevent successful intubation, patients can quickly regain consciousness and resume ventilation and respiration on their own.

The benefits of thiopental in the operating room engender serious risks in the execution chamber. The duration of unconsciousness provided by thiopental is dose dependent. Generally, the larger the dose is, the longer the unconsciousness. If successfully delivered into the circulation, the large doses of thiopental typically given in executions would produce deep anesthesia in essentially all people. However, many foreseeable situations exist in which human or technical errors could result and indeed have resulted in the failure to successfully administer the intended dose and therefore risk inadequate anesthesia or reawakening of the condemned inmate. Sloppy execution procedures, lack of planning for the various ways in which the procedure can go awry, and the absence of qualified personnel who are willing and able to detect and correct problems all conspire to amplify the risks that are already present in the "triple drug cocktail."

Pancuronium Bromide

The second execution drug to be administered is pancuronium bromide, a neuromuscular blocking agent. Such agents paralyze all voluntary muscles, but do not affect sensation, consciousness, cognition, or the ability to feel pain and suffocation. The effect of the pancuronium bromide is to render the muscles (including the diaphragm which moves to permit respiration) unable to contract. It does not affect the brain or the nerves that carry sensory information and pain signals.

Clinically, the drug is used to ensure a patient is securely paralyzed so that surgical procedures can be performed without reflex muscle contraction. Pancuronium bromide is never administered until a patient is adequately anesthetized. Anesthetic drugs are administered before neuromuscular blocking agents so that the patient does not consciously experience the process of becoming paralyzed and losing the ability to breathe. Thus, in any clinical setting where a neuromuscular blocker is to be used, a patient is anesthetized and monitored to ensure anesthetic depth throughout the duration of neuromuscular blocker use. To assess anesthetic depth, a trained medical professional, either a physician anesthesiologist or a nurse anesthetist, provides vigilant surveillance of the patient and his vital signs, using an array of monitoring devices and diagnostic indicators of anesthetic depth. The appropriate procedures for monitoring a patient undergoing anesthesia and who is about to be administered a drug which masks the ability to convey distress are detailed in the American Society of Anesthesiology's recently published *Practice Advisory for Intraoperative Awareness and Brain Function Monitoring*, 104 Anesthesiology 847, 850–851 (April 2006) (describing preoperative and intraoperative measures for gauging anesthetic depth, including close monitoring of sites of IV access). See also *ASA Standards for Basic Anesthetic Monitoring* (Oct. 25, 2005). No state execution protocol, to the extent disclosed, indicates that no one, let alone a properly trained individual, assesses anesthesia prior to the administration of pancuronium bromide.

It is important to understand that pancuronium bromide does not cause unconsciousness in the way that an anesthetic drug does; rather, if administered alone, a lethal dose of pancuronium bromide would cause someone to lose consciousness only after he or she had endured the excruciating experience of suffocation. It would totally immobilize the person by paralyzing all voluntary muscles and the diaphragm, causing the inmate to suffocate to death while experiencing an intense, conscious desire to inhale. Ultimately, consciousness would be lost, but it would not be lost as an immediate and direct result of the pancuronium bromide. Rather, the loss of consciousness would be due to suffocation, which would be preceded by the torment and agony caused by suffocation. This period of torturous suffocation would be expected to last at least several minutes and would only be relieved by the onset of suffocation-induced unconsciousness.

Neuromuscular blocking agents serve no medical function in an execution by lethal injection. Rather, the drugs are administered solely to prevent witnesses from seeing possible body movements of the condemned. They neither advance the judicial goal of the procedure (to cause death) nor serve to render the procedure more humane. Their purpose is purely cosmetic.

Potassium Chloride

Potassium chloride is a compound that contains essential blood ions and is typically administered medically in trace amounts as a necessary electrolyte. While a certain potassium level is important for normal cardiac electrical activity, a rapid increase in blood concentration of potassium causes cardiac arrest. There is no medical dispute that intravenous injection of concentrated potassium chloride solution, such as that administered peripherally during lethal injections, causes excruciating pain because the vessel walls of veins are richly supplied with sensory nerve fibers that are highly sensitive to potassium ions. Although other chemicals exist which can be used to stop the heart and which do not cause pain on administration, no department of corrections in the United States uses such drugs.

Botched Executions

A living person who is to be intentionally subjected to the excruciating pain of potassium injection or the terror of asphyxiation must be provided with adequate anesthesia. This imperative is of the same order as the imperative to provide adequate anesthesia for any person or any prisoner undergoing painful surgery. But because of the combination of problems, IV insertion, and drug delivery, a number of executions have been botched.

There are examples of poorly conducted executions from all over the country. Sometimes, problems arise in mixing and preparing the drugs. Sometimes, the problems arise in achieving IV access. There are too many examples of poorly performed executions to capture in this paper, but there are some examples which stand out as notable.

Ohio

In the May 2006 Ohio execution of Joseph Lewis Clark, a long time intravenous drug abuser, the Department of Corrections had difficulty establishing peripheral intravenous access. Nevertheless, the officials started the execution. It is reported that Mr. Clark then "raised his head from the gurney and repeatedly told the team, 'It don't work.'"[12] The Department of Corrections officials apparently failed to recognize that Mr. Clark's veins had "collapsed," causing the inmate to reawaken during the execution process and plead "Can't you just give me something by mouth to end this."[13] It is clear that the Ohio Department of Corrections was competent neither to correctly place the IV catheter nor to recognize and manage the resulting problem. Clark's autopsy report shows 19 puncture wounds from attempted intravenous access.

Florida

In the December 2006 Florida execution of Mr. Angel Diaz, witnesses reported that, after the execution began, Mr. Diaz tried to speak, his face was contorted, and he grimaced, one eye closed, while the other remained open, and he appeared to gasp for air for 10 to 12 minutes.[14] A witness described a "fish out of water" appearance, which is a classic description of patients who are gasping and straining to draw breath because of partial or near-complete paralysis by neuromuscular blockers.

Statements taken from the execution team reveal that they failed to follow the Florida protocol for drug delivery and when they encountered difficulty in "pushing the lethal chemicals … made a decision to direct the primary executioner to switch from line "A" [the first IV line] to line "B" [the backup IV line] without an assessment of the primary access site."[15] As a result, after finding it hard to administer thiopental into Mr. Diaz's right arm, the execution team switched to the backup line but did not readminister thiopental; instead, the executioners started by administering the neuromuscular blocking agent, pancuronium bromide.

The autopsy of Mr. Diaz revealed "perforations of the cannulated veins" with the cannulae "extend[ing] into vein lumens through punctures in anterior vein walls [which] continue through posterior vein walls and into underlying soft tissue."[16] Chemical burns and blistering were observed on both of Mr. Diaz's arms.[17] It would seem evident that Mr. Diaz suffered as a result of the Florida Department of Corrections' inability to adequately achieve IV access and thoughtless delivery of drugs after switching IV lines.

Oklahoma

Oklahoma has conducted a number of executions in which inmate convulsions have been reported. For example, Scott Carpenter was executed by the State of Oklahoma on May 8, 1997. At 10 minutes after midnight, as lethal drugs entered his body, witnesses reported that Mr. Carpenter "moaned loudly. He exhaled and then his body convulsed. As the drugs began to take effect, [Mr.] Carpenter made loud rasping sounds and continued to convulse his muscles [and] visibly tensed as he struggled to breathe as the color drained from his face."[18] Four minutes after the execution began, Mr. Carpenter "[t]urned a deep shade of blue."[19] Mr. Carpenter "let out a guttural moan, gasped for breath and convulsed violently, stretching the belt that strapped his body to the table as his body arched upward,"[20] and his body "shuddered with 18 violent convulsions, followed by eight lesser ones."[21] Twelve minutes after the execution began, Mr. Carpenter was pronounced dead.

Robyn Parks was executed by the State of Oklahoma on March 10, 1992. At 42 minutes after midnight, the execution began. Mr. Parks said, "I'm still awake."[22] "Less than two minutes after Warden Dan Reynolds ordered the execution to begin, Parks' body began bucking under straps that held him to a gurney. He spewed out all the air in his lungs, spraying a cloud of spit."[23] Witnesses said "[i]t was overwhelming, stunning, disturbing."[24] Eleven minutes after the execution began, Mr. Parks was pronounced dead.

In at least one execution, witnesses reported seeing the infiltration of fluid from the IVs into the tissue surrounding the catheter:

LaFevers simply didn't go right as an execution. ... I remember looking at his left arm and seeing what I thought was some swelling or maybe even some bruising. It didn't look right. And at the time, I wasn't sure exactly what it was, but I felt like he might not be getting something into that arm or that whatever was going through that tube was not getting into his veins because it looked like it was creating swelling to me.[25]

Other witnesses reported that, as the lethal drugs began to flow, Mr. LaFevers "laid his head back, and he began to go into convulsions, gasping for breath, his chest heaving."[26] He "started raising off the bed" and "[t]he rising of his chest and the burst of air happened together over and over, as if he were gasping."[27] "[H]is eyes stayed open."[28] "[H]e appeared to have a bruise and swelling in his left arm ... where he had an IV tube."[29] After 6 minutes of convulsions, Mr. LaFevers was dead.

The medical examiner's office concluded there had been an infiltration in Mr. LaFevers's left arm. The Court concluded "that in the LaFevers case something did go awry and most regrettably so."[30]

It is the inevitable consequence of a complex process which is carried out by ill-trained and poorly proficient personnel that such botched executions have occurred.

Veterinary Standards

Veterinary doctors describe that it is of the utmost importance to maintain close contact with a subject to be euthanized so that they can monitor vital signs and the sites of IV access. These protections are given to any animal euthanized, even when the euthanization drug is one that cannot cause pain or suffering.

Indeed, veterinary anesthesiologists know, as do medical anesthesiologists, that:

"[d]etermining level of consciousness is as much an art as it is a skill, and requires training and experience. There is no one monitor in animals or people that assesses degree of consciousness. Consciousness can be assessed in animals by observing: (1) muscle relaxation, (2) location of the pupils in the orbit, (3) absence or presence of eye movements, (4) respiratory rate, (5) heart rate, (6) blood pressure, (7) response to mildly painful stimulation, and (8) movement. I put my hands on the patient to help me assess these variables, and I rely upon monitors to help provide data such as blood pressure or heart rate."[31]

Veterinary protections for the subject to be euthanized are even greater when the drugs used to cause death can themselves cause pain, as does potassium chloride. Indeed, the American Veterinary Standards on Euthanasia require that, when death is induced by potassium chloride, it is an absolute prerequisite that it be done only after one qualified to assess anesthetic depth has ascertained the subject is deeply asleep and nonresponsive to noxious stimuli:

It is of utmost importance that personnel performing this technique [euthanasia by potassium chloride injection] are trained and knowledgeable in anesthetic techniques, and *are competent in assessing anesthetic depth* appropriate for administration of potassium chloride intravenously. *Administration of potassium chloride intravenously requires animals to be in a surgical plane of anesthesia characterized by loss of consciousness, loss of reflex muscle response, and loss of response to noxious stimuli.*[32]

Executions, on the other hand, take place with no one, let alone a qualified person, to monitor anesthetic depth. Instead, the condemned inmate is left unattended for the process to play out to its end, regardless of whether the condemned is experiencing a problem.

We kill our prisoners in the United States in a way that we would never be allowed to kill a dog.

Technical Issues

The recent review of lethal injection has encouraged prisons and scientists to consider innovative methods to ascertain whether prisoners have reached and are being maintained at an adequate anesthetic depth. In North Carolina, the state department of corrections acquired a Bispectral Index Monitor ("BIS") to ascertain whether the administration of thiopental has produced a deep anesthetic state before the administration of the remaining drugs. This novel approach has been rejected by the manufacturer of the BIS device who stated: "The BIS monitors have never been tested or submitted for approval or approved by the FDA for the use intended [in executions]."[33] Moreover, the manufacturers have said that, had they known North Carolina intended to use a BIS monitor in an execution, they "would have interceded to prevent the sale."[34]

Lawyers for prisoners and state departments of corrections have tried to use serum thiopental levels acquired after death to prove the antemortem depth of consciousness. But the use of such data is complex. As I reported with coauthors Donald Stanski and Derrick Pounder:

It is widely accepted that concentrations of a drug in post-mortem blood might not reflect the concentrations present at the time of death because of post-mortem drug redistribution—ie, site-dependent and time dependent changes in drug concentration that occur after death. These problems are particularly significant with thiopental, a highly lipophilic drug. Thiopental can take many minutes to reach equilibrium in highly perfused compartments, and longer in less well perfused tissues. When death ensues before equilibrium, as is the case during lethal injection, post-mortem passive diffusion from blood into tissues can cause thiopental concentrations in blood to decline. Results of studies on post-mortem drug diffusion effects suggest that this is a likely explanation for low concentrations of thiopental in blood sampled several hours to days after death."[35]

Indeed, recent executions in Connecticut and Montana confirm that thiopental concentrations in blood samples drawn many hours after death are sharply lower than the thiopental concentrations from blood samples drawn shortly after death. But notwithstanding the difficulties in using postmortem thiopental samples, some data from around the country, taken from blood samples drawn shortly after death, show levels of thiopental that are inconsistent with deep anesthesia. These data heighten our already intense concern that departments of corrections cannot reliably induce and maintain the deep level of anesthesia needed for a humane execution.

The Future for Lethal Injection

With states across the country now reconsidering lethal injection as a method of execution, its future as the execution method of choice is unclear. Each of the steps of execution must be performed flawlessly for a humane execution to result. But the evidence shows myriad problems with carrying out each of the steps: (1) achieving IV access, (2) qualifications of personnel carrying out executions, (3) the drugs selected. As U.S. District Judge Fogel said, "the pervasive lack of professionalism in the implementation [of lethal injection] at the very least is deeply disturbing."[36] It is proving to be inherently problematic when "legislatures delegate death to prison personnel and executioners who are not qualified to devise a lethal injection protocol, much less carry one out."[37] We are seeing today the result of putting in place a poorly thought out and poorly executed process—and witnessing the foreseeable and gratuitous suffering of condemned prisoners.

References

1 *Royal Commission on Capital Punishment (1949–1953) Report*, at 261 (Her Majesty's Stationary Office Reprinted 1965) (rejecting lethal injection as a method of execution).

2 At present all but one of the 38 death penalty states, and the federal and military judicial systems, employ lethal injection as either the sole method of execution or, in the cases of some states that were late to adopt, as one of the methods available to be chosen by the condemned prisoner.

3 OKLA. STAT. tit. 22 §1014 (A).

4 Thiopental is also known as sodium thiopental, Sodium Pentothal, and thiopentone. It will be referred to throughout as thiopental.

5 In fact, the legislative debate over lethal injection centered on whether prisoners ought to be executed by a more painful and mutilating method. For example, on April 20, 1977, Representative Converse moved to amend the proposed lethal injection bill to adopt the "biblical procedure of 'eye for eye' i.e. each person convicted shall be executed in the same manner as the death of the victim for the conviction occurred." Legislative History of Oklahoma House Bill 10, An Act Relating To Criminal Procedure; Amending 22 O.S. 1971, Section 1014; And Specifying The Manner Of Inflicting Punishment Of Death.

6 So Long as They Die, Lethal Injection in the United States, Human Rights Watch Vol. 18, No.1(G), at 31 (April 2006) (quoting A. Jay Chapman).

7 California Lethal Injection Protocol, SQ-OP-0-770-31 (March 6, 2006).

8 From the autopsy report on the death of Ricky Rector who was executed by lethal injection by the State of Arkansas on January 24, 1992.

9 Femoral central line placement is an intrusive and painful surgical procedure which must be performed by highly skilled medical practitioners like anesthesiologists or surgeons. There are instances where prison guards have performed such procedures in executions.

10 *Morales v. Tilton, et al.*, Nos. C-06-219, JF RS C-06-926, JF RS __ F. Supp. 2d __, 2006 WL 3699493, at *6 (N.D. Cal. Dec. 15, 2006).

11 Plaintiff's Post Trial Brief, at 85 (Nov. 28, 2006), *Morales v. Tilton, et al.*, Nos. C-06-219, C-06-926 (N.D. Cal.).

12 Jim Provance, *Problematic execution draws questions: Correction official to appear before panel*, TOLEDO BLADE (May 17, 2006).

13 Jim Provance, *Problematic execution draws questions: Correction official to appear before panel*, TOLEDO BLADE (May 17, 2006).

14 Affidavit of Neal A. Dupree, Capital Collateral Regional Counsel for South Florida.

15 Summary of the Findings of the Department of Corrections' Task Force Regarding the December 13, 2006 Execution of Angel Diaz, at 7, Submitted December 20, 2006 to James R. McDonough, Secretary of the Florida Department of Corrections.

16 Medical Examiner Report NE 06–589, Postmortem Examination of the Body of Angel Diaz, at 1–2 (Feb. 8, 2007).

17 Medical Examiner Report NE 06–589, Postmortem Examination of the Body of Angel Diaz, at 1 (Feb. 8, 2007).

18 Carlton M. Lane, *22-year-old executed for Eufala area murder*, MCALESTER NEWS-CAPITAL, May 8, 1997, at 1.

19 *Id.*

20 Michael Smith, *Execution of Killer a Quiet One*, THE TULSA WORLD, May 9, 1997, at A15.

21 Anthony Thornton, *State Fulfills Killer's Wish For Execution*, THE DAILY OKLAHOMAN, May 8, 1997, at 1.

22 Kandra Wells, *Parks Body Taken To OKC After Execution*, MCALESTER NEWS-CAPITAL, Mar. 10, 1992, at 2.

23 Wayne Green, *11 Minutes That Took A Lifetime*, TULSA WORLD, Mar. 2, 1992, at A13.

24 *Id.*

25 Tr. Preliminary Injunction Hearing, at 21, 24, *Patton v. Jones et al.*, No. 06–591 (W.D. Okla. Aug. 8, 2006).

26 Howard Pankratz, *Leadville Senator Witnesses Execution of Aunt's Killer*, DENVER POST, Jan. 31, 2001, at B01.

27 Decl. Catherine M. Burton (Feb. 19, 2004).

28 Decl. Patrick J. Ehlers (Mar. 1, 2004).

29 Decl. Patrick J. Ehlers (Mar. 1, 2004).

30 Tr. Preliminary Injunction Hearing, at 235, *Patton v. Jones et al.*, No. 06–591 (W.D. Okla. Aug. 8, 2006).

31 Oct. 28, 2005, Affidavit of Kevin Concannon, D.V.M., D.A.C.V.A., Page et al. v. Beck, et al., S:04-CT-04-BO (E.D.N.C.).

32 *2000 Report of the American Veterinary Medical Association Panel on Euthanasia*, 218 (5) J. AM. VET. MED. ASS'N 669, 681 (2001) (emphasis added).

33 April 14, 2006, Affidavit of Scott D. Kelley, M.D., para. 12, *Brown v. Beck et al.*, No. 06-CT-3018-H (E.D.N.C.).

34 April 14, 2006, Affidavit of Scott D. Kelley, M.D., para. 22, *Brown v. Beck et al.*, No. 06-CT-3018-H (E.D.N.C.).

35 Mark J. S. Heath, Donald R. Stanski, & Derrick J. Pounder, Correspondence, *Inadequate anaesthesia in lethal injection for execution*, THE LANCET 2005; 366:1073–1074.

36 *Morales v. Tilton, et al.*, Nos. C-06-219, JF RS C-06-926, JF RS __ F. Supp. 2d __, 2006 WL 3699493, at *7 (N.D. Cal. Dec. 15, 2006).

37 Deborah W. Denno, *When Legislatures Delegate Death: The Troubling Paradox Behind States Uses Of Electrocution And Lethal Injection And What It Says About Us*, 63 OHIO STATE L. J. 63, 66 (2002).

Section 2

Communicable Disease

You can't have a book addressing either criminal justice or public health without a section on communicable disease—so we didn't. In the United States, the prevalence of communicable disease among inmates is higher than in almost any other identifiable domestic population. Why is this? To a large extent, it is caused by drug abuse. Among inmates, infection with HIV and viral hepatitis are largely due to injection drug use, although a substantial proportion of female inmates have sexually transmitted HIV infection. Tuberculosis is an infection of poverty and crowding, so it is no surprise that inmates have high rates of latent TB infection. HIV infection accelerates the development of active tuberculosis; HIV and viral hepatitis mutually accelerate; and all the sexually transmitted diseases increase susceptibility to acquiring HIV infection. Thus, the communicable diseases we encounter behind bars are interrelated.

This section begins with Joseph Bick's chapter on HIV and viral hepatitis in corrections. Dr. Bick is an infectious disease physician working behind bars. In the chapter, he explores the epidemiology, screening, health education, treatment, and considerations for aftercare for inmates infected with HIV or viral hepatitis. Among other things, Dr. Bick discusses the medical and economic value of routine HIV testing in inmates, a program that is getting increasing attention nationwide and is now recommended by the Centers for Disease Control and Prevention. In addition, he discusses the value of counseling, partner notification, and transmission behind bars, all of this from the perspective of primary prevention, early detection, and treatment following nationally accepted guidelines.

Cindy Weinbaum and Karen Hennessey, both at the Centers for Disease Control and Prevention, present the most up-to-date information on the epidemiology and prevention of viral hepatitis. With great detail, Drs. Weinbaum and Hennessey summarize current thinking and recommendations of the Centers for Disease Control and Prevention regarding viral hepatitis. Focusing on primary prevention with vaccinations and early detection in inmates can have a great public health yield. Increasingly, correctional systems are adding risk screening and vaccination against viral hepatitis to the scope of their correctional health services and well they should. These authors emphasize the value of prevention and speak strongly for broader attention to prevention of viral hepatitis in correctional facilities.

In his chapter on HIV prevention, Barry Zack details the rationale and the supporting evidence for HIV prevention programs behind bars. Mr. Zack has extensive experience with HIV prevention in the California prison system and he has helped develop public health policy regarding HIV and AIDS.

Farah Parvez, a public health physician with the Centers for Disease Control and Prevention and the New York City Department of Health, provides us with the current status of tuberculosis among inmates, including a summary of the recommendations of the Centers for Disease Control and Prevention for the management of TB infection behind bars. Some of these recommendations have changed in the past few years, due to decreasing incidence of active TB and new diagnostic technology for latent infection. During the 1990s we had large numbers of cases of TB in correctional facilities, including outbreaks of multidrug-resistant strains. Notwithstanding the reduction in the case rate of TB nationwide, in part due to effective treatment for HIV and in part due to public health department diligence, we have to remain alert because up to 25% of prisoners (in some states) are infected with latent TB. Even with the declining case rate for active TB, there is no indication that the rate of latent TB infection has been reduced. As a consequence, there is a reservoir of tubercle bacilli in our communities and in jails and prisons.

Even more has changed with sexually transmitted infections, especially syphilis, gonorrhea, and chlamydia. Charlotte Kent and Gail Bolan, both public health practitioners, explore the epidemiology, etiology, screening, and treatment of these diseases, diseases that are so prevalent among inmates. They discuss the now widely used urine-based testing for gonorrhea and chlamydia which has made detection and timely treatment available to any correctional facility in the nation. Their mapping data from San Francisco, on communities to which inmates return, is provocative in terms of the targeted interventions that can be taken behind bars for a positive effect in the broader community. Drs. Kent and Bolan use the kind of analysis that makes strong arguments for targeted testing and treatment.

Chapter 8

HIV and Viral Hepatitis in Corrections: A Public Health Opportunity

Joseph A. Bick

Inmates are disproportionately impacted by communicable diseases such as HIV and viral hepatitis (Hammett et al., 2002, BOJ Statistics, 2002). Once incarcerated, the conditions that exist in most of the world's jails and prisons create an ideal environment for the transmission of contagious diseases. Overcrowded communal living environments, delays in medical treatment, insufficient access to clean laundry, soap, and water, and prohibitions against the use of harm reduction measures such as condoms and needle exchange increase the probability that infectious diseases will be transmitted from one inmate to another. The transient status of inmates who are frequently and often abruptly moved from one location to another complicates the diagnosis of infection, recognition of an outbreak, interruption of transmission, performance of a contact investigation, and eradication of disease.

While incarcerated, inmates interact with over 500,000 correctional employees and millions of annual visitors (Hammett et al., 2002). Most inmates are eventually released and return to their communities (Zack et al., 2000). Once released, former inmates often do not access health care, and frequently fail to continue treatments that have been initiated during their incarceration (Wohl et al., 2004, Springer et al., 2004). Many jails and prisons have insufficient information technology, and linkages between the different jurisdictions and agencies responsible for the care of inmates are often poor. Many correctional systems inadequately communicate with their public health counterparts in the free world, squandering opportunities for continuity of care.

Definitions

Jails: detention centers operated by city and country governments. Jails serve as detention centers for persons who are either awaiting trial or who have been sentenced to less than 1 year of incarceration.

Prisons: detention centers operated by state and federal governments. Prisons serve as detention centers for persons who have been sentenced to more than 1 year of incarceration.

Inmates: residents of jails and prisons

Prisoners: residents of prisons

Further complicating the appropriate management of contagious illnesses among the incarcerated is the high prevalence of comorbidities such as mental illness and substance abuse. Many inmates are distrustful of authority and reluctant to cooperate with health care providers. Fearful of adverse publicity, some jails and prisons have been slow to ask for assistance from outside agencies when faced with infectious disease outbreaks. Furthermore, published guidelines for diagnosis and treatment of communicable diseases are not always readily applicable to the correctional setting. All of these factors contribute to lost opportunities for diagnosis, treatment, prevention, immunization, and harm reduction education. Consequences include the development of preventable complications of untreated illness and missed opportunities for interrupting transmission of infection to the larger community.

In this chapter, I will explore the disproportionate impact of infectious diseases in jails and prisons on the health of the society at large, discuss some of the unique challenges and opportunities that exist in correctional public health, review the importance of enhanced interjurisdictional cooperation, and advocate for the creation of a more seamless system of health care for individuals as they move throughout the criminal justice system and return to the free world. Furthermore, I will address the importance of linking correctional health care with public health and community health providers, and argue for the importance of correctional settings as frontlines in our national strategies to reduce the prevalence of preventable diseases. These issues will be explored by discussing two illustrative diseases that significantly impact on the incarcerated: HIV and viral hepatitis.

Human Immunodeficiency Virus (HIV)

HIV/AIDS is the fifth leading cause of death among persons aged 25 to 44 in the United States (CDCP, 2003). Over the past decade, the widespread use of highly active antiretroviral therapy (HAART) has led to a marked decline in morbidity and mortality among HIV-infected patients (DHHS, 2006; BOJ Statistics, 2002). To prevent perinatal HIV transmission, a protocol of routine testing of pregnant women, antiretroviral therapy for those found to be infected, elective cesarean section in those with detectable HIV viral loads, antiretroviral therapy for newborns, and avoidance of breast-feeding among HIV-infected women has been adopted in this country. These measures have led to a marked decline in the number of HIV-infected newborns in the United States (CDCP, 2006a; Cooper et al., 2002). Furthermore, effective prophylactic medications are available to prevent the development of opportunistic infections (OIs) such as *Pneumocystis carinii* pneumonia, toxoplasmosis, and disseminated *Mycobacterium avium-intracellulare* complex (USPHS/IDSA, 2002; McNaghten et al., 1999; Bick et al., 1997). The use of these prophylactic treatments has contributed to a marked decrease in OIs and prolonged survival.

The prevalence of AIDS among prison populations is estimated to be at least 5 times higher than that in the general U.S. population, and HIV/AIDS remains one of the most common causes of death among prisoners in the United States (BOJ Statistics, 2002). Although up to 25% of people living with HIV in this country have spent time in a jail or prison, less than half of prison systems and few jails routinely provide HIV testing on entry (Spaulding et al., 2002; Hammett et al., 1999).

Effective treatment of HIV in prisons has brought about a 75% reduction in AIDS-related mortality, a decline mirroring that of nonincarcerated populations (Baham et al., 2002; Bick et al., 1997). HIV testing programs in prison can play an important role in prevention. Identification of HIV-infected persons can prompt partner counseling and referral services, promoting others to be HIV tested and potentially hindering the spread of the virus. Additionally, studies have shown that nonincarcerated individuals reduce their frequency of risk behaviors following HIV diagnosis (CDCP, 2000b; Weinhardt et al., 1999; Wolitski et al., 1997). Inmates who are aware of their HIV-infected status may similarly reduce HIV transmission behaviors both in prison and on returning to their communities. HAART minimizes infectiousness by reducing viral load in genital secretions, reducing the risk of transmission (Chakraborty et al., 2001; Quinn et al., 2000).

There has been incomplete success in this country in identifying all of those who are HIV-infected. Furthermore, many persons do not test until late in the course of their infection, often because of the development of an opportunistic infection or malignancy (Neal and Fleming, 2002; CDCP, 2003b). At the time of diagnosis, up to 40% of those who are HIV-infected have CD4 cell counts of < 200 cells/mm^3 and are therefore candidates for HAART. Because of this late diagnosis, up to 40% of individuals die within a year of learning of their HIV infection (Klein et al., 2003). In an attempt to improve upon the early diagnosis of HIV, the U.S. Preventive Services Task Force (USPSTF) recommended routine HIV counseling and screening for all persons at increased risk for HIV infection (USPSTF, 2005). According to the USPSTF, a person is considered to be at increased risk for HIV infection if he or she reports one or more of the following risk factors:

- men who have had sex with men after 1975
- persons who have had unprotected sex with multiple partners
- past or present injection drug users
- persons who have exchanged sex for money or drugs or who have had a sex partner who has exchanged sex for money or drugs
- persons who have a past or present sex partner who is HIV-infected, bisexual, or an injection drug user
- persons who have had a sexually transmitted disease (STD)
- those who received a blood transfusion between 1978 and 1985

However, HIV testing driven solely by risk factor assessment misses many of those who are HIV-infected. Approximately 25% of HIV-infected persons in the United States report no HIV risk factors (Klein et al., 2003; Alpert et al., 1996; Liddicoat et al., 2004; Jenkins et al., 2006; Chen et al., 1998). Some individuals are reluctant to disclose risk factors, while others may not know that they are at risk (CDCP, 1999a, 2004a, 2005).Therefore, the USPSTF also recommends routine HIV screening of persons seen in high-risk or high-prevalence clinical settings even in the absence of individual risk factors (USPSTF, 2005). The Centers for Disease Control and Prevention (CDCP) defines high-prevalence settings as those known to have a 1% or greater prevalence of HIV infection. High-prevalence settings include sexually transmitted disease (STD) clinics, correctional facilities, homeless shelters, tuberculosis clinics, clinics serving men who have sex with men, and adolescent health clinics with a high prevalence of STDs.

Unfortunately, even HIV testing driven by determination of individual risk factors and high-prevalence settings still fails to reach a sizable number of HIV-infected Americans. Those who are not aware of being HIV-infected cannot benefit from proven HIV treatments. Furthermore, HIV-infected persons who do not know their status may unknowingly transmit HIV to others (Marks et al., 2005). The ongoing HIV epidemic in this country will not be interrupted unless greater successes are achieved in identifying all of those who are infected with HIV. Patients, including the incarcerated, are more likely to accept HIV testing when it is offered routinely to everyone (Baham et al., 2004; Fincher-Mergi et al., 2002; CDCP, 2005). In recognition of this reality, the CDCP has recently taken the important step of recommending that voluntary, opt-out testing for HIV be integrated into the routine health care of all Americans (CDCP, 2006b). Key points of the new recommendations include:

- Routine voluntary HIV screening should be performed for all patients aged 13–64.
- Those who are at high risk for HIV should be retested at least annually. High-risk persons include:
  - injection-drug users and their sex partners
  - persons who exchange sex for money or drugs
  - sex partners of HIV-infected persons
  - MSM
  - persons who themselves or whose sex partners have had more than one sex partner since their most recent HIV test
- Patients should be informed orally or in writing that HIV testing will be performed unless they decline (opt-out screening).
- Patients should be provided an explanation of HIV infection and the meanings of positive and negative test results, and offered an opportunity to ask questions and to decline testing.
- Consent for HIV screening should be incorporated into the patient's general informed consent for medical care. A separate consent form for HIV testing is not recommended.
- Easily understood informational materials should be made available in the language of the patient.

Routine HIV screening has been found to be as cost-effective as other established screening programs for chronic diseases (hypertension, colon cancer, and breast cancer) in settings where the prevalence of HIV is as low as 0.1% (Sanders et al., 2005; Paltiel et al., 2005, 2006). Triple drug combination therapy for HIV has been associated with a near doubling of life expectancy for patients with advanced AIDS, with a cost of $23,000 per quality-adjusted year of life saved. This cost compares favorably with treatment of high blood pressure, and is more cost-effective than treating high cholesterol or breast cancer (Freedberg et al., 2001). Numerous studies have demonstrated that the cost of antiretroviral therapy is more than offset by savings associated with decreased opportunistic infections, cancers, and hospitalizations (Ruane et al., 1997; Torres and Barr, 1997). A recent study in a noncorrectional setting found that annual health care expenditures for HIV-infected patients with advanced disease (CD4 counts <50 cells/mm^3) were 2.63 times greater than those for patients with CD4 counts >350/mm^3 ($36,533 versus $13,885 per patient)

(Chen et al., 2006). Notably, improvement in clinical status associated with increases in CD4+ cell count led to a reduction in health care expenditures. Patients who experienced increases in CD4+ cell counts had lower annual health care expenditures, while those who experienced declines in CD4+ cell counts had higher expenditures. The higher costs in those with advanced disease were due to an increased use of non-antiretroviral medications and hospitalizations. In the correctional setting, expenditures attributable to hospitalization are often significantly higher than among nonincarcerated persons because of the cost of guarding the inmate-patient while out in the community. Therefore, it is likely that the savings associated with earlier treatment would be even more significant in the correctional setting than in the free world.

Mandatory HIV testing programs can increase the yield of new diagnoses, and are in place in 19 state correctional systems. However, this approach has been denounced by the American Public Health Association, the World Health Organization, and the American Civil Liberties Union (World Health Organization, 2006; Lange, 2003). Critics cite the difficulties inherent in preserving confidentiality in prison and the discrimination and stigmatization that HIV-infected prisoners have historically endured, particularly as a result of segregation. In the correctional setting, HIV-infected inmates may face disparate treatment based on their HIV status. Examples include restrictions on job assignments, limitations on potential housing sites, decreased educational opportunities, prohibitions against conjugal visiting, enhanced punishments for in-custody infractions (those who are known to be HIV-infected may be subject to harsher punishments if they are found guilty of being involved in the willful exchange of body fluids), and prolonged sentences (in some states, inmates who work earn time off their sentence for each day worked; if less job opportunities exist for those who are HIV-infected, HIV-infected inmates may in fact end up serving longer sentences).

Some laws may serve to discourage voluntary testing or disclosure of HIV status. Examples in California include:

- Health and Safety Code (HSC) 121015: permits a treating physician to disclose a person's HIV status to that person's spouse and any person reasonably believed to be the sexual or needle sharing partner of the individual.
- HSC 120291: states that if an individual is known to be HIV-infected and engages in unprotected sex, he/she can be charged with a felony.
- HSC 121070: requires medical personnel to disclose the HIV status of all inmates to the "officer in charge" of the detention facility. This officer in charge is then required to notify all employees and volunteers who may have direct contact with the inmate of the inmate's HIV status.
- Penal code (PC) 12022.85: increases by 3 years the sentence of those convicted of rape, unlawful sodomy, or oral copulation if the defendant knew that they were HIV infected.
- PC 647: elevates any subsequent prostitution conviction among those known to be HIV-infected from a misdemeanor to a felony.
- PC 7520: directs correctional officials that they must notify parole and probation officers when an HIV-infected inmate is released.
- PC 7521: allows parole and probation officers to inform the spouse of paroling inmates of their HIV status.

Legislators should carefully consider the potential disincentives to HIV testing and/or disclosure prior to enacting new laws dealing with HIV and other contagious illnesses.

There are two types of routine voluntary testing, "opt-in" and "opt-out." In a voluntary routine opt-in model for HIV testing, HIV testing is routinely offered to all patients but each person must then choose to accept testing. In a voluntary routine opt-out model, HIV testing is offered to all and is then performed unless the individual requests that it not be done. Routine opt-out testing may help to normalize the testing process and decrease test-associated stigma, increasing acceptance of offered testing and potentially increasing new diagnoses. Some inmate advocates suggest that opt-out testing conducted in jail or prison is coercive by nature and akin to mandatory testing. A recent study within the California Department of Corrections and Rehabilitation (CDCR) demonstrated that offering routine one-to-one HIV counseling of all incoming inmates doubled the acceptance of voluntary HIV testing (Baham et al., 2004). This study also concluded that a significant percentage of high-risk individuals had never previously tested for HIV, and that offering multiple testing modalities (blood, urine, and oral fluid) can increase the number of individuals who choose to test.

Clearly, testing is just one important step in addressing the ongoing HIV epidemic. Those who are found to be HIV-infected must be provided access to physicians who have training and experience in the treatment of HIV-infected patients. One definition for HIV specialist put forward by the HIV Medicine Association is a clinician who has had primary responsibility for the care of at least 25 HIV patients during the course of a year. This definition is based on published data demonstrating improved outcomes for patients cared for by clinicians who have at least this number of HIV-infected patients (Kitahata et al., 1996; Volberding et al., 1996). Unfortunately, many HIV-infected inmates do not have ready access to HIV specialists. In a recent survey of correctional health care providers, only 43% reported that an HIV specialist was "often" available to see patients and 38% stated that a specialist was never available (Bernard et al., 2006). Use of inadequately experienced providers increases the risk for the development of resistant HIV, opportunistic infections, and malignancies, and shortens the survival of HIV-infected patients. In addition to access to HIV specialists, the availability of all FDA-approved antiretroviral and preventive medications must be ensured. All HIV-infected persons must be provided access to routine labwork for monitoring treatment, to include determinations of HIV viral load and CD4 counts. Resistance assays are an essential component of HIV treatment and must be readily available (DHHS, 2006).

Confidential partner notification, counseling, and testing can be very useful in interrupting ongoing transmission of HIV (CDCP, 2006c). HIV-infected inmates should be encouraged to disclose their HIV status to their current and past sex and injection drug use partners. Both HIV-positive and -negative individuals should be provided access to education, prevention, and harm reduction programs. The CDCP recommends that HIV prevention efforts in prisons address common HIV risk behaviors such as male–male sex, injection drug use, and nonsterile tattooing (Wohl, 2006). Prevention programs currently operating in U.S. correctional facilities include prevention case management (Bauserman & Richardson, 2003), peer education (Grinstead et al., 1999), and various forms of health education and risk reduction programs (Bryan et al., 2006). HIV prevention programs must acknowledge that risky behavior occurs in correctional settings, and encourage inmates to engage in safer sex and avoid sharing needles both while they are incarcerated *and* after release from prison. Peer-led HIV risk reduction educational programs are well-suited to the correctional environment. Culturally tailored HIV risk reduction activities can be more effective at sensitizing target populations to HIV/AIDS concerns and increasing the likelihood that targeted individuals are tested for HIV and discuss HIV/AIDS with friends (Rucker-Whitaker et al., 2006).

Sexual activity that places inmates at high risk for HIV transmission while incarcerated has been well documented. In a recent report of HIV transmission in Georgia prisons, 54 of 68 inmates who seroconverted during incarceration (79%) reported engaging in male-to-male sex while incarcerated. Most (72%) reported having had consensual sex, while only 30% of these reported using condoms or improvising barrier protection (CDCP, 2006f). Condoms are highly effective at preventing the transmission of HIV and other STDs (NIAID, 2001). The CDCP has recommended that condoms be made available in correctional settings, but resistance to implementation of this simple, cost-effective measure is widespread (Correctional Service Canada, 1999; CDCP, 2003a; Dolan et al., 2004). In the United States, only two state prison systems (Vermont and Mississippi) and five local jail systems (Philadelphia, Los Angeles, New York, San Francisco, and Washington, DC) make condoms available to inmates (Wohl, 2006). Consensual sex between inmates is illegal in most correctional systems in the United States. Concerns that condoms would be used to throw body fluids at employees and that distribution of condoms would be equivalent to encouraging illegal sexual activity have served to limit condom distribution.

Intravenous drug use is a major risk factor for HIV infection. In 1997, 83% of state prisoners admitted to a history of drug use, while 57% admitted to using illicit drugs in the month before their commitment offense (Mumola, 1999). In the same survey, 49% of prisoners reported a history of cocaine or crack use, while 25% admitted to having used heroin or opiates (BJS, 1999). Many inmates continue to abuse drugs during their incarceration. In spite of the tremendous burden of substance abuse among the incarcerated, only 39% of state and 45% of federal inmates who used drugs in the month before the offense reported taking part in drug treatment or other drug programs since admission (BOJ, 2004). No correctional systems in the United States make available needle exchange. Because of the link between HIV infection and drug use, access to drug treatment programs is an essential component of correctional HIV care and planning for release into the community.

Inadequate discharge planning for persons released from jail or prison may lead to resumed HIV risk exposures, HIV transmission, and recidivism (McLean et al., 2006). A study comparing incarcerated and reincarcerated HIV-infected patients on HAART found that the majority of reincarcerated patients did not adhere to their medication on release from prison. Release from prison was found to be associated with a deleterious effect on virologic and immunological outcomes (Stephenson et al., 2005). Planning for the transition of inmates to the community is an essential component of the community reintegration of incarcerated persons, and is associated with lower rates of recidivism during the first year postdischarge (Trupin et al., 2004). Discharge planning programs may prevent treatment interruptions, assist inmates to enter substance abuse treatment programs, identify housing and medical care in the community, enter job training and/or educational programs, and decrease the likelihood of reincarceration (Myers, et al., 2005).

Conclusions

Correctional facilities provide a unique opportunity for HIV diagnosis, treatment, prevention, and harm reduction education. Successful interventions in jails and prisons will not only benefit the health of the incarcerated but also have the potential for advancing this nation's efforts to interrupt the further spread of the HIV epidemic. Early diagnosis of HIV-infected persons followed by initiation of HAART and prophylactic medications keeps patients healthier, decreases HIV-associated deaths, decreases the number of new infections, and saves money that would be spent treating the complications of advanced HIV disease. Specific recommendations include:

1. Implement routine opt-out HIV testing at correctional reception centers during intake medical evaluation to identify new infections among inmates whose HIV status is unknown or has been negative on previous tests.
2. Address any legal and regulatory barriers that may exist to the implementation of routine opt-out HIV testing
3. Perform routine confirmatory HIV testing during intake medical evaluation for inmates who report that they are infected.
4. Provide confidential notification to all tested inmates of their HIV test results.
5. Refer all HIV-infected persons to appropriate antiretroviral care, treatment, and prevention services in the correctional facility, the community, or both.
6. Refer persons at high risk of acquiring HIV to prevention services. Referrals include linkages to available programs and services in both the correctional facility and the community.
7. Conduct partner counseling and referral services.
8. Provide alcohol and substance abuse treatment to all of those who might benefit from it.
9. Make available proven harm reduction measures including education and condom distribution.
10. Develop partnerships among health departments, correctional facilities, and community-based organizations (CBOs) so that individuals can be linked to care, treatment, and prevention services in correctional facilities and in the community.
11. Work with participating CBOs to establish procedures and responsibilities for referral services for inmates as part of release planning.

Viral Hepatitis

National hepatitis immunization efforts targeting infants, children, and adolescents have achieved significant success over the past two decades. As a result, most new cases of viral hepatitis in recent years have occurred among adults. Up to 40% of all Americans with chronic viral hepatitis have been incarcerated, and the prevalence of viral hepatitis among inmates is significantly higher than in nonincarcerated settings (Hammett et al., 2002). Inmates continue to engage in behaviors that place them at risk for viral hepatitis both while incarcerated and after being released to the community. As a result, nonimmune inmates comprise a group who would potentially benefit greatly from hepatitis prevention initiatives. It has become increasingly clear that any effective comprehensive national strategy for the prevention, early diagnosis, and treatment of viral hepatitis must include jails and prisons (Glaser & Greifinger, 1993; Association of State and Territorial Health Officials, 2002).

Immunization of those who are nonimmune, diagnosis and treatment of those who are chronically infected, substance abuse treatment, and harm reduction education in the correctional setting can benefit the free community by decreasing costs associated with chronic viral hepatitis, reducing transmission, and decreasing recidivism (Conklin et al., 1998; Mast et al., 1998; Goldstein et al., 2002). However, significant challenges exist to the implementation of a comprehensive viral hepatitis infection control and prevention program in jail and prison settings. Short stays, transient populations, insufficient interjurisdictional cooperation and communication, inadequate information technology, a shortage of medical expertise, patient distrust, and poor reimbursement all conspire to derail viral hepatitis initiatives in the correctional setting. What follows is a discussion of the burden of viral hepatitis in jails and prisons, and some of the challenges and opportunities that exist for the diagnosis, prevention, and treatment of viral hepatitis among the incarcerated.

Transmission of Viral Hepatitis by Drug Use

Intravenous drug use is a major risk factor for viral hepatitis, especially hepatitis B and C. In 1997, 83% of state prisoners admitted to a history of drug use, while 56% admitted to using illicit drugs in the month immediately preceding their commitment offense (Mumola, 1999). Most correctional systems do not provide comprehensive harm reduction programs. Notably, only 39% of state and 45% of federal inmates who used drugs in the month before their commitment offense reported taking part in drug treatment or other drug programs since incarceration (BJS, 2004). No U.S. correctional facility participates in needle exchange, and proven drug treatment strategies such as methadone maintenance and buprenorphine are not available to the majority of inmates who might benefit from them.

Table 8.1 Drug use by inmates: 1997.

Type of drug	Ever used	Used in the month before commitment offense
Any drug	83%	56%
Marijuana	77	39
Cocaine/crack	49	25
Heroin/opiates	24	9
Depressants	24	5
Stimulants	28	9
Hallucinogens	29	4

BJS, National Substance Abuse and Treatment of State and Federal Prisoners, 1997, NCJ 172871, January 1999.

Sexual Transmission of Viral Hepatitis

Transmission of viral hepatitis can occur through sexual activity. Although consensual and nonconsensual sex are illegal in all correctional systems, up to 30% of inmates admit to having been sexually active while incarcerated (Gaiter & Doll, 1996; Nacci & Kane, 1983; Tewksbury, 1989; Saum et al., 1995). Sexual transmission of HBV has been well documented in correctional facilities (CDCP, 2001; Hull et al., 1985; Decker et al., 1985). Condoms are effective in preventing the transmission of hepatitis (NIAID, 2001). Although the CDCP has recommended that condoms be made available in correctional settings, only two state prison systems (Vermont and Mississippi) and five local jail systems (Philadelphia, Los Angeles, New York, San Francisco, and Washington, DC) make condoms available to inmates (CDCP, 2003a; Wohl, 2006).

Other Risks for Transmission of Hepatitis in the Correctional Setting

Percutaneous exposures to blood due to tattoos, fights, and bites are common in correctional facilities. Studies to date have not demonstrated a significant risk for transmission of viral hepatitis that can be attributed to these mechanisms of exposure (Khan et al., 2002; Gershon et al., 1999; Hessl, 2001).

Hepatitis A Virus (HAV) Infection

Although HAV outbreaks have not been reported from U.S. jails or prisons, many inmates have risk factors for HAV such as injection drug use and/or MSM. The prevalence of chronic liver disease due to HBV, HCV, and/or alcohol ingestion is increased in incarcerated populations. Those who have chronic liver disease are predisposed to develop more severe illness if they subsequently acquire HAV or HBV. Therefore, inmates have the potential to benefit significantly from expanded viral hepatitis immunization programs. HAV vaccination is administered in a two-dose series over 6 months, and is safe and efficacious. In an attempt to decrease the transmission of HAV among the incarcerated and the communities to which they will be released, the CDCP has provided recommendations concerning HAV in correctional facilities (CDCP, 1999c). Key among these are the following:

- All those at risk for HAV should know their HAV status. At-risk individuals include injection drug users, MSM, and persons living in high-prevalence areas of the country.
- Nonimmune individuals who are at risk for HAV and those who have chronic liver disease should be vaccinated for HAV.
- Tracking systems to ensure completion of the vaccine series within the correctional system should be established, and systems should be developed to facilitate completion of the second vaccine dose for those inmates who return to the community.

Hepatitis B Virus Infection

Over 40% of adult inmates have serologic evidence for current or past HBV infection. In most jails and prisons, the prevalence of HBV is markedly higher than that seen in the general U.S. population (CDCP, 1991; McQuillan et al., 1999; Coleman et al., 1998). Approximately 30% of persons with acute hepatitis

B report a history of incarceration (Khan et al., 2000). Studies among inmates in a variety of correctional settings have demonstrated prevalences of chronic active HBV infection as high as 3.7%, compared to a prevalence estimate for nonincarcerated Americans of 0.5% (Koplan et al., 1978; Kibby et al., 1982; Bader, 1983; Kaufman et al., 1983; Decker et al., 1984; Hull et al., 1985; Tucker et al., 1987; Barry et al., 1990; Smith et al., 1991; CDCP, 1991; McQuillan et al., 1999; Ruiz et al., 1999; López-Zetina et al., 2001).

The most common source of HBV infection in the United States is through sexual contact. The prevalence of chronic HBV is increased among MSM, injection drug users, and those who have other STDs (Kunches et al., 1986; Zeldis et al., 1992; Levine et al., 1995; Garfein et al., 1996; Remis et al., 2000). Nonimmune inmates are at high risk for acquiring hepatitis though injection drug use or sexual activity during their incarceration or after release (Macalino et al., 1999).

The national strategy for the elimination of HBV transmission has focused primarily on prevention of perinatal HBV infection through maternal screening and postexposure prophylaxis of newborns of HBsAg-positive mothers, HBV vaccination of all infants to prevent infection in childhood and at later ages, vaccination of all adolescents not previously vaccinated to prevent infection in this age group and at later ages, and vaccination of adults and adolescents in groups at increased risk for infection (CDCP, 1991). HBV vaccination prevents not only acute viral hepatitis, but also the complications of chronic HBV such as cirrhosis, liver cancer, and death. This national strategy has been highly effective, leading to a marked decline in the incidence of acute HBV in the United States between 1990 and 2005. The greatest decline has been seen among children and adolescents. Many adults remain at risk for HBV infection, especially unvac-cinated adults who have risk behaviors for HBV transmission (injection drug users, MSM, and heterosexuals who have multiple sexual partners). Adults now account for the overwhelming majority of new HBV infections in this country. For the past 25 years, the Advisory Committee on Immunization Practices (ACIP) has recommended that at-risk inmates be vaccinated for HBV (CDCP, 1991). However, routine vaccination of at-risk adults has not been widely adopted. In some settings, routine HBV vaccination of adults has been highly successful. For example, requiring employers to provide routine HBV vaccination to health-care workers has contributed to a dramatic decrease in the incidence of new infections among this group (U.S. Department of Labor, 1991; CDCP, 1989; Mahoney et al., 1997). In recognition of this reality, the ACIP has issued a major revision to prior recommendations and has called for a comprehensive strategy that includes providing HBV immunization to all nonimmune at-risk adults (CDCP, 2006e). Key components of these new guidelines include:

- Universal HBV vaccination should be provided to at-risk adults (IDUs, MSM, inmates, and persons seen in STD clinics).
- All inmates who are not known to be immune regardless of their length of stay should be vaccinated for HBV.
- An immunization history should be documented in the inmate's medical record, and the information should be provided to the inmate at the time of their release.
- Standing orders should be implemented to facilitate the routine identification and immunization of at-risk adults.

In high-risk populations, a significant percentage of individuals will have already been infected with HBV. Although immunization of those who have already been infected is not harmful, it provides no additional benefit and leads to unnecessary expenditures. Strategies to reduce unnecessary immunizations include reviewing patient medical records and serologic testing for immunity to HBV infection. The cost of prevaccination testing must be weighed against the potential savings that result from decreased use of immunization. One study in a correctional setting determined that prevaccination serologic testing may be cost-effective when the prevalence of immunity from prior infection and vaccination exceeds 25% (CDCP, 2004b). If prevaccination testing is performed, one of the following approaches should be adopted:

1. Measurement of antibody to hepatitis B core antigen (HBcAb) to identify those who have been infected but not those who have been vaccinated, or
2. Measurement of both antibody to hepatitis B surface antigen (HBsAb) and hepatitis B surface antigen (HBsAg). HBsAg will identify those who have either acute or chronic HBV infection, while HBsAb will be present in the setting of immunity due to either infection or vaccination.

HBV immunization is highly effective, and in most situations postvaccination serologic testing is not indicated (Szmuness et al., 1980; Hadler et al., 1991). HIV-infected persons and those who are receiving chronic hemodialysis are less likely to develop protective antibody titers following HBV vaccination. For these individuals, higher vaccine doses are recommended. In high-risk persons, postvaccination serology to document an adequate antibody response should be obtained and non- or partial responders should be revaccinated according to the manufacturer's directions (Fraser et al., 1994; Collier et al., 1988; Bruguera et al., 1992; Rey et al., 2000). High-risk persons include those who are likely to have repeated ongoing exposures to HBV (health care workers and sexual or injection drug using partners of those who are HBs Ag-positive).

A complete HBV vaccination series requires three doses administered over 4 to 6 months. Many jail inmates are released within days, while both jail and prison inmates are commonly moved from facility to facility, often with little if any advanced notice to clinical staff. Ideally, each at-risk individual will be administered the full immunization series. Even if a complete series cannot be administered, protective levels of antibody will develop after one dose of HBV vaccine in up to 50% of persons and in up to 75% of persons after two doses (Davidson et al., 1986, Jilg & Deinhardt, 1986). Therefore, length of stay in itself should not discourage correctional facilities from implementing HBV vaccination programs.

Immunizations for children and adolescents are reimbursed by the federal Vaccines for Children (VCP) Program, but there is no comparable "Vaccines for Adults" program (CDCP VCP). Although the societal benefits attributable to in-custody vaccination programs could be substantial, all too often the costs of such initiatives must be solely borne by the individual correctional systems (Pisu et al., 2002). Public policy makers should address these issues when planning national viral hepatitis elimination initiatives. Without logistical and financial support, opportunities for impacting on the public health will be squandered.

Management of Chronic Hepatitis B

Approximately 5% of those who become infected with HBV will develop chronic hepatitis. These individuals are at risk for developing cirrhosis, end stage liver disease, and hepatocellular carcinoma. In addition, persons with chronic active HBV serve as a source for ongoing transmission to nonimmune individuals. All of those who are found to be chronically infected with HBV should receive education about the illness. Important topics include:

- How to prevent transmission of the virus to others, including vaccination of nonimmune sexual and injection drug use partners, use of condoms, and avoidance of blood or tissue donation.
- Limiting exposure to medications that are potentially hepatotoxic.
- Minimizing or eliminating the ingestion of alcohol.

Chronically infected persons should be referred to a physician who is knowledgeable in the treatment of HBV. Several medications are useful in the treatment of HBV, and in some cases chronic active disease can be rendered inactive and noncontagious. Medical management and antiviral therapy can reduce the risk for cirrhosis and liver cancer. HAV vaccination of nonimmune persons is important to avoid further liver insult.

Hepatitis C Virus Infection

An estimated 1.8% of the U.S. adult population, or approximately 3.9 million persons, are infected with HCV (NHANES III, 1994). Most of those who have acquired HCV experienced no acute symptoms, and many of those who are infected are unaware of it (CDCP, 1998; Aach et al., 1991; Alter et al., 1991). Up to three-fourths of those who become infected with HCV will develop chronic disease. Untreated, up to one-third of those who have chronic HCV will progress to cirrhosis, end-stage liver disease, and premature death. Persons with chronic HCV are also at risk for hepatocellular carcinoma and a variety of extrahepatic manifestations (Strader & Seeff, 1996; Seeff & Hoofuagle, 2002; Fattovich et al., 1997).

The main mechanism of transmission of HCV is direct percutaneous exposure to infectious blood. Those who are most likely to be infected with HCV include IDUs and those who received transfusions of blood or blood products prior to the implementation of routine processing to inactivate HCV (NHANES III, 1994). In the past, most IDUs became infected with HCV within 2 years of starting to share needles and other injection materials. Over the past two decades, the incidence of acute HCV has declined among IDUs. However, IDUs continue to comprise the group with the highest incidence and prevalence of HCV in this country (Garfein et al., 2000; Murrill et al., 2002; Hagan et al., 1999; Lorvick et al., 2001; Thorpe et al., 2000; Diaz et al., 2001; Williams et al., 2000; Alter, 2002). There is no vaccination for the prevention of HCV. Screening of blood products, deferral of donation from those who are infected, the routine use of HCV inactivation procedures in donated blood products, and improved infection control practices have led to a significant decline in the incidence of HCV in this country. Further reductions in the number of new cases will depend on harm reduction education of those who are at risk for infection.

Studies among the incarcerated have found HCV seroprevalences of up to 40% (Ruiz et al., 1999; Alter et al., 1999; Vlahov et al., 1993; Spaulding et al., 1999). Many inmates who are not infected remain at high risk due to ongoing injection drug use behavior both during incarceration and after release. Most inmates do not have access to proven harm reduction measures such as needle exchange, and many inmates who might benefit from substance abuse treatment do not have access to it. As a result, opportunities to treat addiction are lost, and many inmates continue harmful behaviors.

The first step in the management of HCV is identifying those who are infected. Inmates with unknown HCV serostatus should be screened for HCV risk factors, and those who have risk factors should be offered testing for HCV antibodies. Because of the high prevalence of HCV infection among inmates, a compelling argument can be made for routine testing of all inmates. Alternatively, periodic serostudies could be performed to determine the prevalence of HCV infection in each facility. Routine testing could be reserved for facilities in which self-reported risk factors fail to identify the majority of those who are infected. Local universities and/or public health departments should lend their expertise to correctional facilities in the designing and implementation of epidemiologic studies.

All inmates should be educated regarding HCV. Facilities should utilize a variety of complementary educational methods, including inmate to inmate peer training, clinician-provided education, and written informational pamphlets. In-house cable television systems have been used in jails and prisons with some success. Topics that should be included in risk reduction education include how the virus is transmitted, the importance of utilizing clean needles, syringe exchange, and avoiding needle and drug paraphernalia sharing, and the routine use of barrier methods such as condoms during sex. Those who are HCV-infected should receive additional counseling regarding prevention of transmission to others (CDCP, 1998). Specific recommendations for those who are HCV-infected include:

- Do not share toothbrushes or shaving equipment.
- Cover all bleeding wounds.
- Do not donate blood, semen, body organs, or other tissues.
- Do not use illicit drugs.
- If involved in injection drug use, do not reuse or share syringes, needles, and other drug use paraphernalia.

Patients should also be educated concerning how to prevent further liver damage. Progression to cirrhosis and end stage liver disease is more common in those who drink alcohol (more than 10 g/day for women and 20 g/day for men), those who are obese or have substantial hepatic steatosis, and those with HIV coinfection (Benhamou et al., 1999; Poynard et al., 1997; Harris et al., 2001; Koff & Dienstag, 1995; Di Martino et al., 2001). HAV or HBV infection that occurs in those who are chronically infected with HCV can lead to fulminant life-threatening disease. Therefore, HCV-infected persons who are not immune to HAV and/or HBV should be vaccinated. Many substances can potentiate liver disease, so patients should be advised to limit ingestion of nonessential medications. Inmates who are IDUs should be referred for substance abuse treatment. Jails and prisons should partner with community-based organizations (CBOs) to facilitate the referral of IDUs to community treatment facilities at the time of release.

Chronic HCV can be diagnosed by the presence of a detectable HCV viral load in the blood. Persons found to be chronically HCV infected should be referred to a clinician knowledgeable in the management of chronic viral hepatitis. Correctional facilities should adhere to national consensus guidelines for the treatment of HCV. Collaborations with local public health departments and universities may facilitate the appropriate evaluation and treatment of HCV-infected inmates. The goals of HCV treatment include eradicating HCV, reducing the risk for progression to cirrhosis and end-stage liver disease, and decreasing the incidence of hepatocellular carcinoma (Strader et al., 2004). Patients who are treated with interferon or pegylated interferon (peginterferon) in combination with ribavirin have experienced clearing of HCV and decreased liver fibrosis and inflammation (Poynard et al., 2002).

Treatment of HCV requires 6–12 months of weekly injections and twice daily oral medications. Side effects of treatment are common, and can be disabling and life-threatening. Therefore, not all patients will be suitable for treatment. Potential candidates for treatment must be carefully selected and monitored, and in some cases the risk of treatment may outweigh the potential benefits. A partial list of relative and absolute contraindications to treatment with currently available medications includes:

- Major, uncontrolled depressive illness
- Renal, heart, or lung transplantation recipient
- Autoimmune hepatitis or other condition known to be exacerbated by interferon and ribavirin
- Untreated hyperthyroidism
- Pregnant or unwilling/unable to comply with adequate contraception
- Severe poorly controlled illness such as severe hypertension, heart failure, coronary artery disease, and poorly controlled diabetes

Treatment of HCV is costly, but can yield significant dividends in terms of decreased infectiousness, a lower likelihood for cirrhosis, end-stage liver disease, and hepatocellular carcinoma, and decreased costs associated with the treatment of end-stage liver disease. Public policy makers should recognize the societal benefit that can be derived from HCV treatment of the incarcerated when making decisions concerning allocation of health care resources.

HCV-infected persons who are also HIV-infected have an increased risk for liver fibrosis, cirrhosis, and death due to liver disease compared to those who are HIV-negative (Bonacini & Puoti, 2000; Sulkowski et al., 2002; Sulkowski, 2001; Serfaty et al., 2001; Ragni et al., 2003). Approximately 25% of HIV-infected persons in the United States have chronic HCV, and up to 10% of those with chronic HCV may be HIV-coinfected (Alter et al., 1999; Sherman et al., 2002). As treatments for HIV have improved, liver disease has become an increasingly common cause of significant illness and death among those who are infected with HIV (Baham et al., 2002; Palella et al., 1998; Bica et al., 2001; Monga et al., 2001). Because of the high prevalence of HIV/HCV coinfection and because the management of each infection can differ in coinfected persons, all HIV-infected persons should be tested for HCV, and all HCV-infected persons should be tested for HIV. Treatment of HCV in those are HIV-infected can lead to successful HCV eradication. Patients who are infected with both HCV and HIV should be managed in consultation with specialists knowledgeable in the treatment of coinfected persons.

CBOs, public health departments, and local universities should take an active role in the diagnosis, prevention, and treatment of viral hepatitis in correctional settings. Partnerships with outside agencies can facilitate a wide range of activities, including:

- Performance of seroprevalence studies
- Development of recordkeeping systems that track the treatment and vaccination status of patients
- Assistance with case management as patients move throughout various jurisdictions
- Release planning and referral to outside providers
- Referral for substance-abuse treatment
- Education of correctional staff
- Budgetary advocacy with state and federal governments
- Clinical consultation

Conclusions

The United States incarcerates a larger percentage of its population than any other developed country in the world. Inmates are disproportionately impacted by HIV and viral hepatitis, while those who are not infected remain at risk due to unprotected sex and IDU. Undiagnosed inmates represent a large reservoir of individuals who can serve to transmit illness to other inmates, staff, and persons in the free community. The United States has experienced significant success over the past two decades in increasing the life expectancy of those who are HIV-infected and in decreasing the number of new HAV, HBV, and HCV infections. Continued success will depend on an increased emphasis on those we choose to incarcerate. Early diagnosis, harm reduction education, referral for treatment, and immunizations in jail and prison settings not only improve the health of inmates but also the communities to which most of them will one day return. Although many jails and prisons lack the expertise to effectively manage HIV and viral hepatitis, universities, public health departments, and CBOs can serve as invaluable resources. The costs associated with the appropriate management of HIV and viral hepatitis can be significant. There must be an improved understanding of the important public health role played by correctional clinicians, and a greater appreciation of the necessity for direct interjurisdictional cooperation and communication. Correctional public health issues should be include in the curricula of all clinical and public health training programs. Only through a greater understanding of the health care issues facing inmates can this nation take the necessary steps to effectively impact on the health of inmates and the society at large.

References

Aach, R.D., Stevens, C.E., Hollinger, F.B., et al. (1991). Hepatitis C virus infection in post-transfusion hepatitis: An analysis with first- and second-generation assays. *N Engl J Med*, *325*, 1325–1329.

Alpert, P.L., Shuter, J., DeShaw, M.G., Webber, M.P., & Klein, R.S. (1996). Factors associated with unrecognized HIV-1 infection in an inner-city emergency department. *Ann Emerg Med*, *28*, 159–164.

Alter, M.J. (2002). Prevention of spread of hepatitis C. *Hepatology, 36* (Suppl. 1), S93–98.

Alter, H.J., Jett, B.W., Polito, A.J., et al. (1991). Analysis of the role of hepatitis C virus in transfusion-associated hepatitis. In F.B. Hollinger, S.M. Lemon, & H.S. Margolis (Eds.), *Viral hepatitis and liver disease.* (pp. 396–402). Baltimore: Williams & Wilkins.

Alter, M.J., Kruszon-Moran, D., Nainan, O.V., et al. (1999). The prevalence of hepatitis C virus infection in the United States, 1988 through 1994. *N Engl J Med, 341,* 556–562.

Association of State and Territorial Health Officials. (2002) *Hepatitis C and incarcerated populations: The next wave for correctional health initiatives.* Washington, DC: Author.

Bader, T. (1983). Hepatitis B carriers in the prison population [Letter]. *N Engl J Med, 308,* 281.

Baham, J., Bick, J., Giannoni, D., et al. (2002). *Trends in an HIV infected incarcerated population: An autopsy review.* 40th Annual Meeting of the Infectious Diseases Society of America.

Baham, J., Gavin, J., Mittal, S., Kuniholm, M., Harriss, D., Ruiz, J., & Bick, J. (2004, February). *The effect of various counseling and testing methods on the rate of HIV testing among male Prisoners.* 11th Conference on Retroviruses and Opportunistic Infections.

Barry, M.A., Gleavy, D., Herd, K., et al. (1990). Prevalence of markers for hepatitis B and hepatitis D in a municipal house of correction. *Am J Public Health, 80,* 471.

Bauserman, R.L., & Richardson, D. (2003). HIV prevention with jail and prison inmates: Maryland's Prevention Case Management Program. *AIDS Education and Prevention, 15,* 465–480.

Benhamou, Y., Bochet, M., Di Martino, V., et al. (1999). Liver fibrosis progression in human immunodeficiency virus and hepatitis C virus coinfected patients. *Hepatology, 30,* 1054–1058.

Bernard, K., Sueker, J.J., Colton, E., et al. (2006). Provider perspectives about the standard of HIV care in correctional settings and comparison to the community standard of care: How do we measure up? *Infectious Disease in Corrections Report, 9*(3), 1–6.

Bica, I., McGovern, B., Dhar, R., et al. (2001). Increasing mortality due to end-stage liver disease in patients with human immunodeficiency virus infection. *Clin Infect Dis, 32,* 492–497.

Bick, J., Dewsnup, D. (1997). Successful primary prophylaxis of tuberculosis (TB) in HIV-infected Persons with CD4 <100 in a correctional setting. *35th Annual Meeting of the Infectious Diseases Society of America.*

Bick, J., Dewsnup, D., Humphries, C., et al. (1997). Significant decline in HIV associated death rate in a correctional medical facility. *35th Annual Meeting of the Infectious Diseases Society of America.*

Bonacini, M., & Puoti, M. (2000). Hepatitis C in patients with human immunodeficiency virus infection: Diagnosis, natural history, meta-analysis of sexual and vertical transmission, and therapeutic issues. *Arch Intern Med, 160,* 3365–3373.

Bruguera, M., Cremades, M., Salinas, R., et al. (1992). Impaired response to recombinant hepatitis B vaccine in HIV-infected persons. *J Clin Gastroenterol, 14,* 27–30.

Bryan, A., Robbins, R., Ruiz, M., et al. (2006). Effectiveness of an HIV prevention intervention in prison among African Americans, Hispanics, and Caucasians. *Health Education and Behavior, 33,* 154–177.

Bureau of Justice Statistics. (1999). *National substance abuse and treatment of state and federal prisoners, 1997* (NCJ 172871). Available at http://www.ojp.usdoj.gov/bjs/abstract/satsfp97.htm.

Bureau of Justice Statistics. *HIV in prisons and jails, 2002.* Washington, DC: U.S. Department of Justice, Office of Justice Programs.

Bureau of Justice. *Drug use and dependence, state and federal prisoners, 2004* (NCJ-213530). Available at http://www.ojp.usdoj.gov/bjs/abstract/dudsfp04.htm.

CDCP. (1989). Guidelines for prevention of transmission of human immunodeficiency virus and hepatitis B virus to health-care and public-safety workers. *MMWR, 38* (Suppl. 6).

CDCP. (1991). Hepatitis B virus: A comprehensive strategy for eliminating transmission in the United States through universal childhood vaccination—recommendations of the Immunization Practices Advisory Committee (ACIP). *MMWR, 40* (RR-13), 1–25.

CDCP. (1996). Immunization of adolescents: Recommendations of the Advisory Committee on Immunization Practices, the American Academy of Pediatrics, the American Academy of Family Physicians, and the American Medical Association. *MMWR, 45* (RR-13), 1–16.

CDCP. (1998). Recommendations for prevention and control of hepatitis C virus (HCV) infection and HCV-related chronic disease. *MMWR, 47* (RR-19), 1–39.

CDCP. (1999a). Anonymous or confidential HIV counseling and voluntary testing in federally funded testing sites—United States, 1995–1997. *MMWR, 48,* 509–513.

CDCP. (1999b). Vaccine-preventable diseases: Improving vaccination coverage in children, adolescents and adults: A report on recommendations from the Task Force on Community Preventive Services. *MMWR, 48* (RR-8), 1–15.

CDCP. (1999c). Prevention of hepatitis A through active or passive immunization: Recommendations of the Advisory Committee on Immunization Practices. *MMWR, 48* (RR-12), 1–37.

CDCP. (2000a). National center for health statistics. Deaths, percent of total deaths, and death rates for the 15 leading causes of death in 5-year age groups, by race and sex: United States, 2000. Available at: http://www.cdc.gov/nchs/data/dvs/LCWK1_2000.pdf.

CDCP. (2000b). Adoption of protective behaviors among persons with recent HIV infection and diagnosis—Alabama, New Jersey, and Tennessee, 1997–1998. *MMWR, 49*(23), 512–515.

CDCP. (2001). Hepatitis B outbreak in a state correctional facility, 2000. *MMWR, 50*(25), 529–532.

CDCP. (2003a). Incorporating HIV prevention into the medical care of persons living with HIV—Recommendations of the CDC, the Health Resources and Services Administration, the National Institutes of Health, and the HIV Medicine Association of the Infectious Disease Society of America. *MMWR, 52*(RR-12), 1–24.

CDCP. (2003b). Late versus early testing of HIV—16 sites, United States, 2000–2003. *MMWR, 52*(25), 581–586.

CDCP. (2004a). Voluntary HIV testing as part of routine medical care—Massachusetts, 2002. *MMWR, 53,* 523–536.

CDCP. (2004b). Hepatitis B vaccination of inmates in correctional facilities—Texas, 2000–2002. *MMWR, 53,* 681–683.

CDCP. (2005). HIV prevalence, unrecognized infection, and HIV testing among men who have sex with men—five U.S. cities, June 2004–April 2005. *MMWR, 54,* 597–601.

CDCP. (2006a). *Recommendations for use of antiretroviral drugs in pregnant HIV-1 infected women for maternal health and interventions to reduce perinatal HIV-1 transmission in the United States.* Available at http://aidsinfo.nih.gov/ContentFiles/PerinatalGL.pdf.

CDCP. (2006b). Revised recommendations for HIV testing of adults, adolescents, and pregnant women in health-care settings. *MMWR, 55*(RR-14), 1–17.

CDCP. (2006c). HIV infection: Detection, counseling, and referral. Sexually transmitted diseases treatment guidelines. *MMWR, 55*(RR-11), 10–14.

CDCP. (2006d). Twenty-five years of HIV/AIDS—United States, 1981–2006: Successes in HIV prevention. *MMWR, 55*(21), 585–588.

CDCP. (2006e). A comprehensive immunization strategy to eliminate transmission of hepatitis B virus infection in the United States: Recommendations of the Advisory Committee on Immunization Practices (ACIP) Part II: Immunization of adults. *MMWR, 55*(RR-16), 1–25.

CDCP. (2006f). HIV transmission among male inmates in a state prison system: Georgia, 1992–3005. *MMWR, 55*(15), 421–426.

CDCP Vaccines for Children program, information available at http://www.cdc.gov/nip/vfc/Default.htm.

Chakraborty, H., Sen, P.K., Helms, R.W., et al. (2001). Viral burden in genital secretions determines male to female sexual transmission of HIV-1: A probabilistic empiric model. *AIDS, 15,* 621–627.

Chen, R., Accortt, N., Westfall, A., et al. (2006). Distribution of health care expenditures for HIV-infected patients: *Clinical Infectious Diseases, 42,* 1003–1010.

Chen, Z., Branson, B., Ballenger, A., et al. (1998). Risk assessment to improve targeting of HIV counseling and testing services for STD clinic patients. *Sex Transm Dis, 25,* 539–543.

Coleman, P., McQuillan, G.M., Moyer, L.A., et al. (1998). Incidence of hepatitis B virus infection in the United States, 1976–1994: Estimates from the National Health and Nutrition Examination Surveys. *J Infect Dis, 178,* 954–959.

Collier, A.C., Corey, L., Murphy, V.L., et al. (1988). Antibody to human immunodeficiency virus (HIV) and suboptimal response to hepatitis B vaccination. *Ann Intern Med, 109,* 101–105.

Conklin, T.J., Lincoln, T., & Flanigan, T.P. (1998). Public health model to connect correctional health care with communities. *Am J Public Health, 88,* 1249–1250.

Cooper, E.R., Charurat, M., Mofenson, L., et al. (2002). Combination antiretroviral strategies for the treatment of pregnant HIV-1-infected women and prevention of perinatal HIV-1 transmission. *J Acquir Immune Defic Syndr, 29,* 484–494.

Correctional Service Canada. (1999). *Evaluation of HIV/AIDS harm reduction measures in the Correctional Service of Canada.* Ottawa.

Davidson, M., & Krugman, S. (1986). Recombinant yeast hepatitis B vaccine compared with plasma-derived vaccine: Immunogenicity and effect of a booster dose. *J Infect, 13*(Suppl. A), 31–38.

Decker, M.D., Vaughn, W.K., Brodie, J., et al. (1984). Seroepidemiology of hepatitis B in Tennessee prisoners. *J Infect Dis, 150,* 450–459.

Decker, M.D., Vaughn, W.K., Brodie, J., et al. (1985). The incidence of hepatitis B in Tennessee prisoners. *J Infect Dis, 152,* 214–217.

DHHS: Guidelines for the use of antiretroviral agents in HIV-1-infected adults and adolescents: October 10, 2006. Available at http://aidsinfo.nih.gov/ContentFiles/AdultandAdolescentGL.pdf.

Diaz, T., Des Jarlais, D.C., Vlahov, D., et al. (2001). Factors associated with prevalent hepatitis C: Differences among young adult injection drug users in lower and upper Manhattan, New York City. *Am J Public Health, 91,* 23–30.

Di Martino, V., Ezenfis, J., Tainturier, M., et al. (2001). Impact of HIV coinfection on the long-term outcome of HCV cirrhosis (abstract 567). 8th CROI.

Dolan, K., Lowe, D., & Shearer, J. (2004). Evaluation of the condom distribution program in New South Wales prisons, Australia. *The Journal of Law, Medicine and Ethics, 32,* 124–128.

Fattovich, G., Giustina, G., Degos, F., et al. (1997). Effectiveness of interferon alfa on incidence of hepatocellular carcinoma and decompensation in cirrhosis type C. *J Hepatol, 27,* 201–205.

Fincher-Mergi, M., Cartone, K.J., Mischler, J., et al. (2002). Assessment of emergency department healthcare professionals' behaviors regarding HIV testing and referral for patients with STDs. *AIDS Patient Care STDs, 16,* 549–553.

Fraser, G.M., Ochana, N., Fenyves, D., et al. (1994). Increasing serum creatinine and age reduce the response to hepatitis B vaccine in renal failure patients. *J Hepatol, 21,* 450–454.

Freedberg, K. F., Losina, E., Weinstein, M. C., et al . (2001). The cost-effectiveness of combination antiretroviral therapy for HIV disease. *N Engl J Med, 344,* 824–831.

Gaiter, J., & Doll, L.S. (1996). Editorial: Improving HIV/AIDS prevention in prisons is good public health policy. *Am J Public Health, 86,* 1201–1203.

Garfein, R.S., Vlahov, D., Galai, N., et al. (1996). Viral infections in short-term injection drug users: The prevalence of the hepatitis C, hepatitis B, human immunodeficiency, and human T-lymphotropic viruses. *Am J Public Health*, *86*, 655–661.

Garfein, R.S., Williams, I.T., Monterroso, E.R., et al. (2000). HCV, HBV and HIV infections among young, street-recruited injection drug users (IDUs): The collaborative injection drug users study (CIDUS II) [Abstract 115]. *10th International Symposium on Viral Hepatitis and Liver Disease, Atlanta*.

Gershon, R.R., Karkashian, C.D., Vlahov, D., et al. (1999). Compliance with universal precautions in correctional health care facilities. *J Occup Environ Med*, *41*, 181–189.

Glaser, J.B., & Greifinger, R.B. (1993). Correctional health care: A public health opportunity. *Ann Intern Med*, *118*, 139–145.

Goldstein, S.T., Alter, M.J., Williams, I.T., et al. (2002). Incidence and risk factors for acute hepatitis B in the United States, 1982–1998: Implications for vaccination programs. *J Infect Dis*, *185*, 713–719.

Grinstead, O., Zack,B., & Faigles, B. (1999). Collaborative research to prevent HIV among male prison inmates and their female partners. *Health Education and Behavior*, *26*, 225–238.

Hadler, S.C., Coleman, P.J., O'Malley, P., et al. (1991). Evaluation of long-term protection by hepatitis B vaccine for seven to nine years in homosexual men. In: F.B. Hollinger, S.M. Lemon, & H. Margolis (Eds.), *Viral hepatitis and liver disease: Proceedings of the 1990 International Symposium on Viral Hepatitis and Liver Disease*. (pp. 776–778). Baltimore: Williams & Wilkins.

Hagan, H., McGough, J.P., Thiede, H., et al. (1999). Syringe exchange and risk of infection with hepatitis B and C viruses. *Am J Epidemiol*, *149*, 203–213.

Hammett, T.M., Harmon, P., & Maruschak, L.M. (1999). *1996–1997 update: HIV/ AIDS, STDs, and TB in correctional facilities*. Washington, DC: U.S. Department of Justice, National Institute of Justice.

Hammett, T.M., Harmon, M.P., & Rhodes, W. (2002). The burden of infectious disease among inmates of and releases from US correctional facilities, 1997. *Am J Public Health*, *92*, 1789–1794.

Harris, D.R., Gonin, R., Alter, H.J., et al. (2001). The relationship of acute transfusion-associated hepatitis to the development of cirrhosis in the presence of alcohol abuse. *Ann Intern Med*, *134*, 120–124.

Hessl, S.M., (2001). Police and corrections. *Occup Med*, *16*, 39–49.

Hull, H.F., Lyons, L.H., Mann, J.M., et al. (1985). Incidence of hepatitis B in the penitentiary of New Mexico. *Am J Public Health*, *75*, 1213–1214.

Jenkins, T.C., Gardner, E.M., Thrun, M.W., et al. (2006). Risk-based human immunodeficiency virus (HIV) testing fails to detect the majority of HIV-infected persons in medical care settings. *Sex Transm Dis*, *33*, 329–333.

Jilg, W., & Deinhardt, F. (1986). Results of immunization with a recombinant yeast-derived hepatitis B vaccine. *J Infect*, *13*(Suppl. A), 47–51.

Kaufman, M.L., Faiver, K.L., & Harness, J.K. (1983). Hepatitis B markers among Michigan prisoners [Letter]. *Ann Intern Med*, *98*, 558.

Khan, A., Goldstein, S., Williams, I., et al. (2000). Opportunities for hepatitis B prevention in correctional facilities and sexually transmitted disease treatment settings (Abstract). *Antiviral Therapy*, *5*, 21–22.

Khan, A., Simard, E., Wurtzel, H., et al. (2002). The prevalence, risk factors, and incidence of hepatitis B virus infection among inmates in a state correctional facility [Abstract]. *Program and abstracts of the 130th Annual Meeting of the American Public Health Association, Philadelphia*.

Kibby, T., Devine, J., & Love, C. (1982). Prevalence of hepatitis B among men admitted to a federal prison [Letter]. *N Engl J Med*, *306*, 17.

Kitahata, M.M., Koepsell, T.D., Deyo, R.A., et al. (1996). Physicians' experience with the acquired immunodeficiency syndrome as a factor in patients' survival. *N Engl J Med*, *334*, 701–706.

Klein, D., Hurley, L.B., Merrill, D., et al. (2003). Review of medical encounters in the 5 years before a diagnosis of HIV-1 infection: Implications for early detection. *J Acquir Immun Defic Syndr*, *32*, 143–152.

Koff, R.S., & Dienstag, J.L. (1995). Extrahepatic manifestations of hepatitis C and the association with alcoholic liver disease. *Semin Liver Dis*, *15*, 101–109.

Koplan, J.P., Walker, J.A., & Bryan, J.A. (1978). Prevalence of hepatitis B surface antigen and antibody at a state prison in Kansas. *J Infect Dis*, *137*, 505.

Kunches, L.M., Craven, D.E., & Werner, B.G. (1986). Seroprevalence of hepatitis B virus and delta agent in parenteral drug abusers: Immunogenicity of hepatitis B vaccine. *Am J Med*, *81*, 591–595.

Lange, T. (2003). HIV and civil rights: A report from the frontlines of the HIV/AIDS epidemic. http://www.aclu.org/FilesPDFs/hivcivilrights.pdf.

Levine, O.S., Vlahov, D., Koehler, J., et al. (1995). Seroepidemiology of hepatitis B virus in a population of injecting drug users. *Am J Epidemiol*, *142*, 331–341.

Liddicoat, R.V., Horton, N.J., Urban, R., et al. (2004). Assessing missed opportunities for HIV testing in medical settings. *J Gen Intern Med*, *19*, 349–356.

López-Zetina, J., Kerndt, P., Ford, W., et al. (2001). Prevalence of HIV and hepatitis B and self-reported injection risk behavior during detention among street-recruited injection drug users in Los Angeles County, 1994–1996. *Addiction*, *96*, 589–595.

Lorvick, J., Kral, A.H., Seal, K., et al. (2001). Prevalence and duration of hepatitis C among injection drug users in San Francisco, Calif. *Am J Public Health*, *91*, 46–47.

Macalino, G.E., Salas, C.M., Towe, C.W., et al. (1999). Incidence and community prevalence of HIV and other blood borne pathogens among incarcerated women in Rhode Island [Abstract]. *National HIV Prevention Conference*, Atlanta.

Mahoney, F.J., Stewart, K., Hu, H., et al. (1997). Progress toward the elimination of hepatitis B virus transmission among health care workers in the United States. *Arch Intern Med*, *157,* 2601–2605.

Marks, G., Crepaz, N., Senterfitt, J.W., et al. (2005). Meta-analysis of high-risk sexual behavior in persons aware and unaware they are infected with HIV in the United States: Implications for HIV prevention programs. *J Acquir Immune Defic Syndr*, *39*, 446–453.

Mast, E.E., Williams, I.T., Alter, M.J., et al. (1998). Hepatitis B vaccination of adolescent and adult high-risk groups in the United States. *Vaccine*, *16*, S27–S29.

McLean, R.L., Robarge, J., & Sherman, S.G. (2006). Release from jail: Moment of crisis or window of opportunity for female detainees? *Journal of Urban Health*, *83*, 382–393.

McNaghten, A.D., Hanson, D.L., Jones, J.L., et al. (1999). Effects of antiretroviral therapy and opportunistic illness primary chemoprophylaxis on survival after AIDS diagnosis. Adult/Adolescent Spectrum of Disease Group. *AIDS*, *13*, 1687–1695.

McQuillan, G.M., Coleman, P., Kruszon-Moran, D., et al. (1999). Prevalence of hepatitis B virus infection in the United States: The National Health and Nutrition Examination Surveys, 1976 through 1994. *Am J Public Health*, *89*, 14–18.

Monga, H.K., Rodriguez-Barradas, M.C., et al. (2001). Hepatitis C virus infection-related morbidity and mortality among patients with human immunodeficiency virus infection. *Clin Infect Dis*, *33*, 240–247.

Mumola, C.J. (1999). *Substance abuse and treatment, state and federal prisoners, 1997*. Bureau of Justice Statistics Special Report. Washington, DC: U.S. Department of Justice, Office of Justice Programs. Publication No. NCJ 172871.

Murrill, C.S., Weeks, H., Castrucci, B.C., et al. (2002). Age-specific seroprevalence of HIV, hepatitis B virus, and hepatitis C virus infection among injection drug users admitted to drug treatment in 6 US cities. *Am J Public Health*, *92*, 385–387.

Myers, J., Zack, B., Kramer, K., et al. (2005). Get Connected: An HIV prevention case management program for men and women leaving California prisons. *American Journal of Public Health*, *95*, 1682–1684.

Nacci, P.L., & Kane, T.R. (1983). The incidence of sex and sexual aggression in federal prisons. *Federal Probation, 47*, 31–36.

National Health and Nutrition Examination Survey (NHANES III) 1994. Available at http://origin.cdc.gov/nchs/data/nhanes/databriefs/viralhep.pdf.

Neal, J.J., & Fleming, P.L. (2002). Frequency and predictors of late HIV diagnosis in the United States, 1994 through 1999 [Abstract]. *9th Conference on Retroviruses and Opportunistic Infections*, Seattle, Washington.

NIAID. (2001). Scientific evidence on condom effectiveness for sexually transmitted disease (STD) prevention, Available at http://www3.niaid.nih.gov/NR/rdonlyres/84AF59B3-F28E-4971-8297-775D1C020FE4/0/condomreport.pdf.

Palella, F.J. Jr., Delaney, K.M., Moorman, A.C., et al. (1998). Declining morbidity and mortality among patients with advanced human immunodeficiency virus infection. HIV Outpatient Study Investigators. *N Engl J Med, 338*, 853–860.

Paltiel, A. D., Walensky, R. P., Schackman, et al. (2006). Expanded HIV screening in the United States: Effect on clinical outcomes, HIV transmission, and costs. *Ann Intern Med, 145*, 797–806.

Paltiel, A.D., Weinstein, M.C., Kimmel, A.D., et al. (2005). Expanded screening for HIV in the United States—An analysis of cost-effectiveness. *N Engl J Med, 352*, 586–595.

Pisu, M., Meltzer, M.I., & Lyerla, R. (2002). Cost-effectiveness of hepatitis B vaccination of prison inmates. *Vaccine, 21*, 312–321.

Poynard, T., Bedossa, P., & Opolon, P. (1997). Natural history of liver fibrosis progression in patients with chronic hepatitis C. *Lancet, 349*, 825–832.

Poynard, T., McHutchison, J., Manns, M., et al. (2002). Impact of pegylated interferon alfa-2b and ribavirin on liver fibrosis in patients with chronic hepatitis C. *Gastroenterology, 122*, 1303–1313.

Quinn, T., et al. (2000). Viral load and heterosexual transmission of human immunodeficiency virus type 1. *N Engl J Med, 342*, 921–929.

Ragni, M.V., Belle, S.N., Im, K.A., et al. (2003). Survival of human immunodeficiency virus-infected liver transplant recipients. *J Infect Dis, 188*, 1412–1420.

Remis, R.S., Dufour, A., Alary, M., et al. (2000). Association of hepatitis B virus infection with other sexually transmitted infections in homosexual men. Omega Study Group. *Am J Public Health, 90*, 1570–1574.

Rey, D., Krantz, V., Partisani, M., et al. Increasing the number of hepatitis B vaccine injections augments anti-HBs response rate in HIV-infected patients. Effects on HIV-1 viral load. *Vaccine, 18*, 1161–1165.

Ruane, P.J., Ida, J., Zakowoski, P.C., et al. (1997). Impact of newer antiretroviral (ARV) therapies on inpatient and outpatient utilization of healthcare resources in patients with HIV. *Abstracts from the 4th Conference on Retroviruses and Opportunistic Infections, Washington, DC*. Abstract 262.

Rucker-Whitaker, C., Flynn, K.J., Kravitz, G., et al. (2006) Understanding African-American participation in a behavioral intervention: Results from focus groups. *Contemporary Clinical Trials, 27*, 274–286.

Ruiz, J.D., Molitor, F., Sun, R.K., et al. (1999). Prevalence and correlates of hepatitis C virus infection among inmates entering the California correctional system. *West J Med, 170*, 156–160.

Sanders, G.D., Bayoumis, A.M., Sundaram, V., et al. (2005). Cost-effectiveness of screening for HIV in the era of highly active antiretroviral therapy. *N Engl J Med, 352*, 570–585.

Saum, C.A., Surratt, H., Inciardi, J.A., et al. (1995). Sex in prison: Exploring the myths and realities. *The Prison Journal, 75*, 413–430.

Seeff, L.B., & Hoofnagle, J.H. (2002). National Institutes of Health Consensus Development Conference: management of hepatitis C: 2002. *Hepatology, 36* (Suppl. 1), S1–S2.

Serfaty, L., Costagliola, D., Wendum, D., et al. (2001). Impact of early-untreated HIV: A case control study. *AIDS, 15*, 2011–2016.

Sherman, K.E., Rouster, S.D., Chung, R.T., et al. (2002). Hepatitis C virus prevalence among patients infected with human immunodeficiency virus: A cross-sectional analysis of the US adult AIDS Clinical Trials Group. *Clin Infect Dis*, *34*, 831–837.

Smith, P.F., Mikl, J., Truman, B.I., et al. (1991). HIV infection among women entering the New York State correctional system. *Am J Public Health*, *81*(Suppl. 1), 35–40.

Spaulding, A., Greene, C., Davidson, K., et al. (1999). Hepatitis C in state correctional facilities. *Preventive Medicine*, *28*, 92–100.

Spaulding, A., Stephenson, B., Macalino, G., et al. (2002). Human immunodeficiency virus in correctional facilities: A review. *Clinical Infectious Diseases*, *35*, 305–312.

Springer, S.A., Altice, R., et al. (2004). Effectiveness of antiretroviral therapy among HIV-infected prisoners: Reincarceration and the lack of sustained benefit after release to the community. *Clin Infect Dis*, *38*, 1754–1760.

Stephenson, B.L., Wohl, D.A., Golin, C.E., et al. (2005). Effect of release from prison and re-incarceration on the viral loads of HIV-infected individuals. *Public Health Reports*, *120*, 84–88.

Strader, D.B., & Seeff, L.B. (1996). The natural history of chronic hepatitis C infection. *Eur J Gastroenterol Hepatol*, *8*, 324–328.

Strader, D., Wright, T., Thomas, D., et al. (2004). AASLD practice guidelines: Diagnosis, management, and treatment of hepatitis C. *Hepatology*, *39*, 1147–1171.

Sulkowski, M.S. (2001). Hepatitis C virus infection in HIV-infected patients. *Curr Infect Dis Rep*, *3*, 469–476.

Sulkowski, M.S., Moore, R.D., Mehta, S.H., et al. (2002). Hepatitis C and progression of HIV disease. *JAMA*, *288*, 199–206.

Szmuness, W., Stevens, C.E., Harley, E.J., et al. (1980). Hepatitis B vaccine: Demonstration of efficacy in a controlled clinical trial in a high-risk population in the United States. *N Engl J Med*, *303*, 833–841.

Tewksbury, R. (1989). Measures of sexual behavior in an Ohio prison. *Sociology and Social Research*, *74*, 34–39.

Thorpe, L.E., Ouellet, L.J., Levy, J.R., et al. (2000). Hepatitis C virus infection: Prevalence, risk factors, and prevention opportunities among young injection drug users in Chicago, 1997–1999. *J Infect Dis*, *182*, 1588–1594.

Torres, R., & Barr, M. (1997). Impact of combination therapy for HIV infection on inpatient census. *N Engl J Med*, *336*, 1531–1532.

Trupin, E.W., Turner, A.P., Stewart, D., et al. (2004). Transition planning and recidivism among mentally ill juvenile offenders. *Behavioral Science Law*, *22*, 599–610.

Tucker, R.M., Gaffey, M.J., Fisch, M.J., et al. (1987). Seroepidemiology of hepatitis D (delta agent) and hepatitis B among Virginia state prisoners. *Clinical Therapeutics*, *9*, 622.

US Department of Labor, Occupational Safety and Health Administration. (1991) 29 CFR Part 1910.1030. Occupational exposure to bloodborne pathogens: final rule. *Federal Register*, *56*, 640004–182.

USPHS/IDSA guidelines for the prevention of opportunistic infections in persons infected with human immunodeficiency virus. (2002). Available at http://aidsinfo.nih.gov/Guidelines/GuidelineDetail.aspx?MenuItem=Guidelines&Search=Off&GuidelineID=13&ClassID=4.

U.S. Preventive Services Task Force Guide to Clinical Preventive Services. (2005). http://www.ahrq.gov/clinic/uspstf/uspshivi.htm.

Vlahov, D., Nelson, K.E., Quinn, T.C., & Kendig, N. (1993). Prevalence and incidence of hepatitis C virus infection among male prison inmates in Maryland. *Eur J Epidemiol*, *9*, 566–569.

Volberding, P.A. (2006). Improving the outcomes of care for patients with human immunodeficiency virus infection. *New England Journal of Medicine*, *334*, 729–731.

Weinhardt, L.S., Carey, M.P., Johnson, B.T., et al. (1999). Effects of HIV counseling and testing on sexual risk behavior: A meta-analytic review of published research, 1985–1997. *Am J Public Health*, *89*, 1397–1405.

Williams, I.T., Fleenor, M., Judson, F., et al. (2000). Risk factors for hepatitis C virus (HCV) transmission in the USA: 1991–1998. Abstract 114. *10th International Symposium on Viral Hepatitis and Liver Disease, Atlanta.*

Wohl, D. (2006). Special Report: Transmission of HIV within a state prison. *Infectious Disease in Corrections Report*, *9*(5), 1–2.

Wohl, D.A., Stephenson, B.L., Strauss, R., et al. (2004). Access to HIV care and antiretroviral therapy following release from prison. Abstract 859. *11th Conference on Retroviruses and Opportunistic Infections.*

Wolitski, R.J., MacGowan, R.J., Higgins, D.L., et al. (1997). The effects of HIV counseling and testing on risk-related practices and help-seeking behavior. *AIDS Educ Prev*, Suppl. B, 52–67.

World Health Organization. (2006). *HIV testing and counselling*: *The gateway to treatment, care and support.* Available at http://www.who.int/3by5/publications/briefs/hiv_testing_counselling/en/print.html.

Zack, B., Flanigan, T., & Decarlo, P. What is the role of prisons in HIV, hepatitis, STD, and TB prevention? Available at http://www.caps.ucsf.edu/index.php.

Zeldis, J.B., Jain, S., Kuramoto, I.K., et al. (1992). Seroepidemiology of viral infections among intravenous drug users in northern California. *West J Med*, *156*, 30–35.

Chapter 9

Prevention of Viral Hepatitis

Cindy Weinbaum and Karen A. Hennessey

Introduction

Persons incarcerated in correctional systems comprise approximately 0.7% of the U.S. population and have a disproportionately greater burden of infectious diseases, including infections with hepatitis viruses (National Commission on Correctional Health Care, 2002). Approximately 2% of prison and jail releasees have current or chronic hepatitis B infection compared to 0.4–0.5% in the general population; and at least 17% were infected with hepatitis C compared to 1.8% of the general population (Box 9.1) (McQuillan et al., 1999; Alter et al., 1999).

On incarceration, all adults lose access to their usual public and private health-care and disease-prevention services. Their health care becomes the sole responsibility of either the correctional system (federal, tribal, state, or local) or, less frequently, the public health system (National Commission on Correctional Health Care, 1993). For the majority of persons, entry into the correctional system provides an opportunity to access health care that they could not access before. However, the rapid turnover of the incarcerated population, especially in jails, and the suboptimal funding of correctional health and prevention services, often limits the correctional system in providing both curative and preventive care.

The significance of including incarcerated populations in community-based disease prevention and control strategies is now recognized by public health and correctional professionals (Glaser & Greifinger, 1993; Association of State and Territorial Health Officials, 2002). Improved access to medical care and prevention services for incarcerated populations can benefit communities by reducing disease transmission and associated medical costs (Conklin, Lincoln, & Flanigan, 1998; Mast, Williams, Alter, & Margolis, 1998; Silberstein, Coles, Greenberg, Singer, & Voigt, 2000; Kahn, Scholl, Shane, Lemoine, & Farley, 2002; Goldstein et al., 2002). Inmates who participate in health-related programs while incarcerated have lower recidivism rates and are more likely to maintain health-conscious behaviors (Conklin et al., 1998). Finally, because incarcerated persons have a high frequency of infection with hepatitis viruses, community efforts to prevent and control these infections require inclusion of the correctional population (CDC, 1998a, 2005; Fiore, Wasley, & Bell, 2006).

Box 9.1 Definitions

Adult:	Person aged ≥19 years.
Anti-HAV:	Total antibody to hepatitis A virus (HAV) detected in serum of persons with acute or resolved HAV infection; indicates a protective immune response to infection, vaccination, and passively acquired antibody.
Anti-HBc:	Antibody to hepatitis B core antigen; positive test indicates past or current infection with HBV.
Anti-HBs:	Antibody to hepatitis B surface antigen; indicates immunity to HBV infection, either from HBV infection or from immunization.
Anti-HCV:	Antibody to HCV; positive test indicates past or current infection with HCV.
Arrestee:	Person placed under arrest by law enforcement who has not been formally charged with a crime.
Detainee:	Person arrested and legally charged with a crime who is held in a correctional facility before trial.
HAV:	Hepatitis A virus, the infectious agent that causes HAV infection and hepatitis A.
HBeAg:	Hepatitis B e antigen; positive test correlates with HBV replication and infectivity.
HBsAg:	Hepatitis B surface antigen; positive test indicates an active HBV infection.
HBIG:	Hepatitis B immune globulin; sterile preparation of high-titer antibodies (immunoglobulins) to hepatitis B surface antigen obtained from pooled human plasma of immunized persons and which provides protection against HBV infection.
HBV:	Hepatitis B virus, the infectious agent that causes HBV infection, hepatitis B, and chronic liver disease.
HBV DNA:	Deoxyribonucleic acid from HBV; positive test indicates active infection.
HCC:	Hepatocellular carcinoma; a primary liver cancer caused by chronic HBV or HCV infection that is usually fatal.
HCV:	Hepatitis C virus, the infectious agent that causes HCV infection, hepatitis C, and chronic liver disease.
HCV RNA:	Ribonucleic acid from HCV; positive test indicates active infection.
IDU:	Injection-drug use; injection-drug users are persons who have ever used needles to inject illicit drugs.
IG:	Immune globulin; sterile preparation of antibodies (immunoglobulins) made from pooled human plasma that contains anti-HAV and provides protection against hepatitis A.
IgM anti-HAV:	Immunoglobulin M antibody to HAV; positive test indicates acute HAV infection.
IgM anti-HBc:	Immunoglobulin M antibody to hepatitis B core antigen; positive test indicates acute HBV infection.
Infant:	Person aged ≤1 year.
Inmate:	Incarcerated person.
Jail:	Locally operated correctional facility that confines persons pending arraignment, awaiting trial and sentencing, or serving their sentences (usually ≤1 year).
Juvenile:	Person aged <19 years, in custody of the legal system.
Prison:	Adult correctional facility under the jurisdiction of state or federal authorities that confines persons with a sentence of >1 year.

Background and Epidemiology of Hepatitis Viruses in Correctional Settings

Hepatitis A Virus Infection

Clinical Description of HAV Infection

HAV infection is usually acquired by the fecal–oral route, produces a self-limited disease that does not result in chronic infection or long-term liver disease, and usually produces symptoms of acute viral hepatitis after an average incubation period of 28 days (range: 15–50 days). Signs and symptoms usually last less than 2 months, although 10–15% of symptomatic persons have prolonged or relapsing disease lasting up to 6 months (Glikson, Galun, Oren, Tur-Kaspa, & Shouval, 1992). Peak infectivity occurs during the 2 weeks prior to onset of jaundice or elevation of liver enzymes, when the concentration of virus in stool is highest (Fiore et al., 2006). Persons with chronic liver disease who acquire hepatitis A are at increased risk for fulminant hepatitis (Vento et al., 1998).

Epidemiology of HAV Infection

Following the implementation of routine hepatitis A vaccination of children, overall hepatitis A rates have declined approximately 75% from 1990–1997 to 2004 (Wasley, Samandari, & Bell, 2005; Fiore et al., 2006). In 2004, the rate of hepatitis A case reports was 1.9 cases per 100,000 population (Fiore et al., 2006). The prevalence of HAV infection among persons aged ≥6 years in the United States was estimated to be 31.1% based on data from the National Health and Nutrition Examination Survey III conducted in 1988–1994 (Bell et al., 2005).

In the United States, the majority of cases of hepatitis A occur through person-to-person transmission during communitywide outbreaks (Bell et al., 1998; Fiore et al., 2006). HAV transmission can occur through close personal contact (e.g., household contact, sexual contact, drug use, or children playing), and contaminated food or water (e.g., infected food-handlers or raw shellfish). The most frequently reported source of infection (12–26%) is household or sexual contact with a person with HAV infection. Other risk groups include injection and noninjection drug users and men who have sex with men (MSM). Approximately 50% of persons with hepatitis A have no source identified for their infection.

Up to 15% of nationally reported hepatitis A cases occurred among persons reporting drug use or MSM behaviors (Fiore et al., 2006). In some communities, hepatitis A outbreaks involving users of injected and noninjected methamphetamine have accounted for approximately 30% of reported cases (Bell et al., 1998; Van Beneden et al., 1998; Hutin, Bell, et al., 1999; Fiore et al., 2006). Transmission has been documented to occur from parenteral blood exposure (e.g., blood transfusion or injection-drug use) (Bower, Nainan, Han, & Margolis, 2000). However, the majority of transmission among users of illicit drugs is believed to occur through fecal contamination of drug paraphernalia and subsequent percutaneous inoculation, as well as from close personal contact (Hutin, Sabin, et al., 1999).

Hepatitis A outbreaks among MSM are frequently reported, and cyclic outbreaks occur in urban areas of the United States (Henning, Bell, Braun, & Barker, 1995; CDC, 1998b). HAV-infected MSM report more frequent oral–anal contact, longer duration of sexual activity, and a larger number of sex partners than persons without serologic evidence of infection (Corey & Holmes, 1980; Coutinho et al., 1983; Katz, et al., 1997; Stokes, Ferson, & Young, 1997).

HAV Infection in Correctional Settings

Although inmates are at risk for hepatitis A because of close personal contacts, sexual behaviors, and injection drug use, no hepatitis A outbreaks have been reported from correctional settings. Seroprevalence studies have found prevalence of prior HAV infection among incarcerated persons (22–39%) to be similar to age-adjusted prevalence rates in the general U.S. population (Weinbaum, Lyerla, & Margolis, 2003; Fiore et al., 2006). Employment in a correctional setting has not been identified as a risk factor for HAV infection.

Hepatitis B Virus Infection

Clinical Description of HBV Infection

HBV is a bloodborne pathogen, transmitted by percutaneous or permucosal (e.g., sexual) exposure to infectious blood or body fluids (e.g., semen or saliva). HBV circulates in high titers in the blood and lower titers in other body fluids (e.g., semen, vaginal fluid, or saliva), and is approximately 100 times more infectious than HIV and 10 times more infectious than HCV (CDC, 2001c).

Acute hepatitis B develops in approximately 30–50% of adults at the time of initial infection and is characterized by anorexia, nausea, vomiting, and often jaundice. The risk of progression to chronic infection varies with age, being highest among young children and infants (30–90%) and lowest among adolescents and adults (2–6%) (Lok & McMahon, 2001).

Persons with chronic HBV infection serve as the primary source of infection for others (McQuillan et al., 1999; CDC, 2005). The majority of persons with chronic HBV infection are asymptomatic, and one third have no evidence of liver disease, despite high levels of viral replication (Lee, 1997). Chronic HBV infection can lead to cirrhosis and HCC. Lifetime risk of death from chronic liver disease or HCC is 15–25% (Beasley, Hwang, Lin, & Chien, 1981; Beasley, 1988; Chang et al., 1997; McMahon, 1997; McMahon, Holck, Bulkow, & Snowball, 2001). Rates of progression to cirrhosis and HCC are approximately 25% for persons who acquire infection during childhood and 15% for persons who acquire infection at older ages. Other factors that influence rates of progression include: HBeAg status; coinfection with HDV, HIV, HCV; and alcohol abuse (Rizzetto, 1983; McMahon, 1997; Ockenga et al., 1997; Zarski et al., 1998; Monto & Wright, 2001; Gao, 2002). HBV-related liver disease and HCC cause approximately 4000–5000 deaths in the United States annually (CDC, unpublished data, 2002).

Epidemiology of HBV Infection

An estimated 4.9% of the civilian, noninstitutionalized U.S. population has serologic evidence of past or present HBV infection, and 0.4–0.5% have chronic infection (McQuillan et al., 1999; CDC, 2005). Overall prevalence of HBV infection differs among racial/ethnic populations and is highest among persons who have immigrated from areas with a high endemicity of HBV infection (e.g., Asia, Pacific Islands, Africa, and the Middle East) (Coleman, McQuillan, Moyer, Lambert, & Margolis, 1998). Prevalence of infection among blacks is four times that among whites (11.9% versus 2.6%) (McQuillan et al., 1999).

With the implementation of a comprehensive hepatitis B vaccination strategy since 1991, the incidence of acute hepatitis B has declined 78% during 1990–2005 from 8.5 to 1.9 per 100,000 population (CDC, 2006b). The rate of acute hepatitis B varies by age, sex, and race; the highest rates occur among persons aged 25–44, and males have higher rates than females. Disease incidence continues to be the highest among blacks, the lowest rate was observed among Hispanics whose rate dropped below that of non-Hispanic whites for the first time in 2003.

Sexual contact is the predominant mode of HBV transmission among adults (Goldstein et al., 2002). In a sentinel surveillance project including six U.S. counties during 2001–2004, 30% of persons with acute hepatitis B reported having multiple sexual partners and 24% were MSM (Williams et al., 2005). In addition, injection drug use was reported by 13% of the acute hepatitis B cases and 40% of the persons with acute hepatitis B had no identifiable risks for hepatitis B infection. The percentage of cases reporting occupational exposure to blood continues to be low (approximately 0.5%) as a result of routine hepatitis B vaccination of health care workers and use of standard precautions to prevent exposure to bloodborne pathogens (CDC, 2006b).

HBV Infection in Correctional Settings

Despite laws prohibiting sex between residents of correctional systems (Gaiter & Doll , 1996), 2–30% of inmates have sex while incarcerated (Nacci & Kane, 1983; Decker, Vaughn, Brodie, Hutcheson, & Schaffner, 1984; Tewksbury, 1989; Saum, Surratt, Inciardi, & Bennett, 1995). Only two state prison systems and five city or county correctional systems make condoms available to adult inmates and detainees for use in their facilities (Vermont, Mississippi, New York City, Philadelphia, San Francisco, Washington, DC, Los Angeles). Arrested adults also have a high prevalence of illicit drug use; in 2004 inmate surveys, 83% of state prisoners and 79% of federal prisoners reported past drug use, and 56% of state prisoners and 50% of federal prisoners reported using drugs in the month before their offense (Mumola & Karberg, 2006). Among jail inmates, drug use in the month before incarceration was reported by 55%, and injection-drug use (IDU) was reported by 18% (Wilson, 2000; http://www.ojp.usdoj.gov/bjs/pub/pdf/sdatji02.pdf). IDU during incarceration has been reported by 3–28% of adult inmates (Decker et al., 1984; Zimmerman, Martin, & Vlahov, 1991; CDC, 2001a; Khan et al., 2002). Although certain correctional systems offer substance-abuse treatment and education programs, demand usually exceeds program capacity (Stephan, 1997), and there appear to be no comprehensive risk-reduction programs available within correctional facilities.

Measured prevalence of serologic markers for current or past HBV infection among prison inmates has ranged from 13% to 47%, with variation by region. Prevalence is higher among women (37–47%) than men (13–32%) (Koplan, Walker, & Bryan, 1978; Decker et al., 1984; Hull et al., 1985; Smith, 1986; Tucker et al., 1987; Barry, Gleavy, Herd, Schwingl, & Werner, 1990; Ruiz et al., 1999; Weinbaum et al., 2003). Chronic HBV infection prevalence was 1.0–3.7% among prison inmates in various studies, 2–6 times the national prevalence estimate of 0.4–0.5% (Koplan et al., 1978; Bader, 1983; Kaufman, Faiver, & Harness, 1983; Decker et al., 1984; Bader, 1986; Tucker et al., 1987; Smith et al., 1991; Ruiz et al., 1999; López-Zetina, Kerndt, Ford, Woerhle, & Weber, 2001). The few studies of HBV infection among jail inmates found the prevalence to be similar to that in prisons, ranging from 16% to 21% (Solomon, Flynn, Muck, & Vertefeuille, 2004; Hennessey et al., 2006).

While the majority of HBV infections among incarcerated persons are acquired in the community, incidence rates within correctional facilities have ranged from 0.8% to 3.8% per year (Decker et al., 1984; Hull et al., 1985; Khan et al., 2002;

CDC, 2004a). In one state prison, after identification of a single case of acute hepatitis B, serologic testing identified new HBV infections in 1.2% of the inmate population and serologic testing of susceptible inmates 1 year later identified an additional 3.8% newly infected inmates (CDC, 2001a; Khan et al., 2002). During a 3½-year follow-up period, 92 new HBV infections were identified, with patients housed in multiple facilities, suggesting widespread ongoing transmission throughout the prison system (Khan et al., 2005). As another indication of the risk for HBV transmission, 5.6% of cases with acute hepatitis B reported to CDC's Sentinel Counties Study of Viral Hepatitis have a history of incarceration during the disease incubation period (Goldstein et al., 2002). HBV transmission in the prison setting can occur through sexual activity, IDU, and percutaneous exposures that are not apparent, as it does in households where persons with chronic HBV infection reside (Peters, Purcell, Lander & Johnson, 1976; Bernier et al., 1982).

On release, susceptible inmates are often at increased risk for infection because they resume high-risk behaviors. A study of recidivist women reported an HBV infection seroconversion rate of 12.2/100 person-years between incarcerations (Macalino et al., 1999), compared with an estimated incidence of 0.03/100 person-years for the U.S. population (Weinbaum et al., 2003).

Hepatitis C Virus Infection

Clinical Description of HCV Infection

HCV, a bloodborne pathogen, is most efficiently transmitted by direct percutaneous exposure to infectious blood. Of persons newly infected with HCV, only 20–30% have symptoms of acute hepatitis (Aach et al., 1991; Alter et al., 1991; CDC, 1998a). Chronic infection develops in approximately 75–85% of persons infected as older adults (age >45) and in 50–60% of persons infected as juveniles or young adults (Alter & Seeff, 2000).

The majority of persons with chronic HCV infection are asymptomatic, and approximately 30% have no evidence of liver disease based on serum aminotransferase levels. Among chronically infected persons, evidence of chronic liver disease develops in 70% of those infected as adults (Alter & Seeff, 2000). The risk for progression to cirrhosis varies by age at infection with persons infected as older adults at greater risk of progression than persons infected as juveniles or younger adults. Clinical progression is also accelerated by alcohol intake, chronic coinfection with HBV, and male sex (Alter & Seeff, 2000). Coinfection with HIV increases HCV viral loads, the rate of progression to fibrosis and cirrhosis, and liver-related mortality (Sulkowski, Mast, Seeff, & Thomas, 2000). HCC develops among 1–5% of persons with chronic hepatitis C (CDC, 1998a).

Epidemiology of HCV Infection

Using data from the National Health and Nutrition Examination Survey (NHANES) conducted during 1999–2002, an estimated 4.1 million persons (1.6%) in the civilian, noninstitutionalized U.S. population have been infected with HCV, of whom approximately 3.2 million (1.3%) are chronically infected (Armstrong et al., 2006). Men had a higher prevalence of HCV infection than women (2.1% versus 1.1%) and blacks had a higher prevalence of HCV infection than whites (3.0% versus 1.5%). When considering age, the highest prevalence was among those aged 40–49 which is consistent with a 1990 survey that reported the highest prevalence among those aged 30–39 (Alter et al., 1999).

Substantial or repeated percutaneous exposure to blood (e.g., IDU, exposure to clotting factor concentrates that did not undergo viral inactivation, and transfusions from HCV-positive donors) is the single most important risk factor for HCV infection. Of persons aged 20–59 who were anti-HCV-positive participating in the 1999–2002 NHANES, 48% reported a history of IDU (Armstrong et al., 2006). Data from the early 1990s found HCV antibody prevalence among persons who had been injecting 1 year or less of 77–89% (Thomas et al., 1995; Garfein, Vlahov, Galai, Doherty, & Nelson, 1996). More recent reports have found HCV antibody prevalence from 27% to 38% among injection-drug users less than 30 years of age (Garfein et al., 1998; Hahn et al., 2002, Thorpe et al., 2002). Incidence rates remain high, from 9% to 34% per year (Garfein et al., 1998; Hagan et al., 2001; Hahn et al., 2002; Thorpe et al., 2002; Des Jarlais et al., 2003, 2005).

Moderate prevalence (10%) has been reported among long-term hemodialysis patients, and lower prevalence is reported among persons with high-risk sexual practices (5%) and health care workers (1–2%) (CDC, 1998a). HCV is not transmitted efficiently through occupational exposure to blood. The risk of acquiring HCV infection from a contaminated needle stick is <2%, and transmission rarely has been documented from mucous membrane or nonintact skin exposures (CDC, 2001c).

Incidence of new HCV infections has been declining since the late 1980s, largely the result of a decrease in infections among injection-drug users. The majority of new HCV infections continue to occur in adult age groups (persons >25 years of age) with the greatest decline in incidence among 25- to 39-year-olds, historically the age group with the highest rates of infection. In this age group, incidence has declined by 92% from 1992 to 0.4/100,000 in 2004 (CDC, 2006b). Blacks and whites have the same incidence of new infection (0.2/100,000); rates among males (0.3/100,000) and females (0.2/100,000) are also similar. No association has been found between newly acquired HCV infection and military service, medical, surgical, or dental procedures, tattooing, acupuncture, ear piercing, or foreign travel (Alter et al., 1982, 1989). If transmission from such exposures does occur, the frequency has been too low to detect. However, results from seroprevalence studies of noninstitutionalized populations have been variable (Alter, 2002). Although one small study of IDUs suggested an increased risk for both HBV and HCV infection among those tattooed while in prison (Samuel, Doherty, Bulterys, & Jenison, 2001), limited studies have not confirmed this finding (CDC, 2001a; Bair et al., 2005; Samuel et al., 2001).

Despite the decrease in incidence among injection-drug users, the major risk factor for HCV infection remains IDU, which accounts for 60% of newly acquired infections (Garfein et al., 1996; Alter, 1997; CDC, 1998a; Williams et al., 2000; Garfein, Williams, Monterroso, Valverde, & Swartzendruber, 2000; Murrill et al., 2002). Among injection-drug users, HCV is transmitted by sharing syringes, needles, or other drug paraphernalia contaminated with the blood of an infected person (Koester & Hoffer, 1994; Heimer, Khoshnood, Jariwala-Freeman, Duncan, & Harima, 1996; Hagan et al., 1999). In studies conducted in the 1980s, approximately 80% of newly initiated injection-drug users were infected with HCV within 2 years (Thomas et al., 1995; Garfein et al., 1996; Lorvick, Kral, Seal, Gee, & Edlin, 2001). More recent studies indicate that the rate of HCV acquisition has slowed and approximately one-third of injection-drug users are infected within 2 years after initiating

IDU. Nonetheless, incidence among IDUs remains high at 10–15%/year (Hagan et al., 1999; Garfein et al., 2000; Thorpe, Ouellet, Levy, Williams, & Monterroso, 2000; Diaz et al., 2001).

HCV Infection in Correctional Settings

Inmates are at risk for HCV infection due to past IDU, and other percutaneous exposures (e.g., tattoos, bites, and abrasions) with the potential to transfer infectious blood and transmit bloodborne pathogens are also common in correctional facilities (Gershon et al., 1999; Hessl, 2001; Khan et al., 2002). Among prison inmates, 16–41% have serologic evidence of HCV infection, and 12–35% have chronic HCV infection; rates vary by geographic region (Vlahov, Nelson, Quinn, & Kendig, 1993; Ruiz et al., 1999; Alter et al., 1999; Spaulding, Greene, Davidson, Schneidermann, & Rich, 1999; Weinbaum et al., 2003). Similar prevalence (10–35%) has been detected among jail inmates (Baillargeon et al., 2003; Solomon et al., 2004; Hennessey et al., 2006). Most HCV-infected inmates have a history of IDU. In a Wisconsin study of 1148 inmates, among the 310 (27%) with a history of IDU and serologic evidence of HBV infection or biochemical evidence of liver disease, 91% were determined to be anti-HCV–positive (Weinbaum et al., 2003). Among HCV-positive entering jail inmates in Massachusetts, 85% reported needle-sharing, prior drug use, or a history of hepatitis (Weinbaum et al., 2003).

The risk of HCV acquisition during incarceration is not well-established. The only published study to examine the incidence of HCV infection among prison inmates reported a rate of 1.1 infections/100 person-years of incarceration among males (Vlahov et al., 1993).

Prevention of Viral Hepatitis

Primary prevention of infection with HAV and HBV can be achieved through immunization. For HCV, primary prevention of infection activities includes screening and testing of blood donors, virus inactivation of plasma-derived products, risk reduction counseling and services (e.g., substance abuse treatment) for injection-drug users, and implementation and maintenance of infection control practices to prevent exposure to blood. Identification of persons with chronic HBV and HCV infection provides an opportunity to initiate primary prevention activities including vaccination of household, sex, and needle-sharing contacts of persons with chronic HBV infection and counseling to reduce risks for transmitting HBV and HCV to others. In addition, persons with chronic HBV and HCV infection can be provided medical management that can reduce the progression of chronic liver disease. This section summarizes current information, practices, and recommendations to prevent infection with hepatitis viruses.

Prevention of HAV Infection

Vaccination

Vaccination is the most effective means to prevent HAV infection and reduce disease incidence. Since 2006, hepatitis A vaccination has been recommended for all children at age 1 year (Fiore et al., 2006). In addition, vaccination is recommended for adults at risk (e.g., users of injection and noninjection drugs, MSM) and those who may have a severe outcome after infection (e.g., persons with chronic liver disease) (Table 9.1).

Table 9.1 Viral Hepatitis prevention and control recommendations for inmates in correctional settings.

Activity	HAV	HBV	HCV
Vaccination	• Vaccinate adults at risk of infection (MSM, IDU and non-IDU drug users) and those with chronic liver disease	• All unvaccinated inmates (Table 9.3)	• Not applicable
Screening	• Prevaccination screening for anti-HAV may be considered if cost-effective (Box 3)	• Prevaccination testing may be considered if cost-effective (Box 3) • Consider routine testing for hepatitis B surface antigen of all long-term inmates or at-risk inmates (IDU, HIV infection, persons born in countries with high endemicity of infection)	• All inmates should be assessed for risk factors for HCV infection (IDU, recipients of clotting factors before 1987 and blood transfusions before 1992); those reporting risk factors should be tested for anti-HCV
Preventing transmission	• If a case of acute hepatitis A is identified, conduct an investigation to identify source and to identify persons who need postexposure prophylaxis (Box 2)	• All pregnant women should be tested for HBsAg, infants born to HBsAg-positive mothers should receive postexposure prophylaxis • If a case of acute hepatitis B is identified, conduct investigation to identify source and to identify contacts at risk from the source	• If a case of acute hepatitis C is identified, conduct an investigation to identify the source of infection and to identify contacts at risk from the source
Postexposure prophylaxis	• Unvaccinated or known close contacts of a person with acute hepatitis A should receive postexposure prophlaxis (Box 2)	• Begin postexposure prophylaxis for unvaccinated person after any percutaneous or mucosal exposure to blood or body fluids from an HBsAg-positive source or a source of unknown HBsAg status (Table 9.4)	• After a percutaneous or mucosal exposure to blood, test source person for anti-HCV • If source is anti-HCV-positive, test the exposed person for anti-HCV and ALT at baseline and 4–6 months later or test for HCV RNA at 4–6 weeks
Treatment	• Supportive management of clinical illness	• Evaluate persons with chronic HBV infection for liver disease and eligibility for therapy	• Evaluate persons with chronic HCV infection for liver disease and eligibility for therapy • Administer hepatitis A and hepatitis B vaccine if chronic liver disease is present

Table 9.2 Hepatitis A vaccination dosages and schedule.

Vaccine and recipient ages (years)	Dose	Volume (ml)	No. of doses	Schedule (months)
Havrix[®1]				
1–18	720 EL.U.[2]	0.5	2	0 and 6–12
≥19	1440 EL.U.[2]	1.0	2	0 and 6–12
VAQTA[®3]				
1–18	25 units	0.5	2	0 and 6–18
≥19	50 units	1.0	2	0 and 6–18
Twinrix[®4,5]				
≥18	720 EL.U.[2]	1.0	3	0, 1, and 6

Source: CDC. MMWR 2006;55(No. RR–7)1–23.
[1] Manufactured by GlaxoSmithKline Biologicals, Rixensart, Belgium.
[2] Enzyme-linked immunosorbent assay (ELISA) units.
[3] Manufactured by Merck & Co. Inc., Whitehouse Station, New Jersey.
[4] Manufactured by GlaxoSmithKline Biologicals, Rixensart, Belgium.
[5] Twinrix also contains hepatitis B vaccine antigen.

[†]Sputum smear or culture may be negative in persons with TB disease) (Weinbaum et al., 2003). Hepatitis A vaccination dosages and schedule are shown in Table 9.2. Prevaccination serologic testing for susceptibility is indicated only if the expected prevalence of immunity, cost of vaccination, and cost of testing make such testing cost-effective (Fiore et al., 2006).

Postexposure Prophylaxis

Passive immunization with immune globulin (IG) is 80–90% effective in preventing hepatitis A if administered ≤2 weeks after exposure to HAV (0.02 ml/kg IM) (Fiore et al., 2006). Anti-HAV testing of persons exposed to HAV is not recommended because it would delay IG administration and is likely not cost-effective. Although limited data indicate hepatitis A vaccine might provide protection when administered soon after exposure, an appropriately designed clinical trial has not yet been completed and use of hepatitis A vaccine alone is not recommended for postexposure prophylaxis (Fiore et al., 2006). However, persons who receive IG postexposure prophylaxis, and for whom hepatitis A vaccine is also recommended, should be vaccinated (Fiore et al., 2006).

Diagnosis and Management of HAV Infection

The diagnosis of hepatitis A is based on a positive serologic test for IgM anti-HAV in a person with clinical signs or symptoms of acute viral hepatitis. Serologic confirmation of HAV infection is required because hepatitis A cannot be distinguished from other forms of viral hepatitis on the basis of clinical presentation alone. Management of clinical illness is supportive.

Preventing HAV Transmission

Acute hepatitis A is a reportable condition in all states. After diagnosis of an acute hepatitis A case in a correctional facility, an investigation should be initiated with the assistance of local health authorities if needed, to identify the source of infection and to identify persons who need postexposure prophylaxis. IG is recommended for cellmates, sexual contacts, and persons having ongoing

---

Box 9.2 Contact investigation and postexposure prophylaxis after identification of an acute hepatitis A case

---

- Coordinate the contact investigation with local and state health departments.
- If index patient is a food handler, public health officials should be involved in the investigation to evaluate the risk for transmission and the need for prophylaxis.
- Prophylaxis is single dose of immune globulin (IG) (0.02 ml/kg body weight, intramuscular) administered as soon as possible but not >2 weeks after exposure.
- Candidates for prophylaxis include the following unvaccinated persons who were exposed to an index patient during the 2 weeks before onset of symptoms:

  cellmates or dormitory mates,
  sex contacts,
  other close contacts based on epidemiologic investigation, or
  other food handlers if the index patient was a food handler.

- IG is not routinely indicated when an index case occurs in a school, work setting, or temporary housing unit.
- When a person with hepatitis A is admitted to a hospital, standard and contact precautions are indicated. Staff members are at low risk for infection and prophylaxis is not indicated.

Source: CDC. Guidelines for viral hepatitis surveillance and case management. Atlanta, GA: 2002. Available at http://www.cdc.gov/ncidod/diseases/hepatitis/resource/PDFs/revised%20 GUIDELINES%20formatted4.pdf

---

close personal contact with a person who was serologically confirmed with hepatitis A infection (Box 9.2) (Fiore et al., 2006).

Current Practice

The extent to which hepatitis A policies have been adopted and hepatitis A vaccination recommendations have been implemented in correctional facilities has not been quantified.

Prevention of HBV Infection

Vaccination

Prevention of HBV infection is most effectively achieved through hepatitis B vaccination (CDC, 2005). The national strategy to eliminate HBV transmission has four components: (1) prevention of perinatal HBV infection by screening all pregnant women for active HBV infection and providing immunoprophylaxis to infants born to HBV-infected mothers; (2) hepatitis B vaccination of all infants beginning at birth; (3) vaccination of all adolescents not previously vaccinated; and (4) vaccination of unvaccinated adults in groups at risk for infection (American Academy of Pediatrics, 1997; CDC, 2005, 2006a).

Since 2003, CDC has recommended that all adults who receive a medical evaluation in a correctional facility be administered hepatitis B vaccine, unless they have proof of completion of the vaccine series or serologic evidence of immunity to infection (Table 9.1) (Weinbaum et al., 2003). Hepatitis B vaccination dosages and schedules are shown in Table 9.3. Since each dose of vaccine confers some protection against HBV infection (30–50% after one dose and 75% after two doses) (Davidson & Krugman, 1986; Jilg & Deinhardt, 1986; André, 1989; CDC, 2002b), the vaccine series should be started irrespective of the anticipated length of an inmate's incarceration (Davidson & Krugman,

Table 9.3 Hepatitis B vaccine dosages[1] and schedules.

Age group	Recombivax HB[®2]		Engerix-B[®3]		Twinrix[®3]	
	µg	ml	µg	ml	µg	ml
All children and adolescents ≤19 years	5	0.5	10	0.5	–	–
Adolescents 11–15 years	10	1.0[4]	–	–	–	–
Adults ≥20 years	10	1.0	20	1.0	20[5]	1.0
Adult dialysis patients ≥20 years and other immunocompromised persons	40	1.0[6]	40	2.0[7]	–	–

[1] Recombivax HB and Engerix-B are administered on a three-dose schedule at 0, 1, and 6 months, 0, 2, and 4 months, or 0, 2, and 6 months. Twinrix is administered on a three-dose schedule at 0, 1, and 6 months.
[2] Manufactured by Merck & Co. Inc., Whitehouse Station, New Jersey.
[3] Manufactured by GlaxoSmithKline Biologicals, Rixensart, Belgium.
[4] Adult formulation administered on a two-dose schedule at 0 and 4–6 months.
[5] Twinrix is only licensed for persons aged >17 years, and contains both hepatitis A and hepatitis B vaccine antigens.
[6] Dialysis formulation administered on a three-dose schedule at 0, 1, and 6 months.
[7] Two 1.0-ml doses administered in one or two injections, on a four-dose schedule at 0, 1, 2, and 6 months.

1986; Jilg & Deinhardt, 1986; Cassidy et al., 2001; CDC, 2005). Ensuring vaccine series completion requires that an immunization record is included in the medical record of all inmates, is transferred among correctional facilities if an inmate is transferred, and is provided to the inmate as part of release planning. In correctional settings where written vaccination records are not accessible, an oral history of completing a hepatitis B vaccine series can be used to defer hepatitis B vaccination. Persons who are uncertain about their vaccination status should be vaccinated. Other methods for assessing vaccination history (e.g., assuming a person received hepatitis B vaccine to comply with preschool or middle school-entry requirements or participation in the U.S. military) might be considered, but such methods require further research before they can be recommended as reliable alternatives (CDC, 2006a).

Serologic testing prior to vaccination: When an inmate population has a prevalence of immunity from prior infection and vaccination greater than 25% (Box 9.3), testing for immunity to HBV infection might reduce vaccine cost (CDC, 2004b). Vaccination of a person immune to HBV infection does not increase risk for adverse events.

Serologic testing after vaccination: Testing to determine antibody response to vaccination is not necessary for healthy adults. For immunocompromised persons (e.g., hemodialysis patients or HIV-infected) and persons with continued known exposure to HBV infection (e.g., infants born to HBsAg-positive mothers, sex partners of HBsAg-positive persons, or health care workers), testing for antibody to hepatitis B surface antigen (anti-HBs) is needed to verify response to vaccination and the possible need for revaccination (CDC, 2001b, 2002a, 2005).

Box 9.3 Method to determine cost-effectiveness of prevaccination screening for hepatitis B vaccination[1]

The breakeven point for the cost of prevaccination serologic testing, when first vaccine dose is administered at the time of blood draw, is

$$T = P1 \times [P2 + P2(P3)] \times v$$

T = cost of serologic test (anti-HBc or anti-HBs)

$P1$ = prevalence of past infection/immunization

$P2$ = percentage of recipients of first dose who actually receive a second dose

$P3$ = percentage of recipients of doses 1 and 2 who receive dose 3

$[P2 + P2(P3)]$ = average number of doses for a person starting the series

v = cost per dose of vaccine, including administrative costs

[1] Using this formula for hepatitis A vaccination assumes no vaccination is administered at the time of the blood draw. For hepatitis A vaccination, T = cost of serologic test for anti-hepatitis A virus (HAV); $T = P1 \times v$.

Postexposure Prophylaxis

After exposure of a susceptible individual to HBV, immunization with hepatitis B immune globulin (HBIG) and/or hepatitis B vaccine within ≤24 hours after exposure to HBV can effectively prevent acute and chronic infection (Table 9.4) (CDC, 2006a).

Serologic Testing for Chronic HBV Infection

Correctional facilities should consider routine testing of all long-term inmates for hepatitis B surface antigen, to facilitate rapid vaccination of contacts, direct counseling for preventing secondary transmission, and ensure medical evaluation of infected persons (Weinbaum et al., 2003). If routine testing is not performed, testing should be considered for inmates in groups with risk factors for chronic HBV infection (i.e., IDU, HIV-infected, or persons from countries with a high rate of infection) (map of hepatitis B surface antigen by country: http://www2.ncid.cdc.gov/travel/yb/utils/ybGet.asp?section=dis&obj=hbv. htm&cssNav=browseoyb).

HBsAg testing is recommended for all pregnant women as soon as the pregnancy is recognized, irrespective of hepatitis B vaccination history or previous test results (CDC, 2006a). In addition, women with risk factors for HBV infection during their pregnancy (e.g., intercurrent STDs, multiple sex partners, sex partners and household contacts of HBsAg-positive persons, or clinically apparent hepatitis) need retesting for HBsAg late in pregnancy because of the high risk for HBV infection (CDC, 2002d, 2005).

Management of Chronic HBV Infection

HBsAg-positive persons should be evaluated by a physician experienced in the management of chronic liver disease. Certain patients with chronic HBV infection will benefit from early intervention with antiviral treatment, management of factors that can contribute to disease progression, or screening to detect hepatocellular carcinoma at an early stage. Therapy for hepatitis B is a rapidly changing area of clinical practice. Currently, five therapies are approved by the FDA for the treatment of chronic HBV infection: interferon

Table 9.4 Guidelines for postexposure prophylaxis[1] of persons with nonoccupational exposures[2] to blood or body fluids that contain blood, by exposure type and vaccination status.

Exposure	Treatment	
	Unvaccinated person[3]	Previously vaccinated person[4]
HBsAg[5]-positive source		
Percutaneous (e.g., bite or needlestick) or mucosal exposure to HBsAg-positive blood or body fluids	Administer hepatitis B vaccine series and hepatitis B immune globulin (HBIG)	Administer hepatitis B vaccine booster dose
Sex or needle-sharing contact of an HBsAg-positive person	Administer hepatitis B vaccine series and HBIG	Administer hepatitis B vaccine booster dose
Victim of sexual assault/abuse by a perpetrator who is HBsAg-positive	Administer hepatitis B vaccine series and HBIG	Administer hepatitis B vaccine booster dose
Source with unknown HBsAg status		
Victim of sexual assault/abuse by a perpetrator with unknown HBsAg status	Administer hepatitis B vaccine series	No treatment
Percutaneous (e.g., bite or needlestick) or mucosal exposure to potentially infectious blood or body fluids from a source with unknown HBsAg status	Administer hepatitis B vaccine series	No treatment
Sex or needle-sharing contact of person with unknown HBsAg status	Administer hepatitis B vaccine series	No treatment

Source: CDC. MMWR 2006;55(No. RR-16): 1–33.

[1] When indicated, immunoprophylaxis should be initiated as soon as possible, preferably within 24 hours. Studies are limited on the maximum interval after exposure during which postexposure prophylaxis is effective, but the interval is unlikely to exceed 7 days for percutaneous exposures or 14 days for sexual exposures. The hepatitis B vaccine series should be completed.

[2] These guidelines apply to nonoccupational exposures. Guidelines for management of occupational exposures have been published separately and also can be used for management of nonoccupational exposures, if feasible.

[3] A person who is in the process of being vaccinated but who has not completed the vaccine series should complete the series and receive treatment as indicated.

[4] A person who has written documentation of a complete hepatitis B vaccine series and who did not receive postvaccination testing.

[5] Hepatitis B surface antigen.

alfa-2b, peginterferon alfa-2a, lamivudine, adefovir dipivoxil, and entecavir (American Association for the Study of Liver Diseases, http://www.aasld. org/eweb/?webkey=764aa7a7-0707-4798-bf2c-1e1f38331e50). Therapy is generally recommended for patients who have active disease (i.e., alanine aminotransferase levels >2 times the upper limit of normal), a liver biopsy indicating progressive disease, or both (Hoofnagle, 2006). Treatment of persons coinfected with HIV and HBV requires selection of antivirals with activity against both viruses selected to avoid development of viral resistance (DHHS Panel on Antiretroviral Guidelines for Adults and Adolescents—A Working Group of the Office of AIDS Research Advisory Council. Guidelines for the use of antiretroviral agents in HIV-1-infected adults and adolescents, 2006; http://aidsinfo.nih.gov/ContentFiles/AdultandAdolescentGL.pdf).

Preventing HBV Transmission

Acute hepatitis B is a reportable condition in all 50 states. After diagnosis of an acute hepatitis B case in a correctional facility, a prompt investigation should be initiated with the assistance of local health authorities, if needed, to identify the source of infection and to identify persons who need postexposure prophylaxis (Tables 9.1, 9.4) (Weinbaum et al., 2003). Identification of inmates with chronic HBV infection is needed to prevent HBV transmission to others by vaccinating sexual and social contacts and cellmates (CDC, 2005).

Perinatal HBV infections can be prevented through routine HBsAg testing of pregnant women and timely postexposure immunization of their infants (Beasley et al., 1983; Stevens et al., 1985; Margolis, Alter, & Hadler, 1991). Independent of maternal HBsAg status, hepatitis B vaccination is recommended for all infants beginning at birth (CDC, 2006a). Initiating hepatitis B vaccination soon after birth serves as a safety net to prevent HBV infection in infants whose mothers were not tested (CDC, 2006a).

Current Practices: Prevention of HBV in Correctional Settings

Vaccinating inmates in prisons has been demonstrated feasible and cost-saving from both inside and outside of prisons and jails (Pisu, Meltzer, & Lyerla, 2002). Components of successful vaccination programs in correctional facilities include establishment of policies for vaccination and a source of payment for vaccine (Lofgren, Paul, Kefalos, & Nichol, 1990; Crouse, Nichol, Peterson, & Grimm, 1994; Merkel & Caputo, 1994; Moran, Nelson, Wofford, Velez, & Case, 2000). In a census of state and federal adult correctional facilities conducted in 2000, 65% of facilities reported providing hepatitis B vaccine to all or a subset of inmates (Beck & Manuschak, 2002). Of these, 25% administered at least one dose of vaccine during the 12-month survey period. A 2005 survey of correctional systems (47 federal and state and 33 city and county) found that 82% offered vaccines to all inmates and 11% offered vaccination to all incoming inmates (Kennedy et al., 2006). Three state correctional systems that offered hepatitis B vaccine (Massachusetts, Michigan, and Texas) found that 60–80% of incoming inmates accepted vaccination (Weinbaum et al., 2003).

The 2005 survey of correctional systems found that 60% of facilities have a policy for prevaccination screening (Kennedy et al., 2006). Twenty-six percent of facilities test all inmates to identify persons with chronic hepatitis B infection and 52% test inmates with risk factors for HBV infection.

Prevention of HCV Infection

CDC's national strategy for prevention and control of HCV infection includes both primary prevention activities that reduce risks for acquiring new HCV infections and secondary prevention activities that reduce risks for liver disease in HCV-infected persons (CDC, 1998a). Primary prevention activities include: (1) prevention of transmission during high-risk activities (e.g., IDU and unprotected sex with multiple partners) through risk-reduction counseling of infected persons and persons at risk of infection; (2) donor screening and product inactivation procedures to eliminate transmission from blood, blood products, donor organs, and tissue; and (3) implementation of infection control practices to reduce risk of transmission from percutaneous exposure to blood in health care and other (i.e., tattooing and body piercing) settings. Secondary prevention activities can reduce risks for chronic disease by identifying HCV-infected persons through diagnostic testing and by providing appropriate medical management and antiviral therapy. There are many challenges to HCV prevention and control in correctional settings; however, consensus on best practices is emerging (Spaulding et al., 2006).

Serologic Testing and Screening for HCV Infection

CDC recommends risk-based HCV testing in correctional settings. Incoming inmates should be asked questions regarding risk factors for HCV infection during entry medical evaluations, and all inmates reporting risk factors for HCV infection (IDU or recipient of clotting factors before 1987 or blood transfusions before 1992) should be tested for anti-HCV (Table 9.1, Weinbaum et al., 2003).

Identification of persons with HCV infection should include both an antibody screening assay (e.g., enzyme immunoassay) and a supplemental or confirmatory test (e.g., recombinant immunoblot assay for anti-HCV or nucleic acid testing for HCV RNA) if the screening test's signal-to-cut-off ratio is low (CDC, 2003). Antibody screening tests detect anti-HCV in ≥97% of infected patients but do not distinguish between acute, chronic, or resolved infection (Fiore et al., 2006).

Confirmation of acute hepatitis C requires negative test results for IgM anti-HAV and IgM anti-HBc and a positive test result for anti-HCV, verified by supplemental testing or a high signal-to-cut–off ratio. Among a limited number of patients, onset of symptoms may precede anti-HCV seroconversion, and follow-up antibody testing might be necessary to make the diagnosis. In persons testing positive for anti-HCV, chronic HCV infection can be distinguished by persistence of HCV RNA for >6 months.

Preventing HCV Transmission

A case of hepatitis C is a reportable condition in all 50 states. After diagnosis of an acute hepatitis C case in a correctional facility, an investigation should be initiated with the assistance of local health authorities, if needed, to identify the source of infection and to identify contacts at risk from the source (Tables 9.1, 9.4) (Weinbaum et al., 2003). Identification of persons with chronic HCV infection is also needed to provide counseling on preventing transmission of HCV to others (CDC, 1998a).

Treatment and Management of HCV Infection

HCV-positive persons benefit from evaluation for the presence and severity of chronic liver disease. Antiviral therapy is recommended for persons with persistently elevated ALT levels, detectable HCV RNA, and a liver biopsy that indicates either portal or bridging fibrosis or moderate degrees of inflammation and necrosis (National Institutes of Health, 1997). No clear consensus exists on whether to treat patients with persistently normal serum transaminases.

Information is available on the National Institutes of Health (NIH) website[§] regarding regimens with proven efficacy approved by the FDA for the treatment of chronic hepatitis C (National Institutes of Health, 1997). The FDA has approved three antiviral therapies for treatment of chronic hepatitis C in persons aged >18 years: alpha interferon, pegylated interferon, and alpha or pegylated interferon in combination with ribavirin (National Institutes of Health, 1997; Fried et al., 2002).

Among persons with both HCV and HIV infection, treatment decisions are complicated by consideration of concurrent medications and medical conditions (e.g., hyperthyroidism, renal transplant, or autoimmune disease). If CD4 counts are normal or minimally abnormal (>500/ml), treatment responses to interferon monotherapy are similar to non-HIV–infected persons (Soriano et al., 1994, 1996; Sulkowski et al., 2000). The efficacy of ribavirin/interferon combination therapy among HIV-infected persons has been tested in only a limited number of patients. Ribavirin can have substantial interactions with other antiretroviral drugs (National Institutes of Health, 1997). Patients should be evaluated by a physician familiar with the treatment of patients with HCV/HIV coinfection, and indications for therapy should be reassessed at regular intervals.

Counseling and educational materials should include information concerning reducing further liver damage, as well as treatment options for those with chronic liver disease. Hepatitis A and hepatitis B vaccines are both recommended for HCV-infected persons with chronic liver disease (CDC, 1998a, 2006a; Vento et al., 1998). Persons with hepatitis C should also be counseled to not drink alcoholic beverages, because consumption of >10 g/day for women and >20 g/day for men has been associated with more rapid progression to cirrhosis (Koff & Dienstag, 1995; Poynard, Bedossa, & Opolon, 1997; CDC, 1998a).

Current Practices: Identification and Treatment of HCV-Infected Persons

Serologic testing for anti-HCV of populations with a high proportion of IDUs, including many prison and jail populations, is an efficient strategy for identifying HCV-positive persons (CDC, 1998a). The 2000 census of state and federal adult correctional facilities found that 76% tested inmates for hepatitis C infection; most facilities conducted targeted testing (32% of facilities tested high-risk inmates, 40% tested on request, and 65% tested based on clinical indication) (Beck & Manuschak, 2002). A 2005 survey of correctional facilities found that 33% of facilities tested all or some inmates for HCV infection at intake; 45% of facilities tested in-house inmates with risk factors (Kennedy et al., 2006).

A limited number of studies have examined willingness to be tested, treatment options, compliance, and outcomes among those offered therapy (Spaulding et al., 1999; Allen et al., 2003). A 2005 survey of correctional facilities found that 94% of the 47 state and federal systems and 33% of 33 city or county jails surveyed provide HCV treatment to inmates who meet clinical and administrative criteria (Kennedy et al., 2006). In assessments of other correctional facility screening programs for HIV and STDs, a refusal rate of approximately 50% has been reported (Andrus et al., 1989; Hoxie et al., 1990; Behrendt et al., 1994).

[§]Available at http://www.niddk.nih.gov/health/digest/pubs/chrnhepe/chrnhepc.htm

Limited data from studies in Rhode Island and Pennsylvania indicate approximately 7–27% of all inmates identified with HCV infection ultimately begin treatment (Weinbaum et al., 2003). The majority of inmates were excluded from treatment because of clinical contraindications, short lengths of prison stay, and drug or alcohol use (Spaulding et al., 1999; Allen et al., 2003; Weinbaum et al., 2003). Less-restrictive criteria might increase the number of inmates eligible for treatment (National Institutes of Health, 1997). However, factors contributing to acceptance and completion of treatment regimens need to be identified to improve outcomes.

Juveniles

In 2003, 2.2 million juveniles were arrested and 96,655 were held in residential placement facilities (Snyder & Sickmund, 2006). Limited data are available on burden of viral hepatitis among incarcerated juveniles. The rate of hepatitis A cases among persons aged 14–18 has declined by 95% from 1990 to 2005 (CDC, unpublished data). A study among juvenile detention entrants in Oregon in 1994–1996 found a prevalence of HBV infection (anti-HBc-positive) of 2% and a prevalence of HCV infection (anti-HCV-positive) of 1% (Thomas, Keene, & Cieslak, 2005), and a study of juveniles in Texas found an HCV infection prevalence of 2% (Bair et al., 2005).

In 2001, a national survey of state juvenile correctional systems reported that 36 (86%) of 42 responding systems had a hepatitis B vaccination program in place; 78% used the federally funded Vaccines For Children (VFC) Program to pay for vaccine; and 85% considered vaccination to be a corrections responsibility while a juvenile is in custody. Written hepatitis B vaccination policies were in place in 65% of states, and 27% used a vaccine tracking system or immunization registry (CDC, unpublished data, 2002). In 2006, a survey of state immunization programs found that 80% were registered VFC providers (CDC, unpublished data, 2006). In states with immunization registries and VFC participation, vaccination coverage among incarcerated juveniles has reached levels >90% (Weinbaum et al., 2003). However, where the correctional system does not have legal guardianship of the detained juvenile, the need for parental consent can pose a barrier to vaccination. In certain states, laws enabling minors to consent to their own STD-related treatment and prevention have been implemented to include hepatitis B vaccination, facilitating implementation of vaccination programs (Weinbaum et al., 2003).

Prevention and management of infections with hepatitis viruses for juveniles are similar to those recommended for adults (Weinbaum et al., 2003). However, vaccination recommendations differ. States and communities with existing hepatitis A vaccination programs should administer hepatitis A vaccine to all juveniles, and in areas without existing programs catch-up vaccination of all juveniles can be considered (Weinbaum et al., 2003; Fiore et al., 2006). Such programs might especially be warranted in the context of increasing hepatitis A incidence and outbreaks among children and adolescents. Additionally, hepatitis B vaccination is recommended for all children and adolescents aged <19; therefore, all juveniles without proof of vaccination or immunity should be administered hepatitis B vaccine (Weinbaum et al., 2003; CDC, 2006a).

> **Box 9.4** Elements of viral hepatitis health education for correctional facility inmates
>
> • Routes of transmission
> • Risk factors for infection
> • Disease outcomes, the need for medical management and treatment options
> • Methods to prevent infection, including immunization and harm and risk reduction
> • The importance of substance abuse treatment, when appropriate
> • Sexual precautions including abstinence counseling and condom use
> • Risk-reduction counseling, including not sharing drug paraphernalia
> • Resources in the community available to support and sustain a reduction in risk behaviors

Health Education

During incarceration, numerous educational opportunities exist (e.g., at entry, in HIV-education classes, in other classes). Available education materials include videos, brochures, formal classroom presentations, or informal peer chat sessions, which provide information related to viral hepatitis, routes of transmission, risk factors for infection, methods of prevention, disease outcomes, and treatment options (http://www.cdc.gov/ncidod/diseases/hepatitis/resource/index.htm). Repeated face-to-face sessions have been determined to be the most effective educational strategies with the highest retention of information (Box 9.4) (Jemmott, Jemmott, & Fong, 1992; Magura, Kang, & Shapiro, 1994; Glanz, Saraiya, & Wechsler, 2002). Model programs use peer health educators in workshops for incoming inmates, and community educators to discuss risk assessment, risk reduction, and referrals for soon-to-be released inmates (see http://www.hepprograms.org).

To be effective, risk reduction among the incarcerated population often requires a multidisciplinary approach to address drug use as well as other medical, psychological, social, vocational, and legal problems (CDC, 2002c). Health education programs aimed at reducing risk of infection with hepatitis viruses include discussion of hepatitis A prevention, hygiene practices, and the need for vaccination of persons at risk for infection. Curricula addressing HBV and HCV infections include information concerning modes of transmission and means for prevention, and information about hepatitis B vaccination and risk reduction. Such information can also be incorporated into health-education programs for the prevention of HIV/AIDS.

Release Planning

Release planning is an important, evolving component of health care management for incarcerated persons. The majority of medical release and discharge planning programs in correctional facilities have focused on HIV aftercare (Stephenson et al., 2000; Rich, Holmes, Salas et al., 2001), but management of other chronic infections can also result in beneficial outcomes. A survey of correctional facilities conducted in 2005 found that 34% of the state and federal prisons and 27% of the city and county jails provided discharge planning for inmates with chronic HBV infection (Kennedy et al., 2006). Half of the state and federal facilities and 24% of the city and county facilities provided discharge planning for inmates with HCV infection.

Comprehensive release planning includes transitional housing, continued access to discharge medications and immunizations, and coordination and case-management of long-term specialized care for persons with chronic conditions. Persons diagnosed with chronic HBV infection can benefit from counseling related to preventing transmission to household, sexual, and drug-use contacts. Susceptible contacts of persons diagnosed with chronic HBV infection benefit from hepatitis B vaccination. Persons with chronic hepatitis B or chronic hepatitis C can benefit from (1) counseling regarding ways to reduce further liver damage, (2) referrals to substance abuse treatment and other IDU programs if indicated (http://www.cdc.gov/idu/substance.htm), and (3) medical referrals to specialists for future treatment.

Conclusion

The high prevalence of chronic HBV and HCV infections in correctional facilities and high proportion of inmates with risk factors for acquiring viral hepatitis infections make prevention and control of these infections high priorities for correctional health programs. In addition, because a substantial proportion of releasees to the community continue to acquire or transmit these infections, correctional facility efforts should become part of prevention and control efforts in the broader community.

Highly effective and safe vaccines are available to prevent HAV and HBV infections. Identification of risk factors and infection status, combined with harm- and risk-reduction counseling, and substance-abuse treatment, have the potential to prevent HCV infections in the same manner they have reduced the risk of HIV/AIDS. In addition, identification of persons with chronic HBV and HCV infection provides opportunities for medical evaluation and treatment of chronic liver disease, and measures to prevent further transmission.

The challenges to integration of a comprehensive viral hepatitis prevention and control program in correctional health settings are substantial. They include budgetary and staffing constraints, priorities that compete with preventive health care, and lack of communication among correctional health, public health, and private health-care systems. Despite these challenges a 2005 survey of correctional facilities found that 78% of facilities have written hepatitis policies, 82% offered hepatitis B vaccine to all inmates, and 18% of facilities screen high-risk inmates for HBV infection and 38% of facilities screen high-risk inmates for HCV infection (Kennedy et al. 2006).

Internet Resources

- CDC, viral hepatitis, http://www.cdc.gov/hepatitis
- CDC, immunization, http://www.cdc.gov/nip
- CDC, public health and IDUs, http://www.cdc.gov/idu

- CDC, public health and corrections, http://www.nchstp.cdc.gov/correctional health
- Immunization Action Coalition, immunization resources, http://www.immunize.org
- Immunization Action Coalition, model prevention programs, http//www.hepprograms.org
- National Institutes of Health, National Institute of Digestive Diseases (NIH, NIDDK), HCV treatment consensus statement, http://consensus.nih.gov/cons/116/116cdc_intro.htm
- American Association for the Study of Liver Diseases, viral hepatitis treatment, http://www.aasld.org/eweb/?webkey=764aa7a7-0707-4798-bf2c-1e1f38331e50
- Federal Bureau of Prisons, treatment guidelines, http://www.nicic.org/services/news/bop-medical.htm
- National Commission on Correctional Health Care (NCCHC), http://www.ncchc.org
- American Correctional Association (ACA), http://www.aca.org
- National Institute of Justice (NIJ), Report on the Health Status of Soon-to-Be-Released Inmates, http://www.ncchc.org/pubs_stbr.html

References

Aach, R.D., Stevens, C.E., Hollinger, F.B., et al. (1991). Hepatitis C virus infection in post-transfusion hepatitis: An analysis with first- and second-generation assays. *N Engl J Med, 325*, 1325–1329.

Allen, S.A., Spaulding, A., Osei, A.M., et al. (2003). Treatment of chronic hepatitis C in a state correctional facility. *Arch Intern Med, 138*, 187–190.

Alter, M.J. (1997). Epidemiology of hepatitis C. *Hepatology, 26*(Suppl. 1), 62S–65S.

Alter, M.J. (2002). Prevention of spread of hepatitis C. *Hepatology, 36*(Suppl. 1), S93–S98.

Alter, M.J., Coleman, P.J., Alexander, W.J., et al. (1989). Importance of heterosexual activity in the transmission of hepatitis B and non-A, non-B hepatitis. *JAMA, 262*, 1201–1205.

Alter, M.J., Gerety, R., Smallwood, L., et al. (1982). Sporadic non-A, non-B hepatitis: Frequency and epidemiology in an urban U.S. population. *J Infect Dis, 145*, 886–893.

Alter, M.J., Jett, B.W., Polito, A.J., et al. (1991). Analysis of the role of hepatitis C virus in transfusion-associated hepatitis. In F.B. Hollinger, S.M. Lemon, & H.S. Margolis (Eds.), *Viral hepatitis and liver disease* (pp. 396–402). Baltimore: Williams & Wilkins.

Alter, M.J., Kruszon-Moran, D., Nainan, O.V., et al. (1999). The prevalence of hepatitis C virus infection in the United States, 1988 through 1994. *N Engl J Med, 341*, 556–562.

Alter, M.J., & Seeff, L.B. (2000). Recovery, persistence, and sequelae in hepatitis C virus infection: A perspective on long-term outcome. *Semin Liver Dis, 20*, 17–35.

American Academy of Pediatrics. (1997). Hepatitis B. In G. Peter (Ed.), *1997 red book: Report of the Committee on Infectious Diseases* (24th ed., pp. 247–260). Elk Grove Village, IL: Author.

André, F.E. (1989). Summary of safety and efficacy data on a yeast-derived hepatitis B vaccine. *Am J Med, 87*(Suppl. 3A), 14S–20S.

Andrus, J.K., Fleming, D.W., Knox, C., et al. (1989). HIV testing in prisoners: Is mandatory testing mandatory? *Am J Public Health, 79*, 840–842.

Armstrong, G.L., Wasley, A., Simard, E.P., McQuillan, G.M., Kuhnert, W.L., & Alter, M.J. (2006). The prevalence of hepatitis C virus infection in the United States, 1999 through 2002. *Ann Intern Med, 144*, 705–714.

Association of State and Territorial Health Officials. (2002). *Hepatitis C and incarcerated populations: The next wave for correctional health initiatives.* Washington, DC: Author.

Bader, T. (1983). Hepatitis B carriers in the prison population [Letter]. *N Engl J Med, 308*, 281.

Bader, T.F. (1986). Hepatitis B in prisons. *Biomed Pharmacother, 40*, 248–251.

Baillargeon, J., Wu, H., Kelley, M.J., Grady, J., Linthicum, L., & Dunn, K. (2003). Hepatitis C seroprevalence among newly incarcerated inmates in the Texas correctional system. *Public Health, 117*, 43–48.

Bair, R.M., Baillargeon, J.G., Kelly, P.J., et al. (2005). Prevalence and risk factors for hepatitis C virus infection among adolescents in detention. *Arch Pediatr Adolesc Med, 159*, 1015–1018.

Barry, M.A., Gleavy, D., Herd, K., Schwingl, P.J., & Werner, B.G. (1990). Prevalence of markers for hepatitis B and hepatitis D in a municipal house of correction. *Am J Public Health, 80*, 471–473.

Beasley, R.P. (1988). Hepatitis B virus: The major etiology of hepatocellular carcinoma. *Cancer, 61*, 1942–1956.

Beasley, R.P., Hwang, L.Y., Lin, C.C., & Chien, C.S. (1981). Hepatocellular carcinoma and hepatitis B virus: A prospective study of 22 707 men in Taiwan. *Lancet, 2*, 1129–1133.

Beasley, R.P., Hwang, L.Y., Stevens, C.E., et al. (1983). Efficacy of hepatitis B immune globulin for prevention of perinatal transmission of the hepatitis B virus carrier state: Final report of a randomized double-blind, placebo-controlled trial. *Hepatology, 3*, 135–141.

Beck, A.J., & Manuschak, L.M. (2002). *Hepatitis testing and treatment in state prisons.* Bureau of Justice Statistics. NCJ191702. 2002. Washington, DC: U.S. Department of Justice, Office of Justice Programs.

Behrendt, C., Kendig, N., Dambita, C., Horman, J., Lawlor, J., & Vlahov, D. (1994). Voluntary testing for human immunodeficiency virus (HIV) in a prison population with a high prevalence of HIV. *Am J Epidemiol, 139*, 918–926.

Bell, B.P., Kruszon-Moran, D., Shapiro, C.N., Lambert, S.B., McQuillan, G.M., & Margolis, H.S. (2005). Hepatitis A virus infection in the United States: Serologic results from the Third National Health and Nutrition Examination Survey. *Vaccine, 23*, 5798–5806.

Bell, B.P., Shapiro, C.N., Alter, M.J., et al. (1998). The diverse patterns of hepatitis A epidemiology in the United States—Implications for vaccination strategies. *J Infect Dis, 78*, 1579–1584.

Bernier, R.H., Sampliner, R., Gerety, R., Tabor, E., Hamilton, F., & Nathanson, N. (1982). Hepatitis B infection in households of chronic carriers of hepatitis B surface antigen: Factors associated with prevalence of infection. *Am J Epidemiol, 116*, 199–211.

Bower, W.A., Nainan, O.V., Han, X., & Margolis, H.S. (2000). Duration of viremia in hepatitis A viral infections. *J Infect Dis, 82*, 12–17.

Cassidy, W.M., Watson, B., Ioli, V.A., Williams, K., Bird, S., & West, D.J. (2001). A randomized trial of alternative two- and three-dose hepatitis B vaccination regimens in adolescents: Antibody responses, safety, and immunologic memory. *Pediatrics, 107*, 626–631.

CDC. (1998a). Recommendations for prevention and control of hepatitis C virus (HCV) infection and HCV-related chronic disease. *MMWR, 47*(No. RR-19), 1–39.

CDC. (1998b). Hepatitis A vaccination of men who have sex with men—Atlanta, GA. *MMWR, 47,* 708–711.

CDC. (2001a). Hepatitis B outbreak in a state correctional facility, 2000. *MMWR, 50,* 529–532.

CDC. (2001b). Recommendations for preventing transmission of infections among chronic hemodialysis patients. *MMWR, 50*(No. RR-5), 1–43.

CDC. (2001c). Updated U.S. Public Health Service guidelines for the management of occupational exposures to HBV, HCV, and HIV and recommendations for postexposure prophylaxis. *MMWR, 50*(No. RR-11), 1–42.

CDC. (2002a). Guidelines for preventing opportunistic infections among HIV-infected persons—2002: Recommendations of the U.S. Public Health Service and the Infectious Diseases Society of America. *MMWR, 51*(No. RR-8), 1–46.

CDC. (2002b). Hepatitis B vaccination among high-risk adolescents and adults—San Diego, California, 1998–2001. *MMWR, 51,* 618–621.

CDC. (2002c). Substance abuse treatment and public health: Working together to benefit injection drug users. [Fact sheet series]. US Department of Health and Human Services, CDC, Academy for Educational Development. Available at http://www.cdc.gov/idu/facts/WorkingTogether.htm.

CDC. (2002d). Sexually transmitted diseases treatment guidelines 2002. *MMWR, 51*(No. RR-6), 1–80.

CDC. (2004a). Transmission of hepatitis B virus in correctional facilities—Georgia, January 1999–June 2002. *MMWR, 53,* 678–681.

CDC. (2004b). Hepatitis B vaccination of inmates in correctional facilities—Texas, 2000–2002. *MMWR, 53,* 681–683.

CDC. (2005). A comprehensive immunization strategy to eliminate transmission of hepatitis B virus infection in the United States, Recommendations of the Advisory Committee on Immunization Practices (ACIP), part 1: Immunization of infants, children and adolescents. *MMWR, 54*(No. RR-15), 1–33.

CDC. (2006a). A comprehensive immunization strategy to eliminate transmission of hepatitis B virus infection in the United States. *MMWR, 55*(No. RR-16), 1–33.

CDC. (2006b). Hepatitis Surveillance Report No. 61. Atlanta: US Department of Health and Human Services, Centers for Disease Control and Prevention.

Chang, M.H., Chen, C.J., Lai, M.S., et al (1997). Universal hepatitis B vaccination in Taiwan and the incidence of hepatocellular carcinoma in children. Taiwan Childhood Hepatoma Study Group. *N Engl J Med, 336,* 1855–1859.

Coleman, P., McQuillan, G.M., Moyer, L.A., Lambert, S.B., & Margolis, H.S. (1998). Incidence of hepatitis B virus infection in the United States, 1976–1994: Estimates from the National Health and Nutrition Examination Surveys. *J Infect Dis, 178,* 954–959.

Conklin, T.J., Lincoln, T., & Flanigan, T.P. (1998). Public health model to connect correctional health care with communities. *Am J Public Health, 88,* 1249–1250.

Corey, L., & Holmes, K.K. (1980). Sexual transmission of hepatitis A in homosexual men. *N Engl J Med, 302,* 435–438.

Coutinho, R.A., Albrecht-van Lent, P., Lelie, N., Nagelkerke, N., Kuipers, H., & Rijsdijk, T. (1983). Prevalence and incidence of hepatitis A among male homosexuals. *Br Med J (Clin Res), 287,* 1743–1745.

Crouse, B.J., Nichol, K., Peterson, D.C., & Grimm, M.B. (1994). Hospital-based strategies for improving influenza vaccination rates. *J Fam Pract, 38,* 258–261.

Davidson, M., & Krugman, S. (1986). Recombinant yeast hepatitis B vaccine compared with plasma-derived vaccine: Immunogenicity and effect of a booster dose. *J Infect, 13*(Suppl. A), 31–38.

Decker, M.D., Vaughn, W.K., Brodie, J.S., Hutcheson, R.H., Jr., & Schaffner, W. (1984). Seroepidemiology of hepatitis B in Tennessee prisoners. *J Infect Dis, 150,* 450–459.

Des Jarlais, D.C., Diaz, T., Perlis, T., Vlahov, D., Maslow, C., Latka, M., et al (2003). Variability in the incidence of human immunodeficiency virus, hepatitis B virus, and hepatitis C virus infection among young injecting drug users in New York City. *Am J Epidemiol, 157*, 467–471.

Des Jarlais, D.C., Perlis, T., Arasteh, K., Torian, L.V., Hagan, H., Beatrice, S., et al. (2005). Reductions in hepatitis C virus and HIV infections among injecting drug users in New York City, 1990–2001. *AIDS, 19*(Suppl. 3), S20–S25.

Diaz, T., Des Jarlais, D.C., Vlahov, D., et al. (2001). Factors associated with prevalent hepatitis C: Differences among young adult injection drug users in lower and upper Manhattan, New York City. *Am J Public Health, 91*, 23–30.

Fiore, A.E., Wasley, A., & Bell, B.P. (2006). Prevention of hepatitis A through active or passive immunization: Recommendations of the Advisory Committee on Immunization Practices (ACIP). *MMWR, 55*(No. RR-7), 1–23.

Fried, M.W., Shiffman, M.L., Reddy, K.R., et al. (2002). Peginterferon alfa-2a plus ribavirin for chronic hepatitis C virus infection. *N Engl J Med, 347*, 975–982.

Gaiter, J., & Doll, L.S. (1996). Editorial: Improving HIV/AIDS prevention in prisons is good public health policy. *Am J Public Health, 86*, 1201–1203.

Gao, B. (2002). Interaction of alcohol and hepatitis viral proteins: Implication in synergistic effect of alcohol drinking and viral hepatitis on liver injury. *Alcohol, 27*, 69–72.

Garfein, R.S., Doherty, M.C., Monterroso, E.R., Thomas, D.L., Nelson, K.E., & Vlahov, D. (1998). Prevalence and incidence of hepatitis C virus infection among young adult injection drug users. *J Acquir Immune Defic Syndr Hum Retrovirol, 18*(Suppl. 1), S11–S19.

Garfein, R.S., Vlahov, D., Galai, N., Doherty, M.C., & Nelson, K.E. (1996). Viral infections in short-term injection drug users: The prevalence of the hepatitis C, hepatitis B, human immunodeficiency, and human T-lymphotropic viruses. *Am J Public Health, 86*, 655–661.

Garfein, R.S., Williams, I.T., Monterroso, E.R., Valverde, R., & Swartzendruber, A. (2000). HCV, HBV and HIV infections among young, street-recruited injection drug users (IDUs): The collaborative injection drug users study (CIDUS II) [Abstract 115]. *10th International Symposium on Viral Hepatitis and Liver Disease, Atlanta.*

Gershon, R.R., Karkashian, C.D., Vlahov, D., et al. (1999). Compliance with universal precautions in correctional health care facilities. *J Occup Environ Med, 41*, 181–189.

Glanz, K., Saraiya, M., & Wechsler, H. (2002). Guidelines for school programs to prevent skin cancer. *MMWR, 51*(No. RR-4), 1–18.

Glaser, J.B., & Greifinger, R.B. (1993). Correctional health care: A public health opportunity. *Ann Intern Med,118*, 139–145.

Glikson, M., Galun, E., Oren, R., Tur-Kaspa, R., & Shouval, D. (1992). Relapsing hepatitis: Review of 14 cases and literature survey. *Medicine, 71*, 14–17.

Goldstein, S.T., Alter, M.J., Williams, I.T., et al (2002). Incidence and risk factors for acute hepatitis B in the United States, 1982–1998: Implications for vaccination programs. *J Infect Dis, 185*, 713–719.

Hagan, H., McGough, J.P., Thiede, H., Weiss, N.S., Hopkins, S., & Alexander, E.R. (1999). Syringe exchange and risk of infection with hepatitis B and C viruses. *Am J Epidemiol, 149*, 203–213.

Hagan, H., Thiede, H., Weiss, N.S., Hopkins, S.G., Duchin, J.S., & Alexander, E.R. (2001). Sharing of drug preparation equipment as a risk factor for hepatitis C. *Am J Public Health, 91*, 42–46.

Hahn, J.A., Page-Shafer, K., Lum, P.J., Bourgois, P., Stein, E., Evans, J.L. et al. (2002). Hepatitis C virus seroconversion among young injection drug users: Relationships and risks. *J Infect Dis, 186*, 1558–1564.

Heimer, R., Khoshnood, K., Jariwala-Freeman, B., Duncan, B., & Harima, Y. (1996). Hepatitis in used syringes: The limits of sensitivity of techniques to detect hepatitis B virus (HBV) DNA, hepatitis C virus (HCV) RNA, and antibodies to HBV core and HCV antigens. *J Infect Dis*, *173*, 997–1000.

Hennessey, K.A., Kim, A., Wolf, C., Griffin, V., Tablan, N., Weinbaum, C.W., & Sabin, K. (2006). Prevalence of hepatitis B and hepatitis C virus infections, and HIV co-infection in three jails. *7th Annual Inside Out Summit, CenterForce, San Francisco.*

Henning, K.J., Bell, E., Braun, J., & Barker, N. (1995). A community-wide outbreak of hepatitis A: Risk factors for infection among homosexual and bisexual men. *Am J Med*, *99*, 132–136.

Hessl, S.M. (2001). Police and corrections. *Occup Med*,*16*, 39–49.

Hoofnagle, J.H. (2006). Hepatitis B—preventable and now treatable. *N Engl J Med*, *354*, 1074–1076.

Hoxie, N.J., Vergeront, J.M., Frisby, H.R., Pfister, J.R., Golubjatnikov, R., & Davis, J.P. (1990). HIV seroprevalence and the acceptance of voluntary HIV testing among newly incarcerated male prison inmates in Wisconson. *Am J Public Health*, *80*, 1129–1131.

Hull, H.F., Lyons, L.H., Mann, J.M., Hadler, S.C., Steece, R., & Skeels, M.R. (1985). Incidence of hepatitis B in the penitentiary of New Mexico. *Am J Public Health*, *75*, 1213–1214.

Hutin, Y.J., Bell, B.P., Marshall, K.L., et al. (1999). Identifying target groups for a potential vaccination program during a hepatitis A communitywide outbreak. *Am J Public Health*, *89*, 918–921.

Hutin, Y.J., Sabin, K.M., Hutwagner, L.C., et al. (1999). Multiple modes of hepatitis A virus transmission among methamphetamine users. *Am J Epidemiol*, *152*, 186–192.

Jemmott, J.B., III, Jemmott, L.S., & Fong, G.T. (1992). Reductions in HIV risk-associated sexual behaviors among black male adolescents: Effects of an AIDS prevention intervention. *Am J Public Health*, *82*, 372–377.

Jilg, W., & Deinhardt, F. (1986). Results of immunisation with a recombinant yeast-derived hepatitis B vaccine. *J Infect*, *13*(Suppl. A), 47–51.

Kahn, R.H., Scholl, D.T., Shane, S.M., Lemoine, A.L., & Farley, T.A. (2002). Screening for syphilis in arrestees: Usefulness for community-wide syphilis surveillance and control. *Sex Transm Dis*, *29*, 150–156.

Katz, M.H., Hsu, L., Wong, E., Liska, S., Anderson, L., & Janssen, R.S. (1997). Seroprevalence of and risk factors for hepatitis A infection among young homosexual and bisexual men. *J Infect Dis*, *175*, 1225–1229.

Kaufman, M.L., Faiver, K.L., & Harness, J.K. (1983). Hepatitis B markers among Michigan prisoners [Letter]. *Ann Intern Med*, *98*, 558.

Kennedy, S., Kuck, S., & Nortan, G. (2006). Testing for infectious disease in prisons and large jails: Results of findings from the 10th NIJ/CDC survey of infectious diseases in correctional facilities. Poster at National Conference on Correctional Health Care, Atlanta.

Khan, A.J., Simard, E.P., Bower, W.A., et al. (2005). Ongoing transmission of hepatitis B virus infection among inmates at a state correctional facility. *Am J Public Health*, *95*, 1793–1799.

Khan, A., Simard, E., Wurtzel, H., et al. (2002). The prevalence, risk factors, and incidence of hepatitis B virus infection among inmates in a state correctional facility [Abstract]. *Program and abstracts of the 130th Annual Meeting of the American Public Health Association, Philadelphia.*

Koester, S.K., & Hoffer, L. (1994). "Indirect sharing": Additional HIV risks associated with drug injection. *AIDS & Public Policy Journal*, *9*, 100–105.

Koff, R.S., & Dienstag, J.L. (1995). Extrahepatic manifestations of hepatitis C and the association with alcoholic liver disease. *Semin Liver Dis*, *15*, 101–109.

Koplan, J.P., Walker, J.A., & Bryan, J.A. (1978). Prevalence of hepatitis B surface antigen and antibody at a state prison in Kansas. *J Infect Dis*, *137*, 505–506.

Lee, W.M. (1997). Hepatitis B virus infection. *N Engl J Med*, *337*, 1733–1745.

Lofgren, R.P., Paul, J.M., Kefalos, S.G., & Nichol, K.L. (1990). A multifaceted influenza vaccination program can be exported successfully to a different clinical site. *Clin Res*, *38*, 864A.

Lok, A.S., & McMahon, B.J. (2001). Chronic hepatitis B. *Hepatology*, *34*, 1225–1241.

López-Zetina, J., Kerndt, P., Ford, W., Woerhle, T., & Weber, M. (2001). Prevalence of HIV and hepatitis B and self-reported injection risk behavior during detention among street-recruited injection drug users in Los Angeles County, 1994–1996. *Addiction, 96*, 589–595.

Lorvick, J., Kral, A.H., Seal, K.,Gee, L., & Edlin, B.R. (2001). Prevalence and duration of hepatitis C among injection drug users in San Francisco, Calif. *Am J Public Health, 91*, 46–47.

Macalino, G.E., Salas, C.M., Towe, C.W., et al. (1999). Incidence and community prevalence of HIV and other blood borne pathogens among incarcerated women in Rhode Island [Abstract]. *National HIV Prevention Conference, Atlanta*.

Magura, S., Kang, S.Y., & Shapiro, J.L. (1994). Outcomes of intensive AIDS education for male adolescent drug users in jail. *J Adolesc Health*, *15*, 457–463.

Margolis, H.S., Alter, M.J., & Hadler, S.C. (1991). Hepatitis B: Evolving epidemiology and implications for control. *Semin Liver Dis*, *11*, 84–92.

Mast, E.E., Williams, I.T., Alter, M.J., & Margolis, H.S. (1998). Hepatitis B vaccination of adolescent and adult high-risk groups in the United States. *Vaccine*, *16*, S27–S29.

McMahon, B.J. (1997). Hepatocellular carcinoma and viral hepatitis. In R. A. Willson (Ed.), *Viral hepatitis: Diagnosis, treatment, prevention* (pp. 315–330). New York: Dekker.

McMahon, B.J., Holck, P., Bulkow, L., & Snowball, M. (2001). Serologic and clinical outcomes of 1536 Alaska Natives chronically infected with hepatitis B virus. *Ann Intern Med*, *135*, 759–768.

McQuillan, G.M., Coleman, P., Kruszon-Moran, D., Moyer, L.A., Lambert, S.B., & Margolis, H.S. (1999). Prevalence of hepatitis B virus infection in the United States: The National Health and Nutrition Examination Surveys, 1976 through 1994. *Am J Public Health*, *89*, 14–18.

Merkel, P.A., & Caputo, G.C. (1994). Evaluation of a simple office-based strategy for increasing influenza vaccine administration and the effect of differing reimbursement plans on the patient acceptance rate. *J Gen Intern Med*, *9*, 679–683.

Monto, A., & Wright, T.L. (2001). The epidemiology and prevention of hepatocellular carcinoma. *Semin Oncol*, *28*, 441–449.

Moran, W.P., Nelson, K., Wofford, J.L., Velez, R., & Case, L.D. (2000). Increasing influenza immunization among high-risk patients: Education or financial incentive? *Am J Med*, *101*, 612–620.

Moses, M., Potter, R.H., Hammett, T., Kennedy, S., & Kuck, S. (2007). National survey of infectious diseases in correctional facilities; hepatitis A, B and C, screening, treatment and education. Unpublished data.

Mumola, C.J., & Karberg, J.C. (2006). Drug use and dependence, state and federal prisoners, 2004. Bureau of Justice Statistics Special Report. Washington, DC: US Department of Justice, Office of Justice Programs. Publication No. NCJ 213530.

Murrill, C.S., Weeks, H., Castrucci, B.C., et al. (2002). Age-specific seroprevalence of HIV, hepatitis B virus, and hepatitis C virus infection among injection drug users admitted to drug treatment in 6 US cities. *Am J Public Health*, *92*, 385–387.

Nacci, P.L., & Kane, T.R. (1983). The incidence of sex and sexual aggression in federal prisons. *Federal Probation*, *47*, 31–36.

National Commission on Correctional Health Care. Third party reimbursement for correctional health care. Chicago, IL: National Commission on Correctional Health Care, 1993. Available at http://www.ncchc.org/oldsite/statements/reimbursement.html.

National Commission on Correctional Health Care. (2002). *Health status of soon-to-be-released inmates: A report to Congress*. Vol 1. Washington, DC: Author.

National Institutes of Health. (1997). Management of hepatitis C. *NIH Consensus Statement*, *15*, 1–41.

Noell, J., Rohde, P., Ochs, L., et al. (2001). Incidence and prevalence of chlamydia, herpes, and viral hepatitis in a homeless adolescent population. *Sex Transm Dis*, *28*, 4–10.

Ockenga, J., Tillmann, H.L., Trautwein, C., Stoll, M., Manns, M.P., & Schmidt, R.E. (1997). Hepatitis B and C in HIV-infected patients: Prevalence and prognostic value. *J Hepatol*, *27*, 18–24.

Peters, C.J., Purcell, R.H., Lander, J.J., & Johnson, K.M. (1976). Radioimmunoassay for antibody to hepatitis B surface antigen shows transmission of hepatitis B virus among household contacts. *J Infect Dis*, *134*, 218–223.

Pisu, M., Meltzer, M.I., & Lyerla, R. (2002). Cost-effectiveness of hepatitis B vaccination of prison inmates. *Vaccine*, *21*, 312–321.

Poynard, T., Bedossa, P., & Opolon, P. (1997). Natural history of liver fibrosis progression in patients with chronic hepatitis C. *Lancet*, *349*, 825–832.

Rich, J., Holmes, L., Salas, C., et al. (2001). Successful linkage of medical care and community services for HIV-positive offenders being released from prison. *J Urban Health*, *78*, 279–289.

Rizzetto, M. (1983). The delta agent. *Hepatology*, *3*, 729–737.

Ruiz, J.D., Molitor, F., Sun, R.K., et al. (1999). Prevalence and correlates of hepatitis C virus infection among inmates entering the California correctional system. *West J Med*, *170*, 156–160.

Samuel, M.C., Doherty, P.M., Bulterys, M., & Jenison, S.A. (2001). Association between heroin use, needle sharing and tattoos received in prison with hepatitis B and C positivity among street-recruited injecting drug users in New Mexico, USA. *Epidemiol Infect*, *127*, 475–484.

Saum, C.A., Surratt, H., Inciardi, J.A., & Bennett, R.E. (1995). Sex in prison: Exploring the myths and realities. *The Prison Journal*, *75*, 413–430.

Silberstein, G., Coles, F.B., Greenberg, A., Singer, L., & Voigt, R. (2000). Effectiveness and cost-benefit of enhancements to a syphilis screening and treatment program at a county jail. *Sex Transm Dis*, *27*, 508–517.

Smith, D.A. (1986). Hepatitis B in a general psychiatric hospital [Letter]. *N Engl J Med*, *314*, 1255–1256.

Smith, P.F., Mikl, J., Truman, B.I., et al. (1991). HIV infection among women entering the New York state correctional system. *Am J Public Health*, *81*(Suppl. 1), 35–40.

Snyder, H.N., & Sickmund, M. (2006). *Juvenile offenders and victims: 2006 national report*. Washington, DC: US Department of Justice, Office of Justice Programs, Office of Juvenile Justice and Delinquency Prevention.

Solomon, L., Flynn, C., Muck, K., & Vertefeuille, J. (2004). Prevalence of HIV, syphilis, hepatitis B, and hepatitis C among entrants to Maryland correctional facilities. *J Urban Health*, *81*, 25–37.

Soriano, V., Bravo, R., Garcia-Samaniego, J., et al. (1994). CD4+ T-lymphocytopenia in HIV-infected patients receiving interferon therapy for chronic hepatitis C. HIV–Hepatitis Spanish Study Group. *AIDS*, *8*, 1621–1622.

Soriano, V., Garcia-Samaniego, J., Bravo, R., et al. (1996). Interferon a for the treatment of chronic hepatitis C in patients infected with human immunodeficiency virus. Hepatitis–HIV Spanish Study Group. *Clin Infect Dis*, *23*, 585–591.

Spaulding, A., Greene, C., Davidson, K., Schneidermann, M., & Rich, J. (1999). Hepatitis C in state correctional facilities. *Prev Med*, *28*, 92–100.

Spaulding, A.C., Weinbaum, C.M., Lau, D.T., et al. (2006). A framework for management of hepatitis C in prisons. *Ann Intern Med*, *144*, 762–769.

Stephan, J.J. (1997). *Census of state and federal correctional facilities, 1995. Bureau of Justice Statistics executive summary*. Washington, DC: U.S. Department of Justice, Office of Justice Programs. Publication No. NCJ-166582.

Stephenson, B., Wohl, D., Kiziah, N., et al. (2000). Release from prison is associated with increased HIV RNA at time of re-incarceration [Abstract]. *XIII International AIDS Conference, Durban, South Africa.*

Stevens, C.E., Toy, P.T., Tong, M.J., et al. (1985). Perinatal hepatitis B virus transmission in the United States: Prevention by passive-active immunization. *JAMA, 253,* 1740–1745.

Stokes, M.L., Ferson, M.J., & Young, L.C. (1997). Outbreak of hepatitis A among homosexual men in Sydney. *Am J Public Health, 87,* 2039–2041.

Sulkowski, M.S., Mast, E.E., Seeff, L.B., & Thomas, D.L. (2000). Hepatitis C virus infection as an opportunistic disease in persons infected with human immunodeficiency virus. *Clin Infect Dis, 30*(Suppl. 1), S77–S84.

Tewksbury, R. (1989). Measures of sexual behavior in an Ohio prison. *Sociol Soc Res, 74,* 34–39.

Thomas, A.R., Keene, W.E., & Cieslak, P.R. (2005). Seroprevalence of hepatitis B and C in juvenile detention entrants, Oregon, 1994–1996. *J Adolesc Health, 37,* 410–413.

Thomas, D.L., Vlahov, D., Solomon, L., Cohn, S., Taylor, E., Garfein, R., et al. (1995). Correlates of hepatitis C virus infections among injection drug users. *Medicine (Baltimore), 74,* 212–220.

Thorpe, L.E., Ouellet, L.J., Hershow, R., Bailey, S.L., Williams, I.T., Williamson, J., et al. (2002). Risk of hepatitis C virus infection among young adult injection drug users who share injection equipment. *Am J Epidemiol, 155,* 645–653.

Thorpe, L.E., Ouellet, L.J., Levy, J.R., Williams, I.T., & Monterroso, E.R. (2000). Hepatitis C virus infection: Prevalence, risk factors, and prevention opportunities among young injection drug users in Chicago, 1997–1999. *J Infect Dis, 182,* 1588–1594.

Tucker, R.M., Gaffey, M.J., Fisch, M.J., Kaiser, D.L., Guerrant, R.L., & Normansell, D.E. (1987). Seroepidemiology of hepatitis D (delta agent) and hepatitis B among Virginia state prisoners. *Clin Ther, 9,* 622–628.

Van Beneden, C., Hedberg, K., Zimmerman, P., Gutelius-Johnson, M., Terry, J., & Fleming, D. (1998). Epidemic hepatitis A among illicit drug users in Oregon: Evidence for adult-to-adult transmission [Abstract]. *Program and abstracts of the 1st International Conference on Emerging Infectious Diseases.* Atlanta: American Society for Microbiology.

Vento, S., Garofano, T., Renzini, C., et al. (1998). Fulminant hepatitis associated with hepatitis A virus superinfection in patients with chronic hepatitis C. *N Engl J Med, 338,* 286–290.

Vlahov, D., Nelson, K.E., Quinn, T.C., & Kendig, N. (1993). Prevalence and incidence of hepatitis C virus infection among male prison inmates in Maryland. *Eur J Epidemiol, 9,* 566–569.

Wasley, A., Samandari, T., & Bell, B.P. (2005). Incidence of hepatitis A in the United States in the era of vaccination. *JAMA, 294,* 194–201.

Weinbaum, C., Lyerla, R., & Margolis, H.S. (2003). Prevention and control of infections with hepatitis viruses in correctional settings. Centers for Disease Control and Prevention. *MMWR Recomm Rep, 52,* 1–36.

Williams, I., Boaz, K., Openo, K., et al. (2005). Missed opportunities for hepatitis B vaccination in correctional settings, sexually transmitted disease (STD) clinics, and drug treatment programs. *Annual Meeting of the Infectious Disease Society of America, San Francisco.*

Williams, I.T., Fleenor, M., Judson, F., et al. (2000). Risk factors for hepatitis C virus (HCV) transmission in the USA: 1991–1998 [Abstract 114]. *10th International Symposium on Viral Hepatitis and Liver Disease, Atlanta.*

Wilson, D.J. (2000). *Drug use, testing, and treatment in jails. Bureau of Justice Statistics special report.* Washington, DC: U.S. Department of Justice, Office of Justice Programs. Publication No. NCJ 179999.

Zarski, J.P., Bohn, B., Bastie, A., et al. (1998). Characteristics of patients with dual infection by hepatitis B and C viruses. *J Hepatol*, *28*, 27–33.

Zimmerman, S.E., Martin, R., & Vlahov, D. (1991). AIDS knowledge and risk perceptions among Pennsylvania prisoners. *J Crim Justice*, *19*, 239–256.

Chapter 10

HIV Prevention: Behavioral Interventions in Correctional Settings

Barry Zack

To date, preventive care and prevention services have not been included in our conceptualization or operationalization of prisoners' "right to health care." Given the potential public health impact of focusing on prevention for prisoners, however, the time has come to examine this issue. Although not specifically a right under the Constitution, correctional systems should be obligated to offer comprehensive HIV prevention services to those in custody. The justification for this obligation, at a minimum, has to do with some of the basic tenants of public health disease control: target your prevention dollars on illnesses with high morbidity and mortality rates among populations with the highest rates and whom you can access.

With the prevalence of HIV at least five times higher among the incarcerated compared to those who are not incarcerated, providing effective prevention programs would have a powerful impact on incidence rates in this population. Furthermore, in one well-referenced study, in 1997, 25% of all HIV-positive people in the United States reportedly serve some time in a correctional facility (Hammett et al., 2002) and 90% of prisoners, representing an estimated 7.5 million prisoners annually, return to the free community at some point (Bureau of Justice Statistics Correctional Surveys, 1996). As approximately 51.8% of those individuals are reincarcerated within 3 years (Bureau of Justice Statistics Correctional Surveys, 1996), it is clear that providing effective disease prevention programs to those who are incarcerated would not only help protect them, but would also likely have a synergistic impact on HIV rates in our communities. If departments of corrections were to adopt evidence-based prevention measures, prisoners would simultaneously be returning from incarceration less likely to be infected with HIV and armed with the knowledge and skills to play an important role in reversing the current epidemic trends. This role includes protecting themselves and their loved ones by reducing their own risk behaviors and protecting their communities by educating others and changing norms.

Background

Since its discovery in the early 1980s, more than 25 million people have died worldwide of HIV/AIDS, including more than 500,000 in the United States (World Health Organization, 2005; Centers for Disease Control and Prevention,

2006a). Geographically, this disease has levied its toll most heavily in sub-Saharan Africa. However, in almost every corner of the world, HIV has infiltrated the poorest communities and/or those with the least political power to the greatest degree.

In the United States, HIV/AIDS initially emerged most extensively in the largely white, gay/MSM (men who have sex with other men and do not identify as gay or bisexual) communities of New York City, Los Angeles, and San Francisco. Overall, MSM account for 54% of the cumulative AIDS diagnoses since the start of the epidemic and are estimated to be currently acquiring 45% of incident cases (Centers for Disease Control and Prevention, 2004, 2006c). However, HIV has long since penetrated non-white, gay/MSM communities and is now characterized more by the race and ethnicity of those it has infected than by any single behavior. Although African Americans represent 13% of the U.S. population, they accounted for 51% of newly diagnosed cases of HIV in 2001–2004, resulting in rates 8.5 times higher than for whites. Also at disproportionate risk, Hispanics are infected with HIV at rates 3.3 times higher than for whites (Centers for Disease Control and Prevention, 2006a). The estimated rate of HIV and AIDS among African-American women in 2005 was nearly 24 times and 4 times, respectively, that of white and Hispanic women (Centers for Disease Control and Prevention, 2006d).

The most current information suggests that African-American men who are diagnosed with AIDS are more likely to have been infected by male–male sex than by other behaviors (accounting for 46% of cases compared to 25% and 23%, respectively, for IV drug use and heterosexual sex)(Centers for Disease Control and Prevention, 2006b). Like their male counterparts, African-American women most often contract HIV from their male sexual partners (with heterosexual contact representing 72% of diagnosed AIDS cases among black women in 2003) (Centers for Disease Control and Prevention, 2006b).

In recent years, there has been a great deal of speculation in the scientific as well as lay press suggesting that women are disproportionately burdened with HIV and AIDS as a result of their parterships with currently and formerly incarcerated men (Johnson, 2006). In addition to any contribution that recently released men may make to the HIV epidemics in their communities, there is also the indirect effect of sentencing laws and other policies which disproportionately incarcerate those engaging in behaviors that are associated with both crime and HIV risk (injection drug use and sex work). With so many men in these communities incarcerated, the result of these policies is likely a decreased "pool" of eligible partners thus creating a smaller sexual and drug network and, consequently, a greater opportunity for disease transmission in these communities.

In-Prison Risk

Although less frequent than risk behaviors in the community, in-prison risk behaviors (including sex, use of intravenous drugs, and tattooing) may place the prison population at greater risk for contracting HIV. Compounding the risk inherent in any act that may expose a person to the blood and/or semen/vaginal fluid of another is the fact that in prison, the person to whom one is being exposed is more likely to be infected with HIV, simply due to the higher prevalence rates both among prisoners and in the communities from which the majority of prisoners emerge. With 21% of state prisoners incarcerated for drug-related crimes (Bureau of Justice Statistics, 2000) and the incarceration of a disproportionate number of African Americans, it is not surprising that AIDS and HIV affects state prisoners at rates that are approximately 3 times and 10 times greater, respectively, than the U.S. population as a whole (Hammett et al., 1999; Bureau of Justice Statistics, 2004; Maruschack, 2005). Two percent and 1.1% of state and federal prisoners, respectively, are estimated to be infected with HIV (Hammett et al., 1999; Bureau of Justice Statistics, 2004). Regionally, prison populations in the Northeast have a much higher prevalence of HIV (4.5%) than in other areas of the country (Midwest 1.0%; South 2.2%; West 0.7%)(Bureau of Justice Statistics, 2004).

Regardless of the efforts to prevent sexual activity and drug use inside our prisons and jails, sex and drugs (including intravenous drug paraphernalia) as well as tattooing occur every day in these institutions. Estimates of the percentage of the incarcerated population that engages in sexual activity range from 2 to 65% (Krebs, 2002; Weinbaum et al., 2005). Types of sexual interactions range from romantic, consensual relationships to violent acts of power/domination and rape, and everything in-between. In 2005, there were 2.83 allegations of sexual violence reported to the department of corrections per every 1000 prisoners. More than half of these involved staff (Beck & Harrison, 2005). When including events that are officially reported and those that are not, studies have found that 3–28% of prisoners are sexually assaulted at least once while inside (Krebs & Simmons, 2002) and that 7–12% of male respondents report being raped an average of nine times while doing time (Robertson, 2003).

If a sexual or needle-sharing partner is infected with HIV, the risk of acquisition is greatly reduced by the use of condoms or sterile syringes and/or cleaning needles with bleach. Despite the fact that the WHO and UNAIDS recommend that condoms, bleach, and, possibly, needle exchange programs be made available to prisoners, these items are classified as contraband in most U.S. correctional facilities (Hammett et al., 1999) and therefore are not often used as methods of HIV prevention.

The Evidence for Educational and Behavioral Interventions

Despite the longstanding recognized need for both primary and secondary HIV prevention within the prison system, there have been few quantitative evaluations of HIV prevention interventions with incarcerated populations. In 2006, Bryan and colleagues reviewed this literature and, although the authors did not list their search criteria, they found a total of seven studies published since 1991, only four of which were found to be effective (El-Bassel et al., 1995; Grinstead et al., 1997; St Lawrence et al., 1997; Grinstead, Zack, Faigeles, et al., 2001). In evaluating the quality of these seven studies, the authors used the following criteria: (a) whether it was "a randomized controlled design that compared a theoretically guided HIV prevention intervention to an attention-placebo intervention or standard-of-care control"; (b) the genders included; (c) whether constructs and outcomes were measured immediately prior to the intervention, immediately after the intervention, and a final assessment of behavior after release; (d) and whether the intervention measured constructs that are theoretically and empirically related, and proximal, to HIV prevention behavior. Based on these criteria, the authors came to the following conclusions:

1. Due to the constraints of "working within the corrections systems, only one of the interventions to date (Baxter S. 1991) (which was not found to be effective) has met [the] stringent design requirements";
2. Despite the "disproportionate number of men who are incarcerated as compared to women," only one of the interventions was exclusively among men (Grinstead, et al., 1997);
3. None of the studies collected measures at all of the desired time-points;
4. "Only half of the interventions reviewed assessed changes in intentions, and none specifically asked about post-release intentions" (Grinstead et al., 1997; St Lawrence et al., 1997; West, 2000).

In addition to this literature review of four effective interventions and three interventions with negative findings, Bryan, Ruiz, and O'Neill (2006) also wrote of their own study that influenced beliefs and intentions related to condom use. There are at least four additional published prevention interventions that have shown significant effects (Grinstead et al., 1999b; Bauserman et al., 2001; Ross, Scott, McCann, & Kelley, 2006; Wolitski, 2006) resulting in a total of nine known effective HIV prevention interventions involving prisoners (see Table 10.1). Only one of these interventions was limited to HIV-positive participants (Grinstead, Zack, Faigeles, 2001; Zack et al., 2004). Interventions that were not included in the Bryan et al. (2006) review are highlighted in gray in the table.

In-Prison and Jail Interventions Showing Effect on Postrelease Risk Behavior

Four (El-Bassel et al., 1995; Grinstead, Zack, et al., 1999b; Grinstead, Zack, Faigeles, et al., 2001; Wolitski, 2006) of the nine effective interventions found significant reductions in postrelease HIV risk behavior. These four interventions were equally divided in terms of the format of the interventions, with two providing group sessions and two providing interventions with individuals and centered on the clients' specific challenges, barriers, and concerns. Furthermore, these four interventions were consistent neither in their theoretical approach nor in the amount of "dose" provided, ranging from one 30-minute prerelease session (Grinstead, Zack, et al., 1999b) to 16 sessions lasting 2 hours each (El-Bassel et al., 1995). Three of the four interventions were facilitated by professionals and one by HIV-positive peers and most intervened with participants only during the prerelease period. All four of these interventions were gender-specific and only one included women.

It is important to note that the two individual-level interventions that showed reductions in risk behavior were not exclusively disease or health focused, but emphasized individualized planning for housing, employment

Table 10.1 Behavioral HIV prevention interventions for incarcerated adults with evidence of effectiveness.

Study	N	HIV status	Age	Other participant characteristics	Intervention	Length and location	Delivery	Deliverer	Evaluation design	Outcomes
					Interventions that measured postrelease risk behavior					
El-Bassel et al. (1995)	145	HIV–?	33	Women drug users (within 10 weeks of release)	Skills building and social support enhancement (SS) vs. HIV/AIDS information (AI)	16 sessions, 2 hr/session (SS) vs. 3 sessions, 2hr/session (AI) (all prerelease)	Group	Experienced facilitators with ethnic similarity	Randomized, compared 2 groups 1 month postrelease	No difference between SS and AI in AIDS knowledge, perceived vulnerability to HIV/AIDS, and sexual self-efficacy; SS group had significantly more use of coping skills, emotional support, and safer sex behavior (consistent condom use or abstinence) than AI group
Grinstead, Zack, et al. (1999b)	178	HIV–?	36	Men	Individualized risk assessment and development of a postrelease risk reduction plan	1 session, 30 min; prerelease	Individual	HIV-positive peers	RCT, follow-up surveys completed with 43% of 414 total participants	Men who received intervention were more likely to use a condom the first time they had sex after release and were less likely to use drugs, inject drugs, or share needles within 2 weeks of release
Grinstead, Zack, Faigeles et al. (2001)	123	HIV+	38	Men (within 6 months of release)	HIV information, HIV treatment, HIV and sex, substance use, nutrition, and community service referrals	8 sessions, 2 hr/session (all prerelease)	Group	Community service providers	Compared men who volunteered for the program AND attended (intervention) vs. men who volunteered but were not able to attend due to scheduling problems or transfer (comparison); evaluated at preintervention, postintervention, and 1 month following release	Intervention participants were: more likely to have used a condom the first time they had sex postrelease (81% vs. 68%); less likely to have injected drugs (46% vs. 67%); among those who injected drugs, less likely to have shared injection equipment (6% vs. 25%). All participants reported difficulty obtaining health care and meds after release

Study	N	HIV	Age	Population	Intervention	Sessions	Individual/Group	Interventionists	Design	Significant differences
Wolitski (2006)	522	HIV–	18–29	Men (within 14–16 days of release)	HIV, hepatitis, and other STI education only vs. HIV, hepatitis, and other STI education (comparison) + transitional interventions bridging incarceration and community reentry (e.g., housing, employment) (intervention); both interventions used prevention case management, motivational interviewing, and harm reduction	1 session (prerelease), 60–90 min vs. 6 sessions (2 prerelease and 4 at 1, 3, 6, and 12 weeks postrelease)	Individual		Systematically assigned to the prerelease single session or the pre/postrelease enhanced	Significant differences between the groups were observed at the 24-week assessment (12 weeks after last intervention): the intervention group was significantly less likely to report unprotected intercourse (vaginal or anal) during their most recent sexual encounter. They were also less likely to report any unprotected sex in the reporting period. The observed effects were explained by differences in unprotected intercourse with main, but not nonmain, partners
Interventions that only measured constructs known to be associated with reduced risk behavior										
St Lawrence et al. (1997)	90	HIV–?	32	Women	Social Cognitive Theory vs. Theory of Gender and Power	6 sessions; 90 min/session (all prerelease)	Group	Same gender facilitators	RCT. Baseline assessment, second assessment immediately after intervention, third assessment 6 months after intervention and still inside	Both groups showed increases in self-efficacy, self-esteem, Attitudes Towards Prevention scale scores, AIDS knowledge, communication skills, and condom application skills
Grinstead et al. (1997)	2295	HIV–?	32	Men	HIV education, perceived risk for HIV, intentions to engage in HIV risk behavior	1 session (inside at entry)	Group	Peer vs. professional educators	Randomly assigned to peer-led or professional educator-led or no-treatment control group	Both interventions outperformed control in intention to use condoms and being tested for HIV, and the peer intervention was preferred by participants compared to the intervention led by professional educators

(continued)

Table 10.1 (continued)

Study	N	HIV status	Age	Other participant characteristics	Intervention	Length and location	Delivery	Deliverer	Evaluation design	Outcomes

Interventions that only measured constructs known to be associated with reduced risk behavior

Study	N	HIV status	Age	Other participant characteristics	Intervention	Length and location	Delivery	Deliverer	Evaluation design	Outcomes
Bauserman et al. (2001)	745	HIV–?	32	50% men and 50% women (within 6 months of release)	Prevention Case Management; AIDS Risk Reduction Model (AARM), Health Belief Model (HBM), Social Cognitive Theory (SCT), Information, Motivation, Behavior (IMB)	9 sessions; 11 hr total (all pre-release)	Individual + small group	Staff from local health departments	Pre-Post	Significant changes in condom attitudes, self-efficacy for condom use, for injection drug use risk, and for other substance use risk, and in intentions to practice safer sex post release
Bryan et al. (2006)	196	HIV–?	60% 20–35	90% men and 10% women	Social Cognitive Theory, Health Belief Model, cultural sensitivity, and problem solving	6 sessions, 1x/week, 90 min/ session (all prerelease)	Group	Peers	Pre-Post	Influenced beliefs and behaviors related to peer education and influenced beliefs and intentions related to condom use
Ross et al. (2006)	257	97% HIV–	34–43	84% men and 16% women	Stages of Change	5 sessions; 40 hr total (all inside)	Group	Reps from CBOs	Pre-Post	Total knowledge scale significantly improved; a significantly lower proportion of peer educators reported never having had an HIV test at follow-up compared with baseline.

and education within the context of disease prevention (Grinstead, Zack, et al., 1999b; Wolitski, 2006). Most recently, Wolitski (2006) showed a significant difference in risk behavior at 6 months postrelease as a result of an intervention based on prevention case management, in which the participant and intervention staff created an individualized prevention plan for the postrelease period. Myers, Kramer, Gardner, Rucobo, and Costa-Taylor (2005) also documented that pre- and postrelease case management support can facilitate healthy behaviors.

Interventions Showing Effect on Knowledge, Attitudes, and Beliefs Related to Risk Behavior

Although utilizing different theoretical approaches, five interventions to date have shown that prevention education efforts can impact attitudes, self-efficacy, and intentions among incarcerated individuals (Grinstead et al., 1997; St Lawrence et al., 1997; Bauserman et al., 2001; Bryan et al., 2006; Ross et al., 2006). All five of these interventions intervened, at least in part, in a group setting, but there are no other commonalities. The combinations of genders differ across the interventions, the deliverer of the interventions varied, and the range of dose provided by each intervention is wide, from one to nine sessions.

Despite the variety of approaches, this evidence suggests that both HIV-related risk behavior and factors known to be related to these risk behaviors can be reduced as a result of intervention in these populations. Furthermore, though far from conclusive, there is evidence that prevention programs should not be "disease specific," but rather should focus on multiple health issues and the factors that directly impact prisoners' ability to enact prevention behaviors on the outside. In other words, comprehensiveness increases effectiveness.

Other than the published data, there are numerous community-based organizations, departments of corrections, and county jails implementing programs that address these issues. Since most of these programs are not evaluated and/or published in the public health or criminal justice literature, we remain at a disadvantage in neither being able to summarize their methodologies nor being able to identify their potential effective outcomes.

With only nine studies with evidence of effectiveness in the past 20 years, we need to replicate evidence-based interventions in the field while at the same time incorporating innovative community-based intervention strategies that show great promise and which have not yet been tested or evaluated. The following set of core components is an attempt to combine lessons both from the literature and from the field.

Core Components of Behavioral Interventions

HIV prevention program development and implementation in the correctional setting requires four distinct components to be taken into consideration: (1) type of intervention, (2) the timing of the program, (3) the content, and (4) the messenger.

Type of Intervention

There are multiple vehicles to intervene with this population. Some institutions put up posters or distribute brochures and call it "education," when it is really just "information sharing." Education goes beyond the sharing of information. Education should be initiated through individual, group, or institutional programming. Peer-facilitated, multisession group or individual sessions that are comprehensive and client-centered are most effective. Different learning and literacy capacities should be taken into consideration, as should cultural issues, so that the content and delivery is intellectually appropriate for those receiving it.

Individual-level interventions that are client–centered are increasingly showing evidence and promise of effectiveness (Grinstead, Zack, et al., 1999b; Myers et al., 2005; Wolitski, 2006) . In both individual- and group-level intervention, the deliverer should never assume that the recipient engages/does not engage in certain behaviors nor demand that he or she reveal this behavior either to the program staff or to a group. The participant must choose what to reveal to others. However, providing people with the necessary tools and motivations are keys to success.

Timing

The more HIV prevention can be integrated into other health and related programs, the more effective it will be. HIV-specific programming can be counterproductive as attendance and engagement are affected by stigma, perception of risk, and competing life priorities of the incarcerated population.

As people engage in risk behaviors preincarceration, during their incarceration, and on release, it is important that prevention programs occur on a continual basis. Prevention education must occur on entry at reception centers to inform prisoners of "risks inside," as well as including the institutional/department policies about both behavior risks and screening/testing procedures. This education needs to be ongoing as the population is often shifting. Equally, if not more important is the prerelease period. It is well documented that high-risk behavior occurs at the time period immediately following release (Zack et al., 2000). Optimally, prevention education should be initiated at the onset of incarceration, be reinforced during incarceration, strongly emphasized during prerelease planning, and continued on release.

Transitional case management is one model that is increasingly being implemented. This model creates a "partnership" between the prisoner (prerelease from custody) and a community service provider (often from a nonprofit organization). The intervention, therefore, starts prerelease and continues into the community reentry period. The overarching intervention goal is to "plug" the client (now, ex-prisoner) into community services. Specific goals could include (1) entry into a drug treatment program, (2) mental health counseling, (3) access to partner testing and counseling, (4) syringe exchange information, and (5) ongoing support for prevention services.

Content

Just as the HIV epidemic is not equally distributed throughout the country, neither is the basic knowledge or skills necessary to prevent HIV. For some, basic HIV information is still required before a more in-depth program can be initiated. If the basic information is not there, the perception of risk is nonexistent and the program itself is less likely to be approved or accepted by the institution or the prison population.

The basic information gives the incarcerated population the necessary understanding and options for next steps. At a minimum, efforts must be made to inform the individual of:

- modes of transmission;
- risk reduction (for both pre- and postrelease risks);
- the "window period";
- prison/jail and department/jurisdictional specific policies and procedures;
- counseling and voluntary testing; and
- available treatment options.

This basic information, often called "HIV 101," is a critical first step with those who require this basic knowledge and is typically offered in jails and prisons in reception centers. Although important and necessary, this education does little to impact behavior; for change to occur, health behavior theory posits that other factors and conditions need to be developed (e.g., skills, self-efficacy, access to prevention tools).

Once there is a common knowledge base, the next phase of education includes increasing one's perception of risk and skills specifically around risk behaviors (sexual, injection drug, and other blood-to-blood risk behaviors). Increased perception of risk is achieved by the participant examining his or her own behaviors and understanding the risks involved. Skill development usually focuses on the proper use of condoms, strategies for encouraging condom use with partners, understanding and practicing syringe hygiene, increasing awareness of needle exchange programs, and other methods of prevention activities (including not sharing tattooing equipment). One strategy that has been successful in increasing one's perception of risk are the many prisoner peer education programs that use HIV-positive prisoners as educators; it is very powerful to hear a peer state "last year, I was thinking it's everyone else, not me. Then I tested positive."

It is also critically important that the content is addressed in the context of the prison/jail setting. For example, an institution's condom availability program should be considered in recommending specific prevention behaviors.

The Messenger

The "messenger" of the HIV prevention message is critical in this environment. Mistrust is pervasive in many correctional facilities. This mistrust is rooted in differing priorities between prisoners, correctional custody staff, and other correctional support staff. There may also be mistrust within each of these groups; therefore, a trustworthy messenger viewed as neutral and trustworthy is critical. Examples of messengers include staff from prison medical, local health department, or community agencies. Over the past 10 years, peer education has increased in both acceptability and effectiveness.

By using current prisoners as peer educators, the language is more relevant, trustworthiness is increased, and, as a result, the messages are more easily communicated and more likely to be considered. This methodology is not limited to prisoners; the same peer education approach can be effective with medical, correctional, and custody staff. One study (Grinstead et al., 1997) documented that prisoners prefer peers as educators.

Many prevention programs currently in practice do use peer educators as "the messenger." However, different groups have defined peers differently. Peer education in the prison system could be existing prisoners, staff/volunteers from local community groups who have a history of incarceration, and "near" peers, individuals who are able to personally "relate" to the prison experience. If peers are not available, community support could provide the necessary resources (health educators) to conduct/facilitate these sessions.

Models of prisoner peer education have increased in the past 5 years. Many of the peer education programs of today were developed specifically for the prison population, rather than modifying a community curriculum. Examples include Bedford Hills Women's Prison (ACE: AIDS Counseling and Education), Canadian Federal Penitentiary Model (CAN: Con AIDS Network), AFH (Walk Talk), and Centerforce (Reach One Teach One).

Concluding Thoughts on Behavioral Interventions

There are multiple levels of comprehensiveness in correctional prevention programs. These include assessing health behavior and working together to create a prevention plan that is not disease specific and looking beyond the typical health issues to include family reunification, housing, employment, and education. Disease-specific programming has the potential for stigma and "outing" of those involved. Often times, staff is identified by their work and program involvement. The HIV program coordinator becomes the "AIDS person" and everyone interacting with him or her becomes suspect. This has been shown to prevent individuals from approaching the staff with questions or concerns. By expanding the scope of the topic, this staff could be identified as the "health person" and heighten the degree of accessibility and effectiveness of the prevention program.

On the most basic level, the prevention literature shows that knowledge, although not sufficient, is necessary for behavior change (Institute of Medicine, 1997). Research has also shown that skill-building (van Empelen, van Kesteren, van den Borne, Bos, & Schaalma, 2003), increased normative support (Pedlow & Carey, 2004), and modeling (Albarracin, Klein, Mitchell, & Kumkale, 2003; van Empelen et al., 2003) may also be fundamental to risk reduction. However, experience suggests that transmission takes place in a context and that by intervening more broadly (comprehensively) in that context, new infections are more likely to be prevented. This context goes "beyond the condom" and, indeed, "beyond the body" to include the issues of gender power, economics, and community capacity. HIV has infiltrated the poorest communities and those with the least political power to the greatest degree. Without intervening with respect to the contextual factors that directly impact HIV risk behavior, we cannot hope to have a long term impact on the incidence of this disease. To stem the tide of this epidemic, prevention interventions, whether focused on HIV, STIs, hepatitis, or any other health issue, must address the issues of housing, employment, health care access (including access to substance abuse and mental health treatment), and education.

There is a dearth of information documenting the essential components of effective HIV prevention programs for the incarcerated. The evaluation of the success of these programs should include not only sexual and drug-related risk behaviors, but also recidivism, access and utilization of community health services and case managers, housing, employment, education, and, for those who are HIV-positive, medication adherence and health status.

Other Important Opportunities for HIV Prevention

The focus of this chapter is on educational and behavioral interventions as a method of HIV prevention. Other opportunities are presented below. Each one of these options is a documented form of HIV prevention.

Counseling and Testing

Counseling and testing has been shown to be an effective prevention strategy (Kamb et al., 1998). The intent of testing is to become aware of one's HIV status (taking the "window period" into account). The purpose of the counseling component of HIV testing is to reinforce positive health behaviors, with an emphasis on risk reduction. These risk reduction messages are equally important among those who test positive as among those who test negative. In addition, among those who test positive, information about the options available needs to be provided.

In the correctional setting, both the pre- and posttesting counseling are critical components of HIV prevention. Pretesting counseling is critical in the correctional setting as the setting in which it takes place requires additional attention; before one voluntarily consents to be tested for HIV in a correctional setting, the provider should incorporate "setting" into the consent process. For example, if one tests positive, one may be housed in a different location or transferred to a different institution; if one tests positive, one may have access to treatment opportunities and support both during incarceration and on release.

Condom Distribution and/or Availability

It is well documented that with consistent and proper condom use, HIV transmission can be prevented (National Institutes of Health 2001; Hearst, 2004; Holmes & Weaver, 2004). There have been legislative efforts to pass condom availability programs for correctional settings and many in the public and correctional health communities have advocated for such distribution programs. However, currently, few such programs are available.

The WHO and UNAIDS have recommended for more than a decade that condoms be made available to prisoners. As of February 2007, condoms are banned or unavailable in over 90% of U.S. prisons and jails. Currently, the state prisons in Mississippi and Vermont make condoms available, as do county jails in New York City, Philadelphia, Washington, D.C., San Francisco, and Los Angeles. Of those correctional institutions where a condom availability program exists (in both the United States and elsewhere), there have been no security or custody issue that resulted in closing the program (Dolan & Wodak, 2003).

Studies in Europe have documented the increasing acceptability of condom availability in the correctional setting (these state-sponsored programs increased from 53% in 1989 to 81% in 1997; Nerenberg, 2002). The United

States is one of the few industrialized countries that do not make condoms available to the correctional population (Canadian HIV/AIDS Legal Network, 2005). Human Rights Watch reports that these jurisdictions have distributed condoms for years without violence or other incidents that might compromise security, demonstrating that denying condoms to prisoners cannot be justified on public safety grounds.

Access to Clean Injection Equipment

Though there are no sanctioned in-prison/jail syringe exchange programs in the United States, it is well documented that (1) injection drug use occurs in the correctional setting, (2) sterile IDU paraphernalia is extremely difficult to obtain, and (3) as with sexual activity, the risk is greater on the inside as a result of higher prevalence.

An evaluation of programs in Switzerland, Spain, and Germany that provide sterile needles and syringes found "no increase in drug use, a dramatic decrease in needle sharing, no new cases of infection of HIV or Hep B or C, and no reported instances of needles being used as weapons" (Dolan & Wodak, 2003; Okie, 2007).

If a safe syringe/needle exchange program is not legal or feasible, both the World Health Organization and the U.S. Centers for Disease Control and Prevention are on record as stating that other measures should be made available to prevent further transmission. WHO states that the provision of other cleaning techniques (e.g., bleach) should be used "where there is implacable opposition to NSP (Needle Syringe Programs)." The Centers for Disease Control and Prevention states that bleach should be made available "where no other safer options are available." The WHO and UNAIDS also recommend that drug-dependence treatment and methadone maintenance programs be offered in prisons if they are provided in the community, and that needle-exchange programs be considered (Okie, 2007).

HIV Treatment as Prevention

Treatment of STDs can be a method of HIV prevention (Fleming & Wasserheit, 1999). By suppressing viral load, HIV treatment is also a clinical form of HIV prevention (Porco et al., 2004). Physicians and other medical staff also can play a direct or indirect role in prevention with their patients. If time/resources do not allow for this, correctional medical staff can advocate for others to take on this responsibility.

Treatment of Substance Use (Misuse, Abuse, and Addiction)

Through the documentation of the strong relationship between substance use and sexual risk behavior, and the high percentage of substance use of those in the criminal justice system (Bureau of Justice Statistics, 1997), substance abuse treatment is HIV prevention (and very few correctional systems provide substance abuse treatment) (Rich et al., 2001; Fiscella et al., 2004; World Health Organization, 2005; Okie, 2007).

Though there is ample evidence of the history of drug use and need for drug and alcohol treatment inside our prisons and jails, very few treatment programs exist and many of those do not have the capacity to treat all who voluntarily sign up. There are more substance abusers in our prisons and jails than in alcohol/drug treatment programs in the community. An estimated 42% of state prisoners have the comorbidity of substance dependence and mental health problem (Human Rights Watch, 2006).

Mental Health Treatment

A 2006 Bureau of Justice Statistics report documented the quadrupling of the number of mentally ill prisoners in the past 6 years. Rates of mental health disorders among state prisoners are five times higher than the community rates (Bureau of Justice Statistics, 2006); rates among female prisoners were even greater. Prisoners with mental health disorders are significantly more likely to have been physically and sexually abused, to have had family members with substance abuse problems, and to have a family member with an incarceration history.

There is evidence that a large percentage of those who engage in substance use are "self-medicating" a mental health disorder. This feeds the cycle of mental health disorder to substance use to high-risk sexual behavior.

Prevention Outcomes Measures

Different educational HIV prevention efforts have measured their successes with different outcomes. Though the bottom line outcome is not getting infected, there are a myriad of other outcomes that indirectly impact HIV incidence. Outcomes that should be considered for evaluation of programs include condom use and use of sterile injection equipment both inside and after release. The next "level" of outcomes among those who are released include: decreased alcohol/drug use with sexual activity, and if available, use of needle exchange programs, substance abuse and mental health treatment. Finally, with many prisoners not "connected" with community services, working with community case managers (including parole/probation) to access services and stay out of the criminal justice system should be considered as outcome measures. For someone with HIV, success would also include access and utilization of community health services. A successful community reintegration would also include housing, employment, and education. Finally, social support systems (family and friends) can be the critical link between staying healthy or going back inside.

Conclusion

This chapter advocates for the need for HIV prevention programs in the correctional setting; it should be noted that HIV is but one of many health conditions that are disproportionately impacting the incarcerated population. Comprehensive prevention education should include other infectious diseases such as hepatitis, chlamydia, and gonorrhea, all of which are found at greater rates among the incarcerated populations. These interventions should be available at every level targeting every possible audience in order to build a comprehensive, culturally sensitive and feasible HIV prevention program for each institution.

Most HIV prevention programs focus on encouraging the individual to make behavior changes (i.e., the person engaging in high-risk behavior). This is but one strategy for prevention. Other strategies include structural interventions (e.g., condom and clean needle availability), environmental interventions, and policy-level interventions. These efforts would have a synergistic impact on HIV rates in our communities. By providing effective prevention programs to individual prisoners, the results would be felt not only by the individual program participant/client, but also by other prisoners (through diffusion), prison staff (either through observing the program for security reasons or through osmosis), prison visitors, and volunteers. Most importantly, the family members of the prisoners (Grinstead, Zack, Faigeles, et al., 2001) and the free community would be at decreased risk from the effective behavior change of the individual prisoner.

To improve our efforts we need to be mindful of the context of prevention in the correctional setting. The goal for in-prison/jail prevention must include both in-prison and postrelease prevention behaviors. To have the greatest impact on the HIV/STD/hepatitis rates of prisoners, former prisoners, and the communities to which they are released, we should strive to make our prevention programs as comprehensive as possible.

Available data indicate that prevention works. However, we need a commitment by both correctional and medical administrators to increase and improve our prevention efforts. The courts are not looking at the lack of prevention as "deliberate indifference." This commitment must begin with those of us working in the field of correctional health.

Recommendations for HIV Prevention in the Correctional Setting

The following recommendations are based on the aforementioned review of the literature, current prevention research efforts, and the author's more than 20 years of behavioral research in the correctional setting.

1. Comprehensive prevention education, including behavioral interventions, should be available to all prisoners; whenever possible, this should be integrated into existing educational programs throughout their incarceration (e.g., on entry, at any/all institutional transfers, during the course of their incarceration, and, with an added emphasis, in the prerelease period).
2. Counseling (both pre and post) and testing should be voluntary only, requiring opt-in consent with an additional component to allow the individual to understand the ramifications of testing (either positive or negative) in the correctional setting.
3. Policies should be adopted that will allow for preventive practices and disease prevention (condom availability, syringe exchange, and tattoo cleaning).
4. Comprehensive treatment for HIV/STD infection that includes ongoing monitoring of health status including medication adherence and health status should be available to all prisoners.
5. Substance abuse, alcohol, and mental health treatment must be primary, secondary, and tertiary prevention effort priorities.
6. Comprehensive pre- and postrelease transition support with proactive community reentry efforts, including (1) continuity of any/all treatment,

(2) support with housing, employment, and education, (3) family and social support, (4) "plugging" into the community service network, (5) working with community law enforcement (e.g., parole and/or probation) to understand conditions of one's release, must be offered to all releasing prisoners.

7. All in-custody prevention efforts should have a seamless transition to postrelease community prevention services; this must integrate the specific conditions of parole/probation together with reentry efforts and comprehensive community prevention services.

Acknowledgment

The author acknowledges Julie Lifshay, PhD, MPH for her valuable contribution to this chapter.

References

Albarracin, D., McNatt, P., Klein, C. T., Ho, R. M., Mitchell, A. L., & Kumkale, G. T. (2003). Persuasive communications to change actions: An analysis of behavioral and cognitive impact in HIV prevention. *Health Psychology*, *22*, 166–177.

Bauserman, R. L., Ward, M. A., et al. (2001). Increasing voluntary HIV testing by offering oral tests in incarcerated populations. *Am J Public Health*, *91*, 1226–1229.

Baxter, S. (1991). AIDS education in the jail setting. *Crime and Delinquency*, *37*, 48–63.

Beck, A. J., & Harrison, P. M. (2005). Bureau of Justice Statistics Special Report, July 2006, NCJ 214646. Prison Rape Elimination Act of 2003: Sexual Violence Reported by Correctional Authorities. U.S. Department of Justice.

Bryan, A., Robbins, R. N., Ruiz, M. S., & O'Neill, D. (2006). Effectiveness of an HIV prevention intervention in prison among African Americans, Hispanics, and Caucasians. *Health and Education Behavior*, *33*, 154–177.

Bureau of Justice Statistics. (1997). *Substance abuse and treatment of state and federal prisoners*. U.S. Department of Justice.

Bureau of Justice Statistics. (2000). *Corrections statistics*. U.S. Department of Justice.

Bureau of Justice Statistics. (2004). *HIV in prisons*. U.S. Department of Justice.

Bureau of Justice Statistics. (2006). *Mental health problems of prison and jail inmates*. U.S. Department of Justice, Office of Justice Programs.

Bureau of Justice Statistics Correctional Surveys. (1996). *Correctional populations in the United States*. U.S. Department of Justice.

Canadian HIV/AIDS Legal Network. (2005). *HIV/AIDS and hepatitis C in Prisons: The facts*.

Centers for Disease Control and Prevention. (2004). HIV/AIDS Surveillance report 2003. *US Department of Health and Human Services, CDC*, *15*, 1–46.

Centers for Disease Control and Prevention. (2006a). Epidemiology of HIV/AIDS— United States, 1981–2005. *Morbidity and Mortality Weekly Report*, *55*(21), 589–592.

Centers for Disease Control and Prevention. (2006b). *HIV prevention in the third decade*. Chapter 4: Specific populations: How are they affected?

Centers for Disease Control and Prevention. (2006c). *HIV/AIDS among men who have sex with men. Fact Sheet*. http://www.cdc.gov/hiv/pubs/facts/msm.htm

Centers for Disease Control and Prevention. (2006d). *HIV/AIDS Surveillance Report, 2005. US Department of Health and Human Services, CDC*, *17*, 1–54.

Dolan, K., Rutter, S., & Wodak, A. D. (2003). Prison-based syringe exchange programmes: A review of international research and development. *Addiction*, *98*, 153–158.

El-Bassel, N., Ivanoff, A., et al. (1995). Preventing HIV/AIDS in drug-abusing incarcerated women through skills building and social support enhancement: Preliminary outcomes. *Social Work Research*, *19*, 131–141.

Fiscella, K., et al. (2004). Jail management of arrestees/inmates enrolled in community methadone maintenance programs. *Journal of Urban Health*, *81*, 645–654.

Fleming, D. T., & Wasserheit, J. N. (1999). From epidemiological synergy to public health policy and practice: The contribution of other sexually transmitted diseases to sexual transmission of HIV infection. *Sex Transm Infect*, *75*, 3–17.

Grinstead, O., Faigeles, B., et al. (1997). The effectiveness of peer HIV education for male inmates entering state prison. *Journal of Health Education*, *28*, S31–S37.

Grinstead, O., Zack et al. (2001). Reducing postrelease risk behavior among seropositive prison inmates: The health promotion program. *AIDS Education and Prevention*, *13*, 109–119.

Grinstead, O. A., Zack, B., et al. (1999a). Collaborative research to prevent HIV among male prison inmates and their female partners. *Health Education and Behavior*, *26*, 225–238.

Grinstead, O. A., Zack, B., et al. (1999b). Reducing postrelease HIV risk among male prison inmates: A peer-led intervention. *Criminal Justice and Behavior*, *26*, 453–465.

Grinstead, O., Zack, B., Faigeles. (2001). Reducing postrelease risk behavior among HIV seropositive prison inmates: The health promotion program. *AIDS Education and Prevention*, *13*, 109–119.

Hammett, T. M., Harmon, P., et al. (1999). *1996–1997 update: HIV AIDS, STDs, and TB in correctional facilities*. Washington, DC: U.S. Department of Justice Office of Justice Programs.

Hammett, T. M., Harmon, M. P., et al. (2002). The burden of infectious disease among inmates of and releasees from US correctional facilities, 1997. *American Journal of Public Health*, *92*, 1789–1794.

Hearst, N., & Chen, S. (2004). Condom promotion for AIDS prevention in the developing world: Is it working? *Studies in Family Planning*, *35*, 39–47.

Holmes, K. K., Levine, R., & Weaver, M. (2004). Effectiveness of condoms in preventing sexually transmitted infections. *Bulletin of the World Health Organization*, *82*, 454–461.

Human Rights Watch. (2006). U.S.: Number of mentally ill in prisons quadrupled.

Institute of Medicine. (1997). *The hidden epidemic: Confronting sexually transmitted diseases*.

Johnson, R. C., & Raphael, S. (2006). The effects of male incarceration dynamics on AIDS infection rates among African-American women and men. Public Policy, University of California, Berkeley.

Kamb, M. L., Fishbein, M., et al. (1998). Efficacy of risk-reduction counseling to prevent human immunodeficiency virus and sexually transmitted diseases. *Journal of the American Medical Association*, *280*, 1161–1167.

Krebs, C. P. (2002). High-risk HIV transmission behavior in prison and the prison subculture. *The Prison Journal*, *82*, 19–49.

Krebs, C. P., & Simmons, M. (2002). Intraprison HIV transmission: An assessment of whether it occurs, how it occurs, and who is at risk. *AIDS Education and Prevention*, *14*(5 Suppl. B), 53–64.

Maruschack, L. (2005). *HIV in prisons, 2003*. Bureau of Justice Statistics Bulletin.

Myers, J., Zack, B., Kramer, K., Gardner, M., Rucobo, G., & Costa-Taylor, S. (2005). Get Connected: An HIV prevention case management program for men and women leaving the California prisons. *American Journal of Public Health*, *95*, 1682–1684.

National Institutes of Health. (2001). *Scientific evidence on condom effectiveness for sexually transmitted disease prevention*.

Nerenberg, R. (2002). Spotlight: Condoms in correctional settings. Brown Medical School.

Okie, S. (2007). Sex, drugs, prisons, and HIV. *New England Journal of Medicine*, *356*, 105–108.

Pedlow, C. T., & Carey, M. P. (2004). Developmentally appropriate sexual risk reduction interventions for adolescents: Rationale, review of interventions, and recommendations for research and practice. *Annals of Behavioral Medicine*, *27*, 172–184.

Porco, T. C., Martin, J. N., Page-Shafer, K. A., Cheng, A., Charlebois, E., Grant, R. M., & Osmond, D. H. (2004). Decline in HIV infectivity following the introduction of highly active antiretroviral therapy. *AIDS, 18,* 81–88.

Rich, J. D., Holmes, L., et al. (2001). Successful linkage of medical care and community services for HIV-positive offenders being released from prison. *Journal of Urban Health, 78,* 279–289.

Robertson, J. (2003). Rape among incarcerated men: Sex, coercion and STDs. *AIDS Patient Care and STDs, 17,* 423–430.

Ross, M. W., Harzke, A. J., Scott, D. P., McCann K., Kelley M. (2006). Outcomes of Project Wall Talk: An HIV AIDS peer education program implemented within the Texas state prison system. *AIDS Education and Prevention, 18,* 504–517.

St Lawrence, J., Eldridge, G. D., et al. (1997). HIV risk reduction for incarcerated women: A comparison of brief interventions based on two theoretical models. *Journal of Consulting and Clinical Psycholology, 65,* 504–509.

van Empelen, P., Kok, G., van Kesteren, N. M., van den Borne, B., Bos, A. E., & Schaalma, H. P. (2003). Effective methods to change sex-risk among drug users: A review of psychosocial interventions. *Social Science & Medicine, 57,* 1593–1608.

Weinbaum, C. M., Sabin, K. M., et al. (2005). High-risk HIV transmission behavior in prison and the prison subculture. *AIDS, 19*(Suppl. 3), S41–S46.

West, A. D., & Martin, R. (2000). Perceived risk of AIDS among prisoners following educational intervention. *Journal Offender Rehabilitation, 32,* 75–104.

Wolitski, R., & the Project START, Writing Group for the Project START Study Group. (2006). Relative efficacy of a multisession sexual risk-reduction intervention for young men released from prison in 4 states. *American Journal of Public Health, 96,* 1854–1861.

World Health Organization. (2005). *Status paper on prisons, drugs, and harm reduction.* Copenhagen: WHO Europe.

Zack, B., Flanigan, T., et al. (2000). *What is the role of prisons in HIV, hepatitis, STD and TB prevention?* Fact Sheet: Center for AIDS Prevention Studies and the AIDS Research Institute, University of California at San Francisco.

Zack, B., Grinstead, O., et al. (2004). A health promotion intervention for prison inmates with HIV. In B. P. Bowser, S. I. Mishra, C. J. Reback, & G. F. Lemp (Eds.), *Preventing AIDS: Community–Science collaborations* (pp. 97–112). Binghamton, NY: Haworth Press.

Chapter 11

Prevention and Control of Tuberculosis in Correctional Facilities

Farah M. Parvez, M.D., M.P.H.

Introduction

Tuberculosis (TB) is a contagious infectious disease caused by *Mycobacterium tuberculosis* and is a leading source of preventable morbidity and mortality worldwide (Maher & Raviglione, 2005). In 1993, the World Health Organization declared TB a global health emergency. Over a decade later, despite TB control efforts, TB cases continued to rise. An estimated two billion people, or one-third of the world's population, are believed to be infected with *M. tuberculosis* and are at risk for developing active TB disease during their lifetime. Annually, worldwide, eight to nine million people develop active TB and nearly two million die from the disease. The expanding human immunodeficiency virus (HIV) epidemic and the emergence of multi- and extensively drug resistant TB contribute greatly to the global burden of TB disease (CDC, 2006b, 2007).

TB is a major public health concern in correctional facilities throughout the world. Incarcerated populations are at disproportionately high risk for developing TB infection and disease compared to general populations (MacNeil, Lobato, & Moore, 2005; Hammett, Harmon, & Rhodes, 2002). Numerous TB outbreaks have occurred in correctional facilities and transmission of TB from inmates to persons within such facilities has been well documented (MacIntyre, Kendig, Kummer, Birago, Graham, & Plant, 1999; Jones, Craig, Valway, Woodley, & Schaffner, 1999; Valway, Richards, Kovacovich, Greifinger, Crawford, & Dooley, 1994; & CDC, 2004b). In the past 20 years, the number of ex-offenders released from U.S. prisons has increased fourfold, presenting significant public health challenges to the communities into which they are released (Jones, Woodley, Fountain, & Schaffner, 2003; Bur et al., 2003; Re-Entry Policy Council, 2003). This chapter is intended to provide an overview of current strategies and recommendations for the prevention and control of TB in correctional facilities, with an emphasis on discharge planning for soon-to-be-released inmates. The strengthening of TB prevention and control efforts worldwide is imperative if transmission of TB is to be prevented and elimination of TB is to be achieved (CDC, 1999a).

Background

Etiology of Tuberculosis

M. tuberculosis is a member of the *Mycobacterium tuberculosis* complex, which also includes *M. bovis, M. africanum, M. microti,* and *M. canettii.* Each member of the complex can cause TB disease; however, *M. tuberculosis* is the most prevalent human pathogen of this group. *M. tuberculosis* is a slow-growing, intracellular, acid-fast bacillus (AFB), identified by nucleic acid amplification testing and culture. Though considered an obligate aerobe, *M. tuberculosis* can exist in anaerobic environments within its host (Barclay & Wheeler, 1989).

Transmission of Tuberculosis

M. tuberculosis is spread via airborne transmission. It is passed from person to person via airborne particles called droplet nuclei. When an individual with pulmonary or laryngeal TB coughs, sneezes, shouts, speaks, or sings, *M. tuberculosis* (tubercle) bacilli, located within these droplet nuclei, are expelled into the air. The droplet nucleus forms after the droplet is expelled and most of its water evaporates. Larger, heavier droplets (>5 μm in diameter) quickly settle out of the air, usually within 3 ft of the source. However, smaller droplets (1–5 μm in diameter) are lighter and can remain suspended, and infectious, in the air for hours or days and may be dispersed by air currents or ventilation systems. In healthcare settings, these infectious droplet nuclei can also be generated during aerosolizing procedures such as sputum induction, bronchoscopy, suctioning, irrigation, and autopsy (CDC, 2005a).

Transmission of *M. tuberculosis* occurs when air contaminated with infectious droplet nuclei is inhaled. Infection may occur, in a susceptible host, if inhaled bacilli within the nuclei reach the alveoli of the lungs. Fewer than ten tubercle bacilli may initiate a pulmonary infection (Sherris & Plorde, 1990). A single cough, talking for 5 min, or singing for 1 min can generate 3000 infectious droplets; one sneeze can generate tens of thousands of such droplets (Todar, 2005). Persons at risk of exposure to and infection with *M. tuberculosis* include: close contacts of persons with TB disease; foreign-born persons from areas with a high incidence or prevalence of TB disease (e.g., Africa, Asia, Eastern Europe, Latin America, and Russia) or who frequently travel to such areas; and residents and employees of high-risk congregate settings including correctional facilities, long-term care facilities, and homeless shelters (CDC, 2005a).

The probability of TB transmission depends on three factors: the infectiousness of the person with TB, the environment in which exposure occurs, and the duration of exposure (Golub et al., 2001). Infectiousness of a person with TB is inferred from microscopic examination of sputum. Persons with TB disease who have large concentrations of tubercle bacilli in their sputum (i.e., if sputum is smear-positive) are more infectious than persons with smear-negative sputum. However, evidence of TB transmission from persons who are smear- or even culture-negative has been documented (CDC, 2005b). The environment in which exposure occurs plays an important role – crowded living or recreational spaces and inadequate ventilation can facilitate TB transmission. Likelihood of transmission after exposure to an infectious person is increased with greater frequency and duration of exposure; however, TB transmission after brief or casual encounters with infectious persons has also been documented, albeit rarely (Richeldi et al., 2004; Golub et al.). In general, TB transmission is most likely to occur from persons with pulmonary or laryngeal TB who either are undiagnosed, are not on effective anti-TB therapy, or are not placed in respiratory isolation (CDC, 2005b).

Pathogenesis of Tuberculosis

There are three stages of TB: primary or initial infection with *M. tuberculosis,* latent or dormant *M. tuberculosis* infection, and reactivation or TB disease. The first stage, primary infection, occurs in a susceptible person if inhaled tubercle bacilli reach the alveoli of the lungs and are engulfed by macrophages. Bacilli may survive initial attempts by the macrophages to destroy them and remain viable. These bacilli are transported by the macrophages to regional lymph nodes and, if not able to be contained, enter the bloodstream and widespread dissemination can occur. The most common site where the tubercle bacilli establish an infection is the upper portion of the lungs, but any organ system may also be involved.

The second stage, latent M. tuberculosis infection (LTBI), begins within 2–12 weeks of the primary infection. The tubercle bacilli multiply within the macrophages until they reach 10^3 to 10^4 in number, eliciting a cell-mediated immune response (American Thoracic Society, 2000). Macrophages and other immune cells are activated, creating granulomas and preventing further multiplication and spread of the bacilli. Though contained, the bacilli remain alive and dormant for long periods of time, maintaining the ability to reactivate at any time and cause TB disease (Wayne & Hayes, 1996). Persons with LTBI are asymptomatic and noncontagious; the only evidence of TB infection may be a positive tuberculin skin test (TST) or interferon gamma release assay (IGRA), or other tests for LTBI (Table 11.1).

The third stage, TB disease, can occur at any time after infection. Primary infection can progress to TB disease without any intervening latent period, particularly in immunocompromised persons. Among persons with LTBI, disease occurs when latent bacilli reactivate and produce active symptomatic disease. The most common site of this reactivation is the upper portion of the lungs; however, any previously infected site in the body can become involved. Persons with pulmonary TB disease usually are symptomatic, contagious, and have positive radiographic (e.g., chest radiograph) or diagnostic test findings. However, absence of such findings does not exclude the diagnosis of TB disease and, particularly for extrapulmonary TB, a high index of suspicion must be maintained.

TB disease develops in individuals whose immune system does not successfully contain their primary infection. Certain factors are associated with increased risk of LTBI progressing to TB disease (Table 11.2). In general, persons with LTBI have approximately a 10% likelihood of developing TB disease during their lifetime; the risk is highest during the first two years after primary infection (American Thoracic Society, 2000). The greatest risk for progression is being immunocompromised; persons who are co-infected with M. tuberculosis and HIV have an estimated 8–10% risk *per year* for developing TB disease (CDC, 1994, 1998, 2004a). Persons who use tobacco, alcohol, or certain drugs of abuse, including injection drugs or crack cocaine, may also have a higher risk for progression to TB disease (CDC, 2005a).

Table 11.1 Difference between latent tuberculosis infection and active tuberculosis disease.

Person with latent tuberculosis infection	Person with active tuberculosis disease
Cannot spread tuberculosis to others	Can spread tuberculosis to others
Has no symptoms and does not feel sick	Usually has symptoms that may include: • Cough that lasts 3 weeks or longer • Pain in the chest • Coughing up blood or sputum • Weakness or fatigue • Weight loss • No appetite • Chills • Fever • Sweating at night
Usually has a positive tuberculin skin test or interferon gamma release assay test[a]	Usually has a positive tuberculin skin test or interferon gamma release assay test[a]
Usually has a normal chest radiograph or evidence of previous healed infection	Usually has an abnormal chest X-ray with evidence of acute disease[a]
Has a normal sputum smear and culture	Usually has positive sputum smear or culture[b]

Source: http://www.cdc.gov/nchstp/tb/pubs/tbfactsheets/250101.htm
[a] May be nonreactive or normal in anyone, but especially persons with human immunodeficiency virus (HIV) and select conditions such as chronic renal failure and medical immunosuppression.
[b] Sputum smear or culture may be negative in persons with TB disease.

Table 11.2 Factors associated with increased risk of progression from latent tuberculosis infection to active tuberculosis disease[a].

Factors
Human immunodeficiency virus infection
Recent close contact with a person with tuberculosis disease
History of prior tuberculosis infection or disease
Diabetes mellitus
Chronic renal failure
End-stage renal disease
Prolonged use of immunosuppressive therapy (e.g., equivalent of prednisone >15 mg/day for ≥1 month, use of tumor necrosis factor-alpha antagonists)
Hematologic malignancy (e.g., leukemia or lymphoma)
Cancers of the head, neck, or lung
Silicosis
Low body weight (≥10% below ideal)
Medical conditions associated with substantial weight loss or malnutrition (e.g., malabsorption syndromes)
History of gastrectomy or jejunoileal bypass

Modified from: American Thoracic Society. (2003). Centers for Disease Control and Prevention, and Infectious Diseases Society of America. Treatment of tuberculosis. *MMWR, 52*(RR11), 1–77.
[a] Some of these factors are also associated with direct progression from primary infection to TB disease.

Progression from LTBI to TB disease can be reduced by 90% with completion of preventive antimicrobial therapy (Committee on Prophylaxis, International Union Against Tuberculosis, 1982). Once TB disease has developed, prolonged consistent multidrug therapy is required to achieve a cure. In the absence of effective treatment for TB disease, chronic wasting is usual and death occurs in up to two-thirds of cases (Dye & Floyd, 2006).

TB in Correctional Facilities

Worldwide, on any given day, an estimated ten million persons are incarcerated in correctional facilities and this number appears to be increasing (Coninx, Maher, Reyes, & Grzemska, 2000). In the U.S. alone, the number of incarcerated persons has quadrupled over the past two decades to a census of over two million (Bureau of Justice Statistics, 2005; U.S. Department of Justice, 2004). Incarcerated populations are at disproportionately high risk for LTBI and TB disease compared to general populations (MacNeil et al., 2005). LTBI is present in 12–60% of inmate populations surveyed worldwide (Abrahao, Nogueira, & Malucelli, 2006; Saunders et al., 2001; Adib, Al-Takash, & Al-Hajj, 1999). TB disease (case) rates in correctional facilities can be up to 50 times the reported national rate (Laniado-Laborin, 2001); prison TB case rates in excess of 2000 cases per 100,000 persons have been reported throughout the world in countries such as Moldova, Malawi, Azerbaijan, Georgia, and Ivory Coast (Coninx2000). In the U.S., the prevalence of TB disease is estimated to be at least 4–17 times greater in correctional populations than in general populations (Hammett et al., 2002). While TB case rates in the general U.S. population have remained at <10 cases per 100,000 persons since 1993, rates as high as 184 cases per 100,000 persons have been reported in jails and prisons (CDC, 2006a). In some large U.S. cities, 20–46% of persons with TB disease are ex-inmates of a jail (Jones & Schaffner, 2001; Hammett et al.). In addition to high TB rates, there is considerable evidence of TB transmission within correctional facilities. Numerous outbreaks of TB, including multidrug resistant (MDR) TB, have been documented in jails and prisons worldwide (Coninx, Pfyffer, et al., 1998; Valway, Richards, et al., 1994; CDC, 1992b, 2003a). Limited surveillance for TB disease, delayed diagnosis and isolation, and high turnover of those with unrecognized TB have led to inmates transmitting TB to other inmates and correctional staff, as well as to persons in the community postrelease (MacIntyre et al., 1999; Jones et al., 1999, 2003; Valway, Richards, et al., 1994; Bur et al., 2003; CDC, 2004b).

Several factors contribute to the high rate and transmission of TB among correctional populations. The physical environment of correctional facilities, such as crowded shared living and recreational spaces with inadequate ventilation, can facilitate TB transmission (Jones et al., 1999; Koo, Baron, & Rutherford, 1997; MacIntyre, Kendig, Kummer, Birago, & Graham, 1997; White et al., 2001). Duration of incarceration also plays a role; longer lengths of incarceration increase the risk of inmates acquiring TB infection (Bellin, Fletcher, & Safyer, 1993; Carbonara et al., 2005; CDC, 2003a). Frequent inter- or intrafacility movement of inmates, common in most correctional facilities, may hinder completion of TB treatment and contribute to treatment failure, drug resistance, and transmission of TB (Cummings, Mohle-Boetani, Royce, & Chin, 1998; Laniado-Laborin, 2001). Many incarcerated persons are at high risk for TB secondary to factors such as impaired immune status from HIV infection or therapy with immunosuppressive agents, malnourishment, tobacco use, or substance abuse (CDC, 1999b, 2000a; Laniado-Laborin). Persons with these factors may be more likely to acquire TB infection if exposed to someone with TB disease. In addition, incarcerated persons with TB who are undiagnosed prior to incarceration can transmit TB to other inmates, correctional employees, or members of the community if not diagnosed and properly treated within the correctional setting (CDC, 2006a).

Prevention and Control of TB in Correctional Facilities

The continued transmission of TB in jails and prisons throughout the world signifies a need for improvement in TB control efforts focused on correctional populations, both during incarceration and postrelease (Laniado-Laborin, 2001). For many incarcerated persons, the correctional setting may be the primary source of health information, intervention, and promotion. As such, correctional facilities have a unique opportunity and responsibility to address TB.

The prevention and control of TB in correctional facilities requires the implementation of a TB control program that ensures prompt disease detection, isolation, management, and discharge planning for infectious inmates. Effective programs include assigned personnel responsible for the program, a written TB control plan, periodic facility-specific TB risk assessments, continuing staff education, and collaborations with public health and community partners (Table 11.3). Fundamental TB prevention and control activities in correctional facilities can be categorized as (1) screening for TB disease and LTBI; (2) preventing TB transmission and treating persons with TB and LTBI; (3) collaboration between correction, public health, and community partners; (4) discharge planning; and (5) program evaluation (CDC, 2006a).

Table 11.3 Characteristics of an effective tuberculosis (TB) control program

I. Assignment of responsibility

   A. Assign responsibility for the TB infection-control program to qualified person(s).

   B. Ensure that persons with expertise in infection control, occupational health, and engineering are identified and included.

II. Risk assessment, TB infection-control plan, and periodic reassessment

   A. Initial risk assessments

      1. Obtain information concerning TB in the community.

      2. Evaluate data concerning TB patients in the facility.

      3. Evaluate data concerning tuberculin skin test (TST) conversions among staff in the facility.

      4. Evaluate data for evidence of person-to-person transmission.

   B. Written TB infection-control program

      1. Select initial risk protocol(s).

      2. Develop written TB infection-control protocols.

   C. Repeat risk assessment at appropriate intervals.

      1. Review current community and facility surveillance data and TST results.

      2. Review records of TB patients.

(continued)

Table 11.3 (continued)

3. Observe staff infection-control practices.

4. Evaluate maintenance of engineering controls.

III. Identification, evaluation, and treatment of patients who have TB

A. Screen patients for signs and symptoms of active TB.

1. On initial encounter in new admission/intake area.

2. Before or at the time of admission.

B. Perform radiologic and bacteriologic evaluation of patients who have signs and symptoms suggestive of TB.

C. Promptly initiate treatment.

IV. Managing persons who have possible infectious TB

A. Promptly initiate TB precautions.

B. Place patients in separate waiting areas or TB isolation rooms.

C. Give patients a surgical mask, a box of tissues, and instructions regarding the use of these items.

V. Managing inpatients who have possible infectious TB

A. Promptly isolate patients who have suspected or known infectious TB.

B. Monitor the response to treatment.

C. Follow appropriate criteria for discontinuing isolation.

VI. Engineering recommendations

A. Design local exhaust and general ventilation in collaboration with persons who have expertise in ventilation engineering.

B. Use a single-pass air system or air recirculation after high-efficiency particulate air (HEPA) filtration in areas where infectious TB patients receive care.

C. Use additional measures, if needed, in areas where TB patients may receive care.

D. Design TB isolation rooms in facilities to achieve greater than or equal to 6 air changes per hour (ACH) for existing facilities and greater than or equal to 12 ACH for new or renovated facilities.

E. Regularly monitor and maintain engineering controls.

F. TB isolation rooms that are being used should be monitored daily to ensure they maintain negative pressure relative to the hallway and all surrounding areas.

G. Exhaust TB isolation room air to outside or, if absolutely unavoidable, recirculate after HEPA filtration.

VII. Respiratory protection

A. Respiratory protective devices should meet recommended performance criteria.

B. Repiratory protection should be used by persons entering rooms in which patients with known or suspected infectious TB are being isolated, by staff when performing cough-inducing or aerosol-generating procedures on such patients, and by persons in other settings where administrative and engineering controls are not likely to protect them from inhaling infectious airborne droplet nuclei.

C. A respiratory protection program is required at all facilities in which respiratory protection is used.

VIII. Cough-inducing procedures

A. Do not perform such procedures on TB patients unless necessary.

B. Perform such procedures in areas that have local exhaust ventilation devices (e.g., booths or special enclosures) or, if this is not feasible, in a room that meets the ventilation requirements for TB isolation.

C. After completion of procedures, TB patients should remain in the booth or special enclosure until their coughing subsides.

(continued)

Table 11.3 (continued)

IX. Staff TB training and education
A. All staff should receive periodic TB education appropriate for their work responsibilities and duties.
B. Training should include the epidemiology of TB in the facility.
C. TB education should emphasize concepts of the pathogenesis of and occupational risk for TB.
D. Training should describe work practices that reduce the likelihood of transmitting *M. tuberculosis*.
X. Staff counseling and screening
A. Counsel all staff regarding TB infection and disease
B. Counsel all staff about the increased risk to immunocompromised persons for developing active TB.
C. Perform TSTs on staff at the beginning of their employment, and repeat at periodic intervals
D. Evaluate symptomatic staff for active TB.
XI. Evaluate staff TST conversions and possible transmission of *M. tuberculosis*.
XII. Coordinate efforts with public health department(s) and community partners.

Modified from: Centers for Disease Control and Prevention. (1994) Guidelines for preventing the transmission of *Mycobacterium tuberculosis* in healthcare facilities. *MMWR*, *43*(RR-13), 1–132.

Screening

Early suspicion of TB in isolation of, diagnosis of, and treatment of persons with TB disease remain the most effective means of preventing TB transmission. Inmates with undiagnosed TB disease can expose other inmates and correctional staff, and, when released, can infect persons living in surrounding communities (Bur et al., 2003; Frieden, Fujiwara, Washko, & Hamburg, 1995; Jones et al., 1999, 2003; Mohle-Boetani et al., 2002; Stead, 1978). The primary goal of screening in a correctional facility is to detect TB disease and prevent transmission. The secondary benefit of TB screening is to find inmates with LTBI who are at higher risk of progressing to TB disease and could benefit from treatment (CDC, 2006a).

The type of screening recommended for a facility is determined by an assessment of the TB transmission risk within that facility. CDC guidelines define a facility's risk as being minimal or nonminimal (CDC, 2006a). A facility has minimal TB risk if (1) no cases of TB disease occurred in the facility in the previous year; (2) it does not house substantial numbers of inmates with TB risk factors (e.g., HIV infection); (3) it does not have significant numbers of inmates from areas of the world with high TB rates; and (4) employees of the facility are not otherwise at risk for TB. Any facility that does not meet these criteria should be categorized as a nonminimal TB risk facility. TB risk should be assessed at least annually, with assistance from the local or state health department (CDC, 2006a). A multipronged approach to TB screening is needed and, based on the context and inmate characteristics, includes TB history, symptom review, diagnostic testing (e.g., TST, IGRA), chest radiograph, and a high index of suspicion.

TB History and Symptom Screening
All correctional facilities, regardless of TB risk level, should obtain a TB history from and conduct a symptom screening of all newly incarcerated inmates on intake. Inmates should be asked about history of and treatment for LTBI

or TB disease (CDC, 2006a). In addition, all inmates should be asked about the presence of TB symptoms. Inmate issues such as acute drug withdrawal, mental illness, and fatigue at time of intake, as well as language or cultural barriers, may hinder obtaining a thorough history and symptom screening and should be addressed (Saunders et al., 2001).

Early symptoms of TB resemble other infectious respiratory illnesses such as influenza, acute bronchitis, or pneumonia. Symptoms include low-grade fever, chills, night sweats, fatigue, loss of appetite, weakness, or unintentional weight loss. In pulmonary TB, the most common form of disease, symptoms often include a prolonged cough (i.e., one lasting 3 weeks), production of sputum, hemoptysis (i.e., coughing up blood or blood-tinged sputum), or chest pain. Physical exam may include rales or signs of lung consolidation. In laryngeal TB, hoarseness or sore throat may be present. TB disease in the respiratory tract is associated with a high degree of infectiousness. Extrapulmonary TB, usually noncontagious, can involve virtually any organ system in the body.

Newly incarcerated inmates should not be housed with other inmates in general population until they have been adequately screened for TB disease. Inmates with symptoms suggestive of TB disease or with history of inadequate treatment for TB disease should be placed in an airborne infection isolation (AII) room until they receive a thorough medical evaluation (CDC, 2006a). AII rooms, formerly known as negative pressure isolation rooms, are single-occupancy rooms used for the isolation of persons infected with organisms spread via airborne droplet nuclei <5 μm in diameter. If the facility does not have an AII room, the inmate should be transferred to a location that has one. The absence of physical findings does not exclude active TB disease and a high index of suspicion should be maintained. Evaluation for TB disease among those in whom it is suspected should include a test for infection (e.g., Mantoux TST or IGRA), a chest radiograph, and sputum examination for microscopy and culture for mycobacteria.

Mantoux TST Screening

The TST is the most common method for detection of TB infection. The Mantoux TST involves the intradermal injection of 0.1 ml of 5 tuberculin units (TU) of purified protein derivative (PPD) on the volar surface of the forearm. Multiple puncture tests (e.g., the tine test) and PPD strengths of 1 TU and 250 TU are not sufficiently accurate and should not be used (CDC, 2000b). In addition, anergy testing, in conjunction with TST, is no longer recommended in the United States (CDC, 1996b). The TST is read within 48–72 h after administration, and the transverse diameter of induration, not redness, is recorded in millimeters (mm). In the majority of cases, a TST result of 10 mm induration is considered a positive result for inmates and correctional facility staff (CDC, 2006a). However, an induration of 5 mm is a positive result for the following persons: HIV-infected; recent contacts of a person with TB disease; chest radiograph consistent with prior TB disease; organ transplant recipients; persons receiving prolonged immunosuppressive therapy; and those with findings raising a high suspicion of TB disease. A TST conversion is defined as an increase of 10 mm or more within a 2-year period (CDC, 2000b).

Persons who have a documented history of a positive TST result or TB disease, or a reported history of severe necrotic reaction to tuberculin, should be exempt from a routine TST (CDC, 2006a). Pregnancy, lactation, or prior

Bacille Calmette-Guerin (BCG) vaccination is not a contraindication to receiving the TST. The same criteria for interpretation of TST results are used for BCG-vaccinated persons.

The TST is not particularly sensitive for TB disease and is highly nonspecific; its sensitivity ranges from 75 to 90% (CDC, 2006a) and may be lower in some populations. Asymptomatic persons who have a positive TST reaction should have a chest radiograph performed within 72 h after skin test is read (CDC, 2006a). Persons with either TB symptoms or history of TB exposure and a positive TST reaction should be promptly placed in an AII room for a diagnostic work-up and evaluated immediately.

Two-step testing can reduce the number of positive TSTs that would otherwise be misclassified as recent conversions and should be considered in persons who are likely to undergo future periodic screenings. Certain persons who were infected with *M. tuberculosis* years earlier exhibit waning delayed-type hypersensitivity to tuberculin. When they receive a TST years later, they may have a false negative result, though they are truly infected; however, this test stimulates the body's ability to react to future TSTs and result in a "boosted" reaction. When a TST is repeated and is positive, the results may be misinterpreted as a new infection (e.g., recent conversion). In two-step testing, persons whose baseline TST yields a negative result are retested 1–3 weeks after the initial test. If the second test is negative, they are considered not infected. If the second test result is positive, they are classified as having previous TB infection. Two-step testing may not be practical in jails, given the high turnover rates, but may be useful in prisons or as part of a correctional employee health program.

Interferon Gamma Release Assays

For nearly 100 years, the TST has been the only diagnostic tool available for the detection of TB infection in persons who have no symptoms or findings of TB (Pai, Kalantri, & Dheda, 2006). Recently, IGRAs have been developed as an alternative. IGRAs are a new class of ex vivo diagnostic assays that measure interferon gamma released by T-cells after stimulation by selected antigens. For M. tuberculosis, these antigens include early secreted antigenic target (ESAT)-6 and culture filtrate protein (CFP)-10, which are present in *M. tuberculosis* but absent from all BCG strains and most other non-TB mycobacteria (with the exception of *M. kansasii, M. marinum, and M. szulgai*) (Pai, Riley, & Colford, 2004; Pai et al., 2006). Available data suggest that IGRAs have a higher specificity than TST and are at least as sensitive as TST for detection of TB disease (Pai et al., 2006). Laboratory-based test results are reported as positive (*M. tuberculosis* infection likely), negative (*M. tuberculosis* infection unlikely but cannot be excluded), or indeterminate. Advantages of IGRAs include: (1) only a single visit is required to obtain results; (2) result is unaffected by prior BCG vaccination; and (3) there is no boosting effect on future IGRA testing. Limitations of IGRAs include: (1) the need for phlebotomy; (2) limited availability of laboratories able to conduct the tests; (3) the higher direct cost per test; and (4) lack of clinical experience in interpreting the results. Comparisons of TST vs. IGRAs have been extensively reviewed (Pai et al., 2005).

Two IGRAs are now commercially available worldwide: (1) QuantiFERON®-TB Gold Test (QFT-G) (Cellestis Ltd, Carnegie, Australia) and (2) the T-SPOT™.TB (Oxford Immunotech Ltd, Oxford, UK). In May 2005, the U.S. Food and Drug Administration licensed QFT-G. QFT-G can be used in all circumstances in which TST is currently being used (CDC, 2005c). However, as with a negative TST result, a negative QFT-G result alone should not exclude the possibility of TB infection and should be supplemented with history, chest radiograph, and if indicated, sputum tests. The T-SPOT™.TB is currently licensed and used in other countries and may become available in the U.S. (Pai et al., 2006).

Chest Radiograph Screening

Chest radiographs are essential in the evaluation of TB. Persons with LTBI may have chest radiograph findings that are normal or that suggest healed infection, such as granulomas or calcification. Persons with TB disease will commonly have lesions in the apical or posterior segments of the upper lobes, or in the superior segment of the lower lobes, of the lungs. Pulmonary cavities, atelectasis, or fibrotic scarring may also be evident. Rarely, chest radiographs may be normal in the presence of pulmonary TB, particularly in patients with HIV and those with isolated laryngeal TB. Miliary TB will appear as diffuse, finely nodular lesions (~2 mm in size) on chest radiograph. Unilateral, or rarely bilateral, pleural effusion may be the only abnormality evident for pleural TB. Imaging techniques such as computed tomography or magnetic resonance imaging may assist in defining nodules, cavities, cysts, calcifications, or other lesions that are observed on chest radiograph.

Chest radiographs should be obtained for persons with TB symptoms or positive TST or IGRA test results. HIV-infected persons, or those who are at risk for HIV but whose status is unknown, should receive a chest radiograph, regardless of TST or IGRA results, as these might be falsely negative. In facilities with on-site radiographic screening, the chest radiograph should be performed as part of intake and preferably be read by a physician within 24 h (CDC, 2006a). Inmates with chest radiographs consistent with TB disease should be promptly placed in an AII room and evaluated, regardless of TST or IGRA results.

Screening with chest radiographs can be an effective means of detecting new cases of TB disease at admission to a correctional facility, particularly in facilities with short lengths of stay or high-risk populations (e.g., HIV, intravenous drug use). Screening inmates with chest radiographs has been shown to increase the TB case-finding rate and enable quicker isolation of suspected TB cases when compared with TST or symptom screening (Jones & Schaffner, 2001; Layton et al., 1997; Puisis, Feinglass, Lidow, & Mansour, 1996). However, universal chest radiography at one detention center was no more sensitive in the detection of active TB cases than routine symptom screen and TST; in addition, it led to an eightfold increase in TB-related work-ups without detecting additional cases of TB (Saunders et al., 2001). Moreover, chest radiography screening does not assist in the detection of LTBI. The decision to implement universal chest radiography for TB screening is facility specific and should consider the following factors: local and facility TB epidemiology, suspected frequency of cutaneous anergy to skin testing among incarcerated population, lengths of stay, and cost-effectiveness (Saunders et al.).

Initial TB Screening of Inmates

The following procedures are recommended for initial TB screening of inmates in all correctional facilities (CDC, 2006a). All inmates admitted to correctional facilities (minimal or nonminimal TB risk) should be evaluated on entry for symptoms of TB, preferably by healthcare staff. In facilities where custody staff conduct intake health screenings, trainings should be periodically provided on obtaining medical histories, identifying and referring inmates with TB signs and symptoms, and maintaining patient confidentiality. Any inmate with symptoms suggestive of TB should be promptly placed in an AII room and evaluated for TB disease. If the facility does not have an AII room, the inmate should be transferred to a facility that has one. All inmates admitted to a minimal TB risk facility should be evaluated for clinical conditions that increase the risk for TB infection or the risk for progressing to TB disease if infected (Table 2); persons with any of these conditions should undergo further screening with a TST, IGRA, or chest radiograph within seven days of admission (CDC, 2006a). All inmates admitted to nonminimal TB risk facilities require screening with TST, IGRA, or chest radiograph within 7 days of admission (CDC, 2006a). Inmates with HIV or risk factors for HIV but whose status is unknown, regardless of TST or IGRA result, should receive a chest radiograph at admission to the facility.

Initial TB Screening of Correctional Employees

Correctional employees, such as officers or medical personnel, are at risk for occupational exposure to TB (Steenland, Levine, Sieber, Schulte, & Aziz, 1997). Correctional facilities should have an employee health program, or component of the overall TB control program, dedicated to prevention of TB among its staff. All new employees should have (1) a medical history and physical exam; (2) TST or IGRA; (3) a chest radiograph if indicated; and (4) consideration for LTBI or TB disease treatment if indicated. Additionally, all regular visitors of nonminimal TB risk facilities, including volunteers or service providers, should be considered for TB screening (CDC, 2006a).

Periodic TB Screening

Two-step TST or single-step QFT-G should be considered for the initial testing of all inmates and employees who will receive repeated TSTs as part of a periodic TB screening program (CDC, 2006a). Correctional facilities should strongly consider using two-step TST for long-term inmates, if TST is used. Routine screening of long-term inmates and correctional facility staff (e.g., custody and medical) should be incorporated into the TB control program (National Commission on Correctional Health Care, 2003). Long-term inmates and all employees who have a negative baseline TST or IGRA result should have a follow-up testing at least annually. Inmates or employees with a history of positive TST or IGRA test result should be screened for symptoms of TB disease; annual chest radiographs are not necessary for routine follow-up evaluations of infected persons (CDC, 2006a).

Preventing Transmission of TB and Treating Patients with TB Disease and LTBI

Prevention of TB transmission and treatment of persons with TB and LTBI are fundamental TB prevention and control activities. Prevention of TB transmission in correctional facilities can be accomplished by using environmental controls and respiratory protection, in addition to TB screening. Treatment of persons with TB and LTBI, particularly those with LTBI who are at high risk for progression to disease, can prevent secondary transmission to other inmates, correctional staff, or members of the community upon the inmates' release from the correctional facility.

Environmental Controls

Exposure to *M. tuberculosis* within correctional facilities can be reduced through consistent and effective use of environmental controls, including (1) general and local exhaust ventilation; (2) air cleaning methods; (3) AII; and (4) environmental control maintenance (CDC, 2006a). These environmental controls are detailed in published guidelines for the prevention of TB in healthcare settings and for environmental infection control in healthcare facilities and can be used to educate staff and inform policies and procedures in correctional settings (CDC, 2003b, 2005a).

General and Local Exhaust Ventilation

General ventilation maintains air quality by two processes: (1) dilution and removal of airborne contaminants and (2) control of the airflow direction and pattern within a facility (CDC, 2006a). Uncontaminated air is supplied into an area where the air is contaminated and the mixed air and contaminants are subsequently removed from the area by an exhaust system. The amount of ventilation in an area is expressed by the number of air changes per hour (ACH). Air within a correctional facility should flow to minimize exposure of others within the building to airborne contaminants and should comply with minimum outdoor air supply, ACH, and ventilation design guidance for correctional facilities (American Society of Heating, Refrigerating, and Air-Conditioning Engineers, 2003; CDC, 2006a) (Table 11.4). General ventilation that exhausts air directly to the outside is the most protective ventilation design and should preferentially be used in areas likely to contain infectious aerosols (CDC, 2006a).

Although general ventilation dilutes the concentration of airborne particles, it does not contain them. Local exhaust ventilation (e.g., hoods, tents, booths) is a preferred source-control technique and is used to contain and remove airborne contaminants at their source and prevent their dispersion into the air. Local exhaust ventilation is often used during aerosol-generating procedures such as sputum induction and bronchoscopy. Such ventilation devices typically use hoods, which are of either exterior or enclosing types. Exterior devices are those in which the infectious source is near, but outside, the hood. Enclosing devices, the preferred type, are those in which the hood either partially or fully encloses the infectious source. Enclosing devices such as tents or booths should have sufficient airflow to remove 99% of airborne particles during the interval between the departure of one patient and the arrival of the next (CDC, 2006a). The time interval required to achieve proper level of airborne contaminant removal from enclosing devices varies, in part, according to the ACH. The higher the number of ACH, the shorter the amount of time that is required for removal of contaminated air (Table 11.5). Air from hoods, booths, or tents may either be exhausted directly to the outside or released

Table 11.4 Ventilation recommendations for selected areas in correctional settings

Correctional area	Minimum total air changes per hour	Air movement relative to adjacent areas	All air exhausted directly outdoors[a]
Cell or dormitory housing unit	6	In	No
Airborne infection isolation (AII) cells	12	In	Yes
Anteroom to AII cell	10	Out/In[b]	Yes
Day rooms	6	Out[c]	No
Intake, holding, or processing area	12	In	Yes
Kitchen or food preparation area	6–10	In	Yes[d]
Laundry	10–12	In	Yes[d]
Visitation area	6	Out[c]	No
Courtrooms	6	Out[c]	No

Source: Modified from Centers for Disease Control and Prevention. (2006). Prevention and control of tuberculosis in correctional and detention facilities: Recommendations from CDC. *MMWR*, *55*(RR-9), 1–44.

[a] Single-pass ventilation that directly exhausts air to the outside is the most protective ventilation design approach and should be used for areas likely to contain infectious aerosols.

[b] Anteroom pressurization should be designed to minimize cross-contamination between patient areas and adjacent areas and should comply with local fire smoke management regulations.

[c] This determination should be made on the basis of the risk assessment conducted at each facility and whether a single-pass ventilation design can be used.

[d] Exhausting all air from kitchens and laundry rooms to the outdoors is recommended for contaminant (not TB) and odor control.

Table 11.5 Air changes per hour (ACH) and time required for removal of airborne contaminants, by efficiency percentage[a]

Air changes per hour	Minutes required for removal[b]	
	99.0% efficiency	99.9% efficiency
2	138	207
4	69	104
6	46	69
12	23	35
15	18	28
20	7	14
50	3	6

Source: Modified from Centers for Disease Control and Prevention. (2006). Prevention and control of tuberculosis in correctional and detention facilities: Recommendations from CDC. *MMWR*, *55*(RR-9), 1–44.

[a] Values apply to a room or enclosure in which (1) the generation of aerosols has ceased (e.g., the infectious inmate is no longer present in the room) or (2) the aerosol procedure has been completed and the room or booth is no longer occupied. The times provided assume perfect mixing of the air in the space; removal times will be longer in areas with imperfect mixing or air stagnation. Caution should be exercised in applying the table to such situations and expertise from a qualified engineer or industrial hygienist should be obtained.

[b] Minutes required for removal of airborne contaminants from the time that generation of infectious aerosols has ceased.

back into the room where the device is located. If air is not released directly to the outside, a high-efficiency particulate air (HEPA) filter should be used at the discharge duct or vent of the exhaust device to remove airborne particulates before the air is recirculated into the room (CDC, 1994).

Air Cleaning Methods

Air cleaning technologies are useful adjuncts to general and local exhaust ventilation and include mechanical air filtration (e.g., HEPA filters) to reduce the concentration of airborne contaminants and ultraviolet germicidal irradiation (UVGI) to kill or inactivate microorganisms so that they no longer pose a risk for infection (CDC, 2006a). Air removed from areas likely to contain infectious aerosols should be preferentially exhausted directly to the outdoors. If direct exhaust is not feasible, HEPA filters should be used to clean the air before returning it to the general ventilation system. Whenever possible, such air should be recirculated into the same general area from which it originated. UVGI may also be used as a supplement to direct exhaust or HEPA filtration. UVGI can be used inside the ductwork of existing heating, ventilating, and air-conditioning systems or in the upper area of the room to be treated to ensure that organisms are inactivated. The effectiveness of UVGI depends on the UVGI lamp placement and intensity, air flow patterns and mixing, and relative humidity. Appropriate installation, maintenance, and monitoring of HEPA filters and UVGI equipment are essential. Additionally, staff and inmates should be educated about potential adverse effects of UVGI exposure such as skin erythema and photokeratoconjunctivitis (inflammation of the eye) (CDC, 2005a).

Airborne Infection Isolation

Inmates known or suspected of having TB disease should be placed in an AII room or cell that meets the design and specifications of an isolation room. AII rooms should have all three of the following characteristics: (1) negative pressure, such that the direction of the air flow is from the outside adjacent space (e.g., the corridor) into the room; (2) numerous ACH (12 ACH for new construction as of 2001; 6 ACH for construction before 2001); and (3) air that is directly exhausted to the outside, or recirculated through a HEPA filter (CDC, 1994). The use of personal respiratory protection is indicated for persons entering these rooms when caring for TB patients. Facilities without an AII room should refer inmates with suspected or confirmed TB to a facility that is able to provide such isolation and evaluate TB patients. If transfer to an alternative facility with an AII room is not available, the inmate should be temporarily housed in a room that has been modified to prevent the escape of infectious aerosols outside the TB-holding area. Inmates may be discontinued from AII when infectious TB disease is considered unlikely and either (1) another diagnosis is made that explains the clinical syndrome or (2) the patient has three negative AFB sputum-smear results. Sputum samples should be collected 8–24 h apart with at least one being an early morning specimen. Inmates for whom suspicion of TB remains despite three negative AFB sputum-smear results should not be removed from AII room until they are on standard anti-TB treatment and are clinically improving. Inmates with confirmed TB disease should remain in AII until they have had three consecutive negative AFB sputum-smear results; have received standard multidrug TB treatment for 2 weeks; and have demonstrated clinical improvement. Because transmission of drug-resistant TB can have dire consequences, facilities may choose to keep suspected or confirmed MDR TB cases in AII rooms until both negative smear and culture results are received (CDC, 2006a).

Environmental Control Maintenance

Environmental controls will fail if they are not appropriately operated and maintained. Improperly maintained AII rooms have been associated with transmission of TB within health care facilities (Ikeda et al., 1995; Kenyon et al., 1997). Correctional facilities should work with ventilation engineers and infection control personnel to ensure the proper design and ongoing maintenance of environmental controls. In addition, correctional facilities should schedule routine preventive maintenance that covers all components of the ventilation system, including air-cleaning devices, to verify that environmental controls are operating as designed. Records of preventive maintenance and repairs should be carefully maintained (CDC, 2006a).

Respiratory Protection

All correctional facilities should develop, implement, and maintain a respiratory protection program. The program should include respiratory protection fit testing and training of all correctional employees who may potentially have contact with infectious or potentially infectious inmates. All staff working with infectious patients should be given respiratory protection to wear and be instructed on proper use. For most circumstances in correctional facilities, National Institute for Occupational Health and Safety-approved respirators (e.g., N95 or higher) should provide adequate staff protection (CDC, 2005a). Detailed guidance on respiratory protection has been published (CDC, 1999c; Garner, 1996). Personal respiratory protection is indicated for all persons who (1) enter AII rooms, (2) transport infectious inmates, or (3) participate in aerosol-generating procedures (e.g., suctioning, sputum induction). Drivers or other persons who are transporting patients with suspected or confirmed TB disease in an enclosed vehicle should also wear N95 respirators. If the inmate has signs or symptoms of TB, consideration should be given to having the inmate wear a surgical mask during transport, in waiting areas, or when others are present (CDC, 2006a).

Treatment

Treatment of TB and LTBI is a critical component of TB containment, both in correctional facilities and in the larger community. An untreated person with TB disease is estimated to infect 10–15 persons per year. Effective anti-TB treatment markedly reduces infectivity. Completion of an effective treatment regimen for TB disease is nearly always curative; without proper treatment, TB is often fatal. A completed regimen of treatment for LTBI can reduce the risk of progression from LTBI to TB disease by 90% (Committee on Prophylaxis, International Union Against Tuberculosis, 1982; Institute of Medicine, 2000).

The effectiveness of TB treatment is primarily determined by adherence to and completion of the treatment regimen (American Thoracic Society, 2003). Interrupted or incomplete treatment increases the risk of treatment failure, relapse of disease, and emergence of drug-resistant TB. Patients who often move residences or are residing in correctional facilities have a higher likelihood of defaulting on treatment (Cummings et al., 1998; MacNeil et al., 2005). The most effective method of monitoring treatment compliance is to use directly observed therapy (DOT). DOT involves watching as the patient swallows the medication. DOT can help diminish infectiousness, reduce risk for relapse, and help prevent the development of drug resistance (American Thoracic Society). DOT is the preferred treatment strategy for all persons with (1) TB disease; (2) LTBI who are on intermittent therapy or are at high risk for progression to disease; (3) recent contact of infectious persons with pulmonary TB. When feasible, DOT is also preferred for persons with LTBI who are on daily dosing.

All persons receiving treatment for TB disease or LTBI should (1) undergo clinical monitoring at least monthly to screen for nausea, vomiting, abdominal pain, jaundice, or discolored urine and (2) be educated about potential adverse effects of the drug(s) and the need to promptly discontinue treatment and seek medical evaluation if adverse effects occur. Certain populations, including individuals with HIV infection, pregnant or postpartum females, persons with history of liver disease (or at risk for chronic liver disease), and regular users of alcohol (CDC, 2000b), initiating LTBI treatment should also receive baseline and subsequent periodic laboratory testing (e.g., measurement of serum transaminases).

Treatment of LTBI

Treatment guidelines for LTBI have been previously published (CDC, 2000b). The preferred treatment regimen for LTBI is 9 months of daily isoniazid for a total of 270 doses or biweekly dosing using DOT for a total of 78 doses (CDC, 2000b) (Table 11.6). A 6-month course of isoniazid or a 4-month course of rifampin is an acceptable alternative for HIV-negative persons. In HIV-positive individuals, the 6-month course of isoniazid should be offered only if the other regimens cannot be given. In addition, substitution of rifabutin for rifampin may be indicated in HIV-infected persons taking certain antiviral medications due to less frequent drug–drug interactions when rifabutin is used. Combination therapy with rifampin and pyrazinamide had previously been recommended for treatment of LTBI; however, this regimen is no longer recommended due to subsequent reports of severe hepatotoxicity and death (CDC, 2003c).

Treatment for TB Disease

Treatment regimens for TB disease must consider all clinical, radiographic, and laboratory results, including drug susceptibility testing. Treatment should be implemented in collaboration with local TB experts to select the appropriate regimen based on diagnostic results (American Thoracic Society, 2003). For most persons with TB disease, the preferred treatment regimen is an initial 2-month phase of rifampin, isoniazid, pyrazinamide, and ethambutol, followed by a continuation phase of isoniazid and rifampin for four or more

Table 11.6 Common drug regimens for treatment of latent tuberculosis infection[a]

Drugs	Duration (months)	Dosing interval	Doses (number)	Rating (evidence)[b]	
				HIV-negative	HIV-positive
Isoniazid	9	Daily	270	A (II)	A (II)
		Twice weekly	78	B (II)	B (II)
Isoniazid[c]	6	Daily	180	B (I)	C (I)
		Twice weekly	52	B (II)	C (I)
Rifampin[d]	4	Daily	120	B (II)	B (III)

Source: Modified from Centers For Disease Control and Prevention. (2006). Prevention and Control of Tuberculosis in Correctional and Detention Facilities: Recommendations from CDC. MMWR, 55(RR-9), 1–44.
[a] The combination of rifampin and pyrazinamide had previously been recommended for the treatment of latent tuberculosis infection; however this regimen should not be offered on the basis of subsequent reports of severe hepatotoxicity.
[b] Ratings are based on modification of the U.S. Public Health Service rating system (American Thoracic Society, CDC. (2000). Targeted tuberculin testing and treatment of latent tuberculosis infection. *American Journal of Respiratory and Critical Care Medicine, 161*, S221–S247). A = preferred; B = acceptable alternative; C = offer when A and B cannot be given. I = randomized clinical trial data; II = data from clinical trials that are not randomized or were conducted in other populations; III = expert opinion.
[c] This regimen should only be offered to HIV-infected persons if other regimens cannot be given.
[d] Substitution of rifabutin for rifampin may be indicated in HIV-infected persons taking certain antiretroviral medications because drug–drug interactions may be less frequent when rifabutin is used.

months after drug resistance is excluded (Tables 11.7 and 11.8). Persons with HIV infection may require use of rifabutin rather than rifampin and may need more frequent dosing than HIV-uninfected persons.

Treatment for TB disease should use DOT until completion. Decision to stop treatment should be made in collaboration with TB experts from local or state public health departments and be based on clinical, bacteriological, and radiographic improvement and total number of anti-TB medication doses taken within a maximum period (American Thoracic Society, 2003).

Case Reporting

In the U.S., all states require designated health care professionals, including those from correctional facilities, to report suspected or confirmed TB cases to their local or state health department. Suspected or confirmed cases among both inmates and correctional staff should be reported. This reporting is mandatory and should be conducted regardless of treatment status, even if an inmate has already been released or transferred from the facility (CDC, 2006a).

Contact Investigations

The identification of a potentially infectious case of TB in a correctional facility should trigger a prompt public health response because of the potential for widespread TB transmission. TB contact investigations are initiated on a case-by-case basis with the goal of interrupting the transmission of *M. tuberculosis*. TB transmission is prevented by (1) promptly isolating and treating persons with TB disease and (2) identifying infected contacts of such persons and providing them with treatment for LTBI. Decisions involved in initiating, planning, and

Table 11.7 Initial drug regimens for culture-positive pulmonary tuberculosis caused by drug-susceptible organisms[a]

Regimen	Drug	Dosing interval	Doses (number)	Minimum duration of treatment
1	Isoniazid Rifampin[b] Pyrazinamide Ethambutol[c]	Daily	56	8 weeks
2	Isoniazid Rifampin[b] Pyrazinamide Ethambutol[c]	Daily, then twice weekly[d]	Daily for 14 doses, then twice weekly for 12 doses	2 weeks of daily dosing, then 6 weeks of twice weekly dosing

Source: Modified from Centers For Disease Control and Prevention. (2006). Prevention and Control of Tuberculosis in Correctional and Detention Facilities: Recommendations from CDC. *MMWR, 55*(RR-9), 1–44.

[a]Guidance on dosing, monitoring during treatment, and less commonly used regimens are detailed in American Thoracic Society. (2003). CDC Infectious Diseases Society of America. Treatment of Tuberculosis. *MMWR, 52*(RR-11), 1–80.

[b]Substitution of rifabutin for rifampin may be indicated in HIV-infected patients taking certain antiretroviral medications because drug–drug interactions may be less frequent when rifabutin is used.

[c]May be discontinued if infecting organism is found to be susceptible to isoniazid and rifampin.

[d]Not recommended for HIV-infected patients with CD4 + T-lymphocyte cell counts of < 100 cells/mm3.

Table 11.8 Continuation phase options for initial drug regimens 1 and 2[a]

Regimen	Option	Drugs	Dosing interval	Doses (number)	Minimum duration[b]	Rating (evidence)[c] HIV-negative	Rating (evidence)[c] HIV-positive
1	A	Isoniazid Rifampin[d]	Daily	126	18 weeks	A (I)	A (II)
1	B	Isoniazid Rifampin[d]	Twice weekly[e]	36	18 weeks	A (I)	A (II)
2	A	Isoniazid Rifampin[d]	Twice weekly[e]	36	18 weeks	A (II)	B (II)

Source: Modified from Centers For Disease Control and Prevention. (2006). Prevention and Control of Tuberculosis in Correctional and Detention Facilities: Recommendations from CDC. *MMWR, 55*(RR-9), 1–44.

[a] Guidance on dosing, monitoring during treatment, and less commonly used regimens are detailed in American Thoracic Society. (2003). CDC Infectious Diseases Society of America. Treatment of Tuberculosis. *MMWR, 52*(RR-11), 1–80.

[b] Patients with cavitation on initial chest radiograph and positive cultures at completion of 2 months of therapy should receive a 7-month (31 weeks; either 217 doses [daily] or 62 doses [twice weekly]) continuation phase.

[c] Ratings are based on modification of the U.S. Public Health Service rating system (American Thoracic Society. (2000). CDC, Targeted tuberculin testing and treatment of latent tuberculosis infection. *American Journal of Respiratory and Critical Care Medicine, 161,* S221–S247). A = preferred; B = acceptable alternative; C = offer when A and B cannot be given. I = randomized clinical trial data; II = data from clinical trials that are not randomized or were conducted in other populations; III = expert opinion.

[d] Substitution of rifabutin for rifampin may be indicated in HIV-infected patients taking certain antiretroviral medications because drug–drug interactions may be less frequent when rifabutin is used.

[e] Not recommended for HIV-infected patients with CD4 + T-lymphocyte cell counts of < 100 cells/mm3.

prioritizing contact investigations are complex; a multidisciplinary team of trained professionals, including infection control, medical, nursing, custody, and local or state public health staff, should be convened to plan and conduct the investigations (CDC, 2006a).

Contact investigations should be initiated for the following conditions: (1) suspected or confirmed pulmonary, laryngeal, or pleural TB with cavitary disease on chest radiograph or positive AFB smears (on sputum or other respiratory specimens) and (2) suspected or confirmed pulmonary or pleural TB with negative AFB smears and a decision has been made to initiate TB treatment. Contact investigations generally are not indicated for extrapulmonary TB (excluding laryngeal and pleural TB) unless pulmonary involvement is also diagnosed.

The following steps should be used for contact investigations. Once an inmate with suspected or confirmed TB disease (source patient) is identified, local public health authorities and correctional management officials should be notified. The source patient should be interviewed and medical records should be reviewed to collect information on (1) TB exposure history and symptoms; (2) date of illness onset; (3) results of diagnostic testing for TB; (4) dates and location of housing, employment, and education within the facilities; and (5) names of contacts (both in the correctional facilities and community). The infectious period for the source patient should be determined. The infectious period is typically defined as 12 weeks before the TB diagnosis was made or the onset of TB symptoms (whichever is longer). The presumptive infectious period can be reduced to 4 weeks preceding the date of diagnosis if the source patient is asymptomatic, is AFB smear negative, and has a noncavitary chest radiograph (CDC, 2006a). All living, working, and recreation areas of the source patient within the facilities should be toured to characterize the ventilation system and airflow direction. Contact lists should be developed, grouped according to location (e.g., incarcerated, released, transferred), and prioritized according to duration and intensity of exposure to the source patient (e.g., high, medium, low priority); local public health staff can assist in the prioritization of contacts (CDC, 2005b).

Contact investigations should focus on identifying the contacts at highest risk for TB transmission, screening them completely, and providing them with a complete course of LTBI treatment if they are infected. Persons with the most exposure to the source patient and HIV-infected or immunocompromised persons (regardless of duration of exposure) are of the highest priority. Medical charts should be reviewed for all high-priority contacts to determine TB-exposure history and symptoms. Baseline TST or QFT-G should be performed on all eligible contacts (e.g., excluding those with prior positive tests or those who were tested after 1–3 months of exposure). All HIV-infected contacts should be evaluated for TB disease and LTBI regardless of TST or QFT-G result; LTBI therapy should be initiated once TB has been excluded (CDC, 2005b). Public health authorities should be notified about contacts who have been transferred to another correctional facility or released to the community so that they can be screened. Follow-up TSTs or QFT-G should be performed 8–10 weeks after exposure to the source patient has ended. Decision to expand the contact investigation beyond the high- and medium-priority contacts should be based on calculated infection rates (e.g., total number of inmates whose TST or QFT-G has converted from negative baseline to positive should be divided by the total number of inmates with a TST placed and read and QFT-G performed) and should be compared with infection rates among nonexposed inmates. The contact investigation team should analyze infection rates both at baseline and follow-up to determine the need for expanding the investigation. Once the contact investigation is completed, the investigation team should prepare a summary report of the methods, results, and follow-up plans of the investigation. Reports should be shared with correctional and public health authorities. Detailed guidelines for conducting contact investigations have been published (CDC, 2005b).

Drug Susceptibility Testing

Initial isolates from persons with positive smears or cultures for *M. tuberculosis* should be tested for susceptibility to anti-TB drugs (CDC, 1992c). Drug susceptibility testing is imperative for choosing effective TB treatment regimens. Delays in susceptibility testing result in a longer duration of ineffective treatment and prolonged infectiousness. Susceptibility testing should be repeated if positive sputum smears or cultures persist despite 3 months of anti-TB drug therapy or develop after a period of negative sputum test results. Drug resistance should be reported to the TB control program at the local or state health department, and consultations with TB experts should be made to select a treatment regimen for drug-resistant TB.

MDR TB, defined as resistance to at least isoniazid and rifampin, emerged globally over the past two decades, creating a major challenge to TB management, including in correctional facilities (CDC, 1992a, 2006b; Valway, Greifinger, Papania, Kilburn, Woodley, DiFerdinando, & Dooley, 1994). MDR TB outbreaks in prisons have been documented worldwide and have resulted in the spread of MDR TB beyond the confines of correctional facilities into the community (Coninx, Pfyffer, et al., 1998; Valway, Greifinger, et al., 1994). Treatment of MDR TB requires the use of second-line drugs that are less effective, more toxic, and costlier than first-line isoniazid- and rifampin-based regimens (American Thoracic Society, 2003).

Ineffective treatment of persons with TB disease (e.g., insufficient quality, quantity, or duration of medications) may lead to the progressive development of drug resistance, including extensively drug resistant (XDR) TB. XDR TB has recently emerged as a worldwide threat to TB control and is characterized by a predilection for immunocompromised persons, high mortality, and limited treatment options (World Health Organization, 2006). XDR TB is defined as resistance to isoniazid and rifampin (MDR TB), plus resistance to any fluoroquinolone and at least one of three injectable drugs (i.e., amikacin, kanamycin, or capreomycin). In the U.S., approximately 4% of MDR TB is XDR TB (CDC, 2006b). In the industrialized nations of Australia, Belgium, Canada, France, Germany, Ireland, Japan, Portugal, Spain, Britain, and the U.S., XDR TB increased from 3% of drug-resistant TB cases in 2000 to 11% in 2004 (CDC, 2006b). During 1993–2002, patients with XDR TB in the U.S. were 64% more likely to die during treatment than patients with MDR TB (CDC, 2006b). Ensuring appropriate, uninterrupted continuity of directly observed TB treatment both within and outside of correctional facilities is of utmost importance in the prevention of drug resistance.

Discharge Planning

Comprehensive discharge planning for soon-to-be-released inmates, or reentrants, with TB infection or disease is an essential component of TB control efforts, both within correctional facilities and in the communities to which inmates return (Hammett, Gaiter, & Crawford, 1998). Effective discharge planning facilitates improved postrelease utilization of medical services (Frieden et al., 1995) and reduced recidivism (Flanigan et al., 1996). In addition, continuity of care postrelease is imperative for reducing secondary TB transmission and preventing the development of drug resistance (Glaser & Greifinger, 1993). Failure to complete a diagnostic evaluation for TB disease can result in undiagnosed reentrants exposing their families, friends, and community members to TB. Treatment interruptions or cessation before completion can also have serious consequences. Individuals with LTBI who do not complete their treatment are at risk for developing TB disease, particularly if they are co-infected with HIV or have other risk factors for progression. Inmates with TB disease who are unable to complete their treatment regimen are at risk for developing drug resistance and relapsing to symptomatic and infectious disease. Recidivists with incompletely diagnosed or untreated TB disease can reintroduce TB into a correctional facility upon admission and place other inmates and correctional staff at risk. Thus case management and discharge planning efforts must be made to ensure timely completion of TB diagnostic evaluation and treatment both during and after incarceration, to prevent potential health risks to both reentrants and the larger community.

Correctional facilities should conduct prerelease case management and discharge planning for all inmates with suspected or confirmed TB disease and those with LTBI who are at high risk for progression to TB disease (CDC, 2006a). For inmates with LTBI who are at low risk for progression to TB disease, correctional facilities should collaborate with appropriate public health agencies to develop feasible discharge planning policies. Regardless of risk of progression, all inmates with LTBI who are started on TB preventive therapy during incarceration should receive discharge planning to ensure uninterrupted treatment after release.

Correctional facilities should have designated staff assigned to conduct TB discharge planning and to notify the appropriate public health agency of inmates with suspected or confirmed TB disease and inmates receiving treatment for LTBI or TB disease (CDC, 2006a). Designated staff may be correction personnel, medical or administrative staff working in the facility, or public health department staff that work on-site. Such personnel should also be responsible for communication with other correctional facilities or community service providers if inmates are transferred or released mid-TB evaluation or treatment. Correction and medical staff within correctional facilities should work with the designated discharge planning staff to develop timely and thorough discharge plans. Planning should address TB diagnosis and treatment efforts begun in jails or prisons and provide for their continuation postrelease. Correctional facilities should ensure that their discharge planning process is comprehensive, is tailored to the needs of the individual, and is conducted in collaboration with public health and community partners.

Collaboration between Correction, Public Health, and Community Partners

Both effective TB case management and discharge planning require and benefit from collaboration between correction, public health, and community partners (Lobato, Roberts, Bazerman, & Hammett, 2004). Such collaboration and coordination maximize the effectiveness of TB control efforts begun in correctional facilities (Hammett, Roberts, & Kennedy, 2001). TB diagnostic evaluation or treatment initiated during incarceration can be completed postrelease by public health or community partners, thus ensuring continuity of care and improved health for the inmate and reducing the likelihood of TB transmission in the community. In addition, collaboration with public health and community partners can assist correctional facilities in overcoming barriers encountered during discharge planning such as brief inmate lengths of stay, unscheduled releases or transfers from the facility, and limited available resources for recommended TB prevention, screening, treatment, and discharge planning services (CDC, 2006a). Public health agencies and community-based organizations may have financial, programmatic, or personnel resources that they can offer to correctional facilities. Public health staff can provide TB medical expertise and assistance with case management, contact investigations, administration of DOT, and accessing community TB-related resources (e.g., local TB clinics for follow-up appointments). In addition, public health departments often maintain TB registries containing diagnostic and treatment-related information on all persons with TB within their jurisdictions. Correctional facilities and public health departments can work together to use TB registry data to find inmates with TB infection or disease and obtain the TB history. Registry information including TB diagnostic test results, drug-susceptibility patterns, and treatment history can be helpful to correctional facilities in case management and discharge planning. Use of TB registry data in correctional settings may also enable health departments to locate persons with TB who have been lost to follow up in the community. Correctional facilities can assist public health departments by promptly reporting all inmates with suspected or confirmed TB disease, so that the public health staff can ensure timely performance of case management, contact investigations, and entry of information into the TB registry. Correctional facilities should contact their local or state health departments to identify their designated TB control staff. Likewise, public health departments should make efforts to contact the infection or TB control staff of local correctional facilities. To facilitate effective collaboration, correctional facilities and public health departments should designate liaisons and have regularly scheduled meetings to discuss correctional TB control issues (Lobato et al.).

Community-based partners, including clinical and social service providers and community correction staff (e.g., probation and parole officers), are vital to the success of discharge planning efforts. Recently released inmates have a multitude of health- and nonhealth-related needs and it is imperative to link them with organizations that are interested and experienced in working with these populations; correctional facilities and public health agencies should make efforts to identify and partner with such organizations. Soon-to-be-released inmates often express a need for help in accessing healthcare services after release and have high expectations of the role that community correction staff will play in helping them gain lawful employment, find substance use treatment programs, stay crime free, or otherwise transition into the community (LaVigne, Visher, & Castro, 2004). Parolees meet with their assigned parole officer on a monthly or bimonthly basis; as such, including community correction staff in prerelease TB-discharge planning, with inmate consent, may facilitate continuity of care (Nelson & Trone, 2000). By participating in discharge planning for soon-to-be-released inmates with LTBI or TB, community correction staff become more knowledgeable about TB and can assess TB management-related compliance issues with their parolees; as such, they are better able to protect themselves, their clients, and their communities (Hammett et al., 2001; Wilcock, Hammett, & Parent, 1995). Community correction can also assist public health departments in locating TB cases that are lost to follow-up in the community and are on probation or parole.

Successful TB discharge planning requires correctional facilities to provide timely and thorough TB diagnostic and treatment information to public health agencies (via mandatory TB case-reporting), as well as to community partners involved in postrelease provision of services. Likewise, feedback of postrelease TB follow-up data from public health departments and community partners back to correctional facilities is helpful in maintaining continuity of care, particularly for persons with TB who are reincarcerated. However, there are patient-confidentiality-related restrictions on sharing information across agencies, and local, state, and federal regulations should be followed. Correction, public health, and community partners should inform and reassure inmates of their confidentiality rights. In addition, inmates should be explained the importance and benefits of signing a limited release or consent so that their TB-related information can be shared among appropriate agencies (Hammett et al., 2001). Caution should be taken to share only the information necessary to provide continuity of care.

Components of Discharge Planning

Incarcerated populations have a complexity of discharge planning needs. Following release from correctional facilities, reentrants face urgent housing, employment, financial, and other subsistence needs that often take priority over their healthcare (Hammett et al., 2001). While incarcerated, inmates may lose their employment, housing, eligibility for food stamps, or Medicaid and Social Security benefits. As such, postrelease, reentrants with TB may not have the ability or resources to make or keep follow-up appointments or obtain necessary medications. They may have language, literacy, or cultural barriers, which further complicate their ability to seek care. In addition, reentrants often have mental health or substance use issues that can hinder their ability to access healthcare services. Thus, to be effective, TB discharge planning efforts must be holistic and tailored to the needs of the reentrant. As such, correctional facility discharge planning programs should (1) initiate discharge planning early; (2) provide case management; (3) obtain detailed postrelease contact information; (4) assess and plan for substance abuse, mental health, and social service needs; (5) make arrangements for postrelease follow-up; (6) make provisions for unplanned release and transfers; and (7) provide education and counseling (CDC, 2006a).

Initiate Discharge Planning Early

Discharge planning efforts for inmates diagnosed with TB infection or disease should begin as early as possible during incarceration and continue postrelease to facilitate continuity of care and avoid delays in initiating or resuming TB treatment. Designated discharge planning staff in the correctional facilities should promptly notify the public health department of all inmates with suspected or confirmed TB disease or inmates receiving TB treatment, even if the inmates have been transferred or released from the facility. Inmates diagnosed with TB disease are of the highest priority for discharge planning and should be interviewed by public health (preferred) or correctional discharge planning staff as soon as possible after diagnosis so that the discharge plan can be developed (CDC, 2006a). Whenever possible, correctional facilities should provide the discharge planning staff with advance notice about the inmates' projected release dates; this will enable development of a more individualized and thorough discharge plan. Even in short-term detention facilities, where a significant number of inmates may be released within one to three days of admission, many critical community TB linkages can be made if the discharge planners are promptly notified about an inmate with TB.

Early involvement of the inmate in the planning process is integral to the success of the discharge plan. Inmates may perceive the discharge plan and community linkages as an extension of their punishment in jail or prison and be reluctant or fearful to participate. Discharge planning staff should work to build a rapport and trusting relationship and to educate the inmates on the benefits of discharge planning to their health and well-being. Staff should assess the inmates' perceptions of their postrelease needs and priorities and tailor the discharge plan accordingly; inmates may have received discharge planning before and know what worked or did not work for them in the past. In addition, staff should assess the inmates' expectations of postrelease support from their families, particularly as it relates to their healthcare. Often soon-to-be-released inmates expect that their families will assist them with accessing healthcare, finding housing or employment, and finances in the community; however, postrelease, inmates may find that the expected support is not always available (La Vigne, 1994; Visher, Kachnowski, La Vigne, & Travis, 2004). Whenever possible, staff should attempt to include inmate families early in the discharge planning process and link inmates with additional and varied sources of support (e.g., peer counselors, support groups) (Nelson & Trone, 2000).

Provide Case Management

Comprehensive case management is an essential component of discharge planning and involves identifying, planning, and facilitating the postrelease services required to meet reentrants' health and social service needs. Case management has been demonstrated to support reentrants in utilizing community healthcare services (Rich et al., 2001), modifying risk behaviors (Rhodes & Gross, 1997), and reducing recidivism (Flanigan et al., 1996). In addition, case management for persons with TB has been shown to improve adherence to TB treatment regimens (Marco et al., 1998) and reduce loss to follow-up in the community (Salomon et al., 1997).

Designated discharge planning staff should provide case management for inmates with TB infection or disease and work with public health and community partners to ensure continuity of care postrelease (Klopf, 1998). Prerelease case management should include a thorough assessment of the inmate's TB exposure, diagnosis, and therapy history by interviewing the inmate directly and reviewing pertinent medical records. Case managers should review the TB exposure history to identify potential TB contacts either in the correctional facility or community and should inform facility infection control and local public health partners so that contact investigations can be initiated as needed. Case managers should also review the results of all TB diagnostic testing conducted during incarceration, such as TST or IGRA, chest radiograph, sputum smears and cultures, and drug susceptibilities. In addition, TB treatment and medication compliance history during incarceration should be reviewed. Case managers should request the local or state public health department to review their TB registry data for additional information that might be useful in discharge planning. Co-morbid conditions, such as HIV or viral hepatitis, can complicate the treatment regimen and should be addressed in the overall discharge plan by ensuring linkages with appropriate community clinical providers.

Case managers should work with public health and community partners to determine where soon-to-be-released inmates will receive TB follow-up care and obtain necessary medications. Newly released inmates sometimes choose not to return to the neighborhood they lived in before incarceration either to avoid previous influences which led to their incarceration or because their family moved to another location (La Vigne, Visher, & Castro, 2004). Additionally, released inmates may wish not to receive medical care in the same neighborhood where they live due to a perceived stigma. Case managers should determine where soon-to-be-released inmates would be able and willing to continue their TB follow-up appointments. Case managers should discuss the importance of the follow-up, and identify and address any potential barriers to inmates being able to keep the appointments.

Obtain Detailed Contact Information

Case managers should emphasize the importance of continuity of care in TB treatment and encourage inmates with LTBI or TB disease to provide accurate postrelease contact information. Case managers should request detailed information from soon-to-be-released inmates, such as (1) their expected residence, including shelters; (2) names and contact information for friends or relatives; and (3) community locations usually frequented, in order to enable location of the released inmate in the community (White et al., 2002). In addition, case managers should obtain a signed consent from inmates authorizing the case manager and public health department to contact and share TB-related information with worksites, community clinical or social service providers, or community correction staff if necessary (CDC, 2006a).

Inmates may provide contact information based on their expectations of where they will reside postrelease; however, for many reasons, they may need to change their residence after they return to the community. Alternatively, inmates may intentionally give correctional staff aliases or incorrect contact information because of mistrust or fear of incrimination or deportation (CDC, 2006a). The inability to locate and provide continuity of care for released inmates with LTBI or TB disease can result in incomplete treatment regimens (Nolan, Roll, Goldberg, & Elarth, 1997) and the risk of transmission or drug resistance (Glaser & Greifinger, 1993). In addition, the use of an alias by an inmate with LTBI or TB disease can hinder continuity of care upon reincarceration and potentially place other inmates and correctional staff at risk. Case managers should confirm contact information, including true identity and any aliases, with inmates on a periodic basis throughout incarceration and immediately before release if possible. Correctional facilities should also develop strategies to confirm an inmate's true identity as quickly as possible after admission to the facility (e.g., using fingerprint-based unique identification number).

Assessment and Plan for Substance Abuse, Mental Health, and Social Service Needs

TB case management efforts must include an assessment of substance abuse, mental health, or social service needs that may adversely influence the inmate's ability to adhere to the TB discharge plan. Substance abuse and mental health issues are significant barriers to continuity of care postrelease and should be addressed by discharge planning staff in correctional facilities (Hammett et al., 2001). After release from jail or prison, many reentrants return to their old neighborhoods and are challenged to avoid the same influences or circumstances that led to their recent incarceration, which places them at risk for defaulting on their TB care. Relapse to substance abuse postincarceration often occurs and can impact all aspects of a reentrant's life including his or her health, housing, relationships, employment, parole conditions, and likelihood of reincarceration (Rich et al., 2001). Inmates with mental illness have similar postrelease issues as those with substance abuse problems. Without sufficient postrelease support in the community, reentrants with mental illness may have difficulty in coping or with treatment adherence and may experience acute decompensation of their mental status, thus greatly increasing the chances of nonadherence to TB follow-up or treatment. Reentrants with prior drug offenses or mental illness often have difficulty in obtaining permanent housing and risk becoming homeless (Lindblom, 1991), which is a major barrier to completion of TB therapy (LoBue, Cass, Lobo, Moser, & Catanzaro, 1999). For inmates with a substance abuse history, case managers should provide referrals to or information about convenient substance abuse treatment programs and peer support group meetings (e.g., Alcoholics or Narcotics Anonymous). In addition, inmates with substance abuse histories are at risk for HIV and viral hepatitis, both of which can affect TB management, and would benefit from referrals to community clinical providers experienced in working with these issues. Inmates with TB who have mental illness require community linkages to mental health treatment programs that are integrated with primary care, substance abuse, and social service providers to best facilitate continuity of care.

Incarceration creates several other barriers for released inmates, which can hinder continuity of TB care. During incarceration, inmates may lose their employment or other sources of income. In addition, inmates often lose health insurance or other government benefits, such as Medicaid, Temporary Assistance for Needy Families, Food Stamps, Supplemental Security Income, or Social Security Disability Insurance, while incarcerated and may have to wait several months postrelease to become eligible again (Bazelon Center for Mental Health Law, 2000). This loss of income and services can adversely impact the inmate's ability to adhere to TB follow-up and treatment in the community. Although federal laws require the suspension of certain benefits during the period of incarceration, many states will terminate the benefits and require inmates to reapply for benefits upon release (Human Rights Watch, 2003). The requirement to reapply for benefits postrelease can present difficulties for inmates as they must provide documentation that may have been lost or destroyed (e.g., birth certificates, social security card, passport, driver's license, or other photo identification). Many states will allow inmates to apply for reinstatement of benefits in anticipation of release from jail or prison; case managers should assist inmates in obtaining the necessary documentation and completing the required application forms.

Correctional facilities should assist this process by making the inmates' driver's licenses, Medicaid cards, or other forms of photo identification available to the case managers during incarceration, as needed, and to the inmates with their personal property postrelease. In addition, correctional facilities should create agreements with agency partners to facilitate prompt reactivation of these benefits (e.g., with state Department of Motor Vehicles to provide nondriver's license photo identification cards, with local Social Security Administration offices to expedite processing of applications) (Hammett et al., 2001). Case managers should ensure that inmates requiring TB care in the community have access to free TB follow-up appointments and medications immediately postrelease and for as long as they are needed.

Make Arrangements for Postrelease Follow-Up

One of the most critical components of discharge planning for inmates with LTBI or TB disease is the arrangement of postincarceration follow-up appointments and access to medications. Inmates on LTBI therapy who are released from jail or prison before treatment is completed have low community clinical follow-up and treatment completion rates (Nolan et al., 1997; Tulsky et al., 1998). Inmates with TB are at high risk for not completing their TB treatment regimen (MacNeil et al., 2005). Factors such as homelessness, substance abuse, lack of social support or stability, unemployment, and lower education levels contribute to nonadherence postrelease (Cummings et al., 1998; White et al., 2002). Whenever possible, efforts should be made to have inmates complete their LTBI or TB therapy during incarceration. If this is not feasible, case managers, in collaboration with public health staff, should arrange for postrelease follow-up of inmates with appropriate community-based clinical providers so that treatment can be completed.

Case managers should first create an individualized discharge plan based on interviews with inmates about their perceived postrelease health- and nonhealth-related needs, review of the medical records, and discussions with appropriate correction, public health, and community correction staff. When deciding where to refer inmates for TB care and substance abuse, mental health, or other social services needs, case managers should attempt to find community providers that can best integrate and coordinate all of these areas. To maximize the likelihood of continuity of care, case managers should ensure that the community-based providers are interested and experienced in meeting ex-inmates' needs and provide services in locations convenient to where inmates anticipate living or working postrelease. Case managers should establish relationships and agreements with community partners to facilitate inmates' utilization of services (e.g., enabling "walk-in services," providing phone or mail appointment reminders, or providing transportation for referred inmates).

A variety of models exist in correctional facilities for linking prerelease inmates to community clinical providers (Hammett et al., 2001). Some involve community providers coming into the jail or prison to provide direct clinical services, establish a therapeutic alliance with the inmates and follow them clinically in the community postrelease (Flanigan et al., 1996). Less intensive models include (1) community providers working with inmates for only a few months prerelease; (2) inmates not meeting the provider during incarceration, but receiving a set appointment postrelease; and (3) inmates receiving a prerelease list of clinical providers to contact (Hammett et al.). Correctional facilities that enable community providers to establish a direct therapeutic relationship with inmates during incarceration optimize the likelihood of continuity of care postrelease. Correctional staff should encourage public health and community partners to establish a prerelease relationship with inmates either by providing direct services to inmates during incarceration, or by working closely with the discharge planning staff to assist in prerelease planning. For some correctional facilities, however, the distance between them and likely community providers presents difficulties to meeting with the inmates prerelease (Hammett et al.). Even in such cases, providing the inmate with a set appointment date can improve compliance with community follow-up (Rich et al., 2001). At minimum, soon-to-be-released inmates should be given a list of community clinical and social service providers and resources.

As part of the discharge plan, case managers should ensure that all inmates who have been diagnosed with LTBI or TB disease receive community referrals for initiation or continuation of TB treatment. In particular, inmates started on DOT for TB disease or LTBI while incarcerated should continue to be closely monitored by local public health staff who will arrange for the continuation of DOT postrelease until the treatment regimen is completed. Inmates with LTBI who do not require DOT should have uninterrupted access to TB medications postrelease for the duration of their treatment regimen. At minimum, they should be given a sufficient supply of their TB medications until their next TB follow-up appointment in the community (CDC, 2006a). If the anticipated inmate release date and community follow-up appointment date are known, then the case manager can determine the exact amount of medication to provide. If either of these dates is unknown, case managers should work with correction or public health staff to arrange for at least a 2-week to 1-month supply of the TB medications to be available at discharge (Hammett et al., 2001). Providing soon-to-be-released inmates with the actual medication is preferable to giving them a prescription; suspension of health insurance or benefit programs due to incarceration may prevent inmates from being able to fill the prescription soon enough to avoid missing doses. However, if legal, policy, or financial reasons prohibit correctional facilities from providing sufficient amounts of medication for discharge, inmates should be given a prescription to cover the time period from release to the first TB appointment in the community (Hammett et al.). Case managers should also inform inmates about public hospitals and clinics affiliated with state or local health departments that may provide free or low-cost TB care and medications. Regardless of whether medications or prescriptions are given, case managers should ensure that the inmates understand the proper dosing and administration of the TB medications and provide written instructions in the inmates' preferred languages.

Make Provisions for Unplanned Release and Transfers

Correctional facilities should have policies and procedures in place to address unplanned transfers or releases of inmates with LTBI or TB disease (CDC, 2006a). Correctional clinical or discharge planning staff should create and routinely update a summary health record for all inmates (Re-Entry Policy Council, 2003), particularly those with LTBI or TB disease. The summary health record can be initiated based on the initial health screening and added to as needed. The summary should contain all pertinent medical history; physical examination, radiology, and laboratory results; prescribed medications; scheduled consults or clinical appointments; and postrelease management plans. For inmates with LTBI or TB, the summary health record should contain detailed information on TB exposure history, diagnostic testing results including TST or IGRA, chest radiograph, sputum smear and cultures, TB therapy, drug susceptibility patterns, and planned postrelease follow-up.

The summary record should be updated throughout the case management and discharge planning process, based on collaboration with public health and community partners. It should be part of the inmate's medical record and be easily accessible. In addition, staff should ensure that the summary is as complete and up-to-date as possible prior to inmate transfer or release. All inmates being released or transferred from jail or prison should receive a copy of their summary health record, so that they have documentation of the tests or services provided and can share this information with clinical providers upon release (CDC, 2006a).

Correctional discharge planning staff should promptly notify the public health department of all releases into the community of inmates with TB disease or those on treatment for LTBI, to ensure continuity of care postrelease. Inmates with LTBI or TB disease who are being released into the community and did not yet have a discharge plan, should, at minimum, be given their summary health record and a list of community TB providers where they can follow-up postrelease. If the summary record cannot be provided before release, inmates should be informed on how to obtain a copy postrelease. Inmates with LTBI or TB disease who are being transferred to another correctional facility should have all of their TB diagnosis and management information sent to the receiving facility, to avoid duplication of tests or delays in treatment initiation or continuation. Inmates with TB disease who are infectious but are eligible for release or transfer to another medical or correctional facility should remain in AII precautions until they become noninfectious (CDC, 2006a). If AII precautions cannot be maintained during and after the transfer process, facility administrators can consider using a brief "medical hold," so that a follow-up plan can be initiated.

Provide Education and Counseling

Ongoing education and counseling about TB is an important component of discharge planning and TB control efforts in correctional facilities. Inmates, as well as correctional facility staff, may not fully understand TB transmission, the difference between LTBI and TB disease, and methods of TB prevention and treatment (Woods, Harris, & Solomon, 1997). In addition, some inmates and staff may still perceive a stigma associated with TB, which may be a barrier to seeking or providing proper TB care (Woods et al., 1997).

TB education, to increase knowledge, and counseling, to change attitudes, have been shown to increase perception of self-efficacy (Morisky et al., 2001) and improve adherence to community TB follow-up visits and completion of treatment regimens postrelease (White et al., 2002). Frequent education sessions were shown to be more effective than a single education session at diagnosis or even financial incentives in facilitating improved adherence to clinic visits and completion of treatment postrelease (White et al., 2002). Inmates on TB treatment should receive ongoing supportive education and counseling about the importance of adhering to the treatment plan after release into the community. Education should be provided in the inmate's preferred language and be culturally sensitive with regard to ethnicity, gender, and age (Goldberg, Wallace, Jackson, Chaulk, & Nolan, 2004; Hovell et al., 2003; White et al., 2003). Individual TB counseling should be conducted in a private setting if possible (White et al., 2003), so that inmates feel comfortable discussing their questions or concerns. Case managers should ensure that inmates are active participants in the development of the TB discharge plan and provide feedback into their motivations or challenges regarding treatment and adherence.

Community-Based Case Management After Release

The first 24 h after release from a correctional facility are critical to an ex-inmate's success with reentry into the community (Mitty, Holmes, Spaulding, Flanigan, & Page, 1998). Reentrants returning to the same neighborhood where they lived prior to incarceration may be exposed to the same circumstances and influences that led to their arrest. Additionally, at the time of release from jail or prison, reentrants may not have adequate food, clothing, shelter, or financial resources; thus, healthcare becomes less of a priority than these other urgent needs. Therefore, it is imperative that the case management process begun in the correctional facility be continued after release, particularly for ex-inmates with suspected or confirmed TB disease, LTBI who are at high risk for progression to disease, or those who are on TB treatment (CDC, 2006a). Former inmates may experience a lack of social stability and support after reentry into the community; often they find that their community case manager is a much-needed source of support and encouragement (Rhodes & Gross, 1997). As such, public health and community partners should attempt to make contact with reentrants within the first week of release to assist with general transition issues and ensure continuity of TB care as prescribed in the discharge plan created in the correctional facility. Case management that is culturally sensitive and serves reentrant-defined needs, along with TB control needs, has been shown to improve completion rates for therapy (Goldberg et al., 2004). Public health and community partners should also work with community correction staff to ensure that ex-inmates adhere to their follow-up TB clinic visits and medication regimens.

DOT for active TB or LTBI, both in the correctional setting and postrelease, is a strategy for facilitating adherence to TB treatment regimens. DOT initiated in the correctional facility provides an opportunity for education and counseling and establishes the medication as routine (CDC, 2006a). The continuation of DOT postrelease may enhance compliance and reduce relapse rates and acquired drug resistance (Nolan et al., 1997). Implementation of DOT in conjunction with housing programs has been effective in improving TB therapy outcomes in homeless populations (LoBue et al., 1999).

Incentives and enablers are another strategy that case managers can use to promote adherence to TB treatment. Incentives are items or services that encourage individuals to complete TB treatment by motivating them with something they want or need (e.g., food, money, clothing). Enablers help clients overcome barriers to completing their TB treatment (e.g., transportation, stable housing, service programs). Incentives and enablers, combined with education and counseling, have been shown to improve adherence to TB follow-up appointments and treatment completion in incarcerated populations (Frieden et al., 1995; Tulsky et al., 1998, White, Tulsky, McIntosh, Hoynes, & Goldenson, 1998; White et al., 2002). Financial incentives are believed to be most effective for promoting adherence (Giuffrida & Torgerson, 1997). Recent data suggest that financial incentives may be helpful in adherence to initial follow-up clinic visits, but that ongoing education and counseling may be more effective in facilitating completion of TB treatment regimen (Pilote et al., 1996; White et al., 2002).

Comprehensive discharge planning and community linkages have been shown to reduce recidivism rates (Flanigan et al., 1996). Despite these successes, approximately two-thirds of all parolees are rearrested within three years; most are rearrested within the first 6 months after release. Thus, case management after release is critical for continuity of care in the event of reincarceration, particularly for inmates who are still taking TB treatment when rearrested.

TB Control Program Evaluation

Correctional facilities should conduct a program evaluation of their TB control program to determine if stated and desired TB prevention and control goals are being met. The program evaluation should include a systematic assessment of TB program goals, activities, and outcomes. In addition, local TB epidemiology data (e.g., TB case rates, demographics of TB cases, local drug susceptibility data) should be used to inform the evaluation. Data from the program evaluation should be used to guide program planning and policy. Guidelines on conducting a TB program evaluation in correctional facilities have been published (CDC, 2006a).

Conclusion

TB in any segment of the population endangers every member of society (Laniado-Laborin, 2001). Correctional facilities are part of our communities, not separate from them (Hammett et al., 2001). If the goal of TB elimination is ever to be achieved, increased attention must be given to incarcerated populations in which the prevalence and transmission risk of TB are high. The early screening, diagnosis, isolation, and treatment of inmates with TB must be prioritized. In addition, continuity of care must be provided throughout incarceration and postrelease through effective TB discharge planning and case management. Collaboration between correction, public health, and community partners is essential and this ensures the greatest chance of success in the prevention, control, and ultimately, elimination of TB.

References

Abrahao, R. M., Nogueira, P. A., & Malucelli, M. I. (2006). Tuberculosis in county jail prisoners in the western sector of the city of Sao Paulo, Brazil. *The International Journal of Tuberculosis and Lung Disease, 10*(2), 203–208.

Adib, S. M., Al-Takash, H., & Al-Hajj, C. (1999). Tuberculosis in Lebanese jails: Prevalence and risk factors. *European Journal of Epidemiology, 15*(3), 253–260.

American Society of Heating, Refrigerating, and Air-Conditioning Engineers. (2003). Justice Facilities. *ASHRAE handbook: HVAC applications* (pp. 8.1–8.3). Atlanta, GA: American Society of Heating, Refrigerating, and Air-Conditioning Engineers.

American Thoracic Society. (2000). Diagnostic standards and classification of tuberculosis in adults and children. *American Journal of Respiratory and Critical Care Medicine, 161*, 1376–1395.

American Thoracic Society, Centers for Disease Control and Prevention, and Infectious Diseases Society of America. (2003). Treatment of tuberculosis. *MMWR, 52(RR*-11), 1–77.

Barclay, R., & Wheeler, P. R. (1989). Metabolism of mycobacteria in tissues. In C. Ratledge, J. Stanford, & J. M. Grange (Ed.), *Clinical aspects of mycobacterial disease* (pp. 37–106). London: Academic Press.

Bazelon Center for Mental Health Law. (2000). Finding the key to successful transition from jail to community. Available from URL: http://www.ich.gov/innovations/1/index.html.

Bellin, E. Y., Fletcher, D. D., & Safyer, S. M. (1993). Association of tuberculosis infection with increased time in or admission to the New York City jail system. *The Journal of American Medial Association, 269*, 2228–2231.

Bur, S., Golub, J. E., Armstrong, J. A., Myers, K., Johnson, B. H., Mazo, D., et al. (2003). Evaluation of an extensive tuberculosis contact investigation in an urban community and jail. *The International Journal of Tuberculosis and Lung Disease, 7*, S417–S423.

Bureau of Justice Statistics. (2005). Adult correctional populations, 1980–2004. Washington, DC: U.S. Department of Justice, Office of Justice Programs. Available at http://www.ojp.usdoj.gov/bjs/glance/corr2.htm.

Carbonara, S., Babudieri, S., Longo, B., Starnini, G., Monarca, R., Brunetti, B., et al. (2005). Correlates of *Mycobacterium tuberculosis* infection in a prison population. *The European Respiratory Journal, 25*, 1070–1076.

Centers for Disease Control and Prevention. (1992a). Transmission of multidrug-resistant tuberculosis among immunocompromised persons in a correctional system-New York, 1991. *MMWR, 41*(28), 507–509.

Centers for Disease Control and Prevention. (1992b). Tuberculosis transmission in a state correctional institution – California, 1990–1991. *MMWR, 41*(49), 927–929.

Centers for Disease Control and Prevention. (1992c). National action plan to combat multidrug-resistant tuberculosis. *MMWR, 41*(RR-11), 1–48.

Centers for Disease Control and Prevention. (1994). Guidelines for preventing the transmission of *Mycobacterium tuberculosis* in health-care facilities. *MMWR, 43*(RR-13), 1–132.

Centers for Disease Control and Prevention. (1996a). The role of BCG in the prevention and control of tuberculosis in the United States. *MMWR, 45*(RR-4), 1–18.

Centers for Disease Control and Prevention. (1996b). Anergy skin testing and tuberculosis preventive therapy for HIV-infected persons: Revised recommendations. *MMWR, 46*(RR-15), 1–10.

Centers for Disease Control and Prevention. (1998). Prevention and treatment of tuberculosis among patients infected with Human Immunodeficiency Virus: Principles of therapy and revised recommendations. *MMWR, 47*(RR-20), 1–78.

Centers for Disease Control and Prevention. (1999a). Tuberculosis elimination revisited: Obstacles, opportunities, and a renewed commitment – Advisory Council for the Elimination of Tuberculosis (ACET). *MMWR, 48*(RR-9), 1–13.

Centers for Disease Control and Prevention. (1999b). Tuberculosis outbreaks in prison housing units for HIV-infected inmates – California, 1995–1996. *MMWR, 48*(4), 79–82.

Centers for Disease Control and Prevention. (1999c). TB Respiratory Protection Program in Health Care Facilities. Available at http://www.cdc.gov/niosh/99–143. html.

Centers for Disease Control and Prevention. (2000a). Drug-susceptible tuberculosis outbreak in a state correctional facility housing HIV-infected inmates – South Carolina, 1999–2000. *MMWR, 49*(46), 1041–1044.

Centers for Disease Control and Prevention. (2000b). Targeted tuberculosis testing and treatment of latent tuberculosis infection. *MMWR, 49*(RR-6), 1–54.

Centers for Disease Control and Prevention. (2001). Helping inmates return to the community. Available at http://www.cdc.gov/idu/facts/cj-transition.htm.

Centers for Disease Control and Prevention. (2003a). Rapid assessment of tuberculosis in a large prison system – Botswana, 2002. *MMWR, 52*(12), 250–252.

Centers for Disease Control and Prevention. (2003b). Guidelines for environmental infection control in health-care facilities: Recommendations of CDC and the Healthcare Infection Control Practices Advisory Committee (HICPAC). *MMWR, 52*(RR-10), 1–42.

Centers for Disease Control and Prevention. (2003c). Update: Adverse Event Data and Revised American Thoracic Society/CDC recommendations against the use of rifampin and pyrazinamide for treatment of latent tuberculosis infection – United States, 2003. *MMWR, 52*(31), 735–739.

Centers for Disease Control and Prevention. (2004a). Tuberculosis associated with blocking agents against tumor necrosis factor-alpha – California, 2002–2003. *MMWR, 53*(30), 683–686.

Centers for Disease Control and Prevention. (2004b). Tuberculosis transmission in multiple correctional facilities – Kansas, 2002–2003. *MMWR, 53,* 734–738.

Centers for Disease Control and Prevention. (2005a). Guidelines for preventing the transmission of Mycobacterium tuberculosis in health-care settings. *MMWR, 54*(RR-17), 1–141.

Centers for Disease Control and Prevention. (2005b). Guidelines for the investigation of contacts of persons with infectious tuberculosis: Recommendations from the National Tuberculosis Controllers Association and CDC. *MMWR, 54*(RR-15), 1–37.

Centers for Disease Control and Prevention. (2005c). Guidelines for using the QuantiFERON®-TB Gold test for detecting *Mycobacterium tuberculosis* infection, United States. *MMWR, 54*(RR-15), 49–55.

Centers for Disease Control and Prevention. (2006a). Prevention and control of tuberculosis in correctional and detention facilities: Recommendations from CDC. *MMWR, 55*(RR-9), 1–44.

Centers for Disease Control and Prevention. (2006b). Emergence of M*ycobacterium tuberculosis* with extensive resistance to second-line drugs – Worldwide, 2000–2004. *MMWR, 55*(11), 301–305.

Centers for Disease Control and Prevention. (2007). Extensively drug-resistant tuberculosis – United States, 1993–2006. *MMWR, 56*(11), 250–253.

Committee on Prophylaxis, International Union Against Tuberculosis. (1982). Efficacy of various durations of isoniazid preventive therapy for tuberculosis: Five years of follow-up in the IUAT trial. *Bulletin of the World Health Organization, 60*, 555–564.

Coninx, R., Maher, D., Reyes, H., & Grzemska, M. (2000). Tuberculosis in prisons in countries with high prevalence. *British Medical Journal, 320*, 440–442.

Coninx, R., Pfyffer, G. E., Mathieu, C., Savina, D., Debacker, M., Jafarov, F., et al. (1998). Drug resistant tuberculosis in prisons in Azerbaijan: Case study. *British Medical Journal,* 316, 1423–1425.

Cummings, K. C., Mohle-Boetani, J., Royce, S. E., & Chin, D. P. (1998). Movement of tuberculosis patients and the failure to complete antituberculosis treatment. *American Journal of Respiratory and Critical Care Medicine, 157*(4), 1249–1252.

Dye, C., & Floyd, K. (2006). Tuberculosis. In D. T. Jamison, J. G. Breman, A. R. Measham, G. Alleyne, M. Claeson, D. B. Evans, P. Jha, A. Mills, & P. Musgrove (Eds.), *Disease control priorities in developing countries* (2nd ed., pp. 271–287. The World Bank Group.

Flanigan, T. P., Kim, J. Y., Zierler, S., Rich, J., Vigilante, K., & Bury-Maynard, D. (1996). A prison release program for HIV-positive women: Linking them to health services and community follow-up. *American Journal of Public Health, 86*(6), 886–887.

Frieden, T. R., Fujiwara, P. I., Washko, R. M., & Hamburg, M. A. (1995). Tuberculosis in New York City – turning the tide. *The New England Journal of Medicine, 333*, 229–233.

Garner, J. S. (1996). Guideline for isolation precautions in hospitals. The Hospital Infection Control Practices Advisory Committee. *Infection Control and Hospital Epidemiology, 17*(1), 53–80.

Giuffrida, A., & Torgerson, D. J. (1997). Should we pay the patient? Review of financial incentives to enhance patient compliance. *British Medical Journal, 315*, 703–707.

Glaser, J. B., & Greifinger, R. B. (1993). Correctional health care: A public health opportunity. *Annals of Internal Medicine, 118*(2), 139–145.

Goldberg, S. V., Wallace, J., Jackson, J. C., Chaulk, C. P., & Nolan, C. M. (2004). Cultural case management of latent tuberculosis infection. *The International Journal of Tuberculosis and Lung Disease, 8*(1), 76–82.

Golub, J. E., Cronin, W. A., Obasanjo, O. O., Coggin, W., Moore, K., Pope, D. S., et al. (2001). Transmission of *Mycobacterium tuberculosis* through casual contact with an infectious case. *Archives of Internal Medicine, 161*, 2254–2258.

Hammett, T. M., Gaiter, J. L., & Crawford, C. (1998). Reaching seriously at-risk populations: Health interventions in criminal justice settings. *Health Education & Behavior, 25*(1), 99–120.

Hammett, T. M., Harmon, M. P., & Rhodes, W. (2002). The burden of infectious disease among inmates of and releasees from US correctional facilities, 1997. *American Journal of Public Health, 92*(11), 1789–1794.

Hammett, T. M., Roberts, C., & Kennedy, S. (2001). Health-related issues in prisoner reentry. *Crime & Delinquency, 47*(3), 390–409.

Hovell, M. F., Sipan, C. L., Blumberg, E. J., Hofstetter, C.R., Slymen, D., Friedman, L., et al. (2003). Increasing Latino adolescents' adherence to treatment for latent tuberculosis infection: A controlled trial. *American Journal of Public Health, 93*(11), 1871–1877.

Human Rights Watch. (2003). Ill-equipped: U.S. prisons and offenders with mental illness. Available at http://www.hrw.org/reports/2003/usa1003/.

Ikeda, R. M., Birkhead, G. S., DiFerdinando, G. T., Jr., Bornstein, D. L., Dooley, S. W., Kubica, G. P., et al. (1995). Nosocomial tuberculosis: An outbreak of a strain resistant to seven drugs. *Infection Control and Hospital Epidemiology, 16*, 152–159.

Jones, T. F., Craig, A. S., Valway, S. E., Woodley, C. L., & Schaffner, W. (1999). Transmission of tuberculosis in a jail. *Annals of Internal Medicine, 131*, 557–563.

Jones, T. F., & Schaffner, W. (2001). Miniature chest radiograph screening for tuberculosis in jails: A cost-effective analysis. *American Journal of Respiratory and Critical Care Medicine, 164*, 77–81.

Jones, T. F., Woodley, C. L., Fountain, F. F., & Schaffner, W. (2003). Increased incidence of the outbreak strain of *Mycobacterium tuberculosis* in the surrounding community after an outbreak in a jail. *The Southern Medical Journal, 96*, 155–157.

Kenyon, T. A., Ridzon, R., Luskin-Hawk, R., Schultz, C., Paul, W. S., Valway, S.E., et al. (1997). A nosocomial outbreak of multidrug-resistant tuberculosis. *Annals of Internal Medicine, 127*, 32–36.

Klopf, L. C. (1998). Tuberculosis control in the New York State Department of Correctional Services: A case management approach. *American Journal of Infection Control, 26*(5), 534–537.

Koo, D. T., Baron, R. C., & Rutherford, G. W. (1997). Transmission of *Mycobacterium tuberculosis* in a California state prison, 1991. *American Journal of Public Health, 87*, 279–282.

Laniado-Laborin, R. (2001). Tuberculosis in correctional facilities: A nightmare without end in sight. *Chest, 119*, 681–683.

La Vigne, N. G., Visher, C., & Castro, J. (2004). Chicago prisoners' experiences returning home. Washington, DC: The Urban Institute. Available at http://www.urban.org/url.cfm?ID = 311115.

Layton, M. C., Henning, K., Alexander, T., Gooding, A., Reid, C., Heyman, B., et al. (1997). Universal radiographic screening for tuberculosis among inmates upon admission to jails. *American Journal of Public Health, 87*, 1335–1337.

Lindblom, E. N. (1991). Toward a comprehensive homelessness-prevention strategy. *Housing Policy Debate, 2*(3), 957–1025.

Lobato, M., Roberts, C., Bazerman, L., & Hammett, T. (2004). Public health and correctional collaboration in tuberculosis control. *American Journal of Preventive Medicine, 27*(2), 112–117.

LoBue, P. A., Cass, R., Lobo, D., Moser, K., & Catanzaro, A. (1999). Development of housing programs to aid in the treatment of tuberculosis in homeless individuals: A pilot study. *Chest, 115*, 218–223.

MacIntyre, C. R., Kendig, N., Kummer, L., Birago, S., & Graham, N. M. (1997). Impact of tuberculosis control measures and crowding on the incidence of tuberculosis infection in Maryland prisons. *Clinical Infectious Disease, 24*, 1060–1067.

MacIntyre, C. R., Kendig, N., Kummer, L., Birago, S., Graham, N. M., & Plant, A.J. (1999). Unrecognised transmission of tuberculosis in prisons. *European Journal of Epidemiology, 15*, 705–709.

MacNeil, J., Lobato, M. N., & Moore, M. (2005). An unanswered health disparity: Tuberculosis among correctional inmates, 1993 through 2003. *American Journal of Public Health, 95*, 1800–1805.

Maher, D., & Raviglione, M. (2005). Global epidemiology of tuberculosis. *Clinics in Chest Medicine, 26*(2), 167–182.

Marco, A., Cayla, J. A., Serra, M., Pedro, R., Sanrama, C., Guerrero, R., et al. (1998). Predictors of adherence to tuberculosis treatment in a supervised therapy programme for prisoners before and after release. Study Group of Adherence to Tuberculosis Treatment of Prisoners. *The European Respiratory Journal, 12*, 967–971.

Mitty, J. A., Holmes, L., Spaulding, A., Flanigan, T., & Page, J. (1998). Transitioning HIV-infected women after release from incarceration: Two models for bridging the gap. *Journal of Correctional Health Care, 5*(2), 239–254.

Mohle-Boetani, J. C., Miguelino, V., Dewsnup, D. H., Desmond, E., Horowitz, E., Waterman, S.H., et al. (2002). Tuberculosis outbreak in a housing unit for human immunodeficiency virus-infected patients in a correctional facility: Transmission risk factors and effective outbreak control. *Clinical Infectious Disease, 34*, 668–676.

Morisky, D. E., Malotte, C. K., Ebin, V., Davidson, P., Cabrera, D., Trout, P. T., et al. (2001). Behavioral interventions for the control of tuberculosis among adolescents. *Public Health Reports, 116*(6), 568–574.

National Commission on Correctional Health Care. (2003). Standards for health services in jails. Chicago, IL: National Commission on Correctional Health Care.

National Commission on Correctional Health Care. (2003). Standards for health services in prisons. Chicago, IL: National Commission on Correctional Health Care.

Nelson, M., & Trone, J. (2000). *Why planning for release matters.* Vera Institute for Justice. Available at http://www.vera.org/publication_pdf/planning_for_release.pdf.

Nolan, C. M., Roll, L., Goldberg, S. V., & Elarth, A. M. (1997). Directly observed isoniazid preventive therapy for released jail inmates. *American Journal of Respiratory and Critical Care Medicine, 155*, 583–586.

Pai, M. (2005). Alternatives to the tuberculin skin test: Interferon-γ assays in the diagnosis of Mycobacterium tuberculosis infection. *Indian Journal of Medical Microbiology, 23*(3), 151–158.

Pai, M., Gokhale, K., Joshi, R., Dogra, S., Kalantri, S., Mendiratta, D. K., et al. (2005). *Mycobacterium tuberculosis* infection in health care workers in rural India: Comparison of a whole-blood interferon g assay with tuberculin skin testing. *The Journal of American Medial Association, 293*, 2746–2755.

Pai, M., Kalantri, S., & Dheda, K. (2006). New tools and emerging technologies for the diagnosis of tuberculosis: Part I. Latent tuberculosis. *Expert Review of Molecular Diagnostics, 6*(3), 413–422.

Pai, M., Riley, L. W., & Colford, J. M. (2004). Interferon-γ assays in the immunodiagnosis of tuberculosis: A systematic review. *The Lancet Infectious Disease, 4*, 761–776.

Pilote, L., Tulsky, J. P., Zolopa, A. R., Hahn, J. A., Schecter, G. F., & Moss, A. R. (1996). Tuberculosis prophylaxis in the homeless. A trial to improve adherence to referral. *Archives of Internal Medicine, 156*(2), 161–165.

Puisis, M., Feinglass, J., Lidow, E., & Mansour, M. (1996). Radiographic screening for tuberculosis in a large urban county jail. *Public Health Reports, 111*, 330–334.

Re-Entry Policy Council. (2003). Charting the Safe and Successful Return of Prisoners to the Community. Available at http://www.reentrypolicy.org/reentry/THE_REPORT.aspx.

Rhodes, W., & Gross, M. (1997). Case management reduces drug use and criminality among drug-involved arrestees: An experimental study of an HIV prevention intervention. *NIJ Research Report*, 1–50.

Rich, J. D., Holmes, L., Salas, C., Macalino, G., Davis, D., Ryczek, J., et al. (2001). Successful linkage of medical care and community services for HIV-positive offenders being released from prison. *Journal of Urban Health, 78*(2), 279–289.

Richeldi, L., Ewer, K., Losi, M., Bergamini, B. M., Roversi, P., Deeks, J., et al. (2004). T cell-based tracking of multidrug resistant tuberculosis infection after brief exposure. *American Journal of Respiratory and Critical Care Medicine, 170*, 288–295.

Salomon, N., Perlman, D. C., Rubenstein, A., Mandelman, D., McKinley, F. W., & Yancovitz, S. R. (1997). Implementation of universal directly observed therapy at a New York City hospital and evaluation of an out-patient directly observed therapy program. *The International Journal of Tuberculosis and Lung Disease, 1*(5), 397–404.

Saunders, D. L., Olive, D. M., Wallace, S. B., Lacy, D., Leyba, R., & Kendig, N. E. (2001). Tuberculosis screening in the federal prison system: An opportunity to treat and prevent tuberculosis in foreign-born populations. *Public Health Reports, 116*(3), 210–218.

Sherris, J. C., & Plorde, J. J. (1990). Mycobacteria. In *Medical microbiology* (2nd ed, pp. 443–461).

Stead, W. W. (1978). Undetected tuberculosis in prison: Source of infection for community at large. *The Journal of American Medial Association, 240*, 2544–2547.

Steenland, K., Levine, A. J., Sieber, K., Schulte, P., & Aziz, D. (1997). Incidence of tuberculosis infection among New York State prison employees. *American Journal of Public Health, 87*(12), 2012–2014.

Tenover, F. C., Crawford, J. T., Huebner, R. E., Geitner, L. J., Horsburgh, C. R., & Good, R. C. (1993). The resurgence of tuberculosis: Is your laboratory ready? *Journal of Clinical Microbiology, 31*(4), 767–770.

Todar, K. (2005). Todar's online textbook of bacteriology. Available at http://textbookofbacteriology.net/tuberculosis.html.

Tulsky, J. P., White, M. C., Dawson, C., Hoynes, T. M., Goldenson, J., & Schecter, G. (1998). Screening for tuberculosis in jail and clinic follow-up after release. *American Journal of Public Health, 88*(2), 223–226.

U.S. Department of Justice. Prison and jail inmates at midyear 2003. Bureau of Justice Statistics Bulletin: 2004. NCJ 203947.

Valway, S. E., Greifinger, R. B., Papania, M., Kilburn, J. O., Woodley, C., DiFerdinando, G. T., et al. (1994). Multidrug resistant tuberculosis in the New York State prison system, 1990–1991. *The Journal of Infectious Disease, 170*, 151–156.

Valway, S. E., Richards, S. B., Kovacovich, J., Greifinger, R. B., Crawford, J. T., & Dooley, S. W. (1994). Outbreak of multi-drug-resistant tuberculosis in a New York state prison, 1991. *American Journal of Epidemiology, 140*(2), 113–122.

Vishner, C., Kachnowski, V., La Vigne, N., & Travis, J. (2004). Baltimore prisoners' experiences returning home. Washington, DC: The Urban Institute. Available at http://www.urban.org/UploadedPDF/310946_BaltimorePrisoners.pdf.

Wayne, L. G., & Hayes, L. G. (1996). An in vitro model for sequential study of shift-down of Mycobacterium tuberculosis through two stages of nonreplicating persistence. *Infection and Immunity, 64*(6), 2062–2069.

White, M. C., Duong, T. M., Cruz, E. S., Rodas, A., McCall, C., Menendez, E., et al. (2003). Strategies for effective education in a jail setting: The Tuberculosis Prevention Project. *Health Promotion Practice, 4*(4), 422–429.

White, M. C., Tulsky, J. P., Goldenson, J., Portillo, C. J., Kawamura, M., & Menendez, E. (2002). Randomized controlled trial of interventions to improve follow-up for latent tuberculosis infection after release from jail. *Archives of Internal Medicine, 162*, 1044–1050.

White, M. C., Tulsky, J. P., McIntosh, H. W., Hoynes, T. M., & Goldenson, J. (1998). A clinical trial of a financial incentive to go to the tuberculosis clinic for isoniazid after release from jail. *The International Journal of Tuberculosis and Lung Disease, 2*, 506–512.

White, M. C., Tulsky, J. P., Portillo, C. J., Menendez, E., Cruz, E., & Goldenson, J. (2001). Tuberculosis prevalence in an urban jail: 1994 and 1998. *The International Journal of Tuberculosis and Lung Disease, 5*, 400–404.

Wilcock, K., Hammett, T. M., & Parent, D. G. (1995). *Controlling tuberculosis in community corrections.* National Institute of Justice: Research in Action, 1–11.

Woods, G. L., Harris, S. L., & Solomon, D. (1997). Tuberculosis knowledge and beliefs among prison inmates and lay employees. *Journal of Correctional Health Care, 4*(1), 61–71.

World Health Organization. (2005). Global Tuberculosis Control. *Surveillance, financing, planning. WHO Report 2005.* WHO, Geneva, Switzerland, 1–247.

World Health Organization. (2006). Emergence of XDR-TB. Available at http://www.who.int/mediacentre/news/notes/2006/np23/en/index.html.

Chapter 12

Controlling Chlamydia, Gonorrhea, and Syphilis Through Targeted Screening and Treatment in Correctional Settings

Charlotte K. Kent and Gail A. Bolan

Sexually transmitted infections (STI) include a broad category of bacterial, viral, protozoan, and fungal infections and ectoparasitic infestations. For three of these bacterial infections, chlamydia, gonorrhea, and syphilis, there is substantive evidence that screening and treatment in correctional settings could play a critical role in their control. We will describe the epidemiology of these infections, the appropriate populations to target for screening, methods to increase treatment of identified infections, evidence of the impact of detention screening in controlling them, and the cost-effectiveness of detention screening. Correctional settings might also play a critical role in controlling HIV, another STI, among some populations, as discussed in Chapter 8.

Epidemiology of Chlamydia, Gonorrhea, Syphilis and Corrections: Overlapping Populations

Chlamydia and Gonorrhea

The United States has the highest rates of STIs among developed countries (Eng & Butler, 1997). Chlamydia and gonorrhea are the two most commonly reported infections with 976,445 and 339,593 cases reported in 2005 (CDC, 2006a). Chlamydia and gonorrhea are most common in persons aged 25 and younger, with peak rates among females aged 15–19 and males aged 20–24 (CDC, 2006a). Rates also are substantially elevated in some racial/ethnic minority populations. Compared with whites, chlamydia rates are more than 7 times greater among blacks, nearly 5 times greater among American Indians/Alaskan Natives, and 3 times greater among Hispanics (CDC, 2006a). Even greater disparities exist in gonorrhea rates, with the rates more than 19 times greater among blacks, more than 3 times greater among American Indians/Alaskan Natives, and more than 2 times greater among Hispanics compared with whites (CDC, 2006a). In addition to demographic characteristics, other risk markers for STIs include: multiple sex partners, drug and alcohol abuse, lower educational attainment and socioeconomic status, and poor access to medical care (Aral & Holmes, 1999).

Chlamydia and gonorrhea can lead to serious long-term sequelae in women, including chronic pelvic pain, pelvic inflammatory disease, infertility, and ectopic pregnancy (Hook & Handsfield, 1999; Stamm, 1999). Additionally, these infections increase the susceptibility and transmissibility of HIV infection (Fleming & Wasserheit, 1999). Annual chlamydia screening of sexually active women aged 25 and younger is recommended (CDC, 2006b), but there are no guidelines for screening men. Because most chlamydial and gonococcal infections in both females and males are asymptomatic (Hook & Handsfield, 1999; Stamm, 1999), screening and treatment of asymptomatic infections is essential for disease prevention and control. Large-scale screening programs that have been in place for several years have decreased both community chlamydia prevalence and disease outcomes (Addiss et al., 1993; Mertz et al., 1997). The most effective method to control chlamydia is routine screening in high-volume, high-prevalence settings (Farley et al., 2003).

Syphilis

Syphilis is a genital ulcerative disease that causes significant cardiovascular and neurological complications if untreated (Sparling, 1999). In pregnant women, 40% of untreated early syphilis results in perinatal death (Radolf et al., 1999). If syphilis was acquired during the 4 years preceding pregnancy, it could lead to infection of the fetus in over 70% of cases (Radolf et al., 1999). Like other STIs, syphilis also facilitates the transmission of HIV (Fleming & Wasserheit, 1999). Syphilis infection is staged by symptoms and likely duration of infection. Early infections of less than 1 year's duration (primary, secondary, and early latent) are the most important stages from a public health perspective, because they represent recent infections among persons and sexual networks which should be targeted for intervention to prevent further ongoing transmission within a community.

Syphilis was extremely common until the introduction of penicillin in the 1940s, with up to 25% persons of lower socioeconomic status infected (Sparling, 1999). Syphilis rates reached a nadir in the United States in 2000, and rates continued to decline among women through 2003 (CDC, 2006a). Beginning in 2001, rates increased nationally among men who have sex with men (MSM) (CDC, 2006a). During 2005, there were 33,278 reported cases of syphilis in the United States, 1/10 the number of gonorrhea cases and 1/30 the number of chlamydia cases (CDC, 2006a). The majority of counties (78%) in the United States reported no cases of syphilis, and half of syphilis cases were found in just 19 counties and two cities (CDC, 2006a). During the late 1990s, syphilis elimination in the United States was considered plausible because of the historically low rates of infection, the limited geographic distribution of infection, and the availability of effective and inexpensive diagnostic tests and treatment (St Louis & Wasserheit, 1998).

For reasons that are not totally clear, syphilis affects a slightly older population than chlamydia and gonorrhea; the peak age among women is 20–24, among heterosexual men is 25–29, and among men who have sex with men is 35–39 (CDC, 2006a). Like chlamydia and gonorrhea, there are substantial differences in rates by race/ethnicity. Among women, compared with whites, African American rates are nearly 15 times greater, American Indian/Alaskan Native rates are 5 times greater and Hispanic rates are 3 times greater (CDC, 2006a).

Correctional Populations

Many persons housed temporarily in jails and juvenile detention facilities have risk factors for STIs: unprotected sex with multiple partners before incarceration, poor access to medical care, lack of education, a personal or family history of drug and alcohol abuse, a history of physical and sexual abuse, young age, and racial or ethnic minority status (Beltrami et al., 1997; Aral & Holmes, 1999; James, 2004; Bureau of Justice Statistics, 2004; Margolis et al., 2006). More than 60% of detained persons are racial or ethnic minorities, more than 40% are younger than 30, and more than 85% are male (National Center for Juvenile Justice, 2004; Bureau of Justice Statistics, 2005; Harrison & Beck, 2006). More specifically, 10% of young African-American males, aged 18 to 29, currently are incarcerated (Harrison & Beck, 2006), and a higher proportion have been incarcerated in the past year. The U.S. Bureau of Justice estimates that with current rates of first incarcerations, 32% of African-American males will enter long-term state or federal prisons during their lifetimes, compared to 17% of Hispanic males and 6% of white males (Bureau of Justice Statistics, 2004). A much higher proportion of men will spend at least some time in short-term juvenile detention or jail settings. Most individuals detained in jails and juvenile detention facilities are released and return to their communities within only a few days or weeks, and many subsequently have unprotected sex (Skolnick, 1998; MacGowan et al., 2003). Thus, the cycle of STI transmission can continue once persons are released from periods of short-term incarceration.

Overlapping Populations—Corrections and STIs

The epidemiology of chlamydia, gonorrhea, syphilis, and correctional populations suggest that some of the persons at greatest risk for STIs are those who pass through correctional settings. Figure 12.1 is illustrative of this point. The San Francisco Department of Public Health (SFDPH) has performed targeted chlamydia and gonorrhea screening of women and

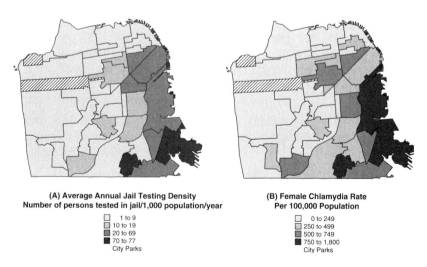

(A) Average Annual Jail Testing Density
Number of persons tested in jail/1,000 population/year

☐ 1 to 9
☐ 10 to 19
▨ 20 to 69
■ 70 to 77
City Parks

(B) Female Chlamydia Rate
Per 100,000 Population

☐ 0 to 249
☐ 250 to 499
▨ 500 to 749
■ 750 to 1,800
City Parks

Figure 12.1 (A) Average annual jail testing density, 1997–2004 and **(B)** female chlamydia rate, 2004 by neighbourhood — San Francisco.

men in the county jails since the fall of 1996. Screening is targeted by age, not by residence. To compare screening in jail by neighborhood, SFDPH calculated jail testing density, which was defined as the average number of persons in the age and sex groups targeted for jail screening who were tested during 1997–2004, divided by the year 2000 census population for these same age and sex groups. In Figure 12.1, the San Francisco map on the left represents jail testing density. It is apparent that the greatest density of testing in jails occurred among residents of the southeastern portion of the city. The map on the right shows 2004 chlamydia rates among women, with the highest rates in the southeast. In San Francisco, there is a significant correlation between the neighborhoods with the greatest jail testing density and the highest rates of chlamydia.

During the second half of 2004, the City of New York Department of Correction began screening men aged 35 and younger for chlamydia at Rikers Island Jail. Prior to this time only men with symptoms were tested (personal communication from Julie Schillinger, New York City Department of Health and Mental Hygiene). Figure 12.2 demonstrates the remarkable number of infections that were detected after this asymptomatic screening program was implemented. The number of infections detected among males in corrections increased 12-fold between the first half of 2004 and 2005. During 2005, there were 40% more infections detected at Rikers Island Jail than in the 10 New York City STD Clinics, and jail screening increased the total number of reported cases of chlamydia among men in the entire city by 60%. The New York City public health surveillance data suggest that there is a tremendous reservoir of asymptomatic chlamydial infection among young adult men in jail.

While incarcerated males are at high risk for chlamydia, the prevalence of infections varied substantially in published studies, from 3% to 25% (Brady et al., 1988; Beltrami et al., 1998; Cromwell et al., 2002; Mertz, Voight, et al., 2002; Chen et al., 2003; Hardick et al., 2003; Bauer et al., 2004; CDC, 2005, 2006a; de Ravello et al., 2005; Kahn et al., 2005; Robertson et al., 2005; Trick

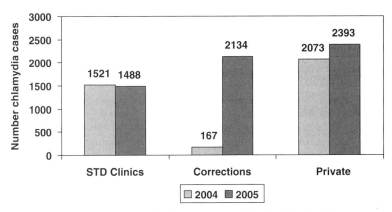

J. Schillinger, New York City Department of Health & Mental Hygiene

Figure 12.2 Reported chlamydia among males by provider type: New York City, Jan – June 2004 compared with Jan – June 2005.

et al., 2006). Among females, the prevalence varied from 1.7% to 24.7% (Bell et al., 1985; Oh et al., 1998; Kelly et al., 2000; Risser et al., 2001; Cromwell et al., 2002; Mertz, Voight, et al., 2002; Hardick et al., 2003; Bauer et al., 2004; Katz et al., 2004; de Ravello et al., 2005; Kahn et al., 2005; Robertson et al., 2005; CDC, 2006a). There was also a wide range found in gonorrhea screening, varying from 0.6% to 18.3% among females and 1.1% to 6.7% among males (Bell et al., 1985; Alexander-Rodriguez & Vermund, 1987; Brady et al., 1988; O'Brien et al., 1988; Ellerbeck et al., 1989; Bickell et al., 1991; Oh et al., 1994, 1998; Beltrami et al., 1998; Pack et al., 2000; Cromwell et al., 2002; Mertz, Voight, et al., 2002; Chen et al., 2003; Hardick et al., 2003; Katz et al., 2004; de Ravello et al., 2005; Kahn et al., 2005; Plitt et al., 2005; Robertson et al., 2005; CDC, 2006a; Trick et al., 2006). The prevalence of these infections varied by geographic region, gender, setting (youth detention, jail or prison), and age of persons screened. The highest prevalence of infections was found in the southeastern United States, reflecting this region's high STI rates (CDC, 2006a).

Data from males and females screened for chlamydia in youth detention and jails in San Francisco illustrate how prevalence varies by gender, age (groupings are by stages of adolescent and adult development), and setting (Figure 12.3). The prevalence of chlamydial infection in San Francisco was consistently higher among females than males, women aged 18–25 had a similar prevalence of infection as younger women, and the highest prevalence of infection among males occurred among men aged 18–25. In San Francisco, SFDPH screens about 90% of females and males in youth detention, but limited resources allow screening of only about 45% of the target population in jails. Despite the limited screening coverage in jails, nearly double the number of infections were detected among young women aged 18–25 in jails than detected in youth detention, and more than four times more infections were detected among young men aged 18–25, than among boys in youth detention (Figure 12.3). The number of infections detected in San Francisco among young adults in jails versus adolescents in youth detention, reflect the prevalence of infection in these settings and the number of persons available for screening in these settings.

The prevalence of syphilis infection detected in corrections also varied by gender, age, and geographic region. The prevalence of reactive serologic tests ranged from 0.0% to 19% (Cohen et al., 1992; Blank et al., 1997, 1999; Silberstein et al., 2000; Wolfe et al., 2001; Kahn et al., 2002; CDC, 2006a). Syphilis was most commonly detected in jails located in communities with high syphilis rates among heterosexuals (Kahn et al., 2004).

Public Health Strategies for Controlling STIs

There are three determinants of the rate of spread (reproductive rate) of STIs: (1) the probability of exposure of infected persons to uninfected persons, which relates to the number of partners an infected person has, (2) the average probability of transmission per partner sexual contact, and (3) the average duration of infectiousness of an infected person (Anderson & May, 1991). The prevalence of STIs in a community is related to the reproductive rate of STIs. While the spread of STIs is based on these three determinants, an individual's risk of acquiring an STI is based on their sexual behavior and the

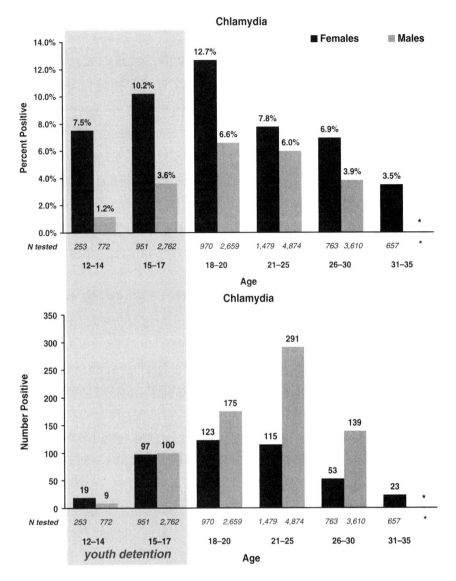

Figure 12.3 Chlamydia percent positive and number positive among persons screened in adult jails and youth detention centers — San Francisco, 2003–2005. Shaded area indicates youth detention. *Males aged 31–35 years not eligible for screening.

probability of having sex with someone who is infectious. For example, given the substantially elevated rates of STIs among African-American women versus white women, a young African-American woman who has the exact same sexual risk behavior as a young white woman but who has an African-American male partner has a much greater risk of acquiring an STI. Therefore, to reduce these racial and ethnic disparities it is critical to prioritize programs that screen and treat members of ethnic and racial populations at highest risk of infection. Screening and treating these populations reduces the duration of infection in the community, which drives down the reproductive rate and the prevalence of infection in the community. This, in turn, lowers the probability of encountering an infected partner. Other strategies to decrease the prevalence of infection in a population include assuring that partners of infected persons are treated (partner management); health education about the importance of accessing care for STI screening, using condoms to prevent STIs (including HIV) and unintended pregnancy, and the risk of multiple partners; and surveillance of emerging STI trends to target intervention resources.

Because many persons detained in jails and youth detention have characteristics that increase their risk for STIs, targeted screening and treatment of STIs in persons entering correctional facilities could prevent medical complications and interrupt transmission to others in the community when they are released. Widespread, targeted screening in short-term correctional facilities, could serve as a public health structural intervention to reduce community rates of STIs.

Targeted STI Screening in Correctional Settings

In order to have the largest impact on the community, targeted STI screening should occur at intake into jails and youth detention because a substantial proportion of detainees are released back to the community within 48 hours (Skolnick, 1998). Screening for STIs in prisons will have much less public health benefit, because generally persons sentenced to prison will be removed from the community for at least 1 year. Thus, they will play only a minor role in ongoing community transmission. In addition, most persons entering prisons will already have been incarcerated for some time prior to their sentencing. Some portion of them will already have cleared their infection, reducing the prevalence of infection and further reducing the cost-effectiveness of screening in the prison setting.

Targeted Chlamydia and Gonorrhea Screening

Because resources for STI screening are limited, screening programs should focus on the highest risk persons in jails and youth detention. Prevalence of infection varies substantially by gender and age. Nationally, the prevalence of chlamydial infection in detention settings among boys younger than 16 was less than 5%, as was the prevalence of infection among men aged 30 and older (CDC, 2006a). Among women aged 35 and older, the prevalence of infection was 5% (CDC, 2006a). The relative ranking of prevalence by gender and age is seen in Figure 12.3. However, because San Francisco has moderate rates of chlamydia among heterosexuals, the observed prevalence of infection is much lower than that observed in much of the country, especially the southeastern United States (CDC, 2006b). Based on San Francisco data and national data (CDC, 2006a), the rank order for targeting chlamydia and gonorrhea screening should be women aged 30 and younger in jails and youth detention, and young adult men aged 18–25 in jails. Currently, the Centers for Disease Control and Prevention (CDC) recommends that all young women in youth detention be screened, and has made screening this population a priority (Kahn et al., 2005). With mounting evidence of the prevalence and number of chlamydial and gonococcal infections among young adults in jails, screening guidelines will likely be expanded to include these populations as well.

Depending on the local prevalence of chlamydia and gonorrhea infection and availability of resources, screening could be expanded to broader age groups. Because the prevalence of infection was high among men aged 26–30 in Chicago, Chicago screening criteria include men in this older age group (Trick et al., 2006). Furthermore, in some communities the prevalence of chlamydia among boys in youth detention is greater than 10% (CDC, 2006a). The prevalence among young men in adult detention in these communities is likely substantially greater, and there are many more young men in jail than youth detention (Bureau of Justice, Justice 2004; Harrison & Beck, 2006), suggesting that screening young men in jails could have an even greater impact on community rates than just screening boys in youth detention. If screening data reported to the CDC are indicative of the national pattern of screening, 45% of chlamydia screening is occurring among boys in youth detention (CDC, 2006a), the population with the lowest priority for limited screening resources.

Because of the ease of specimen collection and the sensitivity and specificity of tests, the CDC recommends nucleic acid amplification technologies for chlamydia and gonorrhea screening in nonclinical settings (CDC, 2002). Collection of specimens for chlamydia and gonorrhea screening is noninvasive (urine) and requires little training. In San Francisco, where screening is part of the routine intake process, health worker staff spend an average of 7 minutes having a brief discussion about STIs, collecting a specimen, and completing paperwork for each person who is screened. Thus, screening can be done quickly and efficiently once established.

Targeted Syphilis Screening

CDC recommends syphilis screening in jails located in communities with a high prevalence of syphilis among heterosexuals (CDC, 2006c). They particularly stress the value of screening women in these settings (CDC, 2006c). Currently there are limited data on the appropriate age to target syphilis screening in corrections. However, given that the peak incidence of syphilis among heterosexuals occurs 5 years later than for chlamydia and gonorrhea (CDC, 2006c), it is likely that screening should target men and women detained in jails to at least age 35. Given the age distribution of infection, syphilis screening in youth detention is likely not warranted except in very limited settings. During 2007, CDC will release written guidelines for the implementation of jail syphilis screening and treatment programs (Beltrami et al., 2007). Regardless of the availability of these guidelines, local public health programs and jails should determine if their communities warrant syphilis screening in jails and what are the appropriate persons to target for screening.

There are several successful models of syphilis screening in jails (Heimberger et al., 1993; Beltrami et al., 1997; Blank et al., 1997; CDC, 1998; Kahn et al., 2002). Programs that used the Rapid Plasma Reagent (Stat RPR), and that had a mechanism to access the local department of health's syphilis case registry to determine the likelihood of reactive RPRs indicating untreated syphilis infection, consistently resulted in a higher treatment rate for arrestees than routine, non-rapid, syphilis testing (Blank et al., 1997; CDC, 1998; Silberstein et al., 2000).

Current syphilis test technology requires the collection of blood specimens (Celum et al., 2002), which requires specimen collection by more highly trained staff than is necessary for chlamydia and gonorrhea screening. CDC and its partners recently have undertaken research and evaluation of noninvasive, point-of-care tests for use in the United States (CDC, 2006c). A sensitive and specific noninvasive, point-of-care test for use in high-prevalence settings in the United States would be a boon to syphilis control, especially in jails.

Methods to Improve Treatment of Persons and their Partners Identified with STIs in Corrections

Identifying persons with STIs in corrections has little public health value unless a high proportion of those with infection are treated. Treatment of persons identified with STIs in corrections varies substantially from a high of 82% to a low of 45% (Heimberger et al., 1993; Beltrami et al., 1997; Blank et al., 1997; Oh et al., 1998; Silberstein et al., 2000; Kahn et al., 2002; Mertz, Schwebke, et al., 2002; Hardick et al., 2003; Barry et al., 2006; Trick et al., 2006). In San Francisco between 2001 and 2004, 81% (1258/1558) of persons with chlamydia and/or gonorrhea identified in the jails were treated (Barry et al., 2006). Among those treated, 79% were treated in the jails, 16% through SFDPH follow-up, and 8% at other treatment venues (Barry et al., 2006).

Factors that SFDPH found to increase treatment in the jails include: assuring that test results are available as quickly as possible, and that patients can be treated as quickly as possible in the jail. Any delay increases the probability that the persons will be released without treatment, which increases the chances they will not be treated because it is frequently difficult to locate people after release. To this end, SFDPH has shortened the laboratory turnaround time as much as possible; developed a mechanism to transmit results to the jail electronic medical record so that results are received as quickly as possible; and generated a list, from laboratory results received that day, alerting Jail Health Staff about who needs treatment. Thus, an electronic jail medical record that can receive test results greatly speeds transmission and notification of results. In order to facilitate quick treatment after results are available, a standing order was developed that allowed nursing staff to treat under the orders of the medical director. Prior to this standing order, treatment in jails was often delayed by 1 to 2 days depending on when a physician was available to see the patient.

To increase treatment after release, SFDPH Jail Health Services and STD Prevention and Control Services have a close working relationship. STD Services receives laboratory results at the same time as Jail Health Services and checks whether a person is still incarcerated. If the person has been released, they immediately assign staff to try to locate the patient. STD Services staff, under the standing order of the STD Services Medical Director, are able to treat persons in the field when they find them, which has increased the proportion of persons treated because many people are reluctant to go to a clinic for treatment (Steiner et al., 2003). In addition, if after 2 weeks, STD Services is unable to find a patient for treatment, an alert is placed in the jail and STD clinic medical record indicating that if the patient should return to either of these settings, they automatically should be treated.

A strategy to increase treatment of partners of infected persons is expedited partner therapy, which includes giving the infected person therapy to provide to their partner(s) (CDC, 2006b) When SFDPH staff provides therapy in the field or at the STD clinic, they offer expedited partner therapy. In addition, SFDPH places expedited partner therapy for two partners into the property of jail patients who are still incarcerated at the time of treatment. The partner therapy is then available for the patient to give to their partner after their release. This partner therapy program in the jails has never been evaluated. However, there is reasonable evidence of the benefit of expedited partner therapy in other settings (Schillinger et al., 2003; Golden, 2005; Golden et al., 2005).

CDC published guidelines about recommended therapies for STIs in 2006 (CDC, 2006b). These guidelines are available at http://www.cdc.gov/mmwr/preview/mmwrhtml/rr5511a1.htm. Generally, in correctional settings, it is preferable to use oral, single dose therapy, even if the treatment might be more expensive, because of the added cost of having inmates brought for treatment multiple times, e.g., a 2-week course of doxycycline versus a single dose of azithromycin for the treatment of chlamydia.

Community Impact of STI Screening in Corrections

The San Francisco jail chlamydia screening program provides evidence of the potential impact STI screening in jails can have on the community (Barry et al., 2006). As mentioned earlier, SFDPH began targeted screening in the jails in the fall of 2006. They compared the prevalence of chlamydia detected among sexually active young women (aged 25 and younger) seen in a community clinic (Clinic S) located in a neighborhood with high jail testing density compared to a community clinic located in a neighborhood with low jail testing density (Clinic O). The prevalence of infection in these two clinics was compared between 1997 and 2004. The initial prevalence at Clinic S was four times higher than at Clinic O. During the evaluation period, the prevalence of infection at Clinic S declined significantly from 16.1% in 1997 to 7.8% in 2004. The prevalence of infection remained stable at Clinic O at 4.7% during the same period with only minor vacillations. No other STD control programs, other than jail screening, could explain the substantial decline in community rates of chlamydia in young women. This decline in community rates of chlamydia among women was seen despite the fact that only about 45% of the target population in the jails was screened and only about 80% of infected persons were treated.

Cost Effectiveness of STI Screening in Corrections

The cost-effectiveness of STI screening in corrections has been examined in a limited fashion with mixed findings due to differences in modeling (Silberstein et al., 2000; Mrus et al., 2003; Blake et al., 2004; Kraut-Becher et al., 2004; Gift et al., 2006). Models have generally shown that the cost-effectiveness improves as the treatment rate before release improves (Kraut-Becher et al., 2004) or as screening men is translated to treatment of cases in women that would otherwise have gone undetected (Blake et al., 2004). Clearly, the higher the prevalence of infection in the population screened, the more cost-effective the screening program will be.

Future Areas for Research and Evaluation

During 2006, a vaccine for the human papillomavirus (HPV) types most commonly associated with cervical cancer and genital warts was introduced for women (Saslow et al., 2007). It remains to be seen whether recommendations will be developed to vaccinate young women in youth detention, as there are recommendations for vaccination of adolescents for other infections in this setting.

As cities, such as New York City, expand corrections screening, there needs to be evaluation of the impact of these massive screening efforts. There should be evaluations of the best methods to increase treatment of persons screened in corrections, because screening without treatment has little impact. Modeling the expected prevalence of chlamydia, gonorrhea, and syphilis detected in corrections based on local disease rates, could provide guidance to local programs about which populations to prioritize and allocate resources for. Because STI disparities are greatest in the southeastern United States, and this is the region with the highest burden of incarceration, it would be useful to model the potential STI burden among incarcerated persons in this region and the impact screening and treatment in corrections could have on regional STI rates. In addition, modeling could suggest how comprehensive screening must be in order to have an impact. In these times of shrinking resources, we must use our limited funds as effectively as possible. Modeling could provide insight into the most effective use of public health and correctional health resources to improve the health of the community.

Summary

There is a heavy burden of STIs among select populations of incarcerated persons. Evidence suggests that targeted screening and treatment of STIs can reduce community rates of infection. Broad-based, national screening of targeted young people in corrections, especially young males in jails, would allow public health programs an opportunity to leverage the alarming racial and ethnic disparities within the incarcerated population to address important subpopulations at greatest risk for STIs. If all young men were screened in jails, over the course of a year more than 10% of black men at greatest risk for chlamydial and gonococcal infection would be screened and treated, presenting a key opportunity for public health impact in the communities these men come from and will return to. Additionally, researchers have attributed the increase in HIV infection among blacks to the rising rate of incarceration among blacks (Johnson & Raphael, 2005). If true, finding and treating STIs among incarcerated adults and their partners will also be increasingly critical as a prevention measure for HIV. Screening and treating young women and men in jails could be an effective method to reduce the burden of STIs, especially among African Americans. The evidence for the public health benefit of targeted STI screening in jails is strong (Cohen et al., 2005), and substantive public health resources should be devoted to targeted jail screening.

Acknowledgments

We thank Jeffrey D. Klausner, MD, MPH, and Pennan Barry, MD, MPH from the San Francisco Department of Public Health, and Julie A. Schillinger, MD, MSc from the New York City Department of Health and Mental Hygiene, for sharing public health surveillance data to be included in the figures.

References

Addiss, D. G., Vaughn, M. L., Ludka, D., Pfister, J., & Davis, J. P. (1993). Decreased prevalence of Chlamydia trachomatis infection associated with a selective screening program in family planning clinics in Wisconsin. *Sex Transm Dis, 20,* 28–35.

Alexander-Rodriguez, T., & Vermund, S. H. (1987). Gonorrhea and syphilis in incarcerated urban adolescents: Prevalence and physical signs. *Pediatrics, 80,* 561–564.

Anderson, R. M., & May, R. M. (1991). *Infectious diseases of humans.* Oxford: Oxford University Press.

Aral, S. O., & Holmes, K. K. (1999). Social and behavioral determinants of the epidemiology of STDs: Industrialized and developing countries. In K. K. Holmes, P. F. Sparling, P.-A. Mardh, S. M. Lemon, W. E. Stamm, P. Piot, & J. N. Wasserheit (Eds.), *Sexually transmitted diseases* (pp. 39–76). New York: McGraw–Hill.

Barry, P., Kent, C. K., Scott, K., Goldenson, J., & Klausner, J. D. (2006). *National STD Prevention Conference, Jacksonville, FL.*

Bauer, H. M., Chartier, M., Kessell, E., Packel, L., Brammeier, M., Little, M., & Bolan, G. (2004). Chlamydia screening of youth and young adults in non-clinical settings throughout California. *Sex Transm Dis, 31,* 409–414.

Bell, T. A., Farrow, J. A., Stamm, W. E., Critchlow, C. W., & Holmes, K. K. (1985). Sexually transmitted diseases in females in a juvenile detention center. *Sex Transm Dis, 12,* 140–144.

Beltrami, J. F., Cohen, D. A., Hamrick, J. T., & Farley, T. A. (1997). Rapid screening and treatment for sexually transmitted diseases in arrestees: A feasible control measure. *Am J Public Health, 87,* 1423–1426.

Beltrami, J. F., Farley, T. A., Hamrick, J. T., Cohen, D. A., & Martin, D. H. (1998). Evaluation of the Gen-Probe PACE 2 assay for the detection of asymptomatic Chlamydia trachomatis and Neisseria gonorrhoeae infections in male arrestees. *Sex Transm Dis, 25,* 501–504.

Beltrami, J. F., Williams, S., & Valentine, J. (2007). STD screening and treatment during jail intake: The national syphilis elimination perspective. *Sex Transm Dis, 34,* 120–121.

Bickell, N. A., Vermund, S. H., Holmes, M., Safyer, S., & Burk, R. D. (1991). Human papillomavirus, gonorrhea, syphilis, and cervical dysplasia in jailed women. *Am J Public Health, 81,* 1318–1320.

Blake, D. R., Gaydos, C. A., & Quinn, T. C. (2004). Cost-effectiveness analysis of screening adolescent males for chlamydia on admission to detention. *Sex Transm Dis, 31,* 85–95.

Blank, S., McDonnell, D. D., Rubin, S. R., Neal, J. J., Brome, M. W., Masterson, M. B., & Greenspan, J. R. (1997). New approaches to syphilis control. Finding opportunities for syphilis treatment and congenital syphilis prevention in a women's correctional setting. *Sex Transm Dis, 24,* 218–226.

Blank, S., Sternberg, M., Neylans, L. L., Rubin, S. R., Weisfuse, I. B., & St Louis, M. E. (1999). Incident syphilis among women with multiple admissions to jail in New York City. *J Infect Dis, 180,* 1159–1163.

Brady, M., Baker, C., & Neinstein, L. S. (1988). Asymptomatic Chlamydia trachomatis infections in teenage males. *J Adolesc Health Care, 9,* 72–75.

Bureau of Justice Statistics. (2004). *Criminal offenders statistics.* In: Bureau of Justice Statistics. Washington, DC: Bureau of Justice Statistics, Office of Justice Programs, U.S. Department of Justice.

Bureau of Justice Statistics. (2005). *Jail statistics.* In: Bureau of Justice Statistics. Washington, DC: Bureau of Justice Statistics, Office of Justice Programs, U.S. Department of Justice.

CDC. (1998). Syphilis screening among women arrestees at the Cook County Jail— Chicago, 1996. *MMWR, 47,* 432–433.

CDC. (2002). Screening tests to detect *Chlamydia trachomatis* and *Neisseria gonorrhoeae* infections—2002. *MMWR, 51*, 1–27.

CDC. (2005). *Sexually transmitted disease surveillance 2004 supplement, Chlamydia Prevalence Monitoring Project*. Atlanta: U.S. Department of Health and Human Services, CDC.

CDC. (2006a). *Sexually transmitted disease surveillance, 2005*. Atlanta: U.S. Department of Health and Human Services, CDC.

CDC. (2006b). Sexually transmitted diseases treatment guidelines, 2006. *MMWR, 55*, 1–94.

CDC. (2006c). *Together we can: The national plan to eliminate syphilis from the United States*. Atlanta: U.S. Department of Health and Human Services.

Celum, C., Marrazzo, J., Ocbamichael, N., Meegan, A., & Stamm, W. (2002). *The practitioner's handbook for the management of sexually transmitted diseases* (3rd ed.). Seattle: University of Washington.

Chen, J. L., Bovee, M. C., & Kerndt, P. R. (2003). Sexually transmitted diseases surveillance among incarcerated men who have sex with men—An opportunity for HIV prevention. *AIDS Educ Prev, 15*, 117–126.

Cohen, D., Scribner, R., Clark, J., & Cory, D. (1992). The potential role of custody facilities in controlling sexually transmitted diseases. *Am J Public Health, 82*, 552–556.

Cohen, D. A., Kanouse, D. E., Iguchi, M. Y., Bluthenthal, R. N., Galvan, F. H., & Bing, E. G. (2005). Screening for sexually transmitted diseases in non-traditional settings: A personal view. *Int J STD AIDS, 16*, 521–527.

Cromwell, P. F., Risser, W. L., & Risser, J. M. (2002). Prevalence and incidence of pelvic inflammatory disease in incarcerated adolescents. *Sex Transm Dis, 29*, 391–396.

De Ravello, L., Brantley, M. D., Lamarre, M., Qayad, M. G., Aubert, H., & Beck-Sague, C. (2005). Sexually transmitted infections and other health conditions of women entering prison in Georgia, 1998–1999. *Sex Transm Dis, 32*, 247–251.

Doherty, I. A., Padian, N. S., Marlow, C., & Aral, S. O. (2005). Determinants and consequences of sexual networks as they affect the spread of sexually transmitted infections. *J Infect Dis, 191*(Suppl. 1), S42–54.

Ellerbeck, E. F., Vlahov, D., Libonati, J. P., Salive, M. E., & Brewer, T. F. (1989). Gonorrhea prevalence in the Maryland state prisons. *Sex Transm Dis, 16*, 165–167.

Eng, T., Butler, W. (Eds.). (1997). *The hidden epidemic: Confronting sexually transmitted diseases*. Washington, DC: Institute of Medicine, National Academy Press.

Farley, T., Cohen, D., & Elkins, W. (2003). Asymptomatic sexually transmitted diseases: The case for screening. *Preventive Medicine, 36*, 502–509.

Fleming, D. T., & Wasserheit, J. N. (1999). From epidemiological synergy to public health practice: The contribution of sexually transmitted disease to sexual transmission of HIV infection. *Sexually Transmitted Infections, 75*, 3–17.

Gift, T. L., Lincoln, T., Tuthill, R., Whelan, M., Briggs, L. P., Conklin, T., & Irwin, K. L. (2006). A cost-effectiveness evaluation of a jail-based chlamydia screening program for men and its impact on their partners in the community. *Sex Transm Dis, 33*, S103–S110.

Golden, M. R. (2005). Expedited partner therapy for sexually transmitted diseases. *Clin Infect Dis, 41*, 630–633.

Golden, M. R., Whittington, W. L., Handsfield, H. H., Hughes, J. P., Stamm, W. E., Hogben, M., Clark, A., Malinski, C., Helmers, J. R., Thomas, K. K., & Holmes, K. K. (2005). Effect of expedited treatment of sex partners on recurrent or persistent gonorrhea or chlamydial infection. *N Engl J Med, 352*, 676–685.

Hardick, J., Hsieh, Y. H., Tulloch, S., Kus, J., Tawes, J., & Gaydos, C. A. (2003). Surveillance of Chlamydia trachomatis and Neisseria gonorrhoeae infections in women in detention in Baltimore, Maryland. *Sex Transm Dis, 30*, 64–70.

Harrison, P. M., & Beck, A. J. (2006). Prison and jail inmates at midyear 2005. In *Bureau of Justice Statistics Bulletin* (pp. 1–12). Washington, DC: Bureau of Justice Statistics, Office of Justice Programs, U.S. Department of Justice.

Heimberger, T. S., Chang, H. G., Birkhead, G. S., DiFerdinando, G. D., Greenberg, A. J., Gunn, R., & Morse, D. L. (1993). High prevalence of syphilis detected through a jail screening program. A potential public health measure to address the syphilis epidemic. *Arch Intern Med*, *153*, 1799–804.

Hook, E. W. I., & Handsfield, H. H. (1999). Gonococcal infections in the adult. In K. K. Holmes, P. F. Sparling, P.-A. Mardh, S. M. Lemon, W. E. Stamm, P. Piot, & J. N. Wasserheit (Eds.), *Sexually transmitted diseases* (pp. 451–466). New York: McGraw–Hill.

James, D. J. (2004). Profile of jail inmates, 2002. In *Bureau of Justice Statistics Special Report* (pp. 1–12). Washington, DC: Bureau of Justice Statistics, Office of Justice Programs, U.S. Department of Justice.

Johnson, R., & Raphael, S. (2005). The effects of male incarceration dynamics on AIDS infection rates among African-American women and men. In *National Poverty Center Working Paper Series #06-22*. Ann Arbor: University of Michigan Gerald R. Ford School of Public Policy.

Kahn, R. H., Mosure, D. J., Blank, S., Kent, C. K., Chow, J. M., Boudov, M. R., Brock, J., & Tulloch, S. (2005). Chlamydia trachomatis and Neisseria gonorrhoeae prevalence and coinfection in adolescents entering selected US juvenile detention centers, 1997–2002. *Sex Transm Dis*, *32*, 255–259.

Kahn, R. H., Scholl, D. T., Shane, S. M., Lemoine, A. L., & Farley, T. A. (2002). Screening for syphilis in arrestees: Usefulness for community-wide syphilis surveillance and control. *Sex Transm Dis*, *29*, 150–156.

Kahn, R. H., Voigt, R. F., Swint, E., & Weinstock, H. (2004). Early syphilis in the United States identified in corrections facilities, 1999–2002. *Sex Transm Dis*, *31*, 360–364.

Katz, A. R., Lee, M. V., Ohye, R. G., Effler, P. V., Johnson, E. C., & Nishi, S. M. (2004). Prevalence of chlamydial and gonorrheal infections among females in a juvenile detention facility, Honolulu, Hawaii. *J Community Health*, *29*, 265–269.

Kelly, P. J., Bair, R. M., Baillargeon, J., & German, V. (2000). Risk behaviors and the prevalence of chlamydia in a juvenile detention facility. *Clin Pediatr (Phila)*, *39*, 521–527.

Kraut-Becher, J. R., Gift, T. L., Haddix, A. C., Irwin, K. L., & Greifinger, R. B. (2004). Cost-effectiveness of universal screening for chlamydia and gonorrhea in US jails. *J Urban Health*, *81*, 453–471.

MacGowan, R. J., Margolis, A., Gaiter, J., Morrow, K., Zack, B., Askew, J., McAuliffe, T., Sosman, J. M., & Eldridge, G. D. (2003). Predictors of risky sex of young men after release from prison. *Int J STD AIDS*, *14*, 519–523.

Margolis, A. D., Macgowan, R. J., Grinstead, O., Sosman, J., Kashif, I., & Flanigan, T. P. (2006). Unprotected sex with multiple partners: Implications for HIV prevention among young men with a history of incarceration. *Sex Transm Dis*, *33*, 175–180.

Mertz, K. J., Levine, W. C., Mosure, D. J., Berman, S. M., & Dorian, K. J. (1997). Trends in the prevalence of chlamydial infections. The impact of community-wide testing. *Sex Transm Dis*, *24*, 169–75.

Mertz, K. J., Schwebke, J. R., Gaydos, C. A., Beidinger, H. A., Tulloch, S. D., & Levine, W. C. (2002). Screening women in jails for chlamydial and gonococcal infection using urine tests: Feasibility, acceptability, prevalence, and treatment rates. *Sex Transm Dis*, *29*, 271–276.

Mertz, K., Voigt, R., Hutchins, K., Levine, W., & Group, J. S. P. M. (2002). Findings from STD screening of adolescents and adults entering corrections facilities: implications for STD control strategies. *Sexually Transmitted Diseases*, *29*, 834–839.

Mrus, J. M., Biro, F. M., Huang, B., & Tsevat, J. (2003). Evaluating adolescents in juvenile detention facilities for urogenital chlamydial infection: Costs and effectiveness of alternative interventions. *Arch Pediatr Adolesc Med*, *157*, 696–702.

National Center for Juvenile Justice. (2004). Census of juveniles in residential placement data-book. In *Census of juveniles in residential placement databook*. Washington, DC: National Center for Juvenile Justice, Office of Juvenile Justice and Delinquency Prevention.

O'Brien, S. F., Bell, T. A., & Farrow, J. A. (1988). Use of a leukocyte esterase dip-stick to detect Chlamydia trachomatis and Neisseria gonorrhoeae urethritis in asymptomatic adolescent male detainees. *Am J Public Health*, *78*, 1583–1584.

Oh, M. K., Cloud, G. A., Wallace, L. S., Reynolds, J., Sturdevant, M., & Feinstein, R. A. (1994). Sexual behavior and sexually transmitted diseases among male adolescents in detention. *Sex Transm Dis, 21*, 127–132.

Oh, M. K., Smith, K. R., O'Cain, M., Kilmer, D., Johnson, J., & Hook, E. W., 3rd. (1998). Urine-based screening of adolescents in detention to guide treatment for gonococcal and chlamydial infections. Translating research into intervention. *Arch Pediatr Adolesc Med, 152*, 52–56.

Pack, R. P., Diclemente, R. J., Hook, E. W., 3rd, & Oh, M. K. (2000). High prevalence of asymptomatic STDs in incarcerated minority male youth: A case for screening. *Sex Transm Dis, 27*, 175–177.

Plitt, S. S., Garfein, R. S., Gaydos, C. A., Strathdee, S. A., Sherman, S. G. & Taha, T. E. (2005). Prevalence and correlates of Chlamydia trachomatis, Neisseria gonorrhoeae, Trichomonas vaginalis infections, and bacterial vaginosis among a cohort of young injection drug users in Baltimore, Maryland. *Sex Transm Dis, 32*, 446–453.

Radolf, J. D., Sanchez, P. J., Schulz, K. F., & Murphy, F. K. (1999). Congenital syphilis. In K. K. Holmes, P. F. Sparling, P.-A. Mardh, S. M. Lemon, W. E. Stamm, P. Piot, & J. N. Wasserheit (Eds.), *Sexually transmitted diseases* (pp. 1165–1190). New York: McGraw–Hill.

Risser, J. M., Risser, W. L., Gefter, L. R., Brandstetter, D. M., & Cromwell, P. F. (2001). Implementation of a screening program for chlamydial infection in incarcerated adolescents. *Sex Transm Dis, 28*, 43–46.

Robertson, A. A., Thomas, C. B., St Lawrence, J. S., & Pack, R. (2005). Predictors of infection with chlamydia or gonorrhea in incarcerated adolescents. *Sex Transm Dis, 32*, 115–122.

Saslow, D., Castle, P. E., Cox, J. T., Davey, D. D., Einstein, M. H., Ferris, D. G., Goldie, S. J., Harper, D. M., Kinney, W., Moscicki, A. B., Noller, K. L., Wheeler, C. M., Ades, T., Andrews, K. S., Doroshenk, M. K., Kahn, K. G., Schmidt, C., Shafey, O., Smith, R. A., Partridge, E. E., & Garcia, F. (2007). American Cancer Society Guideline for human papillomavirus (HPV) vaccine use to prevent cervical cancer and its precursors. *CA Cancer J Clin, 57*, 7–28.

Schillinger, J. A., Kissinger, P., Calvet, H., Whittington, W. L., Ransom, R. L., Sternberg, M. R., Berman, S. M., Kent, C. K., Martin, D. H., Oh, M. K., Handsfield, H. H., Bolan, G., Markowitz, L. E., & Fortenberry, J. D. (2003). Patient-delivered partner treatment with azithromycin to prevent repeated Chlamydia trachomatis infection among women: A randomized, controlled trial. *Sex Transm Dis, 30*, 49–56.

Silberstein, G. S., Coles, F. B., Greenberg, A., Singer, L., & Voigt, R. (2000). Effectiveness and cost-benefit of enhancements to a syphilis screening and treatment program at a county jail. *Sex Transm Dis, 27*, 508–517.

Skolnick, A. A. (1998). Look behind bars for key to control of STDs. *JAMA, 279*, 97–98.

Sparling, P. F. (1999). Natural history of syphilis. In K. K. Holmes, P. F. Sparling, P.-A. Mardh, S. M. Lemon, W. E. Stamm, P. Piot, & J. N. Wasserheit (Eds.), *Sexually transmitted diseases* (pp. 473–478). New York: McGraw–Hill.

St Louis, M. E., & Wasserheit, J. N. (1998). Elimination of syphilis in the United States. *Science, 281*, 353–354.

Stamm, W. E. (1999). *Chlamydia trachomatis* infections of the adult. In K. K. Holmes, P. F. Sparling, P.-A. Mardh, S. M. Lemon, W. E. Stamm, P. Piot, & J. N. Wasserheit (Eds.), *Sexually transmitted diseases* (pp. 407–422). New York: McGraw–Hill.

Steiner, K. C., Davila, V., Kent, C. K., Chaw, J. K., Fischer, L., & Klausner, J. D. (2003). Field-delivered therapy increases treatment for chlamydia and gonorrhea. *Am J Public Health, 93*, 882–884.

Trick, W. E., Kee, R., Murphy-Swallow, D., Mansour, M., Mennella, C., & Raba, J. M. (2006). Detection of chlamydial and gonococcal urethral infection during jail intake: Development of a screening algorithm. *Sex Transm Dis, 33*, 599–603.

Wolfe, M. I., Xu, F., Patel, P., O'Cain, M., Schillinger, J. A., St Louis, M. E., & Finelli, L. (2001). An outbreak of syphilis in Alabama prisons: Correctional health policy and communicable disease control. *Am J Public Health, 91*, 1220–1225.

Section 3

Primary and Secondary Prevention

This section is about preventing morbidity and mortality through health promotion and early detection. Megha Ramaswamy and Nick Freudenberg, correctional health care scholars, begin the section with an intriguing chapter on health promotion. They explain how health promotion is practical and important, using an evidence basis for their rationale. They describe why health promotion activities can help to encourage healthier and safer postrelease behaviors and lifestyles, thus serving a rehabilitative and public safety function in addition to the personal value to the inmate.

Joshua Lee, Marshall Fordyce, and Jody Rich, each a correctional physician, follow with a chapter on evidence-based screening recommendations for incoming inmates. In corrections, we are just learning to use evidence-based medicine to help us with the management of chronic disease and mental illness. These authors give us better insight into how and why to use nationally accepted guidelines to craft our intake protocols.

On the reentry front, Jeff Mellow provides us with more evidence basis for using health education materials as part of discharge planning. Professor Mellow explains the value of using carefully selected and patient-customized materials for more successful reentry.

An expert on suicide prevention, Lindsay Hayes takes the reader on another course in suicide prevention in correctional facilities, through the retrospective lens of a mortality review. The lessons in this chapter are not limited to death by suicide. Mortality review is a critical quality management process, a process that should be taken seriously following all deaths. Mr. Hayes's template is transferable to all mortality reviews.

Dick Grant, a practicing psychiatrist, has written a provocative chapter on psychiatric diagnosis, but not the typical one that would be found in a textbook of correctional psychiatry. Dr. Grant explains the "mad versus bad" dilemma in striking terms. He helps us understand that behavior is not so simplistic and explains how too many correctional health professionals have blinders, especially regarding personality disorders and co-occurring psychiatric diagnoses.

Michelle Staples-Horne, a practitioner and physician executive of a major juvenile justice system, and colleagues Kaiyti Duffy and Michele Rorie provide a broad description of prevention opportunities in juvenile detainees.

In the context of community, family, and juvenile morbidity, these authors review the unique age and gender requirements for a constructive program in adolescent medicine.

Andrea Balis, a historian, also takes a different slant on matters of women's health care. Professor Balis emphasizes the gender-specific issues beyond Pap smears and mammograms, including prior abuse, mental illness, and substance abuse. With this understanding, the author derives the basic elements of a reentry plan for confined women.

Finally, Henrie Treadwell, a social scientist working on correctional health care, with colleagues Mary Northridge and Traci Bethea go into unexplored territory with there treatise on oral health. Using history and evidence, they build a compelling case for the development of comprehensive oral health care services behind bars, a kind of program that we rarely see in prisons and jails across the nation.

Chapter 13

Health Promotion in Jails and Prisons: An Alternative Paradigm for Correctional Health Services

Megha Ramaswamy and Nicholas Freudenberg

According to the Bureau of Justice Statistics, each year about 12 million people, representing 9 million unique individuals, pass through a jail. About 1.5 million individuals are in prison on any given day (Beck, 2006). These individuals include some of the nation's most vulnerable populations, those suffering from or at higher risk of infectious and chronic diseases, addiction and mental illness, and victims and perpetrators of violence (BJS, 2006; Harlow, 1998; National Commission on Correctional Health Care [NCCHC], 2002). Not only are incarcerated populations themselves often unhealthy, but untreated they can also worsen the well-being and impose additional costs on their families and communities (Rogers & Seigenthaler, 2001). Unfortunately, the majority of people leave prison or jail without having their most serious health problems addressed and many correctional health systems see their main responsibility as providing only the most essential medical care to those in their custody. In this chapter, we consider whether the paradigm of health promotion can provide an alternative framework for correctional health and examine the scientific evidence, economic benefits, and legal and moral rationale for this perspective.

According to the World Health Organization, health promotion describes the "process of enabling people to increase control over and to improve their health." Health promotion seeks to bring about changes in individuals, groups, institutions, and policies in order to improve population health. The Ottawa Charter for Health Promotion, adopted by the WHO in 1986, identifies five critical activities for health promotion: developing personal skills for health, creating supportive environments, strengthening community action for health, reorienting health services, and building healthy public policy (Ottawa Charter for Health Promotion, World Health Organization, 1986).

At first sight, this expansive conception of health promotion seems too idealistic to serve as a useful guide for the consideration of its role in prisons and jails. However, in this chapter, we make the case that a comprehensive definition of health promotion can serve as a useful paradigm that links correctional health care to the larger public health system, expands the focus of correctional health services from medical care during custody to preparation for healthy living after release, and provides a rationale for expanding the goals of incarceration to include not only punishment but also rehabilitation.

In this view, correctional health services (CHS) seek to improve population health both by treating the conditions that inmates present to facility providers and by offering the knowledge, skills, and referrals that incarcerated people need to protect their health inside the prison or jail and after release. CHS can also serve as referral sites for both facility-based (during incarceration) and community-based (after release) health education, health care, mental health and social services, and also as resource on health for inmates' partners and children in the free world. In this model, the outcome of incarceration is assessed in part on the extent to which the facility has prepared those in its custody for healthier living after release. Finally, from a criminal justice perspective, health problems such as substance abuse, perpetration of or victimization by violence, mental illness, or chronic or infectious diseases can increase recidivism, encourage dependency, or endanger the well-being of people connected to the returning individual. Health promotion activities that prevent or reduce these problems can help to encourage healthier and safer postrelease behaviors and lifestyles, thus serving a rehabilitative and public safety function.

In this chapter, we consider health promotion as both a set of activities within the five categories identified by the World Health Organization and as a mindset that views CHS as an integral element of public health that is judged by its contribution to improved population health. We distinguish this perspective from the more traditional view that CHS simply provide care that meets minimal legal standards to those in custody.

Rationale and Mandate for Health Promotion in Correctional Facilities

To assist correctional health programs to shift from the current focus on acute care for those in custody to health promotion for populations entering and leaving correctional facilities, it will be necessary to provide a compelling rationale and some external mandate for health promotion. Such arguments can help correctional health staff already interested in this approach to convince their superiors to support such efforts and may persuade policy makers to consider a shift to a health promotion perspective.

Here we review four different approaches to defining standards and models for correctional health care:

1. American Public Health Association's (APHA) Standards for Health Services in Correctional Facilities (2003)
2. National Commission on Correctional Health Care's (NCCHC) Clinical Guidelines (2001, 2003)
3. Re-Entry Policy Council Policy Statements on Physical Health Care (2005)
4. from Europe, the Health in Prisons Project (HIPP), sponsored by the World Health Organization (WHO) (Gatherer, Moiler, & Hayton, 2005; Whitehead, 2006; WHO, 2006)

The APHA guidelines were developed in 1976 and revised in 2003 by correctional health professionals to encourage appropriate health care in correctional facilities that is respectful of patients' rights. The intended audience included medical and nonmedical corrections staff and community-based public health professionals (APHA, 2003).

The NCCHC developed a set of clinical guidelines (2001) to assist health care workers with management of illness in correctional settings and improve incarcerated patient outcomes. The NCCHC also developed a document (2003) that specifically addressed health education within correctional facilities.

The *Report of the Re-Entry Policy Council* (2005) included policy statements drafted from meetings of 100 professionals in workforce, health, housing, public safety, family, community, and victim services. The statement on physical health care addressed prevention, management, and treatment of chronic and infectious disease.

Finally, the Health in Prisons Project (HIPP) was started in Europe in 1995 by the WHO with the goal of improving health in prisons in order to improve public health (Gatherer et al., 2005). Member countries (there are currently 28) have pledged the resources necessary to build a public health infrastructure in prisons and participate actively in the collaboration (Whitehead, 2006).

Together, these documents demonstrate that a wide variety of correctional health and criminal justice professionals and organizations support the inclusion of a health promotion perspective within CHS. In our review of these guidelines, we identified seven program activities that can provide an operational definition of health promotion within correctional facilities. These were counseling, health education, chronic disease management, community follow-up, collaboration, meeting other social needs, and policy advocacy. These activities are not mutually exclusive, e.g., chronic disease management can include counseling, health education, and community follow-up, but each activity has distinct characteristics, as defined in Box 13.1. Table 13.1 summarizes how each of the four standards or guidelines describes these activities. Note that not every standard addresses all seven activities. For example, only HIPP includes policy advocacy as a core activity and the focus on reentry is a more recent development, highlighted by the Re-Entry Policy Council.

In summary, we have so far presented two different approaches to describing health promotion within jails and prisons. The first, using the "key activities" for health promotion developed by WHO, provides a broad framework for an alternative paradigm for the mission of CHS. The second, derived from existing standards for CHS, delineates specific health promotion activities that are described in existing guidelines for CHS. In a later section, we summarize evidence from the literature on existing health promotion interventions in correctional facilities and in the community after release, using the WHO "key activities" as the organizing rubric. First, however, we review contextual and organizational factors that influence health promotion in the correctional system.

Contextual and Organizational Factors

The structure of U.S. jails and prisons offers different opportunities for health promotion. Jails incarcerate individuals who are awaiting adjudication, those sentenced to terms of a year or less, and parole and probation violators (James, 2004). Because of the high volume, short lengths of stay, and rapid

Box 13.1 Definitions of health promotion activities in jails and prisons

Counseling describes one-on-one or small group interactions between health, mental health, social service, or correctional staff and incarcerated or recently released individuals that takes place inside a correctional facility or after release. It provides tailored guidance, emotional support, and information to help individuals address health, psychological, and social problems.

Health education has been defined as "any combination of learning experiences designed to facilitate voluntary actions conducive to health" (Green, Kreuter, Partridge, & Deeds, 1999). Health education is expected to be evidence-based, culturally and linguistically appropriate, and can include multiple modalities such as individual education, peer education, lectures, and role-play.

Chronic disease management assists individuals to manage diseases such as asthma, hypertension, or diabetes. It includes regular screening, counseling and education, skills development, and access to appropriate medical care in the correctional setting and after release.

Community follow-up includes prerelease planning for medical care and social services and postrelease contact to reinforce health education, ensure medical care access and adherence to prescribed regiments and to assist in meeting emerging needs. The interval for community follow-up varies from days to a year or more.

Collaboration describes intersectoral cooperation and coordination among a variety of public and private organizations including correctional, parole and probation, health, mental health, housing, welfare, employment, and other agencies.

Addressing other social needs such as housing, employment, legal assistance, substance use treatment, access to entitlements and family reunification, describes activities designed to assist people returning from jail or prison to create the life circumstances that allow them to make health a higher priority.

Policy advocacy describes activities designed to identify policies that facilitate or impede successful and healthy community reentry after incarceration and to strengthen those policies that assist reentry and modify those that block success.

turnover, jails provide unique opportunities to reach many vulnerable individuals within low-income communities, to link them to community health promotion efforts after release, and, because jails unlike prisons are usually located within high-incarceration communities, to engage family members in health promotion activities (Freudenberg, 2001; Glaser & Greifinger, 1993; Lindquist & Lindquist, 1999; McLean, Robarge, & Sherman, 2006; Rogers & Seigenthaler, 2001). On the other hand, the high turnover, security concerns, dynamic environment, and external demands from elected officials, the media, and the public on jails make them a difficult environment for health promotion This setting requires health staff to have patience, modest goals, and a willingness to balance their desires to address health issues with the custody and control priorities of correctional officials.

Prisons typically house people sentenced to more than a year and include individuals who will never be released from the facility. Longer lengths of stay and a more secure and stable environment sometimes enable prisons to have more opportunities for planned health activities and to have the intensity and duration of contact needed to achieve health goals. On the other hand, prisons have more limited interactions with families and communities, reducing their potential to have an impact on population health (Austin & Hardyman, 2004).

Correctional systems also vary in their support for and commitment to health services. Some jurisdictions have established model programs and CHS, and

Table 13.1 Approaches to health promotion in existing standards and guidelines for correctional health care.

	APHA (2003)	NCCHC (2003, 2001)	Re-Entry Policy Council (2005)	HIPP (Gatherer et al., 2005; Whitehead, 2006; WHO, 2002, 2004, 2006)
Counseling	Individual-level patient education by medical staff for chronic illness and risk behavior for infectious disease	Individual-level patient education by medical staff	Individual-level patient education by medical staff and community-based organizations	—
Health education	Culturally and linguistically appropriate health education provided by trained facilitator for those with chronic/infectious disease and for smoking, nutrition, exercise; use of peer-based, lecture, discussion, and role-play	Culturally and linguistically appropriate health education provided by trained facilitator for those with chronic/infectious disease and for smoking, nutrition, exercise; use of in-house video channels	Culturally and linguistically appropriate health education provided by trained facilitator for those with chronic/infectious disease, smoking, nutrition, exercise, medication adherence, STIs	Education and skill development that emphasize rewards rather than sanctions
Chronic disease management	Medical care (screening, clinic visits, treatment, education) for those with long-term conditions for which self-care is significant	Quality screening, treatment, management, and education for chronic/infectious disease (STIs, tuberculosis, HIV, hepatitis, asthma, high blood cholesterol and pressure, diabetes)	Presence of standardized clinical protocols for evaluation, treatment, and education for those with chronic disease	Quality care provided; address chronic/infectious disease (tuberculosis, HIV) by addressing overcrowding in prisons and using harm reduction approaches
Community follow-up	Prerelease planning and referrals to medical care; postrelease contact for reinforcement of health education and access to medical care and entitlements like Medicaid	Collaboration with community-based organizations to provide prerelease planning for those with chronic/infectious disease	Use services and relationships with community-based organizations prerelease to coordinate care postrelease; seamless and protected medical record transfer	—

(continued)

Table 13.1 (continued)

	APHA (2003)	NCCHC (2003, 2001)	Re-Entry Policy Council (2005)	HIPP (Gatherer et al., 2005; Whitehead, 2006; WHO, 2002, 2004, 2006)
Collaboration	Collaboration with local health departments, government agencies, and community-based organizations to provide corrections-based services and services on reentry	Collaboration with local health departments, government agencies, and community-based organizations to provide corrections-based services and services on reentry	Engagement of community providers to provide effective corrections-based counseling, health education, chronic disease management, and community follow-up	Collaboration among WHO, national departments of justice and health to create a prison health service in participating countries
Other social needs	—	—	Part of transition planning services, especially for those diagnosed with multiple disorders, which can impede successful reentry	Creating alternatives to standard incarceration as part of mental health promotion; use of corrections-based harm reduction services for drug users; focus on rehabilitation
Advocacy	—	—	—	Mandatory policy reports from each participating country to be disseminated widely

wardens, sheriffs, or commissioners/directors are forceful advocates for health (Lincoln et al., 2006; Sinclair & Porter-Williamson, 2004; White et al., 2003). Others, however, view health as a distraction from more traditional custody and control issues and take on health issues mainly in response to litigation (Nathan, 2004). Obviously, health professionals in a supportive environment will have an easier time adding a health promotion perspective into existing CHS, while those in more traditional settings face greater obstacles. Even in challenging environments, however, litigation, new state or federal mandates, or forceful advocacy can stimulate interest in more comprehensive approaches to health, including health promotion.

A third contextual variable of interest is the extent to which existing officials in local or state correctional or health departments or in local or state government as a whole support intersectoral, multilevel approaches to reentry and improved health. The approach to health promotion described here works best if officials, providers, and advocates from multiple systems and agencies are willing to come together to articulate a shared vision , identify and solve problems, exchange resources , and plan comprehensively. Having a high level official who supports and is willing to lead such an effort significantly increases the likelihood of success.

Evidence on Elements of Correctional Health Promotion Programs

While to our knowledge no correctional system has yet implemented a comprehensive and integrated health promotion initiative, in fact all elements of such a program have been implemented in some correctional facilities. Moreover, the evaluation of many such interventions shows that some have been shown to be effective or promising in achieving health outcomes or demonstrating feasibility.

In Box 13.1, we use the WHO key activities to provide an overview of the components of a comprehensive health promotion program for correctional facilities.

Develop Personal Skills

Helping people to develop skills in order to improve their own health is central to the concept of health promotion (O'Donnell, 1989; WHO, 1986). Strategies to develop personal skills include activities such as counseling, health education, and chronic disease management. In recent years, a number of correctional facilities have developed interventions to increase personal skills in the prevention and care of HIV and other sexually transmitted infections (STIs) (Mertz, Voigt, Hutchins, & Levine, 2002; Parece, Herrera, Voigt, Middlekauff, & Irwin, 1999; Robillard et al., 2003; Schady, Miller, & Klein, 2005), tuberculosis (White et al., 2003), violence prevention (Di Placido, Simon, Witte, Gu, & Wong, 2006; Gilligan & Lee, 2005a, 2005b; Greene, Lucarelli, & Shocksnider, 1999), prenatal care and reproductive health (Bell et al., 2004; Bloom, Owen, & Covington, 2003; Clarke et al., 2006; Kyei-Aboagye, Vragovic, & Chong, 2000), and parenting (Bloom et al., 2003;

Table 13.2 Elements of a comprehensive correctional health promotion program.

Health promotion priority	Selected activities/approaches in jails or prisons	Selected health and social outcomes: inmates	Selected health and social outcomes: correctional facilities	Selected health and social outcomes: society as a whole	Selected references
Develop personal skills	Offer chronic disease management, family planning, parenting, violence prevention, harm reduction, peer education, and other health programs	Improved diabetes, asthma, HIV outcomes; lower health care costs; better chances for successful reentry	Improved diabetes, asthma, HIV management; lower health care costs	Reduced transmission of infectious diseases and reliance on health care system for emergency care; improve outcomes for children of inmates	Di Placido et al. (2006), Schady et al. (2005), Bell et al. (2004), Bloom et al. (2003)
Create supportive environments	Reduce overcrowding; improve sanitary conditions; encourage positive social support; reduce physical and sexual assault and intimidation; provide access to healthy food and opportunities for physical activity; encourage family visits	Reduced transmission of infectious diseases; reduced anxiety and depression; lower violence rates; reduced diet; better family functioning postrelease	No overcrowding, lower violence rates and incidences of sexual assault in jails and prisons; lowered anxiety for corrections staff	Reduced transmission of infectious diseases; lower violence rates, including domestic violence; better outcomes for spouses and children of inmates	Olden & White (2005), Leh (1999), Richie et al. (2001), Rich et al. (2001)
Strengthen community action for health	Establish linkages with community organizations, faith organizations, and services providers; organize community coalitions to advocate for policies listed above	Increased access to health care and promotion; access to higher-quality health care	Greater infrastructure and resources for providing health care and health promotion; less reliance on funding from corrections departments and time from staff to provide services	Increased social cohesion in high-incarceration communities and as a result and in addition to, less violence and STIs	Bauserman et al. (2003), Grinstead et al. (2001), Myers et al. (2005)
Reorient health services	Shift from acute episodic treatment to disease management, health promotion, and prevention; develop continuity of care inside and after release; train providers to promote health	Improved control of chronic conditions; lower health care costs after release	Greater infrastructure for providing health care and promotion; lower health care costs; greater efficiency through health promotion	Better community health outcomes; reliance on health care system for emergency care; more seamless medical care inside and on release	Institute of Medicine (2002), Kraut-Becher et al. (2004), Lincoln et al. (2006)
Build healthy public policy	Advocate policies that provide substance abuse, mental health, and other services during incarceration and after release; reduce stigma against people returning; provide job training and education inside and after release	Increased access to and use of substance abuse treatment services, mental health services; increased ability to find employment and reduce dependency after release	Greater infrastructure for substance abuse and mental health treatment and promotion	Lower unemployment rates, illegal activity	Blankenship et al. (2005), Freudenberg et al. (2005a), Holzer et al. (2003)

Harrison, 1997; Thompson & Harm, 2000). While a comprehensive review of the impact of these interventions is beyond the scope of this chapter, a broad generalization is that these programs often demonstrate increases in knowledge and motivation to change; sometimes in health behavior and health beliefs; and less frequently in health status. Program characteristics that have been identified with more successful outcome include use of multiple methods, materials and communications that are culturally and linguistically appropriate, sufficient program intensity and duration, opportunities for practice of skills, and reinforcement of messages (Freudenberg, 2001; Hammett, 2001; Lowenkamp, Latessa, & Smith, 2006; Palmer, 1995). While interventions to improve personal skills are a vital component of correctional health promotion programs, their value is significantly enhanced by interventions at other levels of organization (e.g., family, correctional facility, community, public policy) that help to create a context in which individuals have the opportunity to use the skills they have acquired. For example, several HIPP prisons now make condoms and sterile injection equipment available to people in prison (Gatherer et al., 2005). But while harm reduction initiatives have been successful at providing increased access to clean needles in nonincarcerated populations in the United States (Des Jarlais, McKnight, & Friedmann, 2002; Pouget et al., 2005), no U.S. correctional system distributes clean needles and only a few make condoms available inside the facility (May & Williams, 2002; No authors, 2002). Thus, developing inmates' skills in the use of condoms or sterile injection equipment is only meaningful if these products are in fact available, whether in the correctional facility or after release.

Create Supportive Environments

Research evidence shows that healthy physical and social environments can make important contributions to individual and population health (Berkman, Glass, Brissette, & Seeman, 2000; Brownson, Haire-Joshu, & Luke, 2006; Olden & White, 2005; Yen & Syme, 1999). In correctional facilities, physical environmental factors that have been associated with poor health include overcrowding; lack of privacy; pests; lack of access to showers, hot water, and soap; and exposure to infectious agents (Hoge et al., 1994; Jones, Craig, Valway, Woodley, & Schaffner, 1999; Leh, 1999). Social environmental conditions associated with poor health in correctional facilities include exposure to physical and sexual violence, isolation from family and friends, and stigma (Hairston, 1998; Harner, 2004; Rhodes, 2005).

Creating healthier correctional environments requires making changes in physical conditions, e.g., improving ventilation, reducing overcrowding, or reducing exposure to pests without increasing exposure to harmful pesticides. Often, such changes have been achieved through litigation (Nathan, 2004).

Strategies to improve social environments and increase the positive support that incarcerated people experience include correctional staff training to improve positive interactions with inmates; changes in policies related to visits from partners, family, and children; more vigorous enforcement of laws on sexual violence and inmate bullying, and campaigns against stigma and isolation both inside the facility and after release (Dvoskin & Spiers, 2004; Miller & Metzner, 1994; Nurse, Woodcock, & Ormsby, 2003). For the most part, such interventions have not been described or evaluated in the literature. After release, a variety of reentry program seek to connect people returning from jail to prosocial networks and individuals, strengthen family functions and parenting, and prepare individuals for work and self-sufficiency (McCoy, Roberts, Hanrahan, Clay, & Luchins, 2004; Petersilia, 2003; Richie, Freudenberg, & Page, 2001; Travis, 2005). Often, these programs serve only people with mental illness or HIV infection, rather than the general population. Few of these programs have been systematically evaluated; those that have often show positive but modest results (Grinstead, Zack, & Faigeles, 2001; Needels, James-Burdumy, & Burghardt, 2005; Rich et al., 2001).

Strengthen Community Action for Health

A central tenet of the health promotion literature is that heath professionals alone can achieve only limited improvements in health but in partnership with a variety of community-based organizations more significant gains are possible (Merzel & D'Afflitti, 2003). In correctional settings, community organizations have played a variety of health roles including providing health education and counseling, especially on HIV; seeking referrals for postrelease health care, mental health, and social services; and providing postrelease case management and other services (Bauserman et al., 2003; El-Bassel, Ivanoff, Schilling, Borne, & Gilbert, 1997; Grinstead et al., 2001; Laufer, Jacob Arriola, Dawson-Rose, Kumaravelu, & Krane Rapposelli, 2002; Myers et al., 2005; Rich et al., 2001; Richie et al., 2001).

Negotiating effective partnerships between correctional agencies, health departments, and community organizations presents many challenges, including finding common ground among differing missions, locating the resources that can sustain the collaboration, and choosing priorities among the multiple needs that incarcerated and returning populations face (Freudenberg, Rogers, Ritas, & Nerney, 2005; Robillard et al., 2003).

Reorient Health Services

Most health services in the United States focus on treatment of acute and chronic conditions rather than on primary care and prevention, despite evidence that a shift in emphasis could improve population health and reduce costs (Institute of Medicine, 2002). Reorienting health services requires putting more emphasis on and devoting more resources to health promotion and prevention. In correctional settings, the vast proportion of health care resources is devoted to providing acute care for inmates who present medical problems to correctional health services staff; relatively few resources are devoted to prevention. In jails, correctional health resources are often consumed by performing mandated services such as intake physical examinations, often repeatedly on the same people who reenter the system frequently. While in the free world, extensive routine physical examinations are no longer recommended for young adults, in correctional settings, more effective and economical alternatives to this outdated approach have yet to be developed. In this context, reorienting health services might include:

- expanding prevention and health promotion initiatives,
- providing routine screening for appropriate conditions and ensuring that those testing positive receive appropriate follow-up before or after release,
- devoting more resources to chronic disease management, and
- increasing opportunities for healthier behavior and use of preventive services after release.

Such a reorientation faces significant obstacles in part because many correctional officials believe that their legal mandate is limited to providing acute care to those in their custody. Although the previously cited standards provide a rationale for prevention and health promotion, these activities are usually perceived as a lower priority, even though their potential for improving the health of individuals and populations and reducing the cost of CHS may be greater. Moreover, since most correctional systems do not see health promotion as part of their core mission and most health departments do not rate serving incarcerated populations as a priority, no entity claims leadership in bringing about the reallocation of resources that such a reorientation requires.

To what extent have CHS begun a reorientation of priorities? Examples include the addition of routine chlamydia screening to CHS protocols (Kraut-Becher, Gift, Haddix, Irwin, & Greifinger, 2004), partnerships between CHS and community-based health centers (Lincoln et al., 2006), and stronger linkages between CHS and community-based substance abuse and mental health services (Needels et al., 2005; Rich et al., 2001; Strauss & Falkin, 2000; Tamasino, Swanson, Nolan, & Shuman, 2001; Wilson & Draine, 2006). These examples illustrate the potential for moving on a variety of fronts to shift health care resources from acute care and facility-based services only to a balance of treatment and prevention and facility and community-based care.

Build Healthy Public Policy

In recent years, public health researchers have called attention to the importance to population health of public policies in a variety of sectors, including housing, education, the environment, work, taxation, and criminal justice (Lurie, 2002; McGinnis, Williams-Russo, & Knickman, 2002; Milio, 1998). Recent research on the health of incarcerated populations demonstrates that policies on substance abuse, crime, housing, employment, health care, and other issues can adversely affect their well-being (Blankenship, Smoyer, Bray, & Mattocks, 2005; Freudenberg, Daniels, Crum, & Perkins, 2005; Golembeski & Fullilove, 2005; Holzer, Raphael, & Stoll, 2003; Iguchi et al., 2002; O'Leary & Martins, 2000; Richie et al., 2001). Often these policies impose disproportionate burdens on vulnerable and disenfranchised groups—people of color, women, and drug users, and may thus contribute to growing disparities in health (Freudenberg, 2002; Gaiter, Potter, & O'Leary, 2006; Iguchi, Bell, Ramchand, & Fain, 2005). How have CHS staff taken on advocacy roles? Some have chosen to become active in developing national standards of care that can serve to improve the quality of care in jails and prison (APHA, 2003; NCCHC, 2001). Others have worked to change health insurance policies that barred coverage for people leaving correctional facilities, to provide immunization against hepatitis to people in incarcerated populations, to advocate for laws that require discharge planning for people returning from incarceration, to reduce discrimination against inmates with HIV, and to improve housing options for those coming home from prison or jail (Beck, Sullivan, & Walker, 2001; Freudenberg, Rogers, et al., 2005; Gondles, 2005; Restum, 2005). While the impact of these efforts has not been evaluated, a recent review of litigation on correctional conditions concluded that these lawsuits had led to improvements in the past three decades (Nathan, 2004).

Recommendations

In this section, we suggest actions that could help to move CHS from an acute medical care perspective to a health promotion model. The recommendations are based on our review of the literature and our own experience working in jails and prisons. Once again, we use the activity categories proposed by the World Health Organization's definition of health promotion.

While few correctional systems will have the capacity or resources to adopt all these recommendations, every jail and prison has the potential to expand the repertoire of activities beyond treatment to health promotion. By viewing these two approaches as a continuum with a menu of options, CHS managers can begin to broaden their range of services within the realities of their political and financial constraints. At the same time, by articulating a vision of a correctional system whose mission has widened to include promoting the well-being of those who enter its gates, we offer a more comprehensive view that can contribute more fully to the goals of improved public safety and community health.

Develop Personal Skills

CHS should offer a wide range of health education programs to prevent and manage infectious and chronic diseases; to reduce violence and substance use; and to make healthy decisions about sexuality, intimate relationships, and parenting. Such programs should include cognitive and affective dimensions; tailor interventions to meet the specific needs of various gender, sexual orientation, racial/ethnic, and age groups; and use peer educators as appropriate. Several correctional facilities have developed model peer health education programs (Boudin et al., 1999; Ehrmann, 2002). Experienced correctional administrators have learned that offering services that engage, respect and offer opportunities to incarcerated people contributes to improved security, less violence, and better working conditions for staff.

Create Supportive Environments

Although the public health literature provides strong evidence that supportive environments contribute to improved health, few such interventions have been implemented or evaluated in correctional settings. Specific steps correctional officials can take to improve elements of the prison or jail physical environment that influence health are reduction in overcrowding; comprehensive pest control strategies; adequate lighting and ventilation; and noise control. Improvements in the social environment include increasing opportunities for family visits and telephone calls; staff training and supervision to reduce hostile or violent interactions among inmates or between inmates and staff; clear policies and protocols to prevent sexual violence and coercion among inmates and between inmates and staff; and availability of assistance for those with addictions, especially those going through withdrawal while incarcerated.

Another dimension of the correctional environment that has been inadequately studied is food. While adequate nutrition is an essential component of health, incarcerated populations lose the right to choose their diet. In some facilities, processed, tasteless foods are used as a punishment for inmates who have violated rules. In a few, agricultural programs provide incarcerated individuals with an opportunity to learn gardening or farming skills and to provide fresh produce for the facility and other facilities have offered heart-healthy diets. Few correctional facilities have examined the nutritional quality of food items offered in inmate canteens. Having access to a balanced diet that promotes health would appear to be a basic human right; whether improved nutrition could lead to improved health or criminal justice outcomes has yet to be studied. Given high rates of diabetes and obesity in the low-income communities from which most people in correctional facilities come and return to, using prisons and jails to improve nutritional status could help to control these epidemics.

Similarly, growing evidence points to the short- and long-term benefits of regular physical activity in promoting mental and physical health and preventing weight gain, chronic diseases, and mental health conditions. A healthy correctional facility should ensure that all inmates have access to regular physical activity and avoid depriving inmates of opportunities to exercise as a punishment.

Strengthen Community Action for Health

No correctional health service has the resources to achieve the broad goals outlined here; hence, partnerships with other community organizations are a vital ally in redefining the mission. The reentry programs that have been created in the last several years provide numerous illustrations of the potential for such collaboration. Among the key services that partnerships can provide—each of which enhances and multiplies the benefits from health services—are mental health services, substance abuse treatment, housing, and employment. Community partnerships can provide the essential resources needed for comprehensive approaches to CHS and reentry programs.

Since many community organizations are already funded—albeit sometimes inadequately—to serve vulnerable populations, tailoring their services to people in or returning from correctional facilities may not require major new investments. Moreover, since these organizations are often required to demonstrate their ability to find and engage new clients, partnerships with correctional facilities may help them to meet their funders' mandates.

Developing the organizational framework for community partnerships for correctional health promotion and successful reentry presents significant operational challenges; no single model is likely to suit all jurisdictions. Among the requirements for successful alliances are a clear process for making decisions, accountability mechanisms, a defined vision and mission, and a plan for sustainability.

Reorient Health Services

To shift the mission and services of CHS from acute care only to health promotion will require leadership from correctional managers, public health officials, and advocacy organizations. In our view, an incremental approach is most likely to succeed in which correctional health professionals add more health-promotion-oriented services based on emerging needs, scientific evidence, cost-benefit and cost-effectiveness analyses, and operational capacity. For example, chronic disease management programs for inmates with hypertension or diabetes may prevent hospitalizations of inmates, a disruptive practice for correctional facilities; save correctional health systems and states and municipalities money; and improve the lives of people returning home (Tomlinson & Schechter, 2002). Adding such programs in prisons and for sentenced jail inmates, who will be in the facility long enough to benefit, may reduce health care expenditures as well as improve outcomes. Some studies have provided evidence on the cost-effectiveness or cost benefits of improved CHS, but more such research is needed (National Commission on Correctional Health Care, 2002b).

In addition to the chronic disease management programs previously described, specific CHS that can be added to improve inmate and community health might include:

- routine screening and treatment for infectious diseases such as chlamydia, gonorrhea, hepatitis A, B, and C, and, of course, HIV infection;
- immunizations for hepatitis A and B, influenza, tetanus, and pneumococcus;
- behavioral interventions to reduce violence and aggressive behavior;
- reproductive health services including pregnancy screening, gynecological care, birth control, abortion and prenatal services; new evidence that interconceptional care can improve birth outcomes for women and infants provides a rationale for providing the vulnerable population of incarcerated women with these services;
- nutrition counseling to help individuals lose weight and prevent or control chronic diseases;
- heart-healthy diets and early detection of chronic diseases.

Each correctional health system will need to decide which of these services to add, what standards of quality to achieve, and what mechanisms to use to ensure that available services are distributed equitably according to a public health, rather than a criminal justice, rationale.

Build Healthy Public Policy

Healthy public policy makes it easier for individuals and institutions to choose behaviors that promote health. If we accept the premise that our correctional systems ought to contribute to improved societal well-being and improved public safety, then we need to ask what public policies will enable jails and prisons to realize these goals. To date, few elected officials or correctional systems have systematically considered the mission of prisons and jails from this perspective.

Such an analysis suggests both fundamental and more proximate policy changes that could improve the capacity of correctional systems to improve well-being. For example, incarcerating fewer people would reduce the many unintended consequences of the explosive growth in incarceration of recent decades. These include community and family disruption and a reduction in social cohesion (Rose & Clear, 2003), factors associated with poor public health; increased correctional costs reducing resources available for other needs such as education, health care, and housing; and, perhaps, widening disparities in health due to the long-term negative health consequences of incarceration (Freudenberg, 2002; Gaiter et al., 2006; Iguchi et al., Fain, 2005).

At another level, improved coordination of reentry services including health care, employment, job training, housing, and substance abuse treatment can contribute to improve criminal justice and health outcomes, yet few jurisdictions have established policies that ensure or encourage such coordination.

What role can correctional health professionals play in creating healthier public policies? As in other sectors, they can convene stakeholders to identify policy obstacles, provide evidence to support the value of policy change; advocate for specific policies that will promote health; and help to ensure that healthier policies are in fact implemented. For the most part, health professionals cannot achieve these goals on their own, but in our experience, the participation of health professionals often adds credibility and depth to advocacy efforts to change correctional and reentry policies (Freudenberg, Rogers, et al., 2005).

To support these changes in mission, policies, and practices, correctional health professionals will need to evaluate both incremental and more substantive reforms in order to develop an evidence base that can guide further changes. Other chapters in this volume describe some of the challenges evaluators face in documenting the impact and benefits of CHS.

Conclusion

In this chapter, we have outlined an approach to CHS in which health promotion is a central priority on both sides of the bars. We have argued that the World Health Organization's definition of health promotion as the "process of enabling people to increase control over and to improve their health" provides a useful paradigm for reconsidering the goals of correctional health and that its five activity categories—developing personal skills for health, creating supportive environments, strengthening community action for health, reorienting health services, and building healthy public policy—offer a framework for expanding the scope of CHS. We also presented evidence that existing practice in prisons and jails demonstrates that it is feasible to implement each component of this expanded view and that many such interventions have been shown to be effective or promising.

The challenge ahead is to develop systematic approaches to making prisons and jails settings that improve rather than harm the well-being of the people who enter the front gate and the families and communities to which they return. At one level, this is as simple as recognizing the basic ethical principles that guide health professionals; at another, it will require a transformation of the U.S. correctional system.

References

American Public Health Association. (2003). *Standards for health services in correctional institutions* (3rd ed.). Washington, DC: Author.

Austin, J., & Hardyman, P. (2004). The risks and needs of the returning prisoner population. *Review of Policy Research, 21*, 13–29.

Bauserman, R.L., Richardson, D., Ward, M., Shea, M., Bowlin, C., Tomoyasu, N., & Solomon, L. (2003). HIV prevention with jail and prison inmates: Maryland's Prevention Case Management program. *AIDS Education and Prevention, 15*, 465–480.

Beck, A.J. (2006). The importance of successful reentry to jail population growth. Presented at The Jail Reentry Roundtable, The Urban Institute, Washington, DC, June 27, 2006. Available at http://www.urban.org/projects/reentry-roundtable/round-table9.cfm

Beck, J., Sullivan, P., & Walker, J. (2001). Prisons: Advocates say inmate medical services are public health issue. *AIDS Policy Law, 16*, 1–8.

Bell, J.F., Zimmerman, F.J., Cawthon, M.L., Huebner, C.E., Ward, D.H., & Schroeder, C.A. (2004). Jail incarceration and birth outcomes. *Journal of Urban Health, 81*, 630–644.

Berkman, L.F., Glass, T., Brissette, I., & Seeman, T.E. (2000). From social integration to health: Durkheim in the new millennium. *Social Science and Medicine, 51*, 843–857.

Blankenship, K.M., Smoyer, A.B., Bray, S.J., & Mattocks, K. (2005). Black–white disparities in HIV/AIDS: The role of drug policy and the corrections system. *Journal of Health Care for the Poor and Underserved, 16*(4 Suppl. B), 140–156.

Bloom, B., Owen, B., & Covington, S. (2003). *Gender-responsive strategies: Research, practice, and guiding principles for women offenders,* Washington, DC: U.S. Department of Justice, National Institute of Corrections. http://www.nicic.org/pubs/2003/018017.pdf.

Boudin, K., Carrero, I., Clark, J., Flournoy, V., Loftin, K., Martindale, S., Martinez, M., Mastroieni, R.E., & Richardson, S. (1999). ACE: A peer education and counseling program meets the needs of incarcerated women with HIV/AIDS issues. *J Assoc Nurses AIDS Care, 10*, 90–98.

Brownson, R.C., Haire-Joshu, D., & Luke, D.A. (2006). Shaping the context of health: A review of environmental and policy approaches in the prevention of chronic diseases. *Annual Review of Public Health, 27*, 341–370.

Bureau of Justice Statistics. (2006). Prison statistics. http://www.ojp.usdoj.gov/bjs/prisons.htm

Clarke, J.G., Rosengard, C., Rose, J.S., Hebert, M.R., Peipert, J., & Stein, M.D. (2006). Improving birth control service utilization by offering services prerelease vs. postincarceration. *American Journal of Public Health, 96*, 840–845.

Des Jarlais, D.C., McKnight, C., & Friedmann, P. (2002). Legal syringe purchases by injection drug users, Brooklyn and Queens, New York City, 2000–2001. *Journal of the American Pharmaceutical Association, 42*(6 Suppl. 2), S73–S76.

Di Placido, C., Simon, T.L., Witte, T.D., Gu, D., & Wong, S.C. (2006). Treatment of gang members can reduce recidivism and institutional misconduct. *Law and Human Behavior, 30*, 93–114.

Dvoskin, J.A., & Spiers, E.M. (2004). On the role of correctional officers in prison mental health. *Psychiatric Quarterly, 75*, 41–59.

Ehrmann, T. (2002). Community-based organizations and HIV prevention for incarcerated populations: Three HIV prevention program models. *AIDS Education and Prevention, 14*(5 Suppl. B), 75–84.

El-Bassel, N., Ivanoff, A., Schilling, R., Borne, D., & Gilbert, L. (1997). Skills building and social support enhancement to reduce HIV risk among women in jail. *Criminal Justice and Behavior, 24*, 205–223.

Freudenberg, N. (2001). Jails, prisons, and the health of urban populations: A review of the impact of the correctional system on community health. *Journal of Urban Health*, *78*, 214–235.

Freudenberg, N. (2002). Adverse effects of US jail and prison policies on the health and well-being of women of color. *American Journal of Public Health*, *92*, 1895–1899.

Freudenberg, N., Daniels, J., Crum, M., Perkins, T., & Richie, B.E. (2005). Coming home from jail: The social and health consequences of community reentry for women, male adolescents, and their families and communities. *American Journal of Public Health*, *95*, 1725–1736.

Freudenberg, N., Rogers, M., Ritas, C., & Nerney, M. (2005). Policy analysis and advocacy: An approach to community-based participatory research. In B Israel et al. (Eds.), *Methods in community-based participatory research for health* San Francisco: Jossey–Bass.

Gaiter, J.L., Potter, R.H., & O'Leary, A. (2006). Disproportionate rates of incarceration contribute to health disparities. *American Journal of Public Health*, *96*, 1148–1149.

Gatherer, A., Moiler, L., & Hayton, P. (2005). The World Health Organization European Health in Prisons Project after 10 years: Persistent barriers and achievements. *American Journal of Public Health*, *95*, 1696–1700.

Gilligan, J., & Lee, B. (2005a). The Resolve to Stop the Violence Project: Reducing violence in the community through a jail-based initiative. *Journal of Public Health*, *27*, 143–148.

Gilligan, J., & Lee, B. (2005b). The Resolve to Stop the Violence Project: Transforming an in-house culture of violence through a jail-based programme. *Journal of Public Health*, *27*, 149–155.

Glaser, J., & Greifinger, R. (1993). Correctional health care: A public health opportunity. *Annals of Internal Medicine, 118*, 139–145.

Golembeski, C., & Fullilove, R. (2005). Criminal (in)justice in the city and its associated health consequences. *American Journal of Public Health*, *95*, 1701–1706.

Gondles, E.F. (2005). A call to immunize the correctional population for hepatitis A and B. *The American Journal of Medicine*, *118*(Suppl. 10A), 84S–89S.

Green, L.W., Kreuter, M.W., Partridge, K., & Deeds, S. (1999). *Health education planning: A diagnostic approach* (3rd ed.). Mountain View, CA: Mayfield.

Greene, E., Lucarelli, P., & Shocksnider, J. (1999). Health promotion and education in youth correctional facilities. *Pediatric Nursing*, *25*, 312–314.

Grinstead, O., Zack, B., & Faigeles, B. (2001). Reducing post release risk behavior among HIV seropositive prison inmates: The health promotion program. *AIDS Education and Prevention*, *13*, 109–119.

Hairston, C.F. (1998). The forgotten parent: Understanding the forces that influence incarcerated fathers' relationships with their children. *Child Welfare*, *77*, 617–639.

Hammett, T.M. (2001). Making the case for health interventions in correctional facilities. *Journal of Urban Health, 78*, 236–240.

Harlow, C. (1998). *Profile of jail inmates 1996. Bureau of Justice Statistics Special Report*.

Harner, H.M. (2004). Relationships between incarcerated women: Moving beyond stereotypes. *Journal of Psychosocial Nursing and Mental Health Services*, *42*, 38–46.

Harrison, K. (1997). Parental training for incarcerated fathers: Effects on attitudes, self-esteem, and children's self-perceptions. *Journal of Social Psychology*, *137*, 588–593.

Hoge, C.W., Reichler, M.R., Dominguez, E.A., Bremer, J.C., Mastro, T.D., Hendricks, K.A., Musher, D.M., Elliott, J.A., Facklam, R.R., & Breiman, R.F. (1994). An epidemic of pneumococcal disease in an overcrowded, inadequately ventilated jail. *The New England Journal of Medicine*, *331*, 643–648.

Holzer, H.J., Raphael, S., & Stoll, M.A. (2003). Employment barriers facing ex-offenders. Prepared for the Urban Institute Reentry Roundtable.

Iguchi, M.Y., Bell, J., Ramchand, R.N., & Fain, T. (2005). How criminal system racial disparities may translate into health disparities. *Journal of Health Care for the Poor and Underserved, 16*(4 Suppl. B), 48–56.

Iguchi, M.Y., London, J.A., Forge, N.G., Hickman, L., Fain, T., & Riehman, K. (2002). Elements of well-being affected by criminalizing the drug user. *Public Health Reports, 117*(Suppl. 1), S146–S150.

Institute of Medicine. (2002). *Future of the public's health in the 21st century.* Washington, DC: National Academy Press.

James, D. (2004). *Profile of jail inmates, 2002.* Bureau of Justice Statistics Publication No. NCJ 201932. Washington, DC: U.S. Department of Justice.

Jones, T.F., Craig, A.S., Valway, S.E., Woodley, C.L., & Schaffner, W. (1999). Transmission of tuberculosis in a jail. *Annals of Internal Medicine, 131,* 557–563.

Kraut-Becher, J.R., Gift, T.L., Haddix, A.C., Irwin, K.L., & Greifinger, R.B. (2004). Cost-effectiveness of universal screening for chlamydia and gonorrhea in US jails. *Journal of Urban Health, 81,* 453–471.

Kyei-Aboagye, K., Vragovic, O., & Chong, D. (2000). Birth outcome in incarcerated, high-risk pregnant women. *The Journal of Reproductive Medicine, 45,* 190–194.

Laufer, F., Jacob Arriola, K., Dawson-Rose, C., Kumaravelu, K., & Krane Rapposelli, K. (2002). From jail to community: Innovative strategies to enhance continuity of HIV/AIDS care. *The Prison Journal, 82,* 84–100.

Leh, S.K. (1999). HIV infection in U.S. correctional systems: Its effect on the community. *Journal of Community Health Nursing, 16,* 53–63.

Lincoln, T., Kennedy, S., Tuthill, R., Roberts, C., Conklin, T.J., & Hammett, T.M. (2006). Facilitators and barriers to continuing healthcare after jail: A community-integrated program. *The Journal of Ambulatory Care Management, 29,* 2–16.

Lindquist, C.H., & Lindquist, C.A. (1999). Health behind bars: Utilization and evaluation of medical care among jail inmates. *Journal of Community Health, 24,* 285–292.

Lowenkamp, C.T., Latessa, E.J., & Smith, P. (2006). Does correctional program quality really matter? The impact of adhering to principles of effective intervention. *Criminology and Public Policy, 5,* 201–220.

Lurie, N. (2002). What the federal government can do about the nonmedical determinants of health. *Health Affairs (Millwood), 21,* 94–106.

May, J.P., & Williams, E.L., Jr. (2002). Acceptability of condom availability in a U.S. jail. *AIDS Education and Prevention, 14*(5 Suppl. B), 85–91.

McCoy, M.L., Roberts, D.L., Hanrahan, P., Clay, R., & Luchins, D.J. (2004). Jail linkage assertive community treatment services for individuals with mental illnesses. *Psychiatric Rehabilitation Journal, 27,* 243–250.

McGinnis, J.M., Williams-Russo, P., & Knickman, J.R. (2002). The case for more active policy attention to health promotion. *Health Affairs (Millwood), 21,* 78–93.

McLean, R.L., Robarge, J., & Sherman, S.G. (2006). Release from jail: Moment of crisis or window of opportunity for female detainees? *Journal of Urban Health, 83,* 382–393.

Mertz, K.J., Voigt, R.A., Hutchins, K., Levine, W.C., & Jail STD Prevalence Monitoring Group. (2002). Findings from STD screening of adolescents and adults entering corrections facilities: Implications for STD control strategies. *Sexually Transmitted Disease, 29,* 834–839.

Merzel, C., & D'Afflitti, J. (2003). Reconsidering community-based health promotion: Promise, performance, and potential. *American Journal of Public Health, 93,* 557–574.

Milio, N. (1998). Priorities and strategies for promoting community-based prevention policies. *Journal of Public Health Management and Practice, 4,* 14–28.

Miller, R.D., & Metzner, J.L. (1994). Psychiatric stigma in correctional facilities. *The Bulletin of the American Academy of Psychiatry and the Law, 22,* 621–628.

Myers, J., Zack, B., Kramer, K., Gardner, M., Rucobo, G., & Costa-Taylor, S. (2005). Get Connected: An HIV prevention case management program for men and women leaving California prisons. *American Journal of Public Health, 95,* 1682–1684.

Nathan, V.M. (2004). Taking stock of the accomplishments and failures of prison reform litigation: Have the courts made a difference in the quality of prison conditions? What have we accomplished to date? *Pace Law Review, 24,* 419–425.

National Commission on Correctional Health Care. (2001). Clinical guides. http://www.ncchc.org/resources/clinicalguides.html

National Commission on Correctional Health Care. (2002a). *The health status of soon-to-be-released inmates: A report to Congress.* Vol. 1. Chicago: Author.

National Commission on Correctional Health Care. (2002b). *The health status of soon-to-be-released inmates: A report to Congress* (Vol. 2, pp. 81–166). Chicago: Author.

National Commission on Correctional Health Care. (2003). *Standards for health services in jails.* Chicago: Author.

Needels, K., James-Burdumy, S., & Burghardt, J. (2005). Community case management for former jail inmates: Its impacts on rearrest, drug use, and HIV risk. *Journal of Urban Health, 82,* 420–433.

No authors. (2002). US: Condoms distributed to gay inmates in LA. *Canadian HIV/AIDS Policy & Law Review, 6,* 18–19.

Nurse, J., Woodcock, P., & Ormsby, J. (2003). Influence of environmental factors on mental health within prisons: Focus group study. *British Medical Journal, 327,* 480.

O'Donnell, M.P. (1989). Definition of health promotion: Part III: Expanding the definition. *American Journal of Health Promotion, 3,* 5.

Olden, K., & White, S.L. (2005). Health-related disparities: Influence of environmental factors. *The Medical Clinics of North America, 89,* 721–738.

O'Leary, A., & Martins, P. (2000). Structural factors affecting women's HIV risk: A life-course example. *AIDS, 14,* S68–S72.

Palmer, T. (1995). Programmatic and nonprogrammatic aspects of successful intervention: New directions for research. *Crime & Delinquency, 41,* 100–131.

Parece, M.S., Herrera, G.A., Voigt, R.F., Middlekauff, S.L., & Irwin, K.L. (1999). STD testing policies and practices in U.S. city and county jails. *Sexually Transmitted Disease, 26,* 431–437.

Petersilia, J. (2003). *When prisoners come home: Parole and prisoner reentry.* New York: Oxford University Press.

Pouget, E.R., Deren, S., Fuller, C.M., Blaney, S., McMahon, J.M., Kang, S.Y., Tortu, S., Andia, J.F., Des Jarlais, D.C., & Vlahov, D. (2005). Receptive syringe sharing among injection drug users in Harlem and the Bronx during the New York State Expanded Syringe Access Demonstration Program. *Journal of Acquired Immune Deficiency Syndromes, 39,* 471–477.

Re-Entry Policy Council. (2005). *Report of the Re-Entry Policy Council: Charting the safe and successful return of prisoners to the community.* New York: Author.

Restum, Z.G. (2005). Public health implications of substandard correctional health care. *American Journal of Public Health, 95,* 1689–1691.

Rhodes, L.A. (2005). Pathological effects of the supermaximum prison. *American Journal of Public Health, 95,* 1692–1695.

Rich, J.D., Holmes, L., Salas, C., Macalino, G., Davis, D., Ryczek, J., & Flanigan, T. (2001). Successful linkage of medical care and community services for HIV-positive offenders being released from prison. *Journal of Urban Health, 78,* 279–289.

Richie, B., Freudenberg, N., & Page, J. (2001). Reintegrating women leaving jail into urban communities: A description of a model program. *Journal of Urban Health, 78,* 290–303.

Robillard, A.G., Gallito-Zaparaniuk, P., Arriola, K.J., Kennedy, S., Hammett, T., & Braithwaite, R.L. (2003). Partners and processes in HIV services for inmates and ex-offenders: Facilitating collaboration and service delivery. *Evaluation Review, 27,* 535–562.

Rogers, W., & Seigenthaler, C. (2001). Correctional health care as a vital part of community health. *Journal of Ambulatory Care Management, 24*, 45–50.

Rose, D., & Clear, T. (2003). Incarceration, reentry, and social capital: Social networks in the balance. In J. Travis & M. Waul (Eds.), *Prisoners once removed: The impact of incarceration and reentry on children, families, and communities* (pp. 313–342). Washington, DC: Urban Institute Press.

Schady, F.F., Miller, M.A., & Klein, S.J. (2005). Developing practical "tips" for HIV/AIDS service delivery in local jails. *Journal of Public Health Management and Practice, 11*, 554–558.

Sinclair, C.T., & Porter-Williamson, K. (2004). Health care delivery in the Texas prison system. *Journal of the American Medical Association, 292*, 2212.

Strauss, S., & Falkin, G. (2000). The relationship between the quality of drug user treatment and program completion: Understanding the perceptions of women in a prison-based program. *Substance Use & Misuse, 35*, 2127–2159.

Tamasino, V., Swanson, A., Nolan, J., & Shuman, H. (2001). The Key Extended Entry Program (KEEP): A methadone treatment program for opiate-dependent inmates. *The Mount Sinai Journal of Medicine, 68*(1).

Thompson, P.J., & Harm, N.J. (2000). Parenting from prison: Helping children and mothers. *Issues in Comprehensive Pediatric Nursing, 23*, 61–81.

Tomlinson, D.M., & Schechter, C.B. (2002). Cost-effectiveness analysis of annual screening and intensive treatment for hypertension and diabetes mellitus among prisoners in the United States. In *Health status of soon-to-be-released inmates: A report to Congress*. Vol. 2. Chicago: National Commission on Correctional Health Care.

Travis, J. (2005). *But they all come back: Facing the challenges of prisoner reentry*. Washington, DC: Urban Institute Press.

U.S. Department of Justice, National Institute of Corrections. (2004). Proceedings of the large jail network meeting. http://www.nicic.org/pubs/2004/019466.pdf

White, M.C., Duong, T.M., Cruz, E.S., Rodas, A., McCall, C., Menendez, E., Carmody, E.R., & Tulsky, J.P. (2003). Strategies for effective education in a jail setting: The Tuberculosis Prevention Project. *Health Promotion and Practice, 4*, 422–429.

Whitehead, D. (2006). The Health Promoting Prison (HPP) and its imperative for nursing. *International Journal of Nursing Studies, 43*, 123–131.

Wilson, A.B., & Draine, J. (2006). Collaborations between criminal justice and mental health systems for prisoner reentry. *Psychiatric Services, 57*, 875–878.

World Health Organization. (1986). Ottawa Charter for Health Promotion. 1st International Conference on Health Promotion. Ottawa, Canada.

World Health Organization. (2002). Prevention and promotion in mental health. Mental Health: Evidence and Research, Department of Mental Health and Substance Dependence.

World Health Organization. (2004). Code of good practices for NGOs responding to HIV/AIDS.

World Health Organization. (2006). Health in Prisons Project. World Health Organization Regional Office for Europe. http://www.euro.who.int/prisons

Yen, I., & Syme, S.L. (1999). The social environment and health. *Annual Review of Public Health, 20*, 287–308.

Chapter 14

Screening for Public Purpose: Promoting an Evidence-based Approach to Screening of Inmates to Improve Public Health

Joshua D. Lee, Marshall W. Fordyce, and Josiah D. Rich

Introduction

Jail and prison screening procedures have developed to rapidly identify patients with acute illness or communicable disease to protect the health of other inmates and staff. But the period of incarceration is also an opportune moment to impact public health via evidence-based screening of high-risk individuals who do not otherwise access routine preventive care. Given the dynamic exchange between correctional facilities and medically underserved communities, effective screening in jails and prisons is generally a cost-effective approach to improving population health.

General Considerations Regarding Screening Tests

Approaches to prevention are broadly categorized into levels that reflect the natural history of a disease (Fletcher & Fletcher, 2005; Gorroll & Mulley, 2005). Primary prevention prevents disease before occurrence, for example immunizations and focused health education. Secondary prevention detects disease early and when early treatment impacts progression and transmission. Screening for conditions like hypertension and sexually transmitted diseases are examples of secondary prevention. Tertiary prevention addresses established disease by reducing morbidity and mortality.

The goal of screening is to identify risk factors or disease that can be modified by early intervention. The value of a screening test, then, depends on the value of an early diagnosis. If accurate detection of disease during the asymptomatic phase can meaningfully alter the course of disease and reduce morbidity and mortality or transmission to others, then screening likely has meaningful impact. If an effective screening test is inexpensive relative to the cost of diagnosis and treatment of advanced disease, then the test is likely cost-effective.

Whether a screening test results in better health outcomes depends on the characteristics of the disease, the test, and the patient population. The severity of a disease and its effect on the quality or duration of life, a sufficiently high prevalence, and the availability of acceptable and effective treatment all impact the value of a screening test. Some diseases have an asymptomatic period during which detection and treatment significantly reduces morbidity and mortality. For these diseases, treatment in the asymptomatic phase yields a better therapeutic result than treatment that is delayed until symptoms appear. Other diseases, such as lung cancer, progress very rapidly and have a frustratingly narrow window of asymptomatic disease during which intervention prevents death. Screening does not work without effective early therapy.

The operating characteristics of a screening test are crucial. It must be sufficiently sensitive to detect disease during the asymptomatic period, and sufficiently specific to provide an acceptable positive predictive value. The test should be simple to administer and interpret, low cost, safe, and acceptable to patients and clinicians. "Labeling" and the psychological effects of a positive screen should be anticipated. A positive screening test is not a diagnosis. The diagnosis must be confirmed with further testing. A test's utility can be undermined if false-positive cases are labeled as "diseased" or subsequent workups are intolerably expensive or harmful. Screening should only be undertaken if both clinician and patient will treat a confirmed positive test or otherwise benefit from this new information. Co-morbid conditions can also modulate screening and need to be considered by the physician on an individual basis. For example, there is little value in screening and pursuing a particular diagnosis if a patient has a high likelihood of dying sooner from another cause. Studies evaluating new screening technologies must consider lead-time and time-linked sampling biases. Lead time is the period of time between the detection of disease by screening and when it would ordinarily be diagnosed due to symptoms. Studies that do not account for lead-time bias can overestimate a screening test's impact on survival.

Finally, the characteristics of the patient population are important in critically evaluating a screening program. The prevalence of or harm from the disease must be high. The screening test must have both a high sensitivity so as not to miss cases and a high enough specificity to reduce false-positive tests. For example, in diseases with very low prevalence, a test with a low specificity could produce an unacceptable number of false-positive results. However, by limiting screening to a high-risk population (i.e., universal active TB screening is recommended in certain high-risk jails, but not in a general primary care population), the pretest probability and positive predictive value increases and the rate of false positives decreases. Many of this chapter's recommendations hinge on this principle of targeted screening among a high-risk population.

United States Preventive Services Task Force Recommendations

For the general population, the United States Preventive Services Task Force (USPSTF) reviews the evidence for screening a variety of health issues, and grades the evidence based on the strength of the evidence and the magnitude of net benefit. Recommendations for population-based screening that earned grade A (strongly recommended) or grade B (recommended) in a 2006 review for adult men and women are the following: obesity, depression, and high blood pressure screening for persons of all ages, syphilis screening for "persons at increased risk," colorectal cancer screening at age 50, diabetes type 2 screening for adults with hypertension or hyperlipidemia, and lipid disorder screening per age and gender (men, age 35; women, age 45) ("Guide to Clinical Preventive Services," 2006). Additional procedures are recommended for women: breast cancer screening (mammography) at age 40, cervical cancer screening if sexually active, chlamydial infection screening women 25 and younger or at increased risk, and osteoporosis screening for women 65 or older, postmenopausal, or at increased risk for osteoporotic fractures. Men age 65–75 with a history of ever smoking should be screened for abdominal aortic aneurysm via ultrasonography.

These recommendations are based on a critical review of the evidence for screening in the general population and may need to be reevaluated within correctional settings. For instance, all persons in correctional facilities should be evaluated for syphilis infection, while osteoporosis screening may not be appropriate in many settings (i.e., a central intake facility). None of these conditions, however, are known to occur at lower rates within corrections. Therefore, any facility that provides primary care to the incarcerated should access all of the USPSTF recommended procedures.

Screening in Jail and Prison Populations

Few public institutions are more important to the surveillance and treatment of communicable disease and mental health disorders than jails, prisons, and other detention centers. Due to the concentration and high turnover of high-risk individuals otherwise out of contact with other public and community health systems, correctional institutions are uniquely situated to implement testing, treatment and referrals for chronic diseases, STDs, HIV, and tuberculosis via cost-effective means (Lee, Vlahov, & Freudenberg, 2006). Proper TB control mandates prompt and uniform screening at facility admission. Finally, adequate screening for suicidality and drug and alcohol withdrawal syndromes helps ensure these two leading causes of preventable death among the incarcerated are greatly minimized. Intake and general screening recommendation are summarized in Tables 14.1 and 14.2.

Communicable Disease

Active Tuberculosis Infection
The need to screen for TB on admission to a correctional facility is uncontroversial and based on multiple studies demonstrating higher incidences of active TB in correctional environments and evidence of outbreaks in the setting of poor TB controls (MacNeil et al., 2005; "Prevention and control of tuberculosis in correctional and detention facilities," 2006). Despite this, recommended screening protocols in jails and prisons are not uniformly applied, with only 55% (11 of 20) of large jail systems instituting routine tuberculosis skin testing (TST) at admission in a 1998 survey (Roberts et al., 2006).

Table 14.1 Recommended correctional screening for adults: intake.

Condition	Recommended procedure
Tuberculosis, active infection	Symptom questionnaire and one or more of the following: TST[1] Serum QuantiFERON-Gold Chest X-ray
Syphilis	Nontreponemal serology (RPR, VDRL)
Chlamydia	Urine or swab NAAT[2]
Gonorrhea	Urine or swab NAAT[2]
HIV	Rapid HIV-1 antibody test, blood, or oral swab
Hepatitis C	Serum antibody test
Cervical cancer	Pap smear
Pregnancy	Serum or urine qualitative hCG
Mental illness	Symptom screen, psychiatric history
Suicidality	Symptom and risk factor screening
Alcohol, opioid, and sedative/hypnotic dependence	Drug and alcohol use and withdrawal history

[1] Men age ≥35, women age ≥45.
[2] Persons with HTN and hypercholesterolemia only.

Table 14.2 Recommended correctional screening for adults: general health assessment.

Condition	Recommended procedure
Hypertension	Sphygmomanometery
Cholesterol[1]	Random or fasting serum cholesterol
Diabetes[2]	Fasting serum glucose
Overweight, obesity	Height and weight measurement
Abdominal aortic aneurysm[3]	Ultrasonography
Colon cancer[4]	FOBT[5], flexible sigmoidoscopy, colonoscopy, or barium enema
Breast cancer[6]	Mammography
Osteoporosis[7]	Bone mineral density

[1] Men age ≥35, women age ≥45.
[2] Persons with HTN and hypercholesterolemia only.
[3] Men who have smoked, age 65–75 only.
[4] Persons age ≥50.
[5] Fecal occult blood test.
[6] Women age >40.
[7] Women age >65 or older, postmenopausal, or at increased risk for osteoporotic fractures.

The Centers for Disease Control and Prevention's 2006 document, "Prevention and Control of Tuberculosis in Correctional and Detention Facilities: Recommendations from CDC," provides current consensus guidance for TB screening. This report distinguishes between minimal and non-minimal TB risk facilities when recommending screening strategies. Briefly, minimal TB risk facilities are those with: (1) no infectious TB cases in the last year, (2) the facility does not house substantial numbers of inmates with risk factors for TB including HIV or injection drug use, (3) the facility does not house substantial numbers of new immigrants (emigrated within previous 5 years) from countries with high TB rates, and (4) employees are not otherwise at risk for TB. If any of the four conditions is present, a facility is classified as nonminimal TB risk.

Minimal TB risk facilities should practice universal symptom screening (questionnaires covering pulmonary TB symptoms) and reserve TST, QuantiFERON-TB Gold (QFT-G), or chest radiograph screening for asymptomatic individuals at risk for TB. Risk factors include recent immigration, diabetes, recent contact with a TB case, immunosuppressive therapy, renal failure, or a history of malignancy. Further, minimal TB risk facilities should screen all HIV-positive individuals or those with risk factors for HIV (i.e., IVDU, multiple sexual partners) with chest radiographs, and isolate all suspected active TB cases identified through symptom or chest radiograph screening in an airborne infection isolation (AII) room pending an evaluation for active TB (i.e., consecutive sputum samples sent for acid fast staining).

Nonminimal TB risk facilities, comprising the vast majority of correctional facilities in the United States, should both screen for symptoms via questionnaires *and* offer a universal screening test (TST, QFT-G, or chest radiograph) to all asymptomatic individuals. HIV-positive individuals and those at risk for HIV should be screened using chest radiographs. As in minimal TB risk facilities, any case of suspected active TB following symptom screening or chest radiography should be immediately isolated using AII and prompt sputum examination.

Symptom Screening: All persons entering a correctional facility should receive a standardized questionnaire (with assistance for illiterate individuals) assessing TB-related history and symptoms administered by a trained layperson or, when possible, a health professional. Persons should be asked about any history of active TB or latent TB infection (LTBI), treatment for active TB or LTBI, the main symptoms of active pulmonary TB (prolonged cough [>3 weeks], hemoptysis, or chest pain), and systemic TB symptoms (fever, chills, night sweats, weight loss). Symptoms suggestive of active TB should prompt an immediate medical evaluation and diagnostic testing for TB, including chest radiographs, TST, or QFT-G. Symptom screening has low sensitivity (10–60%) and specificity (70%) compared to the gold standard of sputum examination in cross-sectional studies and is therefore inappropriate as a single screening strategy in nonminimal TB risk facilities (den Boon et al., 2006; Wisnivesky et al., 2005).

Tuberculosis Skin Testing: TSTs are the most common form of mass screening for TB among correctional and other institutionalized populations. The sensitivity of TST using a 15 mm of induration cutoff in immunocompetent LTBI cases approaches 100%. Past BCG vaccination and exposure to nontuberculosis mycobacteria, however, generate considerable rates of false positive tests, which lowers TST specificity and positive predictive value ("Targeted tuberculin testing," 2000) Different cutoffs of induration are recommended to maximize specificity depending on a person's category of risk (Table 14.3). Induration of 10 mm or more in persons admitted to a correctional facility

Table 14.3 Tuberculosis skin testing: Interpretation and cutoffs.

Reaction ≥5 mm	HIV
	Recent TB case contact
	CXR fibrosis c/w prior TB
	Organ transplant
	Immunosuppression
Reaction ≥10 mm	Recent immigrants from high-prevalence countries IVDU
	Residents of high-risk facilities (prisons and jails, nursing homes, hospitals, homeless shelters)
	TB lab personnel
	High-risk medical conditions (silicosis, diabetes, CRF, leukemia or lymphoma, malignancy, weight loss)
Reaction >15 mm	Person with no risk factors for TB

Source: American Thoracic Society. (2000). Targeted tuberculin testing and treatment of latent tuberculosis infection.

without HIV, immunocompromise, prior TB, or recent exposure to an active TB case should prompt a medical evaluation and further testing.

Chest Radiographs: Chest radiographs are the most efficacious means of screening for active pulmonary TB. Sensitivity of radiographs compared to sputum examination in cases of suspected active TB approaches 98%; specificity is lower (60–70%) (den Boon et al., 2006; "Prevention and control of tuberculosis in correctional and detention facilities," 2006). Radiography as universal screening in corrections is limited by cost and logistic considerations, despite data demonstrating that standard, digital, or miniature radiographs increase active TB case-findings, decrease time to isolation, and are cost-effective from a combined health and correctional systems perspective (Jones & Schaffner, 2001; Layton et al., 1997).

QuantiFERON-TB Gold Test: Approved in 2005, QFT-G is as sensitive and more specific a test than TST for detecting TB or LTBI ("Prevention and control of tuberculosis in correctional and detention facilities," 2006). Its chief disadvantages to date are cost and the need for laboratory analysis within 12 hours of sampling. Like TST, it does not distinguish between LTBI or TB. The test measures levels of interferon-gamma present in whole blood cells that have been stimulated by peptides unique to *M. tuberculosis*. CDC guidelines endorse QFT-G as a substitute for TST in all situations, including correctional screening (Mazurek et al., 2005).

Sexually Transmitted Diseases

Serum-based screening for syphilis and urine-based screening for *Chlamydia trachomatis* and *Neisseria gonorrhoeae* infections are cost-effective practices across correctional settings due to high prevalence, underexposure to community-based screening, frequent asymptomatic infections, and end-stage complications including pelvic inflammatory disease and tertiary syphilis (Kahn, Scholl, Shane, Lemoine, & Farley, 2002; Kraut-Becher, Gift, Haddix, Irwin, & Greifinger, 2004) Correctional screening for chlamydia and gonorrhea is particularly cost-effective among adolescents and adult females

(Joesoef, Kahn, & Weinstock, 2006; Mertz, Schwebke, et al., 2002) Reactive syphilis is more likely among men who have sex with men and older adults (Ciesielski et al., 2005) In some localities, STD screening, often for syphilis, is mandated by public health codes.

Syphilis: A 2004 study analyzing national data from 1999 to 2002 demonstrated that 12.5% of all reported early syphilis (primary, secondary, early latent) cases in the United States were identified in correctional facilities, while incarceration rates were on the order of <1% during this period (Kahn, Voigt, Swint, & Weinstock, 2004) U.S. estimates of syphilis prevalence vary by year, population, and region, with higher rates generally reported in both general and correctional populations among adult women, African Americans, HIV-positive individuals, crack cocaine users, sex workers, and those living within urban centers or the Southeast ("Primary and secondary syphilis—United States, 2003–2004," 2006). CDC data from nine adult and five juvenile facilities located in urban counties from 1996 to 1999 showed that the percentage with reactive syphilis tests by county was 8.2% (range, 0.3–23.8%) for women and 2.5% (range, 1.0–7.8%) for men, while the percentage with high-titer tests (^{3}1:8) ranged from 0% to 7.4% for women and from 0.1% to 2.9% for men (Mertz, Voigt, Hutchins, & Levine, 2002).

Serum testing consists of nontreponemal screening followed by treponemal confirmation. Nontreponemal tests include rapid plasma reagent (RPR) and Venereal Disease Research Laboratory test (VDRL). Treponemal tests are the fluorescent treponemal antibody absorbed (FTA-ABS) or *T. pallidum* particle agglutination (TP-PA). Nontreponemal positive results should trigger a confirmatory treponemal test due to high false-positive rates on nontreponemal tests secondary to pregnancy, injection drug use, or unrelated medical conditions (Workowski & Berman, 2006). Sensitivity of nontreponemal tests varies with antibody levels and may be 78–86% in primary syphilis, 100% during secondary syphilis, and 95–98% in latent syphilis (USPSTF, 2004). Treponemal tests have 84% sensitivity in primary syphilis, 100% in other stages, and a specificity of 96%. Alternative methods of syphilis screening, including ELISA and IgG, have not been evaluated in mass screening programs. If follow-up of laboratory results cannot be reasonably assured, point-of-care qualitative syphilis assays present an alternative screening method with comparable sensitivity and specificity to traditional nontreponemal screens (Blank et al., 1997).

Chlamydia: Urethral and cervical infections with chlamydia are the most common sexually transmitted bacterial conditions in the United States. Recent cross-sectional observational trials implementing chlamydia screening in correctional settings have demonstrated infection rates of 15.3–21.5% among women aged 16–74 in Chicago, IL, Birmingham, AL, and Baltimore, MD, 15.6% among adolescent females and 5.9% among adolescent males in 14 U.S. juvenile detention centers, and 4.9% among adult males in Chicago, IL (Kahn et al., 2005; Mertz, Voigt, Hutchins, & Levine, 2002; Trick et al., 2006). Screening tests for chlamydia include nucleic acid amplification tests (NAAT), nucleic acid hybridization assays, culture, and urinalysis for leukesterase. NAAT can be performed on urine samples with minimal compromise of sensitivity as compared to swab samples (91–100 versus 100%). NAAT is the test of choice in males and females in correctional settings where urethral or endocervical swabs are not optimal (Johnson et al., 2002). Because of the high prevalence of chlamydia and the high sensitivities (94–99%) of NAAT, the positive predictive value of NAAT within correctional settings is excellent (Johnson et al., 2002). Thus, positive NAAT screens for chlamydia in correctional populations are presumed evidence of infection and should be treated without further diagnostic testing (i.e., culture).

Gonorrhea. N. gonorrhoeae: cervicitis and urethritis share risk factors and reservoir populations with chlamydia. Rates of gonorrhea-positive screens in corrections have been documented as 5% in adolescent women, 1% in adolescent males, 2–4% in adult females, and 2% in adult males (Mertz, Voigt, Hutchins, & Levine, 2002). Like chlamydia, gonorrhea can also be detected using a NAAT of urine or swab samples. Sensitivities vary by NAAT manufacturer (78–100%) and are decreased but acceptable in urine compared to swab samples (Johnson et al., 2002).

HIV

Routine HIV screening is recommended as a component of general medical care for all persons (Branson et al., 2006). Screening for HIV in correctional facilities is cost-effective and recommended for all patients at all types of facilities given historically elevated HIV prevalence among prisoners and the benefits of early detection. This is a longstanding position of the CDC and USPSTF ("Revised guidelines for HIV counseling," 2001; "Screening for HIV," 2005). Rapid HIV tests of saliva, buccal mucosal cells, or small quantities of blood (derived from a fingerstick) allow same-session availability of test results and make HIV screening a practical addition to most facilities' intake procedures (Branson et al., 2006). While the sensitivity, specificity, and positive predictive value of rapid tests are high (>95%), the results should be considered preliminary and should be accompanied by counseling, medical referrals, and confirmatory testing by Western Blot or immunofluorescent assay. Traditional screening via enzyme-linked immunosorbent assay (ELISA) testing yields high sensitivity and specificity but not point-of-care results. Because of the lag time between infection and seroconversion, persons at risk for recent HIV exposure should be tested at intake and at 4–6 weeks, 3 months, and 6 months (Smith et al., 2005). Persons with ongoing high sexual or other risk should be offered testing at least annually.

Viral Hepatitis

Hepatitis C: Multiple studies have documented rates of chronic viral hepatitis in correctional populations 2–20 times those of the general population, with an estimated one-third of all chronic hepatitis C cases cycling through U.S. jails and prisons in a given year (Hammett, Harmon, & Rhodes, 2002; Macalino, Dhawan, & Rich, 2005; C. M. Weinbaum, Sabin, & Santibanez, 2005). 2003 CDC recommendations call for serologic screening in all incarcerated persons with HCV risk factors, including a history of IVDU, receipt of blood products prior to 1992, receipt of clotting factors prior to 1987, history of hemodialysis, and chronic liver disease or elevated ALT (C. Weinbaum, Lyerla, & Margolis, 2003). Universal HCV screening is recommended when a facility's self-reported history of risk factors alone identifies <75% of anti-HCV-positive inmates, the prevalence of risk factors for HCV infection, including injection-drug use, is known to be high (>75%), or there is a high prevalence (>20%)

of HCV infection among inmates who deny risk factors. However, in a recent screening study, 66% of inmates testing positive for chronic HCV did not report a history of IVDU and most would not have been tested under the 2003 CDC guidelines (Macalino et al., 2005). Given few correctional systems will be able to routinely track and compare rates of HCV and risk factors, it is the authors' recommendation that all persons in correctional facilities be screened for HCV, with positive cases being counseled not to drink alcohol, get vaccinated for HAV and HBV, avoid transmission to others, and consider treatment. Testing should include both an antibody screening assay (e.g., enzyme immunoassay [EIA]) and supplemental or confirmatory testing with an additional, more specific assay (e.g., recombinant immunoblot assay [RIBA] for anti-HCV or nucleic acid testing for HCV RNA).

Hepatitis B: Rates of chronic, treatable HBV infection are lower than those of HCV in correctional populations, though HBV transmission has been shown to be more common than that of HCV or HIV among prisoners (Macalino et al., 2004). Generally, the burden of HBV will decrease due to universal HBV vaccination at birth in the United States begun in 1991. Because acute and chronic HBV is preventable via the HBV vaccination series and vaccinating correctional populations is an efficient way to protect high-risk populations, HBV efforts in jails and prisons have focused on vaccine programs rather than serologic screening (Rich et al., 2003; C. Weinbaum et al., 2003). Pregnant women are the exception and should be screened for HBV at the first prenatal visit.

Hepatitis A: Like HBV, HAV is a preventable infection via vaccination. HAV vaccination is recommended for individuals at high risk for HAV infection or complications (i.e., those in endemic areas and chronic HCV patients). Serologic screening for HAV antibody status is not recommended for general correctional populations.

Mental Health and Substance Use

Mental Health Disorders

Lifetime prevalence estimates of severe mood or psychotic disorders in correctional populations, excluding substance use disorders, are historically much higher than those of the general population and range from 5 to 50% (Abram, Teplin, & McClelland, 2003; Lamb & Weinberger, 1998; Teplin et al., 2005). Universal screening for severe mental illness at admission to a correctional facility is crucial to ensuring adequate treatment, suicide prevention, and discharge planning. There are no national guidelines, however, in selecting validated screens for intake purposes. Instruments used in prevalence studies such as the National Institute of Mental Health Diagnostic Interview Schedule (NIMH-DIS) or the Mini International Neuropsychiatric Interview (MINI) tend to be long in duration and best administered by a trained interviewer. While a two-item PRIME-MD screen for depression has been shown to be both sensitive and specific, it has not been validated in correctional populations, particularly in the moment of a facility intake evaluation (Whooley, Avins, Miranda, & Browner, 1997). Generally, every individual should be asked about a history of psychiatric illness or care, psychotropic medications, past suicide attempts or ideation, and symptoms of mood and psychotic disorders, in addition to assessing current mental status (*Standards for Health Services in Jails*, 1996).

Suicide Prevention and Screening

Identifying risk of self-harm is paramount given the majority of preventable deaths in correctional facilities are from suicide (Lanphear, 1987; Way, Miraglia, Sawyer, Beer, & Eddy, 2005). Risk factors for suicide in correctional settings include a history of mental illness, co-morbid substance use disorders, "stressors" or behavior changes preceding the attempt, and a history of violent crime (Blaauw, Kerkhof, & Hayes, 2005; Way, et al., 2005). Various screening instruments are designed to identify pertinent risk factors for impending suicide attempts, including a 14-item Suicide Screening Inventory or the Scale for Suicidal Ideation (Holi et al., 2005; Kaczmarek, Hagan, & Kettler, 2006). Most validated instruments assess current suicidality (ideation and plans), a history of ideation or attempts, a history of mental illness and treatment, and recent stressors including loss of job, relationships, or deaths of loved ones. Arrest and incarceration is itself a significant stressor, underlining the need for timely suicide screening at admission. Positive screens should trigger comprehensive psychiatric assessments and effective prevention, including hospitalization or protective housing.

Substance Use Disorders

Substance use disorders are the rule in correctional populations. Rates of nicotine dependence approach 90%; alcohol use disorders, 10–30%; and other drug use disorders, 10–60% (Fazel, Bains, & Doll, 2006; *Substance Dependence, Abuse, and Treatment of Jail Inmates,* 2005; Yacoubian, 2003). Alcohol use disorder rates trend higher in men, while drug use disorder rates are higher in women. Given that high rates have been consistent over time and across correctional settings, precise screening for gradations of individual substance use disorders is low yield (e.g., risky use versus abuse versus dependence). Instead, tobacco, alcohol, and drug treatment should be offered universally and independent of an individual's response to intake history items surveying tobacco, alcohol, and drug use. No national guidelines recommend urine toxicology for screening purposes.

Withdrawal Syndromes

Within holding and intake facilities, however, alcohol, sedative-hypnotic, and opioid withdrawal symptoms require targeted screening strategies in order to prevent discomfort and death (*Clinical Practice Guidelines: Detoxification*, 2000; *Standards for Health Services in Jails*, 1996). Despite national guidelines, a minority of U.S. jails report offering detoxification services (Fiscella, Pless, Meldrum, & Fiscella, 2004). All patients should be asked about daily use of alcohol, barbiturates and benzodiazepines, and opioids. Those with chronic, heavy use should be asked about a history of withdrawal syndromes, pharmacologic treatment for withdrawal, and in the case of alcohol and sedative-hypnotics, a history of seizure and delirium tremens (DTs). Clinical Institute Withdrawal Assessment-Alcohol (CIWA) and Clinical Institute Narcotic Assessment (CINA) scores help classify withdrawal severity and chart symptom course, but do not provide cutoffs for screening purposes. In the case of alcohol and sedative-hypnotic withdrawal, the onset of unstable vital signs, altered mental status, or neurologic deficits necessitates prompt treatment and close observation if not hospitalization (*Principles of Addiction*

Medicine, 2003). Opioid withdrawal, while generally not fatal, is marked by severe psychological discomfort and hyperautonomic symptoms. Isolated cases of death related to opioid withdrawal within correctional settings have been noted (Fiscella et al., 2004).

Chronic Disease and Health Maintenance

Cardiovascular and Metabolic Disease

Screening to reduce cardiovascular risk in correctional populations should follow the USPSTF guidelines ("Guide to Clinical Preventive Services," 2006). While cardiovascular disease rates are thought to be higher both within corrections and following release, the burden of CV disease and diabetes is so high in the general population that universal screening should be employed in all health care settings. Blood pressure should be assessed annually in all adults. All smokers should be counseled to quit and offered smoking cessation resources. Random or fasting serum cholesterol is recommended for men aged ³35 and women aged ³45, or beginning at age 20 if other CV risk factors are present. Fasting serum glucose should be used to screen for diabetes and glucose intolerance in persons with hypertension or hyperlipidemia. All persons should be screened for obesity (BMI ³30) and overweight (BMI 25–29.9), though there is insufficient evidence that population-based weight management counseling is effective at achieving weight loss or reduced CV risk. Finally, for those aged 65–75, men who have smoked should be offered one-time ultrasonography screening for abdominal aortic aneurysm.

Cancer

HIV-, smoking-, HCV-, and HPV-related malignancies are thought to occur at higher rates in correctional populations (Baillargeon, Pollock, Leach, & Gao, 2004; Mathew, Elting, Cooksley, Owen, & Lin, 2005). Cervical cancer screening via Pap testing or HPV genetic testing should be offered to all females with an intact cervix at facility admission and then annually. While many clinicians screen for hepatomas via serial ultrasonography or serum alpha fetal protein among patients with liver disease, there is no evidence that this reduces mortality and this is not recommended for general correctional populations. Lung cancer screening via CT scan, CXR, or sputum cytology is thus far ineffective in smokers. Beyond routine HIV primary care and general cancer screening, there are no additional screening tests recommended for HIV-related lymphomas or other malignancies.

USPSTF recommends age-appropriate screening for two other malignancies in addition to cervical cancer. Colon cancer screening begins at age 50 for men and women at average risk via home fecal occult blood testing (FOBT), flexible sigmoidoscopy, the combination of home FOBT and flexible sigmoidoscopy, colonoscopy, and double-contrast barium enema. Women aged ³40 should be offered screening mammography with or without clinical breast examination (CBE) every 1–2 years. Either CBE or breast self-examination without mammography is insufficient.

Given the rates of HCV and smoking among inmates, or the disproportionate numbers of African Americans under correctional supervision, compelling cases could be made to offer routine cancer screening not recommended by USPSTF. For example, many would argue black patients aged ³45 should be screened for prostate cancer via serum prostate-specific antigen or digital rectal examination (Harris & Lohr, 2002). While correctional physicians should certainly discuss with and potentially offer such screening to concerned or high-risk patients, there is insufficient evidence to date for prostate, lung, or hepatocellular carcinoma screening in general correctional populations.

Pregnancy and Diabetes Care

All females on admission to correctional facilities should be screened for pregnancy. If pregnant, women should be offered screening for the following: blood pressure, Rh (D) incompatibility, HIV, chlamydia, gonorrhea, bacterial vaginosis, syphilis, and UTI or asymptomatic bacteriuria ("Guide to Clinical Preventive Services," 2006). They should also be screened for infection with and susceptibility to viral hepatitis B and C. Further discussion of women's health issues is found elsewhere in this text.

Persons with diabetes should be offered blood pressure and cholesterol screening, annual retinal and foot examinations, and screening for microalbuminuria by measurements of urine albumin-to-creatinine ratios. All diabetics should be considered for primary prevention of myocardial infarction with daily aspirin, especially if they are older or have at least one other cardiovascular risk factor (American Diabetes Association, 2007). This is in addition to serial serum glucose measurements among self-reported diabetics following arrest, during the arraignment period, and at facility admission.

Annual Screening Procedures for Long-Term Correctional Populations

There is little evidence for or against specific annual health screening among persons incarcerated for 1 year or more, as distinct from periodic health screening among general adult populations. The USPSTF recommends Pap smears annually or at least every 3 years if there have been three consecutive normal tests. They recommend annual mammography for patients 40 years old and older. Colon cancer screening should be done annually by FOBT, or every 5–10 years if screening is by sigmoidoscopy or colonoscopy. Blood pressure screening is recommended at least every 2 years and cholesterol screening every 5 years, with shorter intervals for those with initial borderline screening results and longer intervals for those with initial low-risk results. It should be noted that these frequencies are suggested based on expert opinion and not grade A or B evidence.

Because prisons and jails are high-risk settings for tuberculosis transmission, annual tuberculosis screening is warranted (symptom questionnaire and TST, QFT-G, or CXR) in facilities that are categorized as nonminimal risk (see the chapter on tuberculosis prevention and control). While prisons and jails are often perceived as high-risk settings for HIV, HCV, HBV and other bloodborne or sexually transmitted diseases, documented intrafacility incidence rates of these conditions are low with the exception of HBV infection rates of 2–4% per year (CDC, 2006; Khan et al., 2005; Macalino et al., 2004). Given any facility's potential for sexual, needle, or other exposures, annual HIV and HCV testing is prudent though not evidence-based. Intrafacility HBV prevention should focus on vaccination rather than repeat screening.

In summary, there are no evidence-based guidelines for annual health screens among inmates excepting yearly Pap testing and mammography. Given high rates of communicable, cardiovascular, and psychiatric disease, however, we

Table 14.4 Recommended correctional screening for adults: annual health screening.

Condition	Recommended procedure
Depression and suicidality	Screening questionnaire
Hypertension	Sphygmomanometry
Cholesterol[1]	Random or fasting serum cholesterol
Diabetes[2]	Fasting serum glucose
Overweight, obesity	Height and weight measurement
Colon cancer[3]	FOBT, flexible sigmoidoscopy, colonoscopy, or barium enema
Breast cancer[4]	Mammography
Cervical cancer	Pap testing
Tuberculosis, active infection	Symptom questionnaire and one or more of the following: TST, Serum QuantiFERON-TB-Gold, Chest X-ray
HIV	Rapid HIV-1 antibody test, blood or oral swab, or ELISA testing
Hepatitis C	Serum antibody test

[1] Men aged ≥ 35, women aged ≥ 45; if other CV risk factors, age ≥20.
[2] Persons with HTN and hypercholesterolemia only.
[3] Persons aged ≥ 50.
[4] Women aged ≥ 40.

recommend the following annual screening procedures: depression and suicidality questionnaires, blood pressure, cholesterol and measurements of body-mass index, fasting serum glucose if the patient has hypertension or hyperlipidemia, Pap testing and mammography (age≥40), FOBT if no colonoscopy or sigmoidoscopy (age≥50), and TB, HIV, and HCV testing. (Table 14.4)

Conclusion

Health screening at admission to a correctional facility and as a routine part of correctional primary care both protects the facility's population and staff and delivers appropriate prevention to the otherwise underserved. Chronic and cardiovascular disease screening in jails and prisons largely conforms to general population guidelines. Mental illness and suicidality, withdrawal symptoms, and communicable diseases, conditions with high prevalences in correctional settings, create opportunities for targeted screening among persons who are otherwise inaccessible to community health systems.

References

Abram, K. M., Teplin, L. A., & McClelland, G. M. (2003). Comorbidity of severe psychiatric disorders and substance use disorders among women in jail. *Am J Psychiatry, 160*, 1007–1010.
American Diabetes Association. (2007). Diabetes management in correctional institutions. *Diabetes Care, 30*(Suppl. 1), S77–S84.

Baillargeon, J., Pollock, B. H., Leach, C. T., & Gao, S. J. (2004). The association of neoplasms and HIV infection in the correctional setting. *Int J STD AIDS, 15*, 348–351.

Blaauw, E., Kerkhof, A. J., & Hayes, L. M. (2005). Demographic, criminal, and psychiatric factors related to inmate suicide. *Suicide Life Threat Behav, 35*, 63–75.

Blank, S., McDonnell, D. D., Rubin, S. R., Neal, J. J., Brome, M. W., Masterson, M. B., et al. (1997). New approaches to syphilis control. Finding opportunities for syphilis treatment and congenital syphilis prevention in a women's correctional setting. *Sex Transm Dis, 24*, 218–226.

Branson, B. M., Handsfield, H. H., Lampe, M. A., Janssen, R. S., Taylor, A. W., Lyss, S. B., et al. (2006). Revised recommendations for HIV testing of adults, adolescents, and pregnant women in health-care settings. *MMWR Recomm Rep, 55*(RR-14), 1–17.

Centers for Disease Control. (2006). HIV transmission among male inmates in a state prison system—Georgia, 1992–2005. *MMWR, 55*(15), 421–426.

Ciesielski, C., Kahn, R. H., Taylor, M., Gallagher, K., Prescott, L. J., & Arrowsmith, S. (2005). Control of syphilis outbreaks in men who have sex with men: the role of screening in nonmedical settings. *Sex Transm Dis, 32*(10 Suppl.), S37–S42.

Clinical practice guidelines: Detoxification of chemically dependent persons. (2000). Washington, DC: National Institute of Corrections.

den Boon, S., White, N. W., van Lill, S. W., Borgdorff, M. W., Verver, S., Lombard, C. J., et al. (2006). An evaluation of symptom and chest radiographic screening in tuberculosis prevalence surveys. *Int J Tuberc Lung Dis, 10*, 876–882.

Fazel, S., Bains, P., & Doll, H. (2006). Substance abuse and dependence in prisoners: A systematic review. *Addiction, 101*, 181–191.

Fiscella, K., Pless, N., Meldrum, S., & Fiscella, P. (2004). Alcohol and opiate withdrawal in US jails. *Am J Public Health, 94*, 1522–1524.

Fletcher, R. H., & Fletcher, S. W. (2005). *Clinical epidemiology: The essentials* (4th ed.). Philadelphia: Lippincott Williams & Wilkins.

Gorroll, A. H., & Mulley, A. G. (2005). *Primary care medicine: Office evaluation and management of the adult patient* (5th ed.). Philadelphia: Lippincott Williams & Wilkins.

Guide to clinical preventive services, 2006: Recommendations of the U.S. Preventive Services Task Force. (2006). AHRQ Publication No. 06-0588. From http://www.ahrq.gov/clinic/pocketgd06/.

Hammett, T. M., Harmon, M. P., & Rhodes, W. (2002). The burden of infectious disease among inmates of and releasees from US correctional facilities, 1997. *Am J Public Health, 92*, 1789–1794.

Harris, R., & Lohr, K. N. (2002). Screening for prostate cancer: An update of the evidence for the U.S. Preventive Services Task Force. *Ann Intern Med, 137*, 917–929.

Holi, M. M., Pelkonen, M., Karlsson, L., Kiviruusu, O., Ruuttu, T., Heila, H., et al. (2005). Psychometric properties and clinical utility of the Scale for Suicidal Ideation (SSI) in adolescents. *BMC Psychiatry, 5*(1), 8.

Joesoef, M. R., Kahn, R. H., & Weinstock, H. S. (2006). Sexually transmitted diseases in incarcerated adolescents. *Curr Opin Infect Dis, 19*, 44–48.

Johnson, R. E., Newhall, W. J., Papp, J. R., Knapp, J. S., Black, C. M., Gift, T. L., et al. (2002). Screening tests to detect Chlamydia trachomatis and Neisseria gonorrhoeae infections—2002. *MMWR Recomm Rep, 51*(RR-15), 1–38.

Jones, T. F., & Schaffner, W. (2001). Miniature chest radiograph screening for tuberculosis in jails: A cost-effectiveness analysis. *Am J Respir Crit Care Med, 164*, 77–81.

Kaczmarek, T. L., Hagan, M. P., & Kettler, R. J. (2006). Screening for suicide among juvenile delinquents: reliability and validity evidence for the Suicide Screening Inventory (SSI). *Int J Offender Ther Comp Criminol, 50*, 204–217.

Kahn, R. H., Mosure, D. J., Blank, S., Kent, C. K., Chow, J. M., Boudov, M. R., et al. (2005). Chlamydia trachomatis and Neisseria gonorrhoeae prevalence and coinfection in adolescents entering selected US juvenile detention centers, 1997–2002. *Sex Transm Dis, 32*, 255–259.

Kahn, R. H., Scholl, D. T., Shane, S. M., Lemoine, A. L., & Farley, T. A. (2002). Screening for syphilis in arrestees: Usefulness for community-wide syphilis surveillance and control. *Sex Transm Dis, 29*, 150–156.

Kahn, R. H., Voigt, R. F., Swint, E., & Weinstock, H. (2004). Early syphilis in the United States identified in corrections facilities, 1999–2002. *Sex Transm Dis, 31*, 360–364.

Khan, A. J., Simard, E. P., Bower, W. A., Wurtzel, H. L., Khristova, M., Wagner, K. D., et al. (2005). Ongoing transmission of hepatitis B virus infection among inmates at a state correctional facility. *Am J Public Health, 95*, 1793–1799.

Kraut-Becher, J. R., Gift, T. L., Haddix, A. C., Irwin, K. L., & Greifinger, R. B. (2004). Cost-effectiveness of universal screening for chlamydia and gonorrhea in US jails. *J Urban Health, 81*, 453–471.

Lamb, H. R., & Weinberger, L. E. (1998). Persons with severe mental illness in jails and prisons: A review. *Psychiatr Serv, 49*, 483–492.

Lanphear, B. P. (1987). Deaths in custody in Shelby County, Tennessee, January 1970–July 1985. *Am J Forensic Med Pathol, 8*, 299–301.

Layton, M. C., Henning, K. J., Alexander, T. A., Gooding, A. L., Reid, C., Heyman, B. M., et al. (1997). Universal radiographic screening for tuberculosis among inmates upon admission to jail. *Am J Public Health, 87*, 1335–1337.

Lee, J., Vlahov, D., & Freudenberg, N. (2006). Primary care and health insurance among women released from New York City jails. *J Health Care Poor Underserved, 17*, 200–217.

Macalino, G. E., Dhawan, D., & Rich, J. D. (2005). A missed opportunity: Hepatitis C screening of prisoners. *Am J Public Health, 95*, 1739–1740.

Macalino, G. E., Vlahov, D., Sanford-Colby, S., Patel, S., Sabin, K., Salas, C., et al. (2004). Prevalence and incidence of HIV, hepatitis B virus, and hepatitis C virus infections among males in Rhode Island prisons. *Am J Public Health, 94*, 1218–1223.

MacNeil, J. R., McRill, C., Steinhauser, G., Weisbuch, J. B., Williams, E., & Wilson, M. L. (2005). Jails, a neglected opportunity for tuberculosis prevention. *Am J Prev Med, 28*, 225–228.

Mathew, P., Elting, L., Cooksley, C., Owen, S., & Lin, J. (2005). Cancer in an incarcerated population. *Cancer, 104*, 2197–2204.

Mazurek, G. H., Jereb, J., Lobue, P., Iademarco, M. F., Metchock, B., & Vernon, A. (2005). Guidelines for using the QuantiFERON-TB Gold test for detecting Mycobacterium tuberculosis infection, United States. *MMWR Recomm Rep, 54*(RR-15), 49–55.

Mertz, K. J., Schwebke, J. R., Gaydos, C. A., Beidinger, H. A., Tulloch, S. D., & Levine, W. C. (2002). Screening women in jails for chlamydial and gonococcal infection using urine tests: Feasibility, acceptability, prevalence, and treatment rates. *Sex Transm Dis, 29*, 271–276.

Mertz, K. J., Voigt, R. A., Hutchins, K., & Levine, W. C. (2002). Findings from STD screening of adolescents and adults entering corrections facilities: Implications for STD control strategies. *Sex Transm Dis, 29*, 834–839.

Prevention and control of tuberculosis in correctional and detention facilities: Recommendations from CDC. Endorsed by the Advisory Council for the Elimination of Tuberculosis, the National Commission on Correctional Health Care, and the American Correctional Association. (2006). *MMWR Recomm Rep, 55*(RR-9), 1–44.

Primary and secondary syphilis—United States, 2003–2004. (2006). *MMWR, 55*(10), 269–273.

Principles of addiction medicine (3rd ed.). (2003). Chevy Chase, MD: American Society of Addiction Medicine.

Revised guidelines for HIV counseling, testing, and referral. (2001). *MMWR Recomm Rep, 50*(RR-19), 1–57.

Rich, J. D., Ching, C. G., Lally, M. A., Gaitanis, M. M., Schwartzapfel, B., Charuvastra, A., et al. (2003). A review of the case for hepatitis B vaccination of high-risk adults. *Am J Med, 114*, 316–318.

Roberts, C. A., Lobato, M. N., Bazerman, L. B., Kling, R., Reichard, A. A., & Hammett, T. M. (2006). Tuberculosis prevention and control in large jails: A challenge to tuberculosis elimination. *Am J Prev Med, 30*, 125–130.

Screening for HIV: recommendation statement. (2005). *Ann Intern Med, 143*, 32–37.

Smith, D. K., Grohskopf, L. A., Black, R. J., Auerbach, J. D., Veronese, F., Struble, K. A., et al. (2005). Antiretroviral postexposure prophylaxis after sexual, injection-drug use, or other nonoccupational exposure to HIV in the United States: Recommendations from the U.S. Department of Health and Human Services. *MMWR Recomm Rep, 54*(RR-2), 1–20.

Standards for health services in jails. (1996). Chicago: National Commission on Correctional Health Care.

Substance dependence, abuse, and treatment of jail inmates, 2002. (2005). Washington, DC: US Department of Justice.

Targeted tuberculin testing and treatment of latent tuberculosis infection. American Thoracic Society. (2000). *MMWR Recomm Rep, 49*(RR-6), 1–51.

Teplin, L. A., Elkington, K. S., McClelland, G. M., Abram, K. M., Mericle, A. A., & Washburn, J. J. (2005). Major mental disorders, substance use disorders, comorbidity, and HIV-AIDS risk behaviors in juvenile detainees. *Psychiatr Serv, 56*, 823–828.

Trick, W. E., Kee, R., Murphy-Swallow, D., Mansour, M., Mennella, C., & Raba, J. M. (2006). Detection of chlamydial and gonococcal urethral infection during jail intake: Development of a screening algorithm. *Sex Transm Dis, 33*, 599–603.

United States Preventive Services Task Force. (2004). *Screening for syphilis infection: Recommendation statement.* Rockville, MD: Agency for Healthcare Research and Quality.

Way, B. B., Miraglia, R., Sawyer, D. A., Beer, R., & Eddy, J. (2005). Factors related to suicide in New York state prisons. *Int J Law Psychiatry, 28*, 207–221.

Weinbaum, C., Lyerla, R., & Margolis, H. S. (2003). Prevention and control of infections with hepatitis viruses in correctional settings. Centers for Disease Control and Prevention. *MMWR Recomm Rep, 52*(RR-1), 1–36.

Weinbaum, C. M., Sabin, K. M., & Santibanez, S. S. (2005). Hepatitis B, hepatitis C, and HIV in correctional populations: A review of epidemiology and prevention. *AIDS, 19*(Suppl. 3), S41–S46.

Whooley, M. A., Avins, A. L., Miranda, J., & Browner, W. S. (1997). Case-finding instruments for depression. Two questions are as good as many. *J Gen Intern Med, 12*, 439–445.

Wisnivesky, J. P., Serebrisky, D., Moore, C., Sacks, H. S., Iannuzzi, M. C., & McGinn, T. (2005). Validity of clinical prediction rules for isolating inpatients with suspected tuberculosis. A systematic review. *J Gen Intern Med, 20*, 947–952.

Workowski, K. A., & Berman, S. M. (2006). Sexually transmitted diseases treatment guidelines, 2006. *MMWR Recomm Rep, 55*(RR-11), 1–94.

Yacoubian, G. S. (2003). Measuring alcohol and drug dependence with New York City ADAM data. *J Subst Abuse Treat, 24*, 341–345.

Chapter 15

Written Health Informational Needs for Reentry

Jeff Mellow

Introduction

In the last 30 years, tools and techniques have been developed and refined to identify, control, and treat inmate health problems, including physical examinations at intake, screening for chronic and communicable diseases, referral of inmates for additional health and behavioral care, peer and community health counseling, health education and risk assessment programs, and comprehensive discharge planning and transitional health care on release. Long-term changes in an inmate's health regimen are nevertheless difficult to implement due to the constant cycling of inmates in and out of correctional institutions. The average time served in state and federal prison is 25 and 47 months, respectively, with jail inmates incarcerated on average between 10 and 20 days (Cunniff, 2002; Ditton & Wilson, 1999; Sabol & McGready, 1999).Though an inmate's stay in a facility may not be for long, correctional health care professionals still have an advantage in combating health and behavioral issues that rarely exists in the community—a controlled setting.

This chapter will discuss the development and assessment of written health education and discharge planning materials as a low-cost and effective tool to supplement the continuation of health care at discharge. In no way is one naive enough to suggest, however, that written information is a cure-all to increase adherence to a discharge plan. Nonadherence to a medical regimen and lack of utilization of community health services on release results both from macro and micro level factors: lack of funds or insurance to pay for health services, inconvenient locations of the health services, adverse effects of medication, ineffective health education, and personal or cultural beliefs (Centers for Disease Control and Prevention [CDC], 1999b). Nevertheless, research also suggests that adherence to treatment and utilization of services is higher when written materials are incorporated in the discharge plan. This chapter will argue that the research is unequivocal on the need for easily understandable discharge plans. This chapter will also provide a template that correctional personnel can use when developing their own written materials for a correctional population.

The Importance of Written Discharge Summaries

Experience from the Medical Field

In a hospital setting, a discharge plan is the process by which health care personnel prepare the patient for taking care of his or her medical needs after release from the hospital. Discharge plans commonly include a discharge summary, which is a "document written by the patient's physician upon discharge; contain a brief summary of all important information from the entire hospitalization or stay in the institution, including the discharge diagnosis and often a plan for follow-up care" (CDC, 1999a, p. 3). Discharge summaries can be brief, stating the patient's diagnosis, medication protocol, and physician to contact if condition worsens. On the other hand, these summaries can be extremely detailed including time and date of follow up appointment, support services in the community to help with the patient's medical need, and even illustrations on how to complete a medical procedure, such as the administration of insulin. Regardless of the format, the goal of written discharge summaries is to make the transition back into the community as healthy as possible.

Believing that inmates will routinely follow their health regime and discharge plan at release may seem implausible when the same individuals keep being readmitted, many times with more severe health and behavioral problems. Correctional personnel may start believing that no type of preparation on the inside will affect how an inmate deals with his or her medical issues on release. The truth is, however, that inmates are not the only ones who have difficulties following a discharge plan. Research conducted on the discharge process in hospital emergency departments indicates that the majority of patients do not comprehend their medical needs and treatment plan at discharge and after their return home (Isaacman, Purvis, Gyuro, Anderson, & Smith, 1992).

In a recent study of patients ($n = 43$) discharged from an urban hospital, 72% could not identify all of their medications at release, 63% did not understand why the medication was prescribed, and more than half (58%) could not articulate their medical diagnosis (Makaryus & Friedman, 2005). This lack of understanding increases emergency room readmissions and becomes a public health matter when the medication regime for communicable diseases is not properly followed. Not understanding their medical protocol is one of the main reasons cited as to why tuberculosis (TB) patients do not adhere to their treatment. This can severely impact their own health, and also increase the probability of spreading TB to others and the development of drug-resistant strains of TB (CDC, 1999b).

Discharge summaries are one tool medical personnel use to increase adherence to discharge plans. According to Moult, Franck, and Brady (2004), written summaries not only increase information retention and adherence to a medical protocol, but also help patients minimize anxiety and improve illness-related communication skills (p. 166). Eames, McKenna, Worrall, and Read (2003, p. 70) further note that health education materials "encourage self-paced learning" and "offer a consistency of message" that individuals cannot receive if the information is solely delivered verbally.

A study by Isaacman et al. (1992) determined that standardized discharge instructions written at the fifth grade level significantly improved the understanding of parents regarding their child's medical needs after being released from the hospital. Based on the above-cited research, it is hypothesized that prisoners who are given "a well-written, organized, and easily understood overview of their conditions, symptoms to expect with their condition, medications they will be taking, how to take the medications, and what side effects to expect" will have a greater rate of adhering to their medical regimen (Makaryus & Friedman, 2005, p. 993). In terms of helping a population adhere to their medical regimen, the effectiveness of discharge summaries in the medical field supports similar uses in corrections.

Most Inmates Don't Receive Discharge Planning

The Centers for Disease Control and Prevention (1999a) defines barrier as "anything that can prevent a patient from being able to adhere to a treatment regimen" (p. 2). One could argue that the increasingly large number of inmates being discharged unconditionally without any community supervision constitutes such a barrier. According to the Bureau of Justice Statistics, "about 112,000 state prisoners were released unconditionally through an expiration of their sentence in 2000, up from 51,288 in 1990" (Hughes & Wilson, 2005). State prisoners being discharged for "maxing out" their sentence now represent approximately 20% of those who are released (Travis, 2005). Jails are even more problematic, with the overwhelming majority of inmates receiving no community supervision. This means that many discharged inmates cannot rely on parole officers to refer them to health and behavioral services to support their reintegration into society. Even when under supervision, enormous caseloads are leaving parole officers stressed and overwhelmed and, consequently, they are not often able to give adequate attention to each and every parolee. In his study which examined the availability and accessibility of resources for ex-inmates, Helfgott (1997) found that inmates often felt that there was nobody to help them. They often did not know what was available, or how to find out.

The fact that so many released prisoners receive no prerelease preparation further supports the creation of written discharge materials, because a pamphlet or a comprehensive resource guide may be the only information on which they can rely. The parallels to the medical field are surprisingly similar. Makaryus and Friedman (2005) note that "after being carefully supervised in the hospital, patients at discharge assume the former responsibilities of the health care team for their own health care" (p. 991). The same can be said for the majority of inmates. However, unlike most patients, inmates must also start from the beginning in finding employment, housing, food, clothing and the development of strong social networks to increase their chance of succeeding in the community. Many times the inmate's family is not there to support him, having given up on the inmate for his past transgressions. The inmate is in a situation where with limited help he has to locate and obtain identification, health care and ongoing treatment for substance abuse, mental illness, and chronic and/or communicable diseases. Written information given to an inmate prior to release may be the only assistance for returning to the community that they receive.

Currently, only a small minority of state prisoners released each year experience a multisession, formalized prerelease program. Angiello (2005) reports that only 10% of prisoners discharged in 1997 were offered any prerelease programs. Also, the majority of the state prison prerelease programs are voluntary, and are available primarily in minimum-secure facilities (Austin, 2001). Furthermore, prisoners with serious mental health issues, gang membership, who are maxing out and who are seriously violent are exempted from participation in specific prerelease programs (Corrections Compendium, 2004). Services are even more limited for the jail population.

Recommendations for the Development of Written Discharge Health Information

Even when the importance of developing health materials as part of a comprehensive discharge plan is acknowledged, correctional personnel must recognize that the majority of inmates have low literacy skills and that written materials must be designed with this in mind. To quote Smith and Smith (1994), who analyzed medical education publications, "information written above patients' reading level is useless and a waste of time and money" (p.1). The criteria for developing easy-to-read, high-quality discharge information vary, but the majority of experts agree that the following must be incorporated for the information to reach its reader: (1) clearly state purpose of the information, (2) write to a fifth or sixth grade literacy level, (3) use short sentences as much as possible, (4) personally address the reader, (5) use a respectful tone, (6) make the design and layout approachable, and (7) describe specific problem-solving strategies (Cotugna, Vickery, & Haefele, 2005; Doak, Doak, & Root, 1996; Fant, Clark, & Kemper , 2005; Irick & Fried, 2001; Moult et al., 2004).

The following recommendations can help correctional personnel develop written health information and discharge summaries for their prerelease population. Several of the following points were first discussed by Mellow and Dickinson (2006) when assessing prisoner reentry guidebooks, but can also be used for any written health information and discharge materials developed for the health needs of inmates being released. When appropriate, examples from health materials from across the country will be used to highlight the recommended style of writing.

Be Considerate of Prevalent Literacy Levels

The educational levels of inmates are below the national average (eighth and ninth grade level) with reading scores on average between the fifth and seventh grade level. A study in 1992 indicated that the majority of prisoners were functionally illiterate with 33% of prisoners performing at level 1 and 37% at level 2 on the National Adult Literacy Survey (Haigler, Harlow, O'Connor, & Campbell, 1994). Individuals with level 1 literacy can sign their name (low level 1 literacy), locate the expiration date on a driver's license, and locate the time of a meeting on a form (high level 1 literacy). They have difficulty, however, locating two features of information in an article, locating an intersection on a street map, and identifying and entering background information on an application for a social security card (Haigler et al., 1994) Those with level 2 literacy cannot use bus schedules to determine the appropriate bus to take, or read a news article and identify a sentence that provides interpretation of a situation (Haigler et al., 1994). Extreme care must be taken to ensure that the complexity and length of text is compatible with the limited literacy levels of many inmates.

Unpublished research by Mellow and Christian (2005) indicates that discharge materials produced for inmates are presently not tested to ensure the appropriate readability level. In a nationwide sample of reentry guides analyzed by Mellow and Christian, no reentry guides were written at the fourth or fifth grade level and the majority of the guides were written at the high school or college level. Information written above an inmate's level increases the frustration they already experience when returning to the community.

It is important, therefore, to evaluate all written materials before they are widely disseminated to the inmates. In essence, this is a "pretesting" of the material to determine if the inmates understand the content and what, if any, changes need to be made prior to a final printing. Converse and Presser (1986) note that the pretest sample should resemble the target population and be no fewer than 25 persons. Therefore, the sample selected should represent different inmate characteristics based on age, sex, race/ethnicity, and educational level.

Depending on the situation within the particular correctional facility, pretesting of inmates can be administered to them alone or in focus groups. Likewise, the pretest can be in an open or closed-ended format. The objective is to find out if the inmates have any problems comprehending the information. One should note, however, that individuals with low literacy levels may feel embarrassed and have a sense of shame about their poor reading skills and will verbally acknowledge they understood the material when asked, even if that is not the case (Safeer & Keenan, 2005). Others will come up with an excuse such as "I forgot my glasses," and ask to take the instructions back to their cell so as not to identify themselves as functionally illiterate. A simple way to evaluate their reading comprehension level of the material is to ask them some basic questions, in a one-on-one situation, about what they read. From this author's experience inmates may need some time to read the materials before responding. Allow them to read the materials for 20 – 30 minutes to reduce their anxiety and elicit a more valid response rate. At a minimum, the following questions should be incorporated into the interview:

- Was the handout/pamphlet/book easy to read?
- Can you show me what words or parts of the handout/pamphlet/book which were hard to read/understand?
- What parts of the handout/pamphlet/book helped you the most?
- What information was not listed that you think should be written down?
- The handout/pamphlet/book talked about _____. Can you tell me in your own words what the handout/pamphlet/book said?

After the interviews, it is advisable to analyze if there was a difference in the comprehension rates of the materials depending on characteristics of the inmates (e.g., age, sex, race/ethnicity, education level).

Another way to measure the readability of written materials produced for inmates is to use readability software, such as the Flesch Reading Ease readability assessment tool available in Microsoft Word. The Flesch Reading Ease Scale is "the most widely used formula to assess such general reading materials as newspapers, magazines, business communications, and other non-technical materials" (Electronic Privacy Information Center, 2006). Many state and federal agencies, including the U.S. Department of Defense, require all training and informational documents to have a Flesch reading scale between a sixth grade and high school level. The following four points outline how to access these readability statistics when using Microsoft Word:

- On the Tools menu, click Options, and then click the Spelling & Grammar tab.
- Select the Check grammar with spelling check box.
- Select the Show readability statistics check box, and then click OK.
- On the Standard toolbar (toolbar: a bar with buttons and options that you use to carry out commands; to display a toolbar, press ALT and then SHIFT+F10), click Spelling and Grammar. When Microsoft Word finishes checking spelling and grammar, it displays information about the reading level of the document.

Like many readability tests, the Flesch Reading Ease score is based on the average number of syllables per word and words per sentence. It rates text on a 100-point scale; the higher the score, the easier it is to understand the document. Though not an exact science, Table 15.1. correlates the Flesch Reading Ease score with the level of reading difficulty and the corresponding grade level of the score (Smith & Smith, 1994, p. 114). Government agencies recommend that all documents be written at the standard difficult level (60–70). However, writing at the fairly easy or easy reading level is recommended for inmates.

A reentry handbook from Washington, DC is a good example of writing to the audience at the literacy level the majority can comprehend. The following are bullet points listed in their handbook on how to improve reading skills, but the format could just as well be used when addressing inmate-related health needs (Sullivan, 2002, p. 5). The Flesch Reading Ease Score of the text is 74 and is written at the sixth grade level.

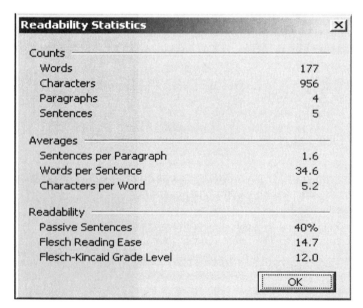

Figure 15.1 The Readability Statistics box of Microsoft Word

Table 15.1 Flesch Reading Ease scores of the first employment paragraph in each reentry guide.

Flesch reading ease score	Reading difficulty	Approx. grade level
0–30	Very difficult	College level up
31–50	Difficult	High school–college
51–60	Fairly difficult	Some high school
61–70	Standard	7th–8th grade
71–80	Fairly easy	6th grade
81–90	Easy	5th grade
91–100	Very easy	4th grade

- If you do not read or write well, enroll in a literacy class.
- If you lack a high school diploma or GED (*General Education Development*), get one.
- If you have enough time to take a basic skills course (*like writing or math*), do it. All of us get rusty in our basic skills when we do not use them for awhile.
- If you have time to take a vocational training class (*like computer repair, word processing, or graphic arts*), do it. It will greatly improve your chances of finding a well-paying job.

Make the Design, Layout, and Information Approachable

Doak, Doak, and Root's (1996) research indicates that the readability of health resource materials increases when the reader finds the text simple and easy to understand. Readability is measured not only by the literacy level of the information, but also by how the material is organized, the writing style, its appearance (e.g., font size and style, spacing, and color contrast of ink and paper), and appeal. An appropriate writing style would have "little or no technical jargon" and use a "conversational style" of writing (p. 43). For example, a TB patient's discharge summary should read "this pill will help you get better" and not "this drug, isoniazid is a bactericidal agent that is highly active against Mycobacterium tuberculosis" (Centers for Disease Control and Prevention [CDC], 1999b, p. 27). The appeal of the material is increased if the information is "culturally, gender and age appropriate" and "matches the logic, language, and experience of the intended audience" (p. 43).

Comic books are a recommended format when communicating health information to inmates. Unlike a static set of facts and figures, comics tell a story using pictures and the written word. Pictures not only aid the reader in understanding the context of the story, but also reduce the anxiety level of reading about health related issues which may impact their personal health. Doak et al., (1996) believe comic books are so popular as a way to disseminate information because "people remember stories better than a set of facts" and "using familiar characters in a familiar setting can help people talk about the real problems in their own lives and community" (p. 110).

The New York City Department of Health and Mental Hygiene [NYC DOHMH] uses the comic book format as one method to help educate

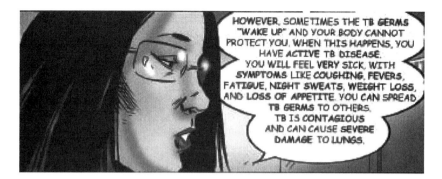

Figure 15.2 Health information comic book *Friends Forever: A Triumph over TB.*

individuals on transmission, diagnosis, and treatment of tuberculosis (NYC DOHMH, 2006). Titled *Friends Forever: A Triumph over TB*, the comic book is 12 pages long, in color, and includes characters of different ethnicities and gender. The last page lists chest center locations in New York City and a phone number to call to make an appointment. The image in Figure 15.2 is of Annie, the public health advisor, telling Joe that he has tested positive for the TB germ and she is answering his questions about TB.

One can also hire companies that specialize in communication solutions for niche markets. Tim Peters and Company (2006), for example, is known for creating comic books to "humanize health information." Tim Peters's *A Sister's Story* uses a prison setting to discuss HIV/AIDS and the importance of getting tested. During the development of the storyline, the artist and writer interviewed current and former inmates and correctional health care providers.

The majority of discharge materials, however, will not be in a comic format. Nevertheless, pictures, even when only a few are dispersed throughout the information, are still one of the best ways to catch a reader's attention and help him understand the information. The Centers for Disease Control and Prevention offers health care providers three different collections of public health images that are free and accessible via the Internet. The CDC's *Public Health Image Library* is a collection of images and multimedia files related to public health. The National Institutes of Health's *National Eye Institute Photo, Image, and Video Catalog* focuses on vision-related images and the CDC's *Division of Diabetes Translation Clip Art* offers 75 diabetes-related illustrations. Figure 15.3, from the Diabetes Clip Art, shows a woman learning to use a blood glucose monitor, a man talking to his doctor, and a bottle of insulin.

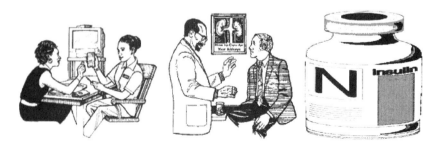

Figure 15.3 Centers for Disease Control Diabetes Clip Art.

Personally Address the Reader

Regardless of whether the written information is given at intake or at discharge, or is 1 page or 60 pages, inmates want the information personalized. *Making It Happen & Staying Home* (Whitaker, 2005) is a 92-page, 4- × 6-inch self-help/resource guide for individuals coming out of New York's jails and prisons. Chapter 3 is titled *What's Up Doc?—Am I OK?* The following are excerpts which highlight a personalized style of writing and are written between the fourth and fifth grade level:

- How's your health? Do you really know? Afraid to ask? Have you had unprotected sex? Shared needles for any reason? Had a forty and a blunt? Swung an episode on the roof, no condom?
- Negative life styles—alcohol, tobacco and other drugs, unhealthy diet, not getting proper rest—are all good reasons to check in and get checked out. Get a physical. Why? To check and deal with the wreckage of your past; you need to know how much damage you've done, if any. (p. 10)
- Have you been tested for STDs, HIV and Hep C? Getting tested can be very personal and stressful. But you still need to know where you stand. You need to know your medical status. Dig this—transmission can also happen in jail. (p. 11)

Describe Specific Problem-Solving Strategies

Written discharge summaries should describe specific problem-solving strategies that inmates can use. Templates of letters, for example, are ideal for inmates preparing for release who will need access to services but may not be able to call these services while incarcerated. The following is an example from Arizona (Tucson Planning Council for the Homeless, 2002, p. 18) of the type of problem-solving strategies and interactive nature of the guides. The beginning of the page describes when the letter should be used and then outlines the letter for the inmate.

Problem-solving strategies which work postrelease in the community may not be feasible inside a correctional facility. A common problem is written information disseminated to inmates which lists only the phone numbers, email addresses, and websites of service providers. The Bazelone Center for Mental Health Law has developed the online brochure *How Can I Apply for Benefits I Did Not Have Before My Arrest?* The following is their description on how to access veterans' benefits while incarcerated.

Veterans Disability Benefits
   If you do not receive these benefits and did not receive them before your arrest, you can begin the application process while you are in jail or prison. You use VA form 21-526,
   Veteran's Application for Compensation and/or Pension, which is available on line.
   You can also apply online using the Veterans On-Line Application (VONAPP), at https://vabenefits.vba.va.gov/vonapp/. (Bazelone Center for Mental Health Law, 2006)

The problem is that the text is written at the 12th grade level (Flesch Reading Ease score 35.9) and recommends inmates access the information online. Only a handful of facilities allow inmates access to the Internet and in all cases only certain websites are available for their use. Even if a phone number was included, most facilities require inmates to make collect calls and

The [following] is a sample letter … to use when writing to halfway houses and other programs before you get out to ask them to reserve a place for you. You should do this about one month to two weeks before your release. Different programs have different rules about how long they are willing to hold a space for someone. They might ask you to write them back closer to your release.

Sample Letter

Pre-Release

Your Name
Your Address
City, State, Zip Code

Today's Date

Agency's Name
Agency's Address
City, State, Zip Code

Dear Sir or Madam,

My name is _____ and I am currently finishing my prison sentence at _____. My release date is _____, and I will have no place to go when I am released.
I am asking that you work with me in advance of my release so that I can have a place to stay and a program to follow instead of becoming homeless. Please send me any necessary paperwork and a list of requirements to qualify for your program so I may collect all that information ahead of time.

I appreciate you assistance, and I eagerly await your reply.

Sincerely,

Your Signature

Source: Tucson Planning Council for the Homeless, 2002

Figure 15.4 Sample letter.

few agencies accept them. The following is an alternative way to write the information, written at the 8th grade level (Flesch Reading Ease score 46.6):

Are you a veteran and need health care?
Call the VA at (877) 222-8387.
Ask for form 21-526 to fill out.
Or write them at:

The Dallas VA Medical Center
4500 South Lancaster Road
Dallas, TX 75216

Highlight the Immediate Needs Crucial to Reentry

Understand that inmates, even with severe chronic or communicable diseases, may not place their health care needs at the forefront on discharge. Therefore, any discharge summary or health care information should also take into consideration what inmates consider as their most pressing needs: obtaining identification, housing, clothing, food, employment, money, and family reunification. Until inmates have their other needs met, the likelihood of them showing up for a medical appointment or adhering to their medical regimen is remote. One way to help is to locate a multipurpose community based organization, otherwise known as a "one-stop center," and highlight in all discharge summaries that this is a good place to go for help and support.

Even when released inmates are committed to their discharge plan, there are numerous barriers which can derail all of their good intentions of maintaining their health protocol. Crick and Potter (2006) conducted five focus groups of former inmates and their families in four cities across the nation to better understand the barriers they face in accessing health and behavioral services. The main concern was the lack of health insurance and money. Therefore, any written discharge information must discuss how to become eligible for health care benefits and focus on how, even if one is not eligible for Medicaid, other benefits may be available to them depending on their special circumstances. Veterans, for example, may be eligible for health care benefits through the Veteran's Administration and people with HIV/AIDS are typically entitled to be part of a state-sponsored AIDS Drug Distribution Program. A list should also be provided of all Federally Qualified Health Centers in the community on their return with an explanation that most health clinics provide primary health care at low cost, sliding scale, or for free. Charity care is also an option offered by hospitals in various states. The following is a template written at the fourth grade level to help released inmates without financial resources obtain health care.

Don't Have Insurance?

- Call the hospital's clinic at _____ and ask when you can see a doctor.
- Get to the hospital early so you can go to the hospital's charity care office.
- Talk with a counselor and tell them you have no money to pay the doctor.
- Ask for a charity care service form to fill out.
- You will know in 10 days if you can receive charity care.
- You do not need to be a citizen or have a green card for charity care.
- Charity care can also be for your family.
- Make sure to bring any doctor bills you get to the counselor.
- They will pay your bill.

Include Only Service Providers with a Steadfast Commitment and Appropriate Accessibility to the Ex-inmate Population and Are Close to Where They Live

"It is common knowledge that nothing frustrates a released ex-offender more than to be referred to a resource that no longer exists" (CSOSA, 2003, p. 16). One could go further and argue that inmates, who have low-frustration tolerance to begin with, also become upset when they are referred to a service that requires fees they cannot afford, does not have an open space for them, has rude personnel, or refuses to work with them because they are a felon. Therefore, all services listed in any discharge summary, reentry guide, or other written material need to be contacted to verify they are willing to work with returning inmates.

Many times, inmates have had such bad experiences with service providers that they are hesitant to interact with them on release. In a reentry guide for prisoners returning to Washington, DC, they acknowledge this issue in their *Where to Get Substance Abuse Treatment or Other Rehabilitation* section.

- All the programs listed here are good programs operated by dedicated people who really want to help you. There are no government programs listed.
- All of these programs are comprehensive. They recognize that there is more than one reason why you have abused drugs and/or alcohol. They recognize that, unless you can change many aspects of your life, you will probably go back to abusing drugs and/or alcohol. So they try to help heal the whole person by assisting you to mend your life and to become a productive citizen. Most have certified substance abuse counselors and licensed social workers. They really do know how to help you. Sullivan (2002, p. 83).

Be Sensitive to Language Barriers

Inmates across the United States are no longer a monolingual English-speaking population. Nineteen percent of the state and federal prison population is Hispanic (Harrison & Beck, 2005). Though not all Hispanics use Spanish as their language of choice, research by Mellow (2001) in a state prison on the East Coast found that 42% of the 122 inmates who identified themselves as Latinos stated they preferred to only speak Spanish, with another 35% preferring to speak Spanish sometimes. In Alaska, similar research found that 32% of the indigenous inmate population preferred to speak their American Indian language all of the time, with 17% stating that they spoke it some of the time.

Murphy, Roberts, Hoffmann, Molina, and Lu (2003) note that "language can be one of the most salient barriers to treatment, especially for first- and second generation migrant families" and therefore bilingual health materials are recommended (p. 218). The benefits are numerous, including:

- Improving clients' comprehension of education materials and instructions;
- Improving clients' ability to follow prescribed treatment and medication schedules;
- Avoiding preventable health crisis and the inappropriate use of health care services;
- Avoiding possible legal liability due to miscommunications;
- Reducing administrative time needed to correct miscommunicated information. (Young, 2000)

It is always recommended to use a professional translator when developing and translating health information, because there are always idiomatic and regionalized expressions which may not be understood by all. Young's (2000) *Developing, Translating and Reviewing Spanish Materials: Recommended Standards for State and Local Agencies* is a good resource to use during the translation process.

Conclusion

Corrections can no longer isolate itself from its public health responsibilities. To quote De Groot and Maddow (2005), "the correctional facility is a publicly funded part of the public health infrastructure in the United States, and it is the ethical and legal responsibility of correctional facilities to respond to the serious medical needs of prisoners" (Chapter 5, p. 15).

The numbers are also just too overwhelming when seen through the prism of individuals with serious health needs and the potential public health risks. Granted, in the short term, developing transitional health care for the 600,000 inmates discharged each year from state prison, with another 8 million (a conservative estimation) inmates released from jails, is unlikely. However, tools must be developed now to begin the slow and arduous process of developing and implementing comprehensive programs for transitioning inmates back to the community. By ignoring the inmates' health needs at release, corrections not only places the public health at risk, but also contributes to millions of dollars in medical costs in years to come for problems that could have been prevented or treated earlier on. Vaccinating an inmate for hepatitis B, in the long run, is less expensive than dealing with chronic liver disease in years to come.

The development and distribution of written health materials and discharge summaries should not be disregarded, just because it has previously not received any attention in the criminal justice field. Every facility should have community specific written discharge materials on inmates with HIV/AIDS, tuberculosis, hepatitis B and C, STDs, substance abuse, diabetes, hypertension, dental care, mental illness, and other chronic and communicable diseases. These health materials would serve the purpose of being an organized, succinct informational resource for inmates returning to their communities, and something they can rely on as a reference even after their release. In addition, it can assist correctional staff in assisting inmates with their prerelease planning.

Though not a comprehensive solution to the health needs of inmates, written health materials have the potential to be a valuable tool to supplement or, if no other alternatives are available, to substitute for a formal medical discharge plan. In addition, and at a low cost, it signals to the correctional staff and the community that corrections is serious about its public health role.

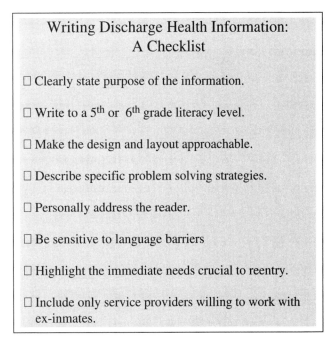

Writing Discharge Health Information:
A Checklist

☐ Clearly state purpose of the information.

☐ Write to a 5th or 6th grade literacy level.

☐ Make the design and layout approachable.

☐ Describe specific problem solving strategies.

☐ Personally address the reader.

☐ Be sensitive to language barriers

☐ Highlight the immediate needs crucial to reentry.

☐ Include only service providers willing to work with ex-inmates.

Figure 15.5 Writing discharge health information checklist.

References

Angiello, E. (2005). Prerelease programs. In M. Bosworth (Ed.), *Encyclopedia of prisons and correctional facilities*. Thousand Oaks, CA: Sage Publications.

Austin, J. (2001). Prisoner reentry: Current trends, practices, and issues. *Crime & Delinquency 47*, 314–334.

Bazelon Center for Mental Health Law. (2006). *How do I obtain other benefits after my release?* Retrieved August 1, 2006, from htttp://www.bazelon.org/issues/criminalization/publications/arrested/obtainother.htm.

Centers for Disease Control and Prevention. (1999a). *Self-study modules on tuberculosis: Glossary*. Atlanta: U.S. Department of Health and Human Services.

Centers for Disease Control and Prevention. (1999b). *Self-study modules on tuberculosis: Patient adherence to tuberculosis treatment*. Atlanta: U.S. Department of Health and Human Services.

Centers for Disease Control and Prevention. (2006). *Publications and products: Diabetes clip art*. Atlanta: U.S. Department of Health and Human Services. Retrieved August 1, 2006, from http://www.cdc.gov/diabetes/pubs/gallery.htm

Converse, J.M., & Presser, S. (1986). *Survey questions: Handcrafting the standardized questionnaire*. Beverly Hills, CA: Sage Publications.

Corrections Compendium. (2004). Re-entry/reintegration: Survey summary. *Corrections Compendium, 29*, 8–24.

Cotugna, N., Vickery, C.E., & Carpenter-Haefele, K.M. (2005). Evaluation of literacy level of patient education pages in health-related journals. *Journal of Community Health, 30*, 213–220.

Crick, C., & Potter, R.H. (2006). The perceptions of mental health services: Benefits and barriers. *Corrections Today, 68*, 34–37.

CSOSA. (2003, October 15). *Comprehensive reentry strategy for adults in the District of Columbia: Action plan*. Washington, DC: Author.

Cunniff, M.A. (2002). *Jail crowding: Understanding jail population dynamics*. Washington, DC: U.S. Department of Justice.

De Groot, A.S., & Maddow, R. (2005). Hepatitis B and hepatitis C among offenders within prisons. In *Managing special populations in jails and prisons*. Kingston, NJ: Civic Research Institute.

Ditton, P.M., & Wilson, D.J. (1999). *Truth in sentencing in state prisons, Bureau of Justice Statistics Special Report*. Washington, DC: U.S. Department of Justice.

Doak, C.C., Doak, L.G., & Root, J.H. (1996). *Teaching patients with low literacy skills*. Philadelphia: Lippincott Williams & Wilkins.

Eames, S., McKenna, K., Worrall, L., & Read, S. (2003). The suitability of written education materials for stroke survivors and their carers. *Topics in Stroke Rehabilitation, 10*, p. 70–84.

Electronic Privacy Information Center. (2006).*Statement of William Lutz*. Retrieved August 2, 2006, from http://www.epic.org/privacy/glba/vtlutz.pdf.

Fant, K. E., Clark, S. J., & Kemper, A. R. (2005). Completeness and complexity of information available to parents from newborn screening programs. *Pediatrics, 115*, 1268–1272.

Haigler, K. O., Harlow, C., O'Connor, P., & Campbell, A. (1994). *Literacy behind walls: Profiles of the prison population from the national adult literacy survey*. Washington, DC: National Center for Education Statistics.

Hammett, T. M., Harmon, M. P., & Rhodes, W. (2002). The burden of infectious disease among inmates of and releases from correctional facilities. In *The health status of soon-to-be-released inmates: A report to Congress* (Vol. 2). Chicago: National Commission on Correctional Health Care.

Harrison, P. M., & Beck, A. J. (2005). *Prisoner in 2004. Bureau of Justice Statistics Bulletin*. Washington, DC: U.S. Department of Justice.

Helfgott, J. (1997). Ex-offender needs versus community opportunity in Seattle, Washington. *Federal Probation*, *61*, 12–24.

Hughes, T., & Wilson, D. J. (2005). *Reentry trends in the United States*. Washinton, DC: Bureau of Justice Statistics.

Irick, K. M., & Fried, S. B. (2001). A content analysis of recent self-help books on caregiving and aging parents. *Clinical Gerontologist*, *23*, 131–144.

Isaacman, D.J., Purvis, K., Gyuro, J., Anderson, Y., & Smith, D. (1992). Standardized instructions: Do they improve communication of discharge information from the emergency department? *Pediatrics*, *89*, 1204–1208.

Makaryus, A.G., & Friedman, E.A. (2005). Patients' understanding of their treatment plans and diagnosis at discharge. *Mayo Clinic Proceedings*, *80*, 991–994.

Mellow, J. (2001). *The development and validation of questionnaire to measure ethnicity*. Ann Arbor, MI: UMI Dissertation Services.

Mellow, J., & Christian, J. (2005, November). *Making discharge planning information accessible*. Paper presented at the annual meeting of the American Society of Criminology, Toronto, Canada.

Mellow, J., & Dickinson, J.M. (2006). The role of prerelease handbooks for prisoner reentry. *Federal Probation*, *70*, 70–76.

Moult, B., Franck, L. S., & Brady, H. (2004). Ensuring quality information for patients: Development and preliminary validation of a new instrument to improve the quality of written health care information. *Health Expectations*, *7*, 165–175.

Murphy, D.A., Roberts, K. J., Hoffman, D., Molina, A., & Lu, M.C. (2003). Barriers and successful strategies to antiretroviral adherence among HIV-infected monolingual Spanish-speaking patients. *AIDS Care*, *15*, 217–230.

New York City Department of Health and Mental Hygiene. (2006). *Friends forever: A triumph over TB*. New York: Author.

Sabor, W.J., & McGready, J. (1999). *Time served in prison by federal offenders, 1986–97*. BJS Special Report. Washington, DC: U.S. Department of Justice.

Safeer, R.S., & Keenan, R. (2005). Health literacy: The gap between physicians and patients. *American Family Physician*, *72*, 463–468.

Smith, C. R., & Smith, C. A. (1994). Patient education information: Readability of prosthetic publications. *Journal of Prosthetics and Orthotics*, *6*, 113–118.

Sullivan, P. (2002). *Starting out, starting over, staying out: A guide for District of Columbia ex-offenders: Housing, food, employment and other resources*. Washington, DC: DC-CURE.

Tim Peters and Company, Inc. (2006). Retrieved August 1, 2006, from http://www.timpetersandcompany.com/niche_markets.htm.

Travis, J. (2005). *But they all come back: Facing the challenges of prisoner reentry*. Washington, DC: Urban Institute Press.

Tucson Planning Council for the Homeless. (2002). *Guidelines on getting out: A handbook to help you prepare for your release in Tucson, Arizona*. Tucson: Author.

Whitaker, W. (2005). *Making it happen & staying home*. New York: NYC Commission on Human Rights.

Young, S.A. (2000). Developing, translating and reviewing Spanish materials: Recommended standards for state and local agencies. State of North Carolina, Department of Health and Human Services. Retrieved June 1, 2006, from http://www.ncpublichealth.com/pdf_misc/DEVSPAN-web.pdf.

Chapter 16

Reducing Inmate Suicides Through the Mortality Review Process

Lindsay M. Hayes

Suicide continues to be a leading cause of death in jails across the country, where well over 400 inmates take their lives each year (Hayes, 1989). The rate of suicide in county jails is estimated to be approximately four times greater than that of the general population (Mumola, 2005). Overall, most jail suicide victims were young white males who were arrested for nonviolent offenses and intoxicated on arrest. Many were placed in isolation and dead within 24 hours of incarceration (Hayes, 1989; Davis & Muscat, 1993). The overwhelming majority of victims are found hanging by either bedding or clothing. Research specific to suicide in urban jail facilities provides certain disparate findings. Most victims of suicide in large urban facilities are arrested for violent offenses and are dead within 1 to 4 months of incarceration (DuRand, Burtka, Federman, Haycox, & Smith, 1995; Marcus & Alcabes, 1993). Due to the extended length of confinement prior to suicide, intoxication is not always the salient factor in urban jails as it is in other types of jail facilities. Suicide victim characteristics such as age, race, gender, method, and instrument remain generally consistent in both urban and nonurban jails.

While suicide is well recognized as a critical problem within jails, the issue of prison suicide has not received comparable attention, perhaps because the number of jail suicides far exceeds the number of prison suicides. Suicide ranks third, behind natural causes and AIDS, as the leading cause of death in prisons (Mumola, 2005). Although the rate of suicide in prison is considerably lower than in jail, it still remains slightly greater than the general population (Mumola, 2005). Most research on prison suicide has found that the vast majority of victims were convicted of personal crimes, housed in single cells (often either administrative or disciplinary segregation), and have histories of prior suicide attempts and/or mental illness (Daniel & Fleming, 2006; He, Felthous, Holzer, Nathan, & Veasey, 2001; Kovasznay, Miraglia, Beer, & Way, 2004; Salive, Smith, & Brewer, 1989; White, Schimmel, Frickey, 2002).

The precipitating factors of suicidal behavior in jail are well established (Bonner, 1992, 2000). It has been hypothesized that two primary causes for jail suicide exist: (1) jail environments are conducive to suicidal behavior and (2) the inmate is facing a crisis situation. From the inmate's perspective, certain features of the jail environment may enhance suicidal behavior: fear of the unknown, distrust of authoritarian environment, lack of apparent control over the future, isolation from family and significant others, shame of incarceration, and the dehumanizing aspects of incarceration. In addition, certain factors are prevalent among inmates facing a crisis situation that could predispose them to suicide: recent excessive drinking and/or use of drugs, recent loss of stabilizing resources, severe guilt or shame over the alleged offense, current mental illness, prior history of suicidal behavior, and an approaching court date. Some inmates simply are (or become) ill-equipped to handle the common stresses of confinement. As the inmate reaches an emotional breaking point, the result can be suicidal ideation, attempt, or completion. During initial confinement in a jail, this stress can be limited to fear of the unknown and isolation from family, but over time (including stays in prison) stress may become exacerbated and include loss of outside relationships, conflicts within the institution, victimization, further legal frustration, physical and emotional breakdown, and problems of coping within the institutional environment (Bonner, 1992). Precipitating factors in prison suicide may include new legal problems, marital or relationship difficulties, and inmate-related conflicts (White et al., 2002).

Despite a declining rate of suicide in county jails throughout the country, there remains the lingering problem of too many preventable suicides occurring alongside the feeble attempt to comprehensively review the deaths through a mortality review process. The thorough examination of an inmate death, encompassing both a mortality review and psychological autopsy, is cited in most national standards. For example, according to National Commission on Correctional Health Care (NCCHC) standards, "a clinical mortality review is an assessment of the clinical care provided and the circumstances leading up to a death" (NCCHC, 2003). In many cases, however, the clinical mortality review is simply a review of the inmate's chart by a physician. A national survey of suicide prevention practices in state prison systems found that only 14% of departments of correction addressed the issue of administrative or mortality reviews in their suicide prevention policy or other administrative directive (Hayes, 1995).

NCCHC standards also recommend a "psychological autopsy," in which a psychologist or other qualified mental health professional conducts "a written reconstruction of an individual's life with an emphasis on factors that may have contributed to the individual's death" (NCCHC, 2003). Although there are various references to psychological autopsies for inmate suicides in the literature (Aufderheide, 2000; Sanchez, 2006), the process is often misunderstood and misused within the correctional environment. Finally, the Joint Commission on Accreditation of Healthcare Organizations (JCAHO) offers guidance through policies and procedures for the "root cause analysis," but it too is rarely found within the correctional facilities (JCAHO, 2005). According to JACHO:

Root cause analysis is a process for identifying the basic and causal factors that underlie variation in performance, including the occurrence or possible occurrence of a sentinel event. A root cause analysis focuses primarily on systems and processes, not on individual performance. It progresses from special causes in clinical processes to common causes in organizational processes and identifies potential improvements in processes or systems that tend to decrease the likelihood of such events in the future, or determines, after analysis, that no such improvement opportunities exist. (p. 2)

In order to fully understand why an inmate committed suicide, as well as whether the correctional facility was in the best possible position to prevent the incident, every suicide and serious suicide attempt (i.e., requiring hospitalization) should be examined through a comprehensive mortality review process. The process is separate and apart from other formal investigations that may be required to determine the cause of death (e.g., medical examiner's autopsy, departmental investigation, state police inquiry, coroner's inquest).

The primary purposes of a mortality review are: What happened in the case under review and what can be learned to help prevent future incidents? Unlike NCCHC requirements which stress only a clinical perspective, the mortality review team must be multidisciplinary and include representatives of both line and management level staff from the corrections, medical, and mental health divisions. Exclusion of one or more disciplines will severely jeopardize the integrity of the review. The multidisciplinary review should include: (1) critical review of the circumstances surrounding the incident; (2) critical review of facility procedures relevant to the incident; (3) synopsis of all relevant training received by involved staff; (4) review of pertinent medical and mental health services/reports involving the victim; (5) review of possible precipitating factors (i.e., circumstances which may have caused the victim to engage in self-injury/suicide) resulting in the incident; and (6) recommendations, if any, for change in policy, training, physical plant, medical or mental health services, and operational procedures (Cox & Hayes, 2003).

Most jail and prison facilities do not embark on a comprehensive and multidisciplinary mortality review process. Why? There are concerns about liability. There is the inherent awkwardness of discussing the circumstances surrounding an inmate's death across various disciplines within an agency. But inevitably, mortality reviews are not conducted because key actors in the process (i.e., the administrators) are afraid of what they may find. Take, for example, the suicide of Edward Vaughn.

According to available records, 45-year-old Edward Vaughn (a pseudonym) was first confined in the Lincoln County Jail on February 8, 2002, for various charges, including alleged criminal attempt at kidnapping, unlawful restraint, and aggravated assault.[1] He was assessed as being both mentally ill and suicidal soon after his confinement. During the intake process, Mr. Vaughn became incoherent and it was determined that he had suffered from an overdose of his psychotropic medication. A razor blade was later found in his clothes. Mr. Vaughn was placed on suicide precautions with the requirement of observation at 15-minute intervals. Two days later on February 10, he was observed to be bleeding from self-inflicted lacerations on his right wrist. He was provided treatment by nursing staff and remained on suicide precautions with observation at 15-minute intervals. The following day, Mr. Vaughn was observed with a noose around his neck and tied to the cell bars. The ligature was removed and he remained on

---

[1] In order to ensure complete confidentiality, certain identifying information regarding the victim, facility, and staff have been changed. No modifications to the facts of the case have been made.

suicide precautions until February 25. On March 30, he was again placed on suicide precautions with the requirement of observation at 15-minute intervals for self-injurious behavior. He was also stripped naked and not provided with any protective clothing (e.g., safety smock, paper gown). Mr. Vaughn was released from the Lincoln County Jail on April 2, 2002.

Mr. Vaughn was again confined in the Lincoln County Jail on October 27, 2002 for charges that included alleged aggravated assault and reckless endangerment. At the scene of arrest, he threatened suicide by placing a knife to his throat. He also appeared depressed ("feeling so bad") and threatened suicide ("can't live anymore") during the intake process. Mr. Vaughn self-reported a history of mental illness, psychiatric hospitalization, and psychotropic medication. He also had observable scars from previous self-inflicted injuries. He was placed on suicide precautions in the reception unit with the requirement of observation at 15-minute intervals. Several hours later, Mr. Vaughn began to engage in self-injurious behavior by repeatedly throwing himself on the floor and wall of his cell causing head trauma, and was placed in a restraint chair and received psychotropic medication. He continued to be observed as "quite tearful and depressed." Mr. Vaughn was subsequently removed from the restraint chair but remained on suicide precautions with the requirement of observation at 15-minute intervals. The following day (October 28), he was found hanging from the cell bars by a blanket that he had torn into strips. Although the arriving nurse declared that "he's gone," Mr. Vaughn remained conscious and was placed in a restraint chair after continuing to threaten suicide. He was subsequently released from the restraint chair, stripped naked without any protective clothing, and remained on suicide precautions. On November 4, Mr. Vaughn was relocated to the mental health unit and remained on suicide precautions until November 14. Although Mr. Vaughn remained housed in the mental health unit, as a result of his suicidal behavior, as well as assaultive behavior to staff, he was punished by receiving a sanction of disciplinary segregation.

During the evening of December 4, 2002, Mr. Vaughn was requested to change cells in the mental health unit. He refused, became very agitated, and was forcefully removed from the unit and relocated in the segregation unit at approximately 8:50 PM. After placement in his segregation cell, Mr. Vaughn remained agitated and began to engage in various forms of self-injurious behavior, including banging his head against the floor, bunk, and wall; climbing on the top bunk and purposely falling off to the concrete floor; attempting to flush his head down the toilet; and trying to hang himself by tying his underwear around his neck and to the towel bar in the cell. He was again placed in a restraint chair.

A few hours later at approximately 12:30 AM on December 5, 2002, Mr. Vaughn was released from the restraint chair and placed on suicide precautions with the requirement of observation at 15-minute intervals. For unexplained reasons, he was reportedly observed at 30-minute intervals during the next several hours. Beginning at approximately 7:30 AM, the officers' logs reflected observation at exact 15-minute intervals. The last documented observation of Mr. Vaughn on suicide precautions occurred at 4:00 PM on December 5, 2002. At approximately 4:16 PM, a correctional officer found Mr. Vaughn hanging from the cell bars by a strip of bed sheet. (According to the videotape recording of the housing unit and the suicide attempt, the last time that an officer was in the housing unit was approximately 3:45 PM and that officer did not walk past Mr. Vaughn's cell. The inmate was seen on the videotape to be tying the sheet to the cell bars at 3:56 PM and the sheet was visible from that time forward until he was found hanging 20 minutes later at 4:16 PM.) The officer called for backup personnel and several correctional staff arrived shortly thereafter and assisted in cutting the sheet away from the bars. The cell door was opened and Mr. Vaughn was placed on the floor. Other correctional personnel arrived in the housing area and stood around the victim. Approximately 3 minutes later at 4:19 PM, medical staff arrived and initiated cardiopulmonary resuscitation (CPR). At approximately 4:29 PM, emergency medical services personnel arrived and continued life-saving measures. Mr. Vaughn was then transported to a local hospital and subsequently pronounced dead.

Why did Edward Vaughn commit suicide? What really happened? Was he ever considered a high risk for suicide? Was he ever considered for hospitalization? Was he on the correct level of observation? Why was he stripped naked without any protective clothing? How was he able to gain access to both a sheet and blanket? Was staff aware that Mr. Vaughn had attempted suicide in the facility several months earlier? Why did correctional officers wait until medical personnel arrived before assisting with CPR? Had any personnel received suicide prevention training prior to the incident? Was Mr. Vaughn's suicide preventable? Were there any similarities between his death and the other prior suicides in the facility? These and many other lingering questions were left unanswered in this case, as well as in several hundred other suicides that occur in correctional facilities each year, simply because many agencies choose not to address them. While verifying the cause of death and ruling out foul play remain the staples of routine investigations, correctional agencies remain reluctant to comprehensively review an inmate suicide, determine whether or not it was preventable, and take corrective action to reduce the opportunity for similar deaths in the future.

What a Mortality Review Would Have Found

A departmental investigation was conducted following Edward Vaughn's suicide and concluded that he was at low to moderate risk for suicide and, based on the facility's adequate policies and procedures, the death was not preventable. Although an NCCHC-accredited facility, a mortality review was not conducted in Mr. Vaughn's case. If a comprehensive mortality review had been conducted, the following issues would have been raised.

First, there was overwhelming evidence to show that Edward Vaughn was at a continuing high risk for suicide in the Lincoln County Jail, and that continuing high risk was known to various medical, mental health, and correctional personnel. This much was known: (1) he had a history of mental illness, psychiatric hospitalization, and psychotropic medication; (2) he was observed to be depressed, agitated, incoherent, "quite tearful" and crying, and displaying numerous self-inflicted injuries and scars; (3) he self-reported both depression ("feeling so bad") and suicidal ideation ("can't live anymore"), as well as requested to remain in the restraint chair when feeling the impulse to engage in suicidal behavior; and (4) he engaged in self-injurious behavior on at least seven separate occasions (immediately prior to or) during his confinement:

- on intake on February 8 when it was suspected that he overdosed on psychotropic medication,
- on February 10 when he was observed to be bleeding from lacerations on his right wrist,
- on February 11 when he was observed with a noose around his neck and tied to the cell bars,
- on March 30 when he was observed engaging in self-injurious behavior,
- on October 27 when he repeatedly threw himself on the floor and wall of his cell causing head trauma,
- on October 28 when he was found hanging from the cell bars by a blanket that he had torn into strips, and
- on December 4 when he observed banging his head against the floor, bunk, and wall; climbing on the top bunk and purposely falling off to the concrete floor; attempting to flush his head down the toilet; and trying to hang himself by tying his underwear around his neck and to the towel bar in the cell.

Despite Mr. Vaughn's continuing high risk for suicide during his confinement in the Lincoln County Jail, the response from staff was the following: placement on 15-minute suicide precautions in various unsafe cells, periodic assessment by contracted medical and mental health staff, psychotropic medication, and periodic placement for a few hours in a restraint chair. These responses were inadequate because Mr. Vaughn was permitted to continue to engage in self-injury and ultimately committed suicide in the facility.

The Lincoln County Jail also had inadequate policies and practices in the area of suicide prevention (particularly levels of observation and safe housing) that were the proximate causes of Mr. Vaughn's suicide. A written suicide prevention policy is a prerequisite for running a correctional facility. The importance of written policy in suicide prevention is clearly stated in the American Correctional Association standards (2004): "A suicide-prevention program is approved by the health authority and reviewed by the facility or program administrator. It includes specific procedures for handling intake, screening, identifying, and supervising of a suicide-prone inmate and is signed and reviewed annually" (p. 64). In addition, the National Commission on Correctional Health Care standards (2003) requires each jail to have a written suicide prevention plan that includes the following components: training, identification, referral, evaluation, housing, monitoring, communication, intervention, notification, reporting, review, and critical incident debriefing.

The Lincoln County Jail's suicide prevention policy stated that the facility will "provide special, housing, increased levels of observation, and medical restraint to those inmates who display self-destructive behavior." Although the policy referenced both ACA and NCCHC standards, it was not consistent with those standards. For example, although national correctional standards required an option for *constant observation* for actively suicidal inmates, the Lincoln County Jail's suicide prevention policy provided two levels of observation for suicidal inmates: *suicide precaution* and *close observation*. A review of the policy indicated little discernible difference between the two supervision levels. In practice, inmates on *suicide precaution* status were stripped naked of their clothing, all items (with the exception of a blanket) were removed from the cell, and they were observed "at irregular 15-minute intervals (no more than 15 minutes between checks). The checks are staggered so that there is no predictable pattern for the inmate to use in planning suicide." Of course, allowing an inmate to be stripped naked without any protective clothing (e.g., safety smock, paper gown) is contrary to all national standards, as well as human decency. Inmates on *close observation* status were allowed to retain their clothing and other possessions and were observed at staggered 15-minute intervals. Thus, the only difference between the two levels was the issue of clothing and possessions. Contrary to Lincoln County Jail policy, Mr. Vaughn was observed for several hours on December 5 at 30-minute intervals, and was rarely observed at staggered or "irregular" 15-minute intervals while on either close observation or suicide precaution status. Instead, the officers' logs were recorded at exact 15-minute intervals.

Despite his continuing high risk for suicide, Mr. Vaughn was never placed on constant observation. Although observation at 15-minute intervals is routinely reserved for inmates assessed as being either at low or moderate risk for suicide, it should never be utilized for a highly suicidal individual. In fact, Lincoln County Jail staff was emphatically warned of Mr. Vaughn's high-risk suicidal behavior when, on his discharge from the emergency room of a local hospital on October 27, 2002, the physician stated: "Be absolutely watchful of his behavior. Consider this patient high-risk for repeated self-injury. Must have someone watching him at all times." A review of the records in this case indicated that facility staff never placed Mr. Vaughn on constant observation nor considered psychiatric hospitalization for his continuing high-risk suicidal behavior.

Further, interviews with jail staff revealed that even the alleged observation of Mr. Vaughn at 15-minute intervals was not always performed by an officer physically walking past his cell, but rather by an officer stationed inside the control booth which was estimated to be between 30 and 40 feet from Mr. Vaughn's cell and partially obstructed by a stairway. A consulting psychiatrist at the Lincoln County Jail later stated it would be improper for a control booth officer to be responsible for the observation of suicidal inmates, and that he was unaware that such a practice was occurring at the Lincoln County Jail. In fact, the last time that an officer was in Mr. Vaughn's housing unit on December 5 was at approximately 3:45 pm, and that officer did not walk past Mr. Vaughn's cell. The inmate was seen on a videotape to be tying the sheet to the cell bars at 3:56 pm and the sheet was visible from that time forward until he was found hanging 20 minutes later at 4:16 pm. It was obvious that none of the officers assigned to the housing unit (including the control officer) adequately observed Mr. Vaughn prior to his death, the proximate cause of which was his ability to successfully commit suicide. In essence, had jail staff followed standard correctional practices and national correctional standards, Mr. Vaughn would have been observed on constant observation following his most recent high-risk self-injurious behavior on December 4 and not had the ability to successfully commit suicide the following day.

With regard to housing of suicidal inmates, consistent with national correctional standards and standard practices in correctional facilities throughout the country, housing assignments should be based on the ability to maximize staff interaction with the inmate, avoiding assignments that heighten the depersonalizing aspects of incarceration. Ideally, suicidal inmates should be housed in the general population, mental health unit, or medical infirmary, located close to staff. All cells designated to house suicidal inmates should be suicide-resistant, free of all obvious protrusions, and provide full visibility. These cells should contain tamperproof light fixtures and ceiling air vents that are protrusion-free. No cell housing a suicidal inmate should have open-faced bars. Rather, each cell door should contain a heavy gauge Lexan (or equivalent grade) glass panel that is large enough to allow staff a full and unobstructed view of the cell interior. Cells housing suicidal inmates should not contain any electrical switches or outlets, bunks with holes and ladders, towel racks on desks and sinks, radiator vents, corded telephones of any length, clothing hooks (of any kind), or any other object that provides an easy anchoring device for hanging (Hayes, 2003). As reiterated in the NCCHC standards, "All cells or rooms housing suicidal inmates are as suicide-resistant as possible (e.g., without protrusions of any kind that would enable the inmate to hang himself/herself)" (p. 102).

Although Lincoln County Jail's suicide prevention policy required "special housing" for suicidal inmates, the policy did not contain any description as to the specific type of housing provided to such inmates. As such, suicidal inmates could be placed in a variety of housing units, each of which contained open-faced bars, shelves with clothing hooks, metal bunks with holes, and towel racks attached to desks. In Mr. Vaughn's case, he was placed on suicide precautions in the reception, mental health, and segregation units, and he was able to attempt suicide in each of these units. For example, he was found hanging from the cell bars in the reception unit on October 28, tried to hang himself from the towel bar attached to the desk in his cell in the segregation unit on December 4, and successfully committed suicide by hanging himself from the cell bars on December 5. For inexplicable reasons, Mr. Vaughn was also able to attempt (and commit) suicide with ligatures that were prohibited from being in his cell, including a blanket and sheet. The communication between corrections, medical, and mental health personnel at the facility was so poor that an officer gave Mr. Vaughn a blanket and sheet because he did not realize the inmate was on suicide precautions.

Given the fact the inmates have historically attempted and/or committed suicide in the Lincoln County Jail utilizing a variety of dangerous anchoring devices (including a successful suicide by hanging of an inmate utilizing a shelf with clothing hooks in July 1995 and a hanging attempt of an inmate utilizing the open-faced bars in February 2000), it is particularly troubling that Mr. Vaughn was placed in a cell on suicide precautions that contained protrusions that were obvious and previously known to be dangerous by jail officials. In fact, the Lincoln County Jail had a policy that required a suicidal inmate to be placed in a dangerous cell (i.e., "Suicide Precaution: This involves the inmate in an open-barred cell").

Although heavy gauge Lexan (or equivalent grade) glass paneling is commonly known and utilized in jail and prison facilities throughout the country to cover bars of cells housing suicidal inmates, when Lincoln County Jail officials were subsequently asked why Lexan paneling was not installed on the barred doors of cells in the facility, they offered inadequate responses, ranging from not having heard of Lexan paneling to the belief that inmates would smear feces on the paneling thus obstructing visibility.

Jail officials had several options to safely house suicidal inmates, including the placement of Lexan (or equivalent grade) glass paneling on selective cells, housing suicidal inmates in cells that did not have open-barred doors, and ensuring that actively suicidal inmates were provided with constant observation of a correctional officer who was stationed directly outside the cell. Instead, jail officials chose none of these or other options and simply continued to allow these obviously dangerous cells to be utilized for housing suicidal inmates.

Finally, although the Lincoln County Jail's 4-hour "In-Custody Suicide Prevention" training lesson plan appeared comprehensive, a review of personnel files revealed that the workshop was offered at 1-hour (not 4-hour) durations and, contrary to both ACA and NCCHC standards, most personnel who interacted with Mr. Vaughn either never received suicide prevention training or received it infrequently from 1995 through 2002.

Conclusion

Although national standards address the issue of mortality reviews in varying degrees, practical guidelines for conducting meaningful reviews are absent. Based on the critical components of a comprehensive suicide prevention program (Hayes, 2005), detailed below is a recommended format and areas of inquiry for conducting a morbidity–mortality review.

1. Training
   - Had all correctional, medical, and mental health staff involved in the incident received both basic and annual training in the area of suicide prevention prior to the suicide?
   - Had all staff who responded to the incident received training (and were currently certified) in standard first aid and cardiopulmonary resuscitation (CPR) prior to the suicide?

2. Identification/Referral/Assessment
   - Upon this inmate's initial entry into the facility, were the arresting/ transporting officer(s) asked whether they believed the inmate was at risk for suicide? If so, what was the response?
   - Had the inmate been screened for potentially suicidal behavior on entry into the facility?
   - Did the screening form include inquiry regarding: past suicidal ideation and/or attempts; current ideation, threat, plan; prior mental health treatment/ hospitalization; recent significant loss (job, relationship, death of family member/close friend, etc.); and history of suicidal behavior by family member/close friend?
   - If the screening process indicated a potential risk for suicide, was the inmate properly referred to mental health and/or medical personnel?
   - Had the inmate received a postadmission mental health screening within 14 days of his/her confinement?
   - Had the inmate previously been confined in the facility/system? If so, had the inmate been on suicide precautions during a prior confinement in the facility/system? Was such information available to staff responsible for the current intake screening and mental health assessments?

3. Communication
   - Was there information regarding the inmate's prior and/or current suicide risk from outside agencies that was not communicated to the correctional facility?
   - Was there information regarding the inmate's prior and/or current suicide risk from correctional, mental health, and/or medical personnel that was not communicated throughout the facility to appropriate personnel?
   - Did the inmate engage in any type of behavior that might have been indicative of a potential risk of suicide? If so, was this observed behavior communicated throughout the facility to appropriate personnel?

4. Housing
   - Where was the inmate housed and why was he/she assigned to this housing unit?
   - If placed in a "special management" (e.g., disciplinary and/or administrative segregation) housing unit at the time of death, had the inmate received a written assessment for suicide risk by mental health and/or medical staff on admission to the special unit?
   - Was there anything regarding the physical design of the inmate's cell and/or housing unit that contributed to the suicide (e.g., poor visibility, protrusions in cell conducive to hanging attempts)?

5. Levels of Supervision
   - What level and frequency of supervision was the inmate under immediately prior to the incident?
   - Given the inmate's observed behavior prior to the incident, was the level of supervision adequate?
   - When was the inmate last physically observed by correctional staff prior to the incident?
   - Was there any reason to question the accuracy of the last reported observation by correctional staff?
   - If the inmate was not physically observed within the required time interval prior to the incident, what reason(s) was determined to cause the delay in supervision?
   - Was the inmate on a mental health and/or medical caseload? If so, what was the frequency of contact between the inmate and mental health and/or medical personnel?
   - When was the inmate last seen by mental health and/or medical personnel?
   - Was there any reason to question the accuracy of the last reported observation by mental health and/or medical personnel?
   - If the inmate was not on a mental health and/or medical caseload, should he/she have been?
   - If the inmate was not on a suicide watch at the time of the incident, should he/she have been?

6. Intervention
   - Did the staff member(s) who discovered the inmate follow proper intervention procedures, i.e., surveyed the scene to ensure the emergency was genuine, called for backup support, ensured that medical personnel were immediately notified, and initiated standard first aid and/or CPR?

- Did the inmate's housing unit contain proper emergency equipment for correctional staff to effectively respond to a suicide attempt, i.e., first aid kit, gloves, pocket mask, mouth shield, or Ambu bag, and rescue tool (to quickly cut through fibrous material)?
- Were there any delays in either correctional or medical personnel immediately responding to the incident? Were medical personnel properly notified as to the nature of the emergency and did they respond with appropriate equipment? Was all the medical equipment working properly?

7. Reporting
- Were all appropriate officials and personnel notified of the incident in a timely manner?
- Were other notifications, including the inmate's family and appropriate outside authorities, made in a timely manner?
- Did all staff who came into contact with the inmate prior to the incident submit a report and/or statement as to their full knowledge of the inmate and incident? Was there any reason to question the accuracy and/or completeness of any report and/or statement?

8. Follow-Up/Morbidity–Mortality Review
- Were all affected staff and inmates offered critical incident stress debriefing following the incident?
- Were there any other investigations conducted (or that should be authorized) into the incident that may be helpful to the morbidity–mortality review?
- As a result of this review, were there any possible precipitating factors (i.e., circumstances which may have caused the victim to commit suicide) offered and discussed?
- Were there any findings and/or recommendations from previous reviews of inmate suicides that are relevant to this morbidity–mortality review?
- As a result of this review, what recommendations (if any) are necessary for revisions in policy, training, physical plant, medical or mental health services, and operational procedures to reduce the likelihood of future incidents?

References

American Correctional Association. (2004). *Performance-based standards for adult local detention facilities* (4th ed.). MD: Author.

Aufderheide, D. (2000). Conducting the psychological autopsy in correctional settings. *Journal of Correctional Health Care, 7,* 5–36.

Bonner, R. (1992). Isolation, seclusion, and psychological vulnerability as risk factors for suicide behind bars. In R. Maris et al. (Eds.), *Assessment and prediction of suicide* (pp. 398–419). New York: Guilford Press.

Bonner, R. (2000). Correctional suicide prevention in the year 2000 and beyond. *Suicide and Life Threatening Behavior, 30,* 370–376.

Cox, J., & Hayes, L. (2003). A framework for preventing suicides in adult correctional facilities. In B. Schwartz (Ed.), *Correctional psychology: Practice, programming, and administration* (pp.4-1–4-20). Kingston, NJ: Civic Research Institute.

Daniel, A., & Fleming, J. (2006). Suicides in a state correctional system: 1992–2002: A review. *Journal of Correctional Health Care, 12,* 1–12.

Davis, M., & Muscat, J. (1993). An epidemiologic study of alcohol and suicide risk in Ohio jails and lockups, 1975–1984. *Journal of Criminal Justice*, *21*, 277–283.

DuRand, C., Burtka, G., Federman, E., Haycox, J., & Smith, J. (1995). A quarter century of suicide in a major urban jail: Implications for community psychiatry. *American Journal of Psychiatry*, *152*, 1077–1080.

Hayes, L. (1989). National study of jail suicides: Seven years later. *Psychiatric Quarterly*, *60*, 7–29.

Hayes, L. (1995). National and state standards for prison suicide prevention: A report card. *Journal of Correctional Health Care*, *3*(1), 5–38.

Hayes, L. (2003). Suicide prevention and protrusion-free design of correctional facilities. *Jail Suicide/Mental Health Update*, *12*(3), 1–5.

Hayes, L. (2005). Suicide prevention in correctional facilities. In C. Scott & J. Gerbasi (Eds.), *Handbook of correctional mental health* (pp. 69–88). Washington, DC: American Psychiatric Publishing.

He, X., Felthous, A., Holzer, C., Nathan, P., & Veasey, S. (2001). Factors in prison suicide: One year study in Texas. *Journal of Forensic Sciences*, *46*, 896–901.

Joint Commission on Accreditation of Healthcare Organizations. (2005). *Sentinel event policy and procedures*. Oakbrook Terrace, IL: Author.

Kovasznay, B., Miraglia, R., Beer, R., & Way, B. (2004). Reducing suicides in New York State correctional facilities. *Psychiatric Quarterly*, *75*, 61–70.

Marcus, P., & Alcabes, P. (1993). Characteristics of suicides by inmates in an urban jail. *Hospital and Community Psychiatry*, *44*, 256–261.

Mumola, C. (2005). *Suicide and homicide in state prisons and local jails*. Washington, DC: Bureau of Justice Statistics.

National Commission on Correctional Health Care. (2003). *Standards for health services in jails*. Chicago: Author.

Salive, M., Smith, G., & Brewer, T. (1989). Suicide mortality in the Maryland state prison system, 1979 through 1987. *Journal of the American Medical Association*, *262*, 365–369.

Sanchez, H. (2006). Inmate suicide and the psychological autopsy process. *Jail Suicide/Mental Health Update*, *8*(2), 5–11.

White, T., Schimmel, D., & Frickey, R. (2002). A comprehensive analysis of suicide in federal prisons: A fifteen-year review. *Journal of Correctional Health Care*, *9*, 321–343.

Chapter 17

Blinders to Comprehensive Psychiatric Diagnosis in the Correctional System

Richard L. Grant

Introduction

There are challenges in providing adequate mental health services to prisoners, but the task is not insurmountable. This chapter focuses on the issues related to full and accurate psychiatric diagnoses as an underpinning to comprehensive treatment. Another focus is on the attitudes and biases about mental disorders held by correctional staff, health professionals, and the inmates themselves. These are inextricably bound to a contemporary understanding of the complexities of multiple coexisting psychiatric diagnoses in a given individual These attitudes can lessen the acceptance of mental disorders as disorders of brain function. The reality of budgetary constraints is an additional difficulty that needs to be redressed, but not here. This chapter aims at the importance of accurate delineation of the mental disorders that bring suffering to those patients and the correctional staff in the form of inner mental anguish and outwardly disordered and disruptive behavior. I posit that a fuller awareness, understanding, and acceptance of this issue could provide an impetus for change in the allocation of resources toward accurate mental health diagnosis leading to more effective treatment.

Going beyond the correctional system to any psychiatric care setting, accurate psychiatric diagnosis in each mental health care recipient is the gateway to comprehensive and effective treatment. Throughout this chapter, the term *psychiatry*, unless otherwise specified, is used in its broadest context to include all mental health care personnel involved in the process of screening, assessment, and treatment of individuals with mental disorders. Secondarily involved are all health care providers in any system where mental disorders are prevalent. All may be blinded to varying degrees from a truly comprehensive view of the impact of mental disorders on the behavior and emotional distress of the persons for whom they have clinical responsibility. These blinders may prevent appropriate referral for a psychiatrist's scrutiny.

The concept of "blinders" refers to the metaphorical difficulty one has, when looking directly at the headlight of a train at night, in seeing what the rest of the train is like. Is it just what you see or is there something more behind it? What explosive dangers lurk in what it carries? How safe and clear-headed is the engineer? Are there defective components that could lead to derailment? Looking at the train's headlight does not give us complete knowledge of what lies behind the train. Likewise, looking at the surface symptoms and behaviors of people with mental disorders yields an incomplete picture. Human Rights Watch (2003) indicates that

- inadequate knowledge,
- negatively biased attitudes,
- insufficiently trained personnel, and
- inadequate financial resources

constitute the source of blinders for psychiatry behind bars. Each of these blinders contributes to an erosion of thorough, comprehensive, and effective management of the mental disorders found in the inmate populations of our jails and prisons. The first three are the subjects of this chapter.

Knowledge: Psychiatric Diagnostic Comorbidity and Modern Neuropsychiatry

Comorbidity

A full understanding of the mental disorders present in a given patient is critical for creating an effective plan for intervention. The first step in delineating the blinders present in the mental health and medical care delivery at correctional institutions is the concept of psychiatric diagnoses. An unknown but very high number of today's physicians were trained under the prevailing "law of parsimony" principle: *Don't make two diagnoses when one diagnosis is adequately explanatory for the symptom presentation.* While this is a useful general rule, modern neuropsychiatric research and practice suggests that it oversimplifies the complexities of brain function and dysfunction. Central to understanding the impact of today's conceptualization of mental disorders is the term *comorbidity*.

Variously, comorbidity can mean:

1. mental disorders that occur related to body disorders such as stroke and depression, hyperthyroidism and anxiety, or traumatic brain injury and personality change,
2. mental disorders that occur in the presence of substance abuse and dependence that are also DSM-IV-TR defined mental disorders (American Psychiatric Association & Task Force on DSM-IV, 2000), and
3. mental disorders co-occurring with each other exclusive of substance disorders.

All three types of comorbidity are significant in correctional populations, although in the literature, comorbidity is often not fully defined. Too often, the third type of comorbidity is little recognized by psychiatrists and psychologists. The separation of Axis I and Axis II diagnoses fosters a dismissal of personality disorders as not amenable to change, and arguably having a strongly if not exclusively volitional component. This contention is not valid but is often strongly held and staunchly defended.

This DSM multiaxial system permits the presence of multiple coexisting psychiatric diagnoses if criteria are met for them. Nevertheless, common psychiatric practice often functions simplistically, as if the law of parsimony has not been spurned by modern research. There is ample literature to support the presence of psychiatric comorbidity (Abram, Teplin, McClelland, & Dulcan, 2003; Abram, Teplin, & McClelland, 2003; Andersen, 2004; Chitsabesan et al., 2006; Compton, Conway, Stinson, Colliver, & Grant, 2005; Comtois, Cowley, Dunner, & Roy-Byrne, 1999; Friedman et al., 2005; Goodwin & Hamilton, 2003; Hawley & Maden, 2003; Herrman, McGorry, Mills, & Singh, 1991; Howerton et al., 2007; Kessler, Chiu, Demler, Merikangas, & Walters, 2005; Kessler, Berglund, et al., 2005; Max et al., 2000; McGough et al., 2005; Oldham et al., 1995; Rosen, Miller, D'Andrea, McGlashan, & Woods, 2006; Slaughter, Fann, & Ehde, 2003; Soderstrom, Sjodin, Carlstedt, & Forsman, 2004; Soderstrom, Nilsson, Sjodin, Carlstedt, & Forsman, 2005; Teplin, Abram, & McClelland, 1996; Torres et al., 2006)

Given the reported significant degree of comorbidity in the general population and in the correctional system, and the higher rate of mental disorders in the latter over the former, it is incumbent for jail and prison psychiatry to have an increased index of suspicion for coexisting mental disorders from both Axis I and Axis II. In pursuit of such comprehensive diagnostic understanding, a number of questions can be posed:

- Does a person with a substance abuse history have other underlying mental disorders?
- Does having a criminal history, unless flagrantly psychotic, preclude major underlying mental disorders needing treatment?
- Does a high psychopathy score on the PCL-R (Hare, 2006) mean that there are no treatable mental disorders?
- Is a person who is "bad" automatically excluded from also being "mad" (Tucker, 1999)?
- Does the judgment that a person is "manipulative" mean that there is no mental disorder present?
- Does the judgment about the presence of manipulativeness say more about the person making the judgment than about the person being described?
- How does the presence of an antisocial or borderline personality disorder, legitimate DSM Axis II disorders, rule out the existence of Axis I disorders? Where is the justification for saying that these two personality disorders may not be *really* mental disorders as is sometimes held?
- Is brain trauma more frequent in people with prior existing mental disorders?

The predicate conditions in these questions often constitute one or another type of blinder for those responsible for optimal biopsychosocial treatment of persons inflicted with mental disorders.

Accuracy in Psychiatric Diagnosis

Whether in prison, in a psychiatric hospital, or in the community, the person with one or several mental disorders deserves the same form of assessment and treatment, ethically and legally. What then are the essential elements for arriving at comprehensive psychiatric diagnoses? Unfortunately, the term *comprehensive* is widely used—and greatly misunderstood. As a working definition, I propose in principle that the process of arriving at a comprehensive psychiatric diagnosis would mean that each and every major diagnostic category on Axis I and Axis II should either be ruled in or ruled out within a clear and convincing degree of medical/psychiatric certainty, understanding that, with increasing data, diagnoses may change. For example, diagnoses are changed from Major Depression to Bipolar Disorder, or from Impulse Control Disorder to Attention Deficit Hyperactivity Disorder (ADHD), or from Schizophrenia to Bipolar Disorder as new information, not previously known or not yet seen, accumulates over time. This new information is often the occasion to make additional comorbid diagnoses as well.

The key to greatest accuracy in diagnosis lies in the history. We are therefore left with, just as with psychological tests, diagnoses as probability statements inexorably tied to the accuracy and completeness of the history or subject responses.

The history of a given individual is complex and multifaceted. In its most thorough application, a detailed history is taken from (1) the individual, (2) whenever possible from one or several significant others, (3) past outpatient and inpatient mental health treatment episodes, (4) general medical treatment records, and (5) if relevant, school records. My usual clinical practice is to tell patients that I expect we will spend two to four hours just collecting the initial verbal history and we will send for prior academic, medical, and psychiatric records. Biopsychosocial treatment may begin in the first meeting but a full understanding of the diagnoses present often comes only later. (It took 2 years working with a 50-year-old woman with ADHD and narcolepsy to establish the presence of a low-level Bipolar II disorder which responded favorably to mood stabilizers.) Routine laboratory work is always done, and, if indicated, specialized laboratory studies as well as psychological and neuropsychological testing should be done. Brain imaging studies such as brain SPECT scanning (Amen, Stubblefield, Carmicheal, & Thisted, 1996) have proved useful in the search for evidence of brain injury secondary to closed head injuries or exposure to toxins. The Society of Nuclear Medicine approved SPECT for the evaluation of suspected brain trauma or toxic injury in 1999 (Society of Nuclear Medicine, 2002).

While not every case needs all of this information, complex cases with hints of or flagrant presentations of not one but two or more coexisting psychiatric disorders need extensive data collection and high-level clinical judgment. My personal clinical observations in the last two decades suggest that a presentation of substance abuse/dependence or ADHD in adults carries a high comorbidity for anxiety spectrum disorders (such as generalized anxiety, obsessive compulsive disorder, panic disorder, and/or posttraumatic stress disorder), bipolar disorder, major depression, and a history of traumatic brain injury (TBI). Conversely, a history of TBI means one must rule out any and all of these Axis I disorders. These details of history cannot be done by questionnaires or screening instruments in the hands of persons unschooled in the complexities of psychiatric diagnosis. A detailed history by experts well versed at making DSM diagnoses is required. Master's-level people and even some doctorate-level psychiatrists and psychologists are not trained for this task leaving the job for psychiatrists, psychologists, or other mental health professionals explicitly trained and closely supervised.

Prevalence of Mental Illness

There is a case to be made that the prison system is the new *de facto* last mental hospital (Gilligan, 2001; Lamb & Weinberger, 2005). The prevalence of mental disorders, Axis I and II, in jail and prison inmates here and in other countries is estimated to be in the range of 40% to 90% (Andersen, 2004; Brooke, Taylor, Gunn, & Maden, 1996; Butler, Allnutt, Cain, Owens, & Muller, 2005; Diamond, Wang, Holzer, Thomas, & des Anges Cruser, 2001; Duggan, Bradshaw, Mitchell, Coffey, & Rogers, 2005; Forrest, 2005; Fryers, Brugha, Grounds, & Melzer, 1998; He, Felthous, Holzer, Nathan, & Veasey, 2001; Herrman et al., 1991; Langeveld & Melhus, 2004; Smith, Sawyer, & Way, 2002; Tucker, 1999). With such high mental disorder prevalence, compounded by TBI or substance abuse, and a high prevalence of coexisting mental disorders, it is no wonder that the correctional system is burdened.

Yet, prisoners and detainees have a constitutional right to receive comprehensive treatment. In systems with simple screening at intake (level I), midlevel screening (level II) by referral from level I, and very limited time spent by psychiatrists by referral from level II, far less than what is needed is known about each inmate to fully understand the multiple dimensions of treatable disorders present and to provide the mandated treatment. One blinder therefore is inadequate knowledge about each inmate that would lead to a full diagnostic picture. To this obfuscation of full understanding, simply based on inadequate knowledge about a person's history and diagnoses, is the further blinder of lack of contemporary neuropsychiatric information about what we have come to know of brain functioning and its role in mental disorders.

There is a much higher proportion of antisocial personality disorder (ASPD), psychopathy, and borderline personality disorder (BPD) in our prison inmate population than in the general population (Blair, 2005). Yet having any one of these diagnoses does not necessarily predict criminal behavior unless criminal behavior is one of the necessary categories for the diagnosis. With the latter we have a tautology. Both of these categorizations carry a pejorative onus and almost universally reflect an accusatory epithet rather than a truly dispassionate diagnostic opinion. Conventional clinical wisdom, certainly *conventional* and *clinical* but not necessarily *wisdom*, has it that these personality disorders are not amenable to change. What then shall we make of Martens's (2004) use of the concept of "remitted psychopaths" but to hold out hope for change in this condition that is not even a DSM disorder?

It is clear that psychopathy, in all its richness and diversity of manifestations, is truly a spectrum disorder (Hare, 2006; Lykken, 2006; Patrick, 2006) with impairments in both behavior and handling emotions. *Psychopathy* is a term for a type of personality disturbance assessed by the Psychopathy Checklist-Revised (PCL-R) (Hare, 2006). This instrument has 20 behavioral items falling in two factors. Factor 1 subsumes glib/superficial charm, grandiose sense of self-worth, pathological lying, conning/manipulative, lack of remorse or guilt, shallow affect, callous/lack of empathy, and failure to accept responsibility for own actions. Factor 2 covers need for stimulation/proneness to boredom, parasitic lifestyle, poor behavioral controls, early behavioral problems, lack of realistic, long-term goals, impulsivity, irresponsibility, juvenile delinquency, and revocation of conditional release (Lykken, 2006). It is not synonymous with ASPD or conduct disorder. Blair (2005) and

Hare (2006) estimate that about one-quarter of ASPD inmates meet criteria for psychopathy. Psychopathy is not viewed as a mental disorder in DSM, probably because it cuts across mental disorders and is arrived at solely from a checklist score equal to or greater than 30 (where possible scores range from 0 to 40). It is important, however, in that it highly predicts aggression, violence, and recidivism—important behaviors in a jail or prison population. The brains of persons with psychopathy perform differently from nonpsychopathic individuals on a rich array of psychological and behavioral tests. This denotes that the brains of these two groups are different. Support for this conclusion can be found, for example, in Brower and Price's (2001) meta-analytic study contention that "[c]linically significant focal frontal lobe dysfunction is associated with aggressive dyscontrol" as determined by (1) linkages of clinical focal frontal lobe disorders to violence, (2) neuropsychologically revealed deficits, (3) clinical neurological findings, and (4) neuroimaging studies using PET, MRI, and SPECT protocols (Amen et al., 1996; Bufkin & Luttrell, 2005; Hawley & Maden, 2003; Slaughter et al., 2003). The common denominator in this sample of the literature is that aggression and violence are usually related to frontal lobe dysfunction (Brower & Price, 2001).

Crocker et al. (2005), in a longitudinal analysis of ASPD, psychopathy, and violence in persons with comorbid severe mental disorders, found that the Self-Report Psychopathy Scale-II "had limited associations with criminality and violence, whereas ASPD, thought disorder, negative affect, and earlier age at psychiatric hospitalization were predictive of aggressive behavior" for the 203 subjects over 3 years. This is further confirmation of the prevalence of comorbidity and speaks to a reversal of the concept that psychopathy alone is more predictive of aggressive violence.

But addressing a knowledge deficit alone is not enough. Exposure to new information or conceptualizations must occur in the presence of accepting attitudes and open minds ready to use that information. The example of professionals who don't "believe" in ADHD is not the most egregious example of how attitudes affect the incorporation and use of information. Holding that people who commit criminal acts are simply immoral or evil by choice is a much more pervasive and destructive belief that often precludes any attempt to understand the underlying disorders of brain function that could be treated. Another example that forecloses on full treatment is thinking that if a person has schizophrenia, she or he cannot have obsessive compulsive disorder or generalized anxiety disorder (or other Axis I disorders). Thus, I turn to what we know about attitudes and biases about mental disorders in prisoners.

Attitudinal Bias

Overall, the range of attitudes about disordered behavior, criminality, and mental disorders held by the general public vary across a continuum anchored at one end by conservative and moralistic views and at the other end by more liberal views. In a study of probation officers and law and criminology students, Carroll, Perkowitz, Lurigio, and Weaver (1987) described the conservative view as a "punitive stance toward crime, belief in individual causality for crime, high scores on authoritarianism, dogmatism, and internal locus of control." The liberal view included "rehabilitation, belief in economic and other external determinants of crime, higher moral stage, and belief in the powers and responsibilities of government to correct social problems." The specific topic of mental illnesses and their neurobiological substrates was not examined. Inferentially, however, it would not be too much of a speculation to surmise that support for the thesis that disordered behavior comes from disordered brains would probably cluster toward the liberal end of this continuum. Scientific information does not fall uniformly and fertilely across this conservative-to-liberal continuum. Hence, attitudes are an important dimension along with knowledge in attempting to forge a greater understanding of mental disorders.

In Israel, Rubinstein (2006) studied right-wing authoritarianism in border police officers, career soldiers, airport security guards, and controls. In general, scores fell significantly from the border police officers to the soldiers and guards (who had similar scores), to the controls. To the extent one can extrapolate from these subjects to the correctional system, I predict that high authoritarianism should be the mode in that setting. This presents further blinders for assimilating modern knowledge about mental disorders.

From an evolutionary perspective, humans have a well-tuned propensity to suspect, or look closely for cheaters. Arguably, those in the criminal justice system may be overselected for this bias when dealing with persons incarcerated for already having tried to "cheat" or act immorally. Our evolutionary environment knew nothing of brain disorders lying behind socially deviant or aberrant behavior. The later development of laws, existing to the current day, codifies unacceptable behavior with little regard for understanding how aberrant brains may underwrite such behavior.

Thus, in a simplistic world where choosing dichotomies over continua is the path of least resistance, the only two choices are to view deviant behavior as either bad or mad in its origins. In the correctional system only those with flagrant psychosis are considered mad. The rest are labeled as bad. They are deemed to cheat, manipulate, malinger, or be factitious.

In support of such thinking, Miresco and Kirmayer (2006) studied 127 psychiatrists and psychologists in a department of psychiatry concerning the presence of mind–body dualism (meaning the mind is distinct from the brain) in their views about patients. They found that if a behavioral problem (or set of symptoms) was deemed to originate "psychologically," the patient was viewed as more blameworthy for the symptoms, and if a neurobiological cause was posited, the patient was considered less responsible and blameworthy. If academic psychiatrists and psychologists still retain this atavistic dualism, which is rife in the general population, we can only expect that the correctional and medical staff of correctional institutions would reveal an even more malignant version concerning the prisoners for whom they have responsibility.

Would that more jurisdictions could join the movement to specialized psychiatric treatment in designated units. The program at Central New York Psychiatric Center (Smith et al., 2002) represents a cutting edge in recognizing comorbidity and the need for specialized and thorough treatment. Peters, LeVasseur, and Chandler (2004) reported 20 co-occurring disorder treatment programs in 13 state correctional systems in 2004.

Long before our current knowledge of neurobiology, Grant and Saslow (1971) proffered a set of principles for psychiatric treatment on an inpatient university psychiatric unit. These were guidelines for staff "attitude and approach" to patients. The first principle still stands as relevant in understanding and dealing with human behavior in general and symptomatic behavior in particular. It is also consistent with modern neuropsychiatric understanding of the underlying brain mechanisms and dysfunctions. The principle is that *each person does the best he can at any given moment*. This means that in any setting with its myriad influences at a given moment in time, a person will use the state of his/her brain at the time, strongly and jointly influenced by both genetic heritage and previous learning (as well as ingested substances) to react more deterministically than choicefully with a given behavior. Whether that behavior is moral or immoral, symptomatic or not, it is the result of a final common pathway for dealing with the instant situation. Such a dispassionate understanding maximizes the possibility of attempting to understand the person and his/her behavior most fully and to best deal with it.

To hold this principle foremost runs diametrically opposed to the mad versus bad or "behavioral" versus "organic" dichotomies. Because of our evolutionary heritage, this principle requires learning and practice. It deals less with motives and more with acceptance and understanding in order to deal most humanely with repetitive excesses, deficiencies, inappropriatenesses, or inconsistencies of behavior that either makes the person or those around her/him miserable. The bias in this principle runs counterintuitively for most people but is consistent with our modern understanding of brain function.

In a study of United Kingdom prison officers working with dangerous and severe personality disorders, Bowers et al. (2006) assessed staff attitudes toward personality disorders using the Attitude to Personality Disorder Questionnaire (APDQ). Over the 16 months of the study those staff with a more positive attitude toward personality disorder had improved general health and job performance, less burnout, and a more favorable impression of managers. This supports the contention that positive attitudes toward any category of inmates vary across prison personnel. However, without a full diagnostic picture of the inmates, there could exist Axis I disorders or histories of toxic brain damage or TBI with attendant symptoms that might unknowingly shape staff attitudes beyond the given singular personality disorder description.

Yet the stigma of mental illness also acts as a brake on the willingness of inmates to seek help with medical or mental disorders. Howerton et al. (2007) indicate that *distrust* constitutes a major barrier to health care seeking in inmates during and after incarceration. They think that a positive precedent could be set by prison health care providers "to help de-stigmatize mental illness" and they recommend "awareness training for health providers." Yet the attitudes, biases, and the philosophy now rife in correctional institutions play a major role in the current configuration of mental health care which discourages mental health care seeking by inmates in prison and afterwards. The conservative approach with high authoritarianism is a blinder for perceiving the need for and implementation of a modern approach to mental health services in jails and prisons.

Conclusions

"No one should want people with serious mental illnesses to be punished for their symptoms." By the use of the plural it is not clear these authors mean this collectively in a population or the presence of comorbid disorders in an individual inmate. However, this is the theme of Metzner and Dvoskin's (2006) recent review of mental health care in supermax settings. The specter of constitutionally mandated mental health treatment ending at the door is not one they relish or support. Rather, they think that more therapeutic and safe management should occur in mental health treatment environments such as are being developed slowly. Supermax settings should not make people more dangerous. Only with accurate assessment and treatment can this be accomplished. More research is needed based on scientific and objective, not attitudinally driven, approaches.

Most prisoners will be paroled after serving their sentence to return to a world they left or worse with their brains better or worse able to deal with it. Much has been written about how this transition should be accomplished best particularly in the linkages to community health and mental health services. Hoge in this volume addresses details about this issue. For optimal success after discharge, rapid access to community services is needed. The referral process should be fortified with clear and detailed documentation of the health care received by inmates during incarceration. If the inmate has not received full and comprehensive treatment in the general and mental health arenas, this compromises significantly the desired seamless transfer of treatment responsibilities to the receiving services.

The blinders to successful mental health treatment beyond budgetary constraints and sufficient personnel have been described as (1) insufficient knowledge about modern neuropsychiatric research and (2) an unfavorable attitudinal bias that inhibits the use of that knowledge. Indeed, a shift in the paradigm of mental health care has occurred in the knowledge area and it may take a generation for the full acceptance of a new view about mental illness and disorders of brain function. More research is in progress.

But the attitudinal blinders may be the more formidable barrier. We need a new *zeitgeist*. The spirit and mood of our current time appears inimical to making the kind of changes needed to deliver effective and thorough, statutorily mandated mental health care to our incarcerated fellow citizens. Such a change is good for us as well as for the parolees as they will soon be among us with our desire for greater public safety. Truly effective mental health treatment may reduce recidivism which means, bottom line, less crime.

There is hope for a two-pronged approach. First is the dissemination of knowledge about the role of brain dysfunction as it affects behavior. Second, the attitude and approach to handling mental illnesses in the correctional system needs to move from its current state, by example, from the top down. This could be done through education at all levels from the public at large, through the legislature to correctional leadership and staff, indeed to the inmates themselves. Such an education could stress this important dimension for humane care without loss of control or the appearance of losing the primary goal of appropriate punishment for crime.

Recommendations for Improving Psychiatric Diagnosis

The goals of these recommendations are to improve access to appropriate mental health treatment interventions and to expedite reentry at parole.

- Conduct institutionwide medical and mental health care continuous quality improvement programs with appropriate medical/psychiatric approval and oversight.
- Institute continuing education programs for medical/psychiatric staff specifically aimed at both diagnostic complexity and the harmful effects of authoritarian bias.

- Institute continuing education programs for medical/psychiatric staff and prison staff and their hierarchy with the goal of reducing stigma concerning psychiatric disorders.
- Increase greater availability of specialized psychiatric units within the prison system.
- Engage in humane, nonpunitive management of suicidality to help reduce the high suicide rate.
- Use dictated psychiatric records, perhaps problem-oriented, and perhaps computerized, so important data and assessments can be read easily, and disseminated.
- Institute preparole transfer of existing psychiatric records to follow-up clinics.
- Make implementation of earliest possible postparole follow-up appointments a high priority.
- Discharge with sufficient medications to last until the known postparole follow-up appointment.
- Do rapid or expedited reenrollment in available Medicare, Medicaid, or Public Assistance to avoid a gap in coverage from parole to follow-up.
- With appropriate confidentiality safeguards, preparole, do consultation with family or significant others about the existing medical and psychiatric disorders.

References

Abram, K. M., Teplin, L. A., & McClelland, G. M. (2003). Comorbidity of severe psychiatric disorders and substance use disorders among women in jail. *Am.J.Psychiatry, 160,* 1007–1010.

Abram, K. M., Teplin, L. A., McClelland, G. M., & Dulcan, M. K. (2003). Comorbid psychiatric disorders in youth in juvenile detention. *Arch.Gen.Psychiatry, 60,* 1097–1108.

Amen, D. G., Stubblefield, M., Carmicheal, B., & Thisted, R. (1996). Brain SPECT findings and aggressiveness. *Ann.Clin.Psychiatry, 8,* 129–137.

American Psychiatric Association & Task Force on DSM-IV. (2000). *Diagnostic and statistical manual of mental disorders: DSM-IV-TR.* Washington, DC: American Psychiatric Association.

Andersen, H. S. (2004). Mental health in prison populations. A review—with special emphasis on a study of Danish prisoners on remand. *Acta Psychiatr.Scand.Suppl.,* 5–59.

Blair, J. (2005). *The psychopath: emotion and the brain.* Malden, MA: Blackwell.

Bowers, L., Carr-Walker, P., Allan, T., Callaghan, P., Nijman, H., & Paton, J. (2006). Attitude to personality disorder among prison officers working in a dangerous and severe personality disorder unit. *Int.J.Law Psychiatry, 29,* 333–342.

Brooke, D., Taylor, C., Gunn, J., & Maden, A. (1996). Point prevalence of mental disorder in unconvicted male prisoners in England and Wales. *BMJ, 313,* 1524–1527.

Brower, M. C., & Price, B. H. (2001). Neuropsychiatry of frontal lobe dysfunction in violent and criminal behaviour: A critical review. *J.Neurol.Neurosurg.Psychiatry, 71,* 720–726.

Bufkin, J. L., & Luttrell, V. R. (2005). Neuroimaging studies of aggressive and violent behavior: Current findings and implications for criminology and criminal justice. *Trauma Violence Abuse, 6,* 176–191.

Butler, T., Allnutt, S., Cain, D., Owens, D., & Muller, C. (2005). Mental disorder in the New South Wales prisoner population. *Aust.N.Z.J.Psychiatry, 39,* 407–413.

Carroll, J. S., Perkowitz, W. T., Lurigio, A. J., & Weaver, F. M. (1987). Sentencing goals, causal attributions, ideology, and personality. *J.Pers.Soc.Psychol., 52,* 107–118.

Chitsabesan, P., Kroll, L., Bailey, S., Kenning, C., Sneider, S., MacDonald, W., et al. (2006). Mental health needs of young offenders in custody and in the community. *Br.J.Psychiatry, 188,* 534–540.

Compton, W. M., Conway, K. P., Stinson, F. S., Colliver, J. D., & Grant, B. F. (2005). Prevalence, correlates, and comorbidity of DSM-IV antisocial personality syndromes and alcohol and specific drug use disorders in the United States: Results from the national epidemiologic survey on alcohol and related conditions. *J.Clin. Psychiatry, 66,* 677–685.

Comtois, K. A., Cowley, D. S., Dunner, D. L., & Roy-Byrne, P. P. (1999). Relationship between borderline personality disorder and Axis I diagnosis in severity of depression and anxiety. *J.Clin.Psychiatry, 60,* 752–758.

Crocker, A. G., Mueser, K. T., Drake, R. E., Clark, R. E., McHugo, G. J., Ackerman, T. H., et al. (2005). Antisocial personality, psychopathy, and violence in persons with dual disorders. *Criminal Justice and Behavior, 32,* 452–476.

Diamond, P. M., Wang, E. W., Holzer, C. E., III, Thomas, C., & des Anges Cruser (2001). The prevalence of mental illness in prison. *Adm. Policy Ment.Health, 29,* 21–40.

Duggan, S., Bradshaw, R., Mitchell, D., Coffey, M., & Rogers, P. (2005). Modernising prison mental health care. *Prof.Nurse, 20,* 20–22.

Forrest, E. (2005). Mental health. Inside job. *Health Serv.J., 115,* 28–30.

Friedman, S. H., Shelton, M. D., Elhaj, O., Youngstrom, E. A., Rapport, D. J., Packer, K. A., et al. (2005). Gender differences in criminality: Bipolar disorder with co-occurring substance abuse. *J.Am.Acad.Psychiatry Law, 33,* 188–195.

Fryers, T., Brugha, T., Grounds, A., & Melzer, D. (1998). Severe mental illness in prisoners: A persistent problem that needs a concerted and long term response. *BMJ, 317,* 1025–1026.

Gilligan, J. (2001). The last mental hospital. *Psychiatr.Q., 72,* 45–61.

Goodwin, R. D., & Hamilton, S. P. (2003). Lifetime comorbidity of antisocial personality disorder and anxiety disorders among adults in the community. *Psychiatry Res., 117,* 159–166.

Grant, R., & Saslow, G. (1971). In Abroms, G. M., Greenfield, N. S. (Eds.) *Maximizing responsible decision-making; or how do we get out of here?* Academic Press Proceedings: The New Hospital Psychiatry, 27–55.

Hare, R. D. (2006). Psychopathy: A clinical and forensic overview. *Psychiatr.Clin. North Am., 29,* 709–724.

Hawley, C. A., & Maden, A. (2003). Mentally disordered offenders with a history of previous head injury: Are they more difficult to discharge? *Brain Inj., 17,* 743–758.

He, X. Y., Felthous, A. R., Holzer, C. E., III, Nathan, P., & Veasey, S. (2001). Factors in prison suicide: One year study in Texas. *J.Forensic Sci., 46,* 896–901.

Herrman, H., McGorry, P., Mills, J., & Singh, B. (1991). Hidden severe psychiatric morbidity in sentenced prisoners: An Australian study. *Am.J.Psychiatry, 148,* 236–239.

Howerton, A., Byng, R., Campbell, J., Hess, D., Owens, C., & Aitken, P. (2007). Understanding help seeking behaviour among male offenders: Qualitative interview study. *BMJ, 334,* 303–306.

Human Rights Watch. (2003). *Ill-equiped: U.S. prisons and offenders with mental illness.*

Kessler, R. C., Berglund, P., Demler, O., Jin, R., Merikangas, K. R., & Walters, E. E. (2005). Lifetime prevalence and age-of-onset distributions of DSM-IV disorders in the National Comorbidity Survey Replication.[see comment][erratum appears in *Arch. Gen. Psychiatry*, 2005 Jul;62(7):768 Note: Merikangas, Kathleen R [added]]. *Arch. Gen. Psychiatry*, 62(6), 593–602.

Kessler, R. C., Chiu, W. T., Demler, O., Merikangas, K. R., & Walters, E. E. (2005). Prevalence, severity, and comorbidity of 12-month DSM-IV disorders in the National Comorbidity Survey Replication.[see comment][erratum appears in *Arch. Gen. Psychiatry*, 2005 Jul;62(7):709 Note: Merikangas, Kathleen R [added]]. *Arch. Gen. Psychiatry*, 62(6), 617–627.

Lamb, H. R., & Weinberger, L. E. (2005). The shift of psychiatric inpatient care from hospitals to jails and prisons. *J.Am.Acad.Psychiatry Law, 33,* 529–534.

Langeveld, H., & Melhus, H. (2004). [Are psychiatric disorders identified and treated by in-prison health services?]. *Tidsskr.Nor. Laegeforen., 124,* 2094–2097.

Lykken, D. T. (2006). *Psychopathic personality.* New York: Guilford Press.

Martens, W. H. J. (2004). Involvement of remitted psychopaths in the therapy of psychopaths. *American Journal of Forensic Psychiatry, 25,* 53–58.

Max, J. E., Koele, S. L., Castillo, C. C., Lindgren, S. D., Arndt, S., Bokura, H., et al. (2000). Personality change disorder in children and adolescents following traumatic brain injury.[erratum appears in J Int Neuropsychol Soc 2000 Nov;6(7):854]. *Journal of the International Neuropsychological Society, 6,* 279–289.

McGough, J. J., Smalley, S. L., McCracken, J. T., Yang, M., Del'Homme, M., Lynn, D. E., et al. (2005). Psychiatric comorbidity in adult attention deficit hyperactivity disorder: Findings from multiplex families. *American Journal of Psychiatry, 162,* 1621–1627.

Metzner, J., & Dvoskin, J. (2006). An overview of correctional psychiatry. *Psychiatr. Clin.North Am., 29,* 761–772.

Miresco, M. J., & Kirmayer, L. J. (2006). The persistence of mind–brain dualism in psychiatric reasoning about clinical scenarios. *American Journal of Psychiatry, 163,* 913–918.

Oldham, J. M., Skodol, A. E., Kellman, H. D., Hyler, S. E., Doidge, N., Rosnick, L., et al. (1995). Comorbidity of Axis I and Axis II disorders. *Am.J.Psychiatry, 152,* 571–578.

Patrick, C. J. (2006). *Handbook of Psychopathy* New York; Guilford Press.

Peters, R. H., LeVasseur, M. E., & Chandler, R. K. (2004). Correctional treatment for co-occurring disorders: Results of a national survey. *Behav.Sci.Law, 22,* 563–584.

Rosen, J. L., Miller, T. J., D'Andrea, J. T., McGlashan, T. H., & Woods, S. W. (2006). Comorbid diagnoses in patients meeting criteria for the schizophrenia prodrome. *Schizophr.Res., 85,* 124–131.

Rubinstein, G. (2006). Authoritarianism among border police officers, career soldiers, and airport security guards at the Israeli border. *J.Soc.Psychol., 146,* 751–761.

Slaughter, B., Fann, J. R., & Ehde, D. (2003). Traumatic brain injury in a county jail population: Prevalence, neuropsychological functioning and psychiatric disorders. *Brain Inj., 17,* 731–741.

Smith, H., Sawyer, D. A., & Way, B. B. (2002). Central New York Psychiatric Center: An approach to the treatment of co-occurring disorders in the New York State correctional mental health system. *Behav.Sci.Law, 20,* 523–534.

Society of Nuclear Medicine. (2002). Society of Nuclear Medicine guidelines for brain perfusion single photon emission computerized tomography (SPECT) using Tc-99m radiopharmaceuticals. In Society of Nuclear Medicine (Ed.), *Society of Nuclear Medicine procedure guidelines manual* (pp. 113–118). Reston, VA.

Soderstrom, H., Nilsson, T., Sjodin, A. K., Carlstedt, A., & Forsman, A. (2005). The childhood-onset neuropsychiatric background to adulthood psychopathic traits and personality disorders. *Compr.Psychiatry, 46,* 111–116.

Soderstrom, H., Sjodin, A. K., Carlstedt, A., & Forsman, A. (2004). Adult psychopathic personality with childhood-onset hyperactivity and conduct disorder: A central problem constellation in forensic psychiatry. *Psychiatry Res., 121,* 271–280.

Teplin, L. A., Abram, K. M., & McClelland, G. M. (1996). Prevalence of psychiatric disorders among incarcerated women. I. Pretrial jail detainees. *Arch.Gen.Psychiatry, 53,* 505–512.

Torres, A. R., Prince, M. J., Bebbington, P. E., Bhugra, D., Brugha, T. S., Farrell, M., et al. (2006). Obsessive-compulsive disorder: Prevalence, comorbidity, impact, and help-seeking in the British national psychiatric morbidity survey of 2000. *Am.J.Psychiatry, 163,* 1978–1985.

Tucker, W. (1999). The "mad" vs. the "bad" revisited: Managing predatory behavior. *Psychiatr.Q., 70,* 221–230.

Chapter 18

Juvenile Corrections and Public Health Collaborations: Opportunities for Improved Health Outcomes

Michelle Staples-Horne, Kaiyti Duffy, and Michele T. Rorie

Most juveniles behind bars move in and out of facilities with short lengths of stay. Relatively few have longer sentences for more serious crimes; they all return to the community. In 2003, law enforcement agencies reported 2.2 million arrests of persons under age 18 (Snyder & Sickmund, 2006). The most serious charges in almost half of all juvenile arrests were for larceny-theft, simple assault, drugs, disorderly conduct, or liquor law violations (Snyder & Sickmund, 2006). The brevity and frequency of these contacts with correctional institutions create challenges and opportunities for health promotion and intervention during incarceration and in preparation for reentry. As the character of juvenile populations varies by region, the services must be customized to the developmental, cultural, and linguistic needs of the local inmate population. To do this, it is essential to understand the background of these young men and women, where they come from, and what circumstances contributed to their incarceration.

Antecedents of Juvenile Detention

In 2006, children under the age of 19 represented approximately 26% of the U.S. population; almost half of these were adolescents (U.S. Census Bureau, 2007). Though the percentage of the total population will remain stable, by 2050 the number of children in the United States will be approximately 36% larger than it was in 2000 (U.S. Census Bureau, 2004). As this population grows, successful transition from adolescence to adulthood becomes more important to the development of a healthy society. There are many forces that shape adolescents' development and treatment, not the least of which are race, ethnicity, socioeconomic status, family structure, and sexual identity. Though incarcerated young men and women come from diverse backgrounds, the majority share the common experience of economic and social disadvantage.

The racial makeup of the juvenile justice population varies by region of the country. In 2002, of all incarcerated U.S. juveniles, 77.9% self-identified as white, 16.4% as black, 1.4% as American Indian, and 4.4% as Asian. Hispanic ethnicity, aside from race, was 18% overall. Ninety-two percent of Hispanic juveniles identified racially as white. These percentages varied significantly by region, however. In the West, a much larger percent of juveniles identified as Hispanic, for example, 51% in New Mexico, 45% in California, 42% in Texas, 37% in Arizona, 30% in Nevada, and 24% in Colorado (Snyder & Sickmund, 2006).

Additionally, states with large native populations (Alaska, South Dakota, New Mexico, and Oklahoma) had juvenile populations with more than 10% American Indian or Alaska Natives. In the District of Columbia, a predominantly African-American city, 72% of the juvenile inmates were black. This is replicated in many southern states including: Mississippi (45%), Louisiana (40%), South Carolina (37%), Georgia (34%), Maryland (33%), and Alabama (32%) (Snyder & Sickmund, 2006).

As with adults, racial minorities have been overrepresented in juvenile justice systems across this country. Black youth, who accounted for 16% of the incarcerated juvenile population in 2003, were involved in a disproportionate number of juvenile arrests for robbery (63%), murder (48%), motor vehicle theft (40%), and aggravated assault (38%) (Snyder & Sickmund, 2006).

Though race and ethnicity are important factors affecting the development of a young person's identity and experiences of prejudice and discrimination, data suggest that socioeconomic status and family structure have a far greater influence on the risk of juvenile incarceration. In 2002, 17% of persons under 18 lived in poverty (based on the poverty threshold of income and family size, adjusted for inflation, using federal government standards), with many living in extreme poverty (U.S. Census Bureau, 2004). Lower socioeconomic status disproportionately affects young men and women of color. Almost one-third of black, 28.6% of Hispanic, and 11.7% of Asian juveniles live in poverty compared to 9.2% of whites.

Research indicates a link between poverty and juvenile delinquency (Snyder & Sickmund, 2006). Because of lack of resources, many lower income communities cannot provide the social supports needed for youth to reach their full potential, including adequate schools, community centers, and hospitals and clinics (Zigler, Taussig, & Black, 1992). Youth in these communities are much more likely to experience violent crime. A study by Lauritsen (2003) indicated that juveniles were more likely to be victims of violent crime if they lived in a disadvantaged community (i.e., high percentages of persons living in poverty, single-parent families with children, unemployment, and households receiving public assistance).

Family structure is also associated with a young person's likelihood of living in poverty and relying on public assistance for sustenance. More than half (52%) of all children living below the poverty level in 2002 were living in single-mother families. Although a greater proportion of children of color live in single-parent households, the proportion of incarcerated juveniles, regardless of race, living in single-parent households increased from 9% in 1960 to 27% in 2002. In 2002, 62% of all children receiving public assistance and 61% receiving food stamps lived in single-mother families (Fields, 2003).

McCurley and Snyder (2006) report that family structure is a better predictor of self-reported problem behaviors, such as running away from home, sexual activity, major theft, assault, and arrest, than race or ethnicity. One reason for this may be that children living in single-parent homes are often at greater risk of abuse and/or neglect. Research (Lauritsen, 2003) indicates that juveniles in single-parent families experienced a 50% greater risk of violence than those in two-parent families. Additionally, young people in single parent families often lack supervision, making them susceptible to risk behaviors.

Though disadvantaged and lower income youth are at higher risk for incarceration, their social misfortune provides increased opportunities for intervention. A large number of juveniles in families receiving public assistance and food stamps will interact with public health facilities and providers by virtue of their Medicaid eligibility for health services. Health professionals should be better trained to assess physical, psychological, and behavioral risk during these encounters.

Medical Needs of Incarcerated Juveniles

Often, the public perceives juveniles as "well enough to get in trouble." Ironically, it is often the behaviors that got them into trouble that increase their risk for morbidity and mortality. For instance, juvenile detainees are more likely to have experimented with smoking, alcohol, and drug use; engaged in risky sexual behaviors with multiple sex partners and lack of condom use; used weapons; and experienced violence and other risk taking behaviors (Crosby et al., 2003). These behaviors increase their likelihood of trauma, accidents, and disease.

A classic study conducted by Hein, Cohen, and Litt (1980) remains the largest study of health status of detainees. The study was conducted at the Spofford Juvenile Detention Center in New York between July 1968 and June 1979, during which 88,106 youth were admitted to the facility; 40,818 received a brief screening since they remained in the facility less than 24 hours. Of the 47,288 adolescents examined more fully, medical problems were diagnosed in 46%. The population demographics were 80% male, 60% African-American, and 25% Hispanic surnamed. The average age was 15 with an average length of stay of 14 days. In this study, the most commonly diagnosed conditions were upper respiratory infections (17%), minor dermatological problems (14%), minor trauma (21%), and psychosomatic states (18%).

Anderson and Farrow (1998) described health services provided for incarcerated adolescents in Washington State. For short-term detention centers with a mean daily population of 47.2, the most common reasons for sick call visits were for substance use (36.6%), trauma (30.8%), psychiatric (21.8%), dermatological (19.2%), respiratory (15.5%), and sexually transmitted diseases (15.3%). For long-term facilities with a mean daily population of 161.7, the most common complaints were for dental care (65.9%), psychiatric (44.9%), dermatological (44.1%), respiratory (35.6%), trauma (35.4%), and substance use (33.7%).

Feinstein et al. reported (1998) the medical status and history of health care utilization of juvenile offenders on admission to an 80-bed detention center in Birmingham, Alabama. African Americans made up 74.5%, while white non-Hispanic males made up 15.4% of the population. Only 7.3% of the juveniles were African-American females and 2.8% white non-Hispanic females. The most common condition was asthma. Other common conditions included: orthopedic problems, mental illness, hearing-related problems, and pregnancy. Almost one-fifth (16.5%) reported a history of hospitalization, the majority of these resulting from trauma-related injuries. Despite these findings, only a third of these youth reported a source of regular medical care, and only 20% reported having a private physician.

The provision of health care to adolescents in an incarcerated environment presents a challenge to health care providers, as well as administration and security staff. The health care model is often perceived as contradictory in a correctional setting. Custody staff, medical providers, and public health agencies have different goals. Fulfilling security requirements and protecting the public safety are the correctional facility's primary goals. In contrast, assuring that the juveniles receive unimpeded access to appropriate medical care is the primary goal of the facility medical provider. The public health agency's goal is to provide disease surveillance and protect the health of the free-world community through risk reduction, disease identification, and treatment. On the surface, it may seem that these goals conflict, but they need not, especially if the mission of the agency includes access to appropriate medical care and continuity of care with community practitioners.

Collaboration is the key to success. A 1997 NIJ/CDC study (Hammett, 1998) analyzed data from a prison and jail survey to identify elements of successful collaboration in the prevention and treatment of HIV/AIDS, STDs, and TB. The key recommendations of the study were:

- Public health agencies should collect and disseminate data on the burden of infectious disease in inmate populations.
- Correctional agencies should be represented on all HIV Prevention Planning groups
- Public health agencies should initiate or expand funding for services and staff in correctional facilities
- Public health and correctional agencies should recognize the importance and potential benefits of interventions in correctional settings to the health of the larger community

Oral Health

Oral health is an important part of overall health and self-esteem. In a review by Treadwell and Formicola (2005), no data were found on the oral health needs of incarcerated juveniles. However, in the general population, 80% of tooth decay occurs among 25% of children 5–17 years of age, primarily in minority and low-income families and in children with low educational levels. These are the children who are disproportionately represented in juvenile justice facilities. For incarcerated adolescents, there are few preventive services and often failure to access dental services, even when covered by Medicaid.

Immunizations

The federally funded Vaccine for Children Program may be used to provide free vaccine to incarcerated juveniles. Public health agencies should be aggressive in enrolling all juvenile correctional facilities in this program and assist them in meeting program requirements.

Routine vaccine for hepatitis B has been recommended for high-risk groups since 1982 and for adolescents generally since 1996. Since risk behaviors for the spread of hepatitis B are highly prevalent in the juvenile population, this vaccine in particular should be strongly promoted. As hepatitis B can be a sexually transmitted infection, juveniles can receive the vaccine without a parent or guardian's consent.

Between November 2001 and March 2004, the Georgia Department of Juvenile Justice, in collaboration with the Georgia Department of Human Resources, Division of Public Health, immunized 16,182 juvenile offenders across 30 detention and long-term secure facilities with hepatitis B vaccine. The Department has continued this aggressive immunization program. The long-term implications of this initiative with regards to decreased morbidity and mortality, reduced medical costs for adult corrections and community health care, increased productivity, and overall reduction in infection rates will likely be significant.

Many states have implemented systems to electronically track immunizations. These systems allow for immunization data to be both retrieved and entered by all registered health providers. Public health agencies have taken the lead in this effort, working with community health care providers. Juvenile justice agencies should gain access to these databases, review immunization status on intake to facilities, and assure that patients are fully immunized prior to release. Where full immunization is not possible because of length of stay, public health agencies can follow up on any remaining dosages required on release.

Providing Comprehensive, Adolescent-Friendly Health Care to Incarcerated Juveniles

Health care and prevention efforts within the juvenile justice system should address the extant risks and conditions of incarcerated youth, focusing on treatment and guidance on healthier living on release. As adolescents are different from children and adults, emotionally, physically, and mentally, their health care services should reflect these differences. Services should be developmentally appropriate and adolescent specific, paying particular attention to the many factors affecting health decisions and behaviors.

Juvenile justice facilities detain youth of varying ages. The needs of these youth differ by stage of development and mental ability. The early adolescent (usually ranging from 10 to 13 years old) is mostly very concrete in his/her thought process. Therefore, counseling and behavioral interventions must reflect this concrete thinking. For instance, a tobacco prevention/cessation program for a young person in this age group should focus on the physical unpleasantness associated with smoking, i.e., bad breath and yellowing teeth, instead of the later health complications that may resound with an older teenager. At this age, the majority of young people will begin the process of physical sexual maturation but this does not mean that the individual has not already initiated sexual activity.

In middle adolescence (ranging from age 14 to 16), the physical changes of puberty are complete and thought processes become more abstract. In this stage, the individual develops a stronger sense of identity and is more susceptible to the influences of peer groups. Counseling and interventions for these teens should incorporate the role of friends and peers in risk-taking behaviors.

Late adolescence encompasses 17 years old and above. In this stage, the body continues to take on adult form and the process of identity development continues. These young men and women, on the verge of becoming legal adults, are of particular concern for juvenile justice authorities and the public health community. Though they might look and often act like adults, these young men and women are still in need of counseling, care, and intervention.

The major causes of morbidity and mortality in these adolescents are unintentional injuries, many of which are related to alcohol and drug use. Other causes of morbidity include unintended pregnancy, sexually transmitted diseases, eating disorders, and depression (Eaton et al., 2006). These factors are not easily discernable from the traditional patient provider model of health interviewing. An alternative model, the HEADSS Model, was developed in 1972 by Dr. Harvey Berman of Seattle and refined by Dr. Eric Cohen and Dr. John M. Goldenring. An acronym for Home, Education/Employment, Activities, Drugs, Depression, Safety, and Sexuality, this model can be particularly useful in the juvenile justice system as health care practitioners explore the complex forces affecting an adolescent's behavior and health outcomes (Goldenring & Cohen, 1988).

In addition to being adolescent specific, services provided to juvenile justice detainees should be culturally and linguistically competent. This includes sensitivity to the ways that culture and health interact. An individual's culture can have profound impact on how pain and illness manifest and when and how individuals seek care. Youth from cultures with stoic attitudes toward illness, may not present for treatment. Also, the acknowledgment and treatment of mental illness may not be acceptable in some cultures which could prevent those youth from seeking treatment for symptoms. As the juvenile justice system is so diverse, professionals need to be trained to assess the effect of culture (including aculturization and cultural isolation) on a detainee's health and risk behavior. Youth may be the first generation in their family to be born in the United States, or may have immigrated recently. These youth may be trapped between the health perceptions of two cultures during the already difficult period of adolescence. Additionally, care must be taken when communicating with youth who do not speak English proficiently. Efforts to address this can include the use of translators and hiring health professionals who are fluent in different languages.

Medical professionals in the juvenile justice system should be aware that insensitive attitudes on the part of practitioners, lack of knowledge and skills regarding reproductive and sexual health, insufficient or inadequate communication, and clinician discomfort with different cultures or the discussion of risk behaviors with adolescents can prevent a young person from disclosing vital health information (Huppert & Adams Hillard, 2003). The final important factor in providing adolescent-friendly health services involves discussing and assuring confidentiality wherever possible. Concerns regarding confidentiality keep many young people from disclosing crucial health information and from seeking care. For instance, a recent study of girls younger than 18 attending family planning clinics found that 47% would no longer attend if their parents had to be notified that they were seeking prescription birth control pills or devices, and another 10% would delay or discontinue STI testing or treatment (Reddy, Fleming, & Swain, 2002).

In the juvenile justice system, parents and/or guardians are not present but concerns about confidentiality still exist and detainees should be assured that their disclosures will be kept confidential. There are times when the provider may need to contact a parent and times when the law allows such contact, but the bias should be toward confidentiality. If a patient appears to be a danger to him/herself or to another person, state laws mandate that a provider inform parents or authorities. Laws governing minors' access and confidentiality to services differ state by state, and many health care providers are unaware of minors' ability to consent to certain confidential health services. Title X dictates that family planning services must be confidential. In many states, confidentiality is decided by the provider but because Title X is federal, it preempts state statutes. Medicaid provides for confidential services to minors, along with Title X.

Federal Medical Privacy Regulations also apply. There is variation across the country among juvenile correctional facilities regarding federal HIPAA compliance. There is a general HIPAA exclusion for correctional facilities; however, if any part of a juvenile justice system is billing electronically for medical services such as Medicaid, they should be HIPAA compliant. It is also advisable that public health and juvenile justice both be HIPAA compliant, so that medical information can pass freely between agencies for improved continuity of care, allowing for appropriate consents from youth and parents/guardians to be utilized. Memoranda of Understanding (MOUs) between agencies can address any HIPAA concerns regarding sharing of confidential medical information.

Reproductive Health Needs of Incarcerated Juveniles

Adolescents in correctional facilities report becoming sexually active at earlier ages and partaking in risky sexual behaviors more frequently than their nonincarcerated peers (Strack & Alexander, 2000). In one study of juvenile offenders aged 14–18, 87% of the sample reported being sexually active. Over one-third reported having sex *before* they were 12 years old and 57% before they were 13 years old. The median age for first sex was 12 for males and 13 for females. Of those who reported having sexual intercourse, half (49%) had had 6 or more partners in their lifetimes, including 22% with 6–10 partners and 16% with more than 20 partners. Of all the sexually active youth, over half had had sex in the past month and 42% reported having *multiple* partners in the past 3 months (Strack & Alexander, 2000). In another study of sexual debut among female juvenile offenders, results showed that the mean age of sexual debut was 13. The mean number of sex partners (lifetime) was 8.8 (Crosby et al., 2004).

Though incarcerated juveniles report greater sexual risk-taking behavior, many do not use condoms consistently (Morrison, Baker, & Gillmore, 1994). Strack and Alexander (2000) found that 44% of the youth reported using condoms only about half the time or less and nearly one fifth of the youth indicating that they *never use* a condom. Among those youth who have had anal intercourse, 70% have had anal sex at least once without a condom. Another study of incarcerated juveniles found that although 96% of female and male respondents were sexually active, only 4% used a condom consistently (Crosby et al., 2004).

Although sexual activity is prohibited within juvenile correctional facilities, it may be occurring either consensually or by sexual assault. The Prison Rape Elimination Act (PREA) was enacted by Congress and will require all correctional facilities, including those serving juveniles, to implement policies and procedures to eliminate prison rape.

Because the majority of detainees have had sex, the discussion of sexual behaviors, including risk and protection, should be included in every preventive medical encounter. Providers should include questions about age at first vaginal, oral, and anal intercourse, current sexual practices, number of partners within the last 3 months, and gender(s) of partners. Though same-sex sexual relations between juvenile detainees are officially prohibited, many detainees may have had same-sex sexual experiences in the past. Additionally, same-sex sexual contact may be occurring within the facility. (See section on Special Populations: GLBTQ Youth.) When questioning all youth about sexual behaviors, it is important to use the word *partner* and not *boyfriend* or *girlfriend* so as not to assume heterosexuality and behaviors. Many youth may be having sex with casual partners or sex work clients who they would not consider as a "boyfriend" or "girlfriend." They may use these terms in reference to a regular partner with whom there may be an emotional attachment.

Additionally, all reproductive health clinical interviews should include discussions on condoms. Though juvenile justice systems often have restrictions on displaying and dispensing condoms within the facility, medical providers and health educators can educate inmates regarding correct and consistent use of condoms so they will be better equipped to protect themselves after incarceration. On release, detainees should either be given (depending on institutional policy) or told where condoms can be purchased or are given out for free.

Due to the high rates of sexual risk behaviors and low rates of condom use, it is not surprising that juvenile detainees experience higher rates of sexually transmitted infections (STIs), including HIV. In one study, 20% of juvenile detainees tested positive for an STI (Crosby et al., 2004). Rates of chlamydia among juvenile detainees range between 2.4, and 27% in females and 1 and 8% in males (Lofy, Hofmann, Mosure, Fine, & Marrazzo, 2006; Kahn et al., 2005; Robertson & Thomas, 2005). Because these rates are so much higher than in the general population, chlamydia screening is recommended for *both* males and females. Gonorrhea rates are also disproportionately high for juvenile detainees—from 0 to 17% in females and 0 to 18% in males (Kahn et al., 2005; Robertson & Thomas, 2005).

In addition to chlamydia and gonorrhea, other STIs affect incarcerated youth, although these are the most common. A 1996 study assessed the prevalence of genital herpes in a sample of detained juveniles and found that 15% of the males and 20% of the females tested positive (Huerta et al., 1996). HPV prevalence has not been defined in this population, but can be extrapolated as being high, based on the other STI data available, low condom use, early sexual debut, and abnormal Pap smears among female juvenile offenders.

The public health implications of these data are overwhelming. Though statistics demonstrate that incarcerated young men and women are at high risk for STIs, many are still not tested. Recent data are limited, but in 1994, 53% of incarcerated juveniles were screened for STIs. In 33% of the surveyed facilities, nonmedical personnel did the screening (Parent et al., 1994). The detention and confinement period for juveniles is a golden opportunity for screening and treatment of STIs by juvenile justice and public health agencies, which should develop the resources to implement effective screening and treatment programs.

New urine-based tests can improve compliance for testing and may be easily incorporated into the intake process of the juvenile correctional facility. The urine-based nucleic acid amplification tests (NAATs) are highly sensitive and specific. Self-collected genital specimens can be used to accurately diagnose chlamydia and gonorrhea infections. In many cases, use of urine specimens can reduce the necessity for a pelvic examination on females and urethral swabs for males, thus extending the diagnostic capability for detecting these infections in nonclinic screening venues (CDC, 2006).

Public health agencies must consider partnering with juvenile justice agencies to promote and facilitate STI screening and treatment of juvenile offenders prior to their return to the community. Partnerships may be informal with staff communicating regarding treatment and follow up and partner notification or may become formalized with the development of an agreement such as a Memorandum of Understanding (MOU). An MOU can allow sharing of information across agencies and define all parties' responsibilities whether in kind or with some fiscal responsibility.

HIV infection rates are growing among this population based on risk behaviors. Adult correctional populations have at least six times the prevalence of HIV than the general population (CDC, 1996). The prevalence of HIV within juvenile correctional facilities is not documented well, as many juvenile systems do not have universal or mandatory testing. Also, adults may be presenting medically with AIDS while infected juveniles may not be symptomatic yet. Juvenile justice facilities should be encouraged to implement the latest CDC recommendations of opt-out testing for HIV incorporated into the routine health care admission process. However, the agency should be prepared for positive HIV test results and develop a mechanism to provide treatment while the youth is still incarcerated and appropriate follow-up on release into the community.

Young men and women confined in the juvenile justice system are also more likely to have been pregnant or involved in a pregnancy. A 2004 study indicated that 32.2% of juveniles had ever been pregnant (Crosby et al., 2004). Another study found that more half (52.3%) of the sexually active youth in out-of-home care reported that they thought they or their partners were pregnant at one time, but found out that they were not. Twenty-five percent indicated two or more such instances (Strack & Alexander, 2004).

A substantial number of young women are pregnant upon their confinement in the juvenile justice system. A 1995 study of 261 juvenile detention facilities found that 68% of the respondents estimated that they were holding one to five pregnant adolescents on a given day, with a reported yearly census of 2000 pregnant teenagers and 1200 teenaged mothers. Nearly half of the facilities (45%) continue to incarcerate after it is determined that a youth is pregnant. Of those institutions that incarcerate pregnant adolescents, 31% provide no prenatal services and 70% provide no parenting classes. Of these facilities, 60% reported at least one obstetric complication in their pregnant population (Breuner & Farrow, 1995).

Pregnancy testing should be a routine part of medical intake for all females entering juvenile correctional facilities. As more than half of all rapes (54%) of women occur before age 18, juvenile justice health professionals should assess for sexual trauma on diagnosis of pregnancy (Tjaden & Thoennes, 2000). Additionally, detainees should be provided with unbiased and comprehensive options counseling regarding their choices, including parenthood, adoption, and pregnancy termination. Juvenile corrections, public health, and other child serving agencies should partner to provide the best outcome for the young offender whatever her choice. If the pregnancy is continued, prenatal care can be provided through coordination with public health agencies. Many females will be discharged from the facility prior to delivery, so follow up into the community for obstetric care is essential. If the young woman decides to terminate the pregnancy, the detention center, while acting within the confines of state law, should see to it that the termination is obtained at the earliest gestation possible.

Although the juvenile justice system is predominately male, pregnancy prevention interventions are needed in this population. Information on pregnancy prevention, particularly contraception, should be provided to males as well as females in the clinical setting. For instance, many young men and women are unaware of emergency contraception. In the event of forced intercourse or contraceptive failure, emergency contraception provides a second chance to prevent pregnancy. Though commonly referred to as "the morning-after pill," the drug regimen has reasonable effectiveness up to 120 hours after unprotected intercourse. Discussion of emergency contraception should be incorporated into the medical intake process. If the young woman has had unprotected intercourse in the last 5 days, juvenile justice medical personnel should be prepared to administer emergency contraception. Young women and men should be educated regarding emergency contraception before release to prevent future pregnancies.

As noted, young men and women run significant reproductive health risks before incarceration. These risks persist and even increase after release. In a 2003 study of the sexual behaviors of young men on release from incarceration, results indicated that 36% men reported having had risky sex (≥two female sex partners and unprotected vaginal sex) in the months following reentry (MacGowan et al. 2003). Therefore, the period of incarceration is an excellent time to initiate pregnancy and STI prevention interventions for both young women and men. In addition to clinical counseling, these can include programs that focus on the antecedents of risky sexual behavior: knowledge of reproductive physiology, condoms, and contraception; and programs that focus on the nonsexual antecedents such as self-efficacy and communication skills.

One final step in public health efforts to reduce pregnancy on release is to partner with juvenile justice agencies in the provision of family planning services during incarceration. Contraception should be provided on release or initiated while the youth is still incarcerated. There are many advantages to the latter. Even though detained young women are not sexually active, initiating a method of contraception will allow for adjustment to the medication and resolution of any related problems while the individual has full access to a medical provider.

Mental Health and Substance Abuse

Nearly one-third of teens report episodes of sadness, depression, and hopelessness (Eaton, 2006). Depression is defined as an illness when the feelings of sadness, hopelessness, and despair persist and interfere with a teen's ability to function. It is more than the normal, everyday ups and downs or the "blues," as some may refer to them. It also is not just situational, relating solely to the fact that the youth is incarcerated. The term *clinical depression* is used when this mood persists for more than a couple of weeks. Clinical depression is a serious health problem that can change behavior, physical health and appearance, academic performance, social activity, and the ability to handle everyday decisions and pressures (DSM-IV, 1994). These feelings may prevent youth from seeking preventive health care and complying with health regimens which can affect behavioral problems and eventual incarceration.

Between two-thirds and three-quarters of detained youths have one or more psychiatric disorders (Wasserman, McReynolds, Lucas, Fisher, & Santos, 2002). Federal courts have affirmed that under the U.S. Constitution's Eighth and Fourteenth Amendments, which bar cruel and unusual punishment and assure the right to substantive due process for youth in the juvenile justice system, detainees with serious mental disorders have a right to receive needed treatment as part of the state's obligation to provide needed medical care (*Estelle v. Gamble*, 1976; *Ruiz v. Estelle*, 1980; *Madrid v. Gomez*, 1995; *Bowring v. Godwin*, 1977). In addition to this argument that all children with mental illness are deserving of care, to ignore this major affliction may contribute to public health and legal problems such as continuation of antisocial behavior, higher health care use, and criminal recidivism.

Despite these known risks, this population remains largely underserved. According to a study done by Teplin, Abram, McClellan, Washburn, and Pikus (2005), there are two reasons juvenile justice youth may receive even fewer services than youth in the general population. The first is that juvenile justice youth (as previously discussed) are disproportionately poor, as well as undereducated; these characteristics limit the type and scope of mental health services that are sought and provided. Second, as many as 75% of detainees with mental disorders also have substance use disorders, which is a higher rate than found in the community. Capitated mental health care also affects service utilization by youth in the juvenile justice and child welfare systems. The Teplin et al. (2005) research suggested that as many as 13,000 detained youths with major mental disorders do not receive treatment every day. It was also noted that the juvenile courts may process more than 139,000 youths per year whose major mental disorders go untreated.

Many factors may influence service utilization, such as family pressure, environmental stress, having a primary care doctor, health insurance, and experiences with past services. These factors may be seen as hindrances or can conversely aid in recovery. The RWJ report found a greater distance from traditional support systems for teens who experience symptoms of depression (Bethell, Lansky, & Fiorillo, 2001). These juveniles were 12 to 21% less likely to report feeling connected to people in their school and are significantly less likely to report involvement in community activities. Forty-eight percent of adolescents with depressive symptoms said they could talk openly with providers compared to 65% without depressive symptoms.

A range of mental health and substance abuse treatment services are needed in criminal justice settings, as the problem of substance use is more pronounced within the detained population. Survey results among juvenile arrestees provide evidence of illegal drug use with more than half of the males testing positive for at least one drug; marijuana was the most frequently detected drug (National Institute of Justice, 1999). Another study concluded that 60 to 87% of female offenders need substance abuse treatment (Prescott, 1998). Substance abuse treatment services are often among the first to be cut during budget reductions. Security and supervision measures are seen as more important obligations than treatment plans when it comes to allocating funds.

Substance abuse treatment is not legally mandated in most correctional settings although it has been proven to have a tremendous effect on reducing the rate of recidivism among inmates. Treatment partnerships within the criminal justice system are time-consuming, and those involving mental health and substance abuse services require additional work. The decision to cut those services without regard to long-term outcomes usually has a detrimental effect (Chandler, Peters, Field, & Juliano-Bult, 2004).

Mental health and substance abuse were perceived as such a major problem among incarcerated juveniles that in 1997, the New York State Office of Children and Family Services (OCFS) implemented a statewide diversion initiative. The Mental Health Juvenile Justice (MH/JJ) Diversion Project has 10 county sites involving county probation and a mental health provider. While each site has its own structured program tailored to the needs of the youth in their community, there are some areas that are common to all 10. Each site is required to provide, at a minimum, the following: screening; assessment; direct services, including individual, group, and family counseling; and referral to mental health, substance abuse, and other community-based services. The variability is seen when it comes to the type of services available, when the youth is diverted, voluntary or mandatory participation, and treatment models. It has also been noted that youth in community-based treatment fared better than youth whose treatment was provided in institutions (Lipsey, 1992).

Special Populations: Gay, Lesbian, Bisexual, and Transgender Youth

It is difficult to ascertain the actual percentage of youth who are grappling with questions regarding their sexuality and gender identity. The majority of the states do not include questions regarding these issues on their Youth Risk Behavior Surveys. The limited data that we do have regarding sexual orientation indicate that between 2 and 4.5% of high school students self-identify as gay, lesbian, or bisexual (Garofalo, Wolf, Kessel, Palfrey, & Durant, 1999; Ries & Saewyc, 1999). These data are definitely underestimates, as many youth have difficulty understanding complexity of sexual attractions or fear disclosure. There are virtually no data on transgenderism in the adolescent population. *Transgender* is an umbrella term that refers to the range of individuals whose gender identity does not match anatomic or chromosomal sex. Transgendered individuals can live as full- or part-time members of another gender and can be heterosexual, homosexual, or bisexual (ACOG, 2005).

What is known, however, is that sexual minority youth face disproportionate risk of family, school, and community violence. After coming out to their families or being discovered, many gay, lesbian, bisexual, transgender, and questioning (GLBTQ) youth can be thrown out of their homes or mistreated. Service providers estimate that 25 to 40% of homeless youth may be GLBTQ (Savin-Williams, 1994). Additionally, these young people often experience greater rates of school violence. In one nationwide survey, over 84% of GLBTQ students reported verbal harassment at school. Over 39% of all gay, lesbian, and bisexual youth reported being punched, kicked, or injured with a weapon at school because of their sexual orientation while 55% of transgender youth reported physical attacks because of their gender identity or gender expression. The consequences of physical and verbal abuse directed at GLBTQ students include truancy, dropping out of school, poor grades, and having to repeat a grade. In one study, 28% of gay and bisexual youth dropped out of school due to peer harassment (Savin-Williams, 1994). Juvenile correctional facilities must consider the potential for violence against these youth and make appropriate security considerations.

Most likely a result of isolation caused by societal homophobia, a disproportionate number of GLBTQ youth turn to drugs or alcohol, suffer from depression, and engage in risky sexual behavior, including survival sex (Garofalo et al., 1998). These factors can increase the risk of juvenile incarceration. Though very little data exist regarding the actual number of GLBTQ youth in the system, it is estimated these youth make up between 4 and 10% of detainees (Feintein et al., 2001). Few juvenile justice facilities have policies prohibiting discrimination on the basis of sexual orientation or gender identity or provide training for staff on how to create safe environments for these youth (Feintein et al., 2001).

Juvenile justice centers can maintain a ban on same-sex sexual contact while maintaining policies that are affirming to all sexual minority youth. This includes implementing training for staff on sensitivity issues and respecting differences. Additionally, if sexual minority youth are experiencing harassment within the facility, appropriate action must be taken to assure their safety. Juvenile justice authorities can also partner with the public health community to secure successful reentry for GLBTQ youth. This includes addressing family counseling needs, locating proper shelter and interventions to limit risk behavior including survival sex.

Incarcerated Juveniles: An Opportunity for Public Health

The period of incarceration for a juvenile presents an opportunity for public health to access a population they may not routinely serve. The catalogue of services available through public health can augment the health care provided by the juvenile facility whether in the form of direct services or through support services for the health program. A strong collaboration with juvenile justice agencies can support the primary goal of public health to prevent the spread of communicable diseases and benefit the overall health of the youth when they return to the greater community. The Georgia Department of Juvenile Justice has just such a collaborative agreement between the Georgia Department of Human Resources Division of Public Health, Division of Family and Children's Services and the Division of Mental Retardation, Developmental Disabilities and Addictive Diseases, and the Juvenile Courts. This interagency program has a formalized MOU. It allows sharing of relevant health information between agencies for the continued medical and mental health care of juveniles on release from a detention center into the community. Youth with health needs are referred to the appropriate agency; tracking of appointments and follow-up is shared among the agencies, so youth will not fall between the cracks. It is hoped that this safety net will assure greater continuity of care in the community and ultimately reduce recidivism of these youth. The I CAN Program is a model program between juvenile corrections and public health that will have a positive impact on the outcome of the lives of many young people.

References

American College of Obstetricians and Gynecologists. (2005). Health care for transgendered individuals. In *Special issues in women's health* (pp. 75–88). Washington, DC: Author.

Anderson, B., & Farrow, J.A. (1998). Incarcerated adolescents in Washington State, health services and utilization. *Journal of Adolescent Health, 22*, 363–367.

Bethell, C., Lansky, D., & Fiorillo, J. (2001). *A portrait of adolescents in America, 2001*. FACCT—Foundation for Accountability. Princeton, NJ: Robert Wood Johnson Foundation.

Bowring v Godwin, 551 F2d 44, 47 (4th Circuit 1977).

Breuner, C.C., & Farrow, J.A. (1995). Pregnant teens in prison: Prevalence, management, and consequences. *Western Journal Medicine, 162*, 328–330.

Centers for Disease Control and Prevention. (1996). HIV/AIDS education and prevention programs for adults in prisons and jails and juveniles in confinement facilities—United States, 1994. *MMWR, 45*, 268–271.

Centers for Disease Control and Prevention. (2006). Sexually transmitted diseases treatment guidelines, 2006. *MMWR Recommendations and Reports, 55*, 1–94.

Chandler, R., Peters, R., Field, G., & Juliano-Bult, D. (2004). Challenges in implementing evidence-based treatment practices for co-occurring disorders in the criminal justice system. *Behavioral Sciences and the Law, 22*, 431–448.

Crosby, R., Salazar, L.F., Diclemente, R.J., Yarber, W.L., Caliendo, A.M., & Staples-Horne, M. (2004). Health risk factors among detained adolescent females. *American Journal of Preventive Medicine, 27*, 404–410.

Crosby R., DiClemente R.J., Staples-Horne M. (2003). *Health issues of juvenile offenders*. In Moore J. (Ed.). Management and Administration of Correctional Health Care: Policy, Practice, and Administration, Kingston, New Jersey: CRI, Inc; 11.1–11.15.

Diagnostic and statistical manual of mental disorders, 4th ed. (1994) Washington, DC: American Psychiatric Association.

Eaton D.K., Kann, L., Kinchen, S., Ross, J., Hawkins, J., Harris, W.A., Lowry, R., McManus, T., Chyen, D., Shanklin, S., Lim, C., Grunbaum, J.A., & Wechsler, H. (2006). Youth risk behavior surveillance—United States 2005. *MMWR Surveillance Summaries, 55*, 1–108.

Estelle v Gamble, 429 US 97 (1976).

Feinstein, R., Greenblatt, A., Hass, L., Kohn, S., & Rana, J. (2001*). Justice for all? A report on lesbian, gay, bisexual, and transgendered youth in the New York juvenile justice system*. New York: Lesbian and Gay Project of the Urban Justice Center.

Feinstein, R.A., Lampkin, A., Lorish, C.D., Klerman, L.V., Maisiak, R., & Oh, M.K. (1998). Medical status of adolescents at time of admission to a juvenile detention center. *Journal of Adolescent Health, 22*, 190–196.

Fields, J. (2003). Children's living arrangements and characteristics: March 2002. *Current Population Reports*. Washington, DC: Census Bureau.

Garofalo, R., Wolf, R.C., Kessel, S, Palfrey, J., & Durant, R.H. (1998). The association between health risk behaviors and sexual orientation among a school-based sample of adolescents. *Pediatrics, 5*, 895–902.

Gavdos, C. (2005). Nucleic acid amplification tests for gonorrhea and chlamydia: Practice and applications. *Infectious Diseases Clinics of North America, 19*, 367–386.

Goldenring, J., & Cohen, E. (1988). Getting into adolescents heads. *Community Pediatrics, 5,* 75–90.

Hammett, T.M. (1998). *Public health/corrections collaborations: Prevention and treatment of HIV/AIDS, STDs and TB.* National Institute of Justice Centers for Disease Control and Prevention. Research in Brief.

Hein, K., Cohen, M.I., & Litt, I.F. (1980). Juvenile detention: Another boundary issue for physicians. *Pediatrics, 66,* 239–245.

Huerta, K., Berkelhamer, S., Klein, J., Ammerman, S., Chang, J., & Prober, C.G. (1996). Epidemiology of herpes simplex virus type 2 infections in a high-risk adolescent population. *Journal of Adolescent Health, 18,* 384–386.

Huppert, J.S., & Adams Hillard, P.K. (2003). Sexually transmitted disease screening in teens. *Current Women's Health Report, 2,* 451–458.

Kahn, R.H., Mosure, D.J., Blank, S., Kent, C.K., Chow, J.M., Boudov, M.R., Brock, J., Tulloch, S., & Jail STD Prevalence Monitoring Project. (2005). Chlamydia trachomatis and Neisseria gonorrhoeae prevalence and coinfection in adolescents entering selected US juvenile detention centers, 1997–2002. *Sexually Transmitted Diseases, 32,* 55–59.

Lauritsen, J. (2003). *How families and communities influence youth victimization.* OJJDP Juvenile Justice Bulletin. Washington, DC: U.S. Department of Justice, Office of Justice Programs, Office of Juvenile Justice and Delinquency Prevention.

Lipsey, M.W. (1992). *Juvenile delinquency treatment: A meta-analytic inquiry into the variability of effects.* In T. Cook et al. (Eds.), Meta-analysis for explanation: A casebook (pp. 83–127). New York: Sage.

Lofy, K.H., Hofmann, J., Mosure, D.J., Fine, D.N., & Marrazzo, J.M. (2006). Chlamydial infections among female adolescents screened in juvenile detention centers in Washington State, 1998–2002. *Sexually Transmitted Diseases, 33,* 63–67.

MacGowan, R.J., Margolis, A.D., Gaiter, J., Morrow, K., Zack, B., Askew, J., McAuliffe, T., Sosman, J.M., Eldridge, G., & the Project START Study Group. (2003). Predictors of risky sex of young men after release from prison. *International Journal of STDs and AIDs, 14,* 519–523.

Madrid v Gomez, 889 F Supp 1146, 9617277v2. US 9th Circuit Court of Appeals (ND CA 1995).

McCurley, C., & Snyder, H. (2006). *Risk, protection, and family structure.* OJJDP Juvenile Justice Bulletin.Washington, DC: U.S. Department of Justice, Office of Justice Programs, Office of Juvenile Justice and Delinquency Prevention.

Morrison, D.M., Baker, S.A., & Gillmore, M.R. (1994). Sexual risk behavior, knowledge, and condom use among adolescents in juvenile detention. *Journal of Youth and Adolescence, 23,* 271–288.

National Center for Health Statistics. (2003). Estimates of the July 1, 2000 and July 1, 2001, United States resident population from the Vintage 2001 postcensal series by year, age, sex, race, and Hispanic origin, prepared under a collaborative arrangement with the U.S. Census Bureau.

National Institute of Justice. (1999). *Arrestee Drug Abuse Monitoring Program: 1998 Annual Report on Drug Use Among Adult and Juvenile Arrestees,* Washington, DC: Author.

Parent, D., Leiter, V., Kennedy, S., Livens, I., Wentworth, D., & Wilcox, S. (1994). *Conditions of confinement: Detention and corrections facilities.* Washington, DC: U.S. Department of Justice, Office of Juvenile Justice and Delinquency Prevention.

Prescott, L. (1998). *Improving policy and practice for adolescent girls with co-occurring disorders in the juvenile justice system.* Delmar, NY: National GAINS Center.

Reddy, D.M., Fleming, R., & Swain, C. (2002). Effect of mandatory parental notification on adolescent girls' use of sexual health care services. *Journal of the American Medical Association, 288,* 710–714.

Ries, B., & Saewyc, E. (1999). Selected finding of eight population-based studies as they pertain to anti-gay harassment and the safety and well-being of sexual minority students. Safe Schools Coalition of Washington, 1–29.

Robertson, A.A., & Thomas, C.B. (2005). Predictors of infection with chlamydia or gonorrhea in incarcerated adolescents. *Sexually Transmitted Diseases, 32*, 15–22.

Ruiz v Estelle, 503 F Supp 1265 (SD Tex 1980).

Savin-Williams, R.C. (1994). Verbal and physical abuse as stressors in the lives of lesbian, gay male and bisexual youths: Associations with school problems, running away, substance abuse, prostitution, and suicide. *Journal of Consulting and Clinical Psychology, 62,* 261–269.

Snyder, H., & Sickmund,M. (2006*). Juvenile offenders and victims: 2006 National Report*. Washington, DC: U.S. Department of Justice, Office of Justice Programs, Office of Juvenile Justice and Delinquency Prevention.

Strack, R., & Alexander, C. (2000). *Report of the Monitoring of Adolescents in Risky Situations (MARS) Project: Findings from the 1999 Out-of-Home Youth Survey*. Baltimore: Department of Health and Mental Hygiene.

Teplin, L., Abram, K., McClellan, G., Washburn, J., & Pikus, A. (2005). Detecting mental disorders in juvenile detainees who receive services. *American Journal of Public Health, 95*, 1773–1780.

Tjaden, P., & Thoennes, N. (2000). Full report of the prevalence, incidence, and consequences of violence against women: Findings from the National Violence Against Women Survey. Washington, DC: National Institute of Justice Report NCJ 183781.

Treadwell, H., & Formicola, A. (2005). Improving the oral health of prisoners to improve overall health and well-being. *American Journal of Public Health, 95*, 1677–1678.

U.S. Census Bureau. (2004). *Annual demographic survey, March supplement, 2004. POV01, age and sex of all people, family members and unrelated individuals iterated by income-to-poverty ratio and race*.

U.S. Census Bureau. (2004). *U.S. Interim Projections by Age, Sex, Race, and Hispanic Origin*. http://www.census.gov/ipc/www/usinterimInternet Release Date: March 18, 2004.

U.S. Census Bureau. (2007). *Annual Estimates of the Population by Five-Year Age Groups and Sex for the United States: April 1, 2000 to July 1, 2006*. (NC-EST2006-01)

Wasserman, G.A., McReynolds, L.S., Lucas, C.P., Fisher, P., & Santos, L. (2002). The voice DISC-IV with incarcerated male youths: Prevalence of disorder. *Journal of the American Academy of Child and Adolescent Psychiatry, 41*, 314–321.

Zigler, E., Taussig, C., & Black, K. (1992) Early childhood intervention. A promising preventative for juvenile delinquency. *American Psychologist, 47*, 997–1006.

Chapter 19

Female Prisoners and the Case for Gender-Specific Treatment and Reentry Programs

Andrea F. Balis

The rapidly rising prison, jail, and probation population is clearly a concern for the entire criminal justice system, but this is especially true in the case of female prisoners. Arrests over the last 20 years have increased for the general population, but the increase is significantly larger among females. A 1998 Justice Department study reported that since 1990 the female adult jail population grew 7.0% while the male adult jail population grew 4.5% during the same time period (BJS, 1999b). Between midyear 2004 and midyear 2005 the number of women under the jurisdiction of the state and federal prison systems grew by 3.4% while the number of men grew by 1.3% (BJS, 2006) Despite these significant changes in the incarcerated population, there has not been a commensurate increase in research devoted to the needs of these women, nor in designing discharge and reentry programs specifically for female prisoners.

There are significant demographic and statistical differences between male and female inmates. Women's needs are different because they are much more likely to have been physically and/or sexually abused then men, both as adults and as children. (BJS 1999; Bloome, Owen, Schenes, & Rosenbaum, 2002; Grey, Mays, & Stohr, 2005; Green, Miranda, Daroowalla, & Siddique, 2005). They are much more likely than men to be responsible for the supervision of children (BJS, 2000; Dalley, 2002; Freudenberg, 2002; Radosh, 2002; Grella & Greenwell, 2006) . They are more likely to be addicted to drugs and to have committed their offense while under the influence of drugs and/or alcohol than men. They are much more likely to suffer from mental illness than men. They have a higher prevalence of HIV/AIDS, sexually transmitted diseases, and chronic illness than men (Blank et al., 1999; Farley et al., 2000; Hogben & Lawrence, 2000, BJS, 2001a; Staton, & Webster, 2003). They are more likely to have been unemployed before their arrest (BJS, 2004). Women who have been in jail or prison are more likely to be stigmatized than men (Richie, Freudenberg, & Page, 2001). Their crimes are somewhat different than men's, including commercial sex work and less violent crime and burglary.

The sharp rise in the number of women who are arrested, convicted, and jailed is, at least in part, a reflection of tougher drug laws and mandatory sentencing practices. Under those laws, women whose drug offenses were relatively minor are punished as severely as more serious offenses committed by men, a situation compounded by the fact that women generally have less information to trade for reduced charges (Radosh, 2002).

The percentage of incarcerated women serving drug sentences has risen from 15% in 1979 to 45% in 1999 (BJS, 1999b). Furthermore, 64% of the females arrested for any reason in 1996 tested positive for illegal drugs at the time of arrest (BJS, 2001a). For a variety of reasons, drug use and dependency is higher among women in the criminal justice system; one study reported that 52% of females have a history of dependency on illicit drugs, versus 44% of males (BJS, 2005b).

While in nondrug cases adult women are generally sentenced to less time than men for the same crime, in the case of juveniles the opposite is true. Teenage girls are detained for less serious offenses than are boys. One study reported that 29% of females versus 19% of males were detained for minor offenses such as public disorder, traffic violation, and status offenses. Underage girls were much more likely to be returned to detention for probation violations or technical violations. They are particularly disproportionately punished for running away, perhaps because they are seen as more vulnerable, or more in need of social control (American Bar Association, 2001).

As concern over this growing population within the criminal justice system has increased, it has become clear that there need to be different institutional practices, treatment programs, and systems of discharge planning. Because of less research on women than men, there is still little specific information on the effectiveness of rehabilitation and reentry programs for women. Without addressing these issues, it is unlikely that there will be significant reductions in recidivism statistics. In addition, if these numbers keep on increasing, whole communities, especially children, will suffer from the loss of these women.

Prior Abuse

Female inmates have a shockingly high incidence of being abused. Bureau of Justice statistics suggest that well over half of female prisoners were physically and/or sexually abused, while only about 15% of male prisoners had been abused. These findings indicate that between 23 and 27% of female offenders were abused before the age of 18, about twice as high as the rate in the general female population (BJS, 1999a). Other studies put the percentage of female prisoners who have been abused even higher. A 1995 study reported that 75.1% of female prisoners had been physically abused during the year before their arrest. Sixty-eight percent claimed they had been forced to have sexual activity as adults. Forty-eight percent of female prisoners said they had been sexually abused under the age of 18 (Singer, Bussey, Song, & Lunghofer, 1995). Among 14 to 18-year-old girls who are already in the criminal justice system, between 75 and 90% report having been abused. Abused and neglected girls and women are twice as likely to be arrested, both as juveniles and as adults, as those who were not abused. This is in contrast to boys and men, where abuse is not as clearly a predictor of future incarcerations.

Not only do girls and women suffer more serious victimization than men and boys, they often react differently to that abuse. Women are much more likely than men to respond with self-blame and depression. Male abuse victims are more likely than women to engage in aggression or violence Women who have been abused are more likely to turn to alcohol and drugs than to respond with violent behavior. As adults, men report that they feel less vulnerable to sexual abuse, but women feel more vulnerable (McClellan, Farabee, & Crouch, 1997). Eighty-nine percent of women who reported that they were abused used drugs regularly.

Girls are more likely to be abused if they grow up in foster care than if they live with at least one parent. They are twice as likely to have been abused if they grew up in a family where there is drug abuse, and a third more likely to be abused if a member of the family was incarcerated. Childhood sexual abuse has been linked to a variety of high–risk behaviors, including unprotected sex with multiple partners and sharing needles. Those who have been abused are more likely to exhibit these behaviors. Neglected children who grow up with little supervision are less likely to learn coping skills. They are less likely to learn to plan. They are more likely to turn to prostitution than girls who have not been abused, and are younger at their first incarceration (Mullings, Marquart, & Hartley, 2003).

Clearly then, childhood abuse and trauma set the stage for later criminal behavior. The children of incarcerated parents, especially mothers, who are more likely to have been living with their children prior to arrest than fathers, are more likely to be victimized in turn.

Substance Abuse and Mental Health Statistics

It is difficult to assess the prevalence of mental illness and substance abuse in many correctional systems with any certainty since in many women's prisons there is inadequate screening when inmates arrive making it impossible to determine the severity of some of these problems. A 2001 survey of services found only 72% of jails for women screen for substance abuse, only 70% screen for mental health problems, 60% screen for physical problems, and fewer than 30% screen for math and reading ability, childhood abuse, spousal abuse, or parenting needs. Worse still, only 10% of women prisoners who are drug abusers are offered treatment (BJS, 2000; Richie et al., 2001).

Justice Department figures indicate that in 2002, more than two-thirds of female jail inmates were dependent on or abused alcohol or drugs. Inmates who were dependent were more likely to have previous criminal records (Staton et al., 2003). A 1993 study, published in the *American Journal of Public Health*, reported that 80% of New York City's female detainees had cocaine in their urine at the time of arrest (Blank et al., 1999).

One study of female prisoners in Kentucky found that 90% of inmates had a history of substance abuse problems, 62% reported symptoms of depression, 53% reported anxiety disorders, and 43% reported difficulty in concentration. Women's drug use differs from that of men in many ways. There are gender differences in the etiology of substance abuse, and in the relative success of various treatment modalities. The fact that women are more likely to have histories of physical and sexual abuse, as well as coexisting psychiatric disorders, and have measurably lower self-esteem than men clearly needs to be taken into account when developing resources.

Illicit drug use can be a way of coping with past or present abuse. It is often a behavior that is embedded in social relationships. Drug use is frequently initiated by a sex partner; continued use becomes part of the fabric of primary relationships (Messina, Burdon, Hagopian, & Prendergast, 2006). These statistics are themselves disturbing, but they take on even more meaning when they are considered in the broader context of substance abuse programs and mental health treatment. A 1995 series of interviews in municipal jails found that according to the Global Severity Index of the Brief System Inventory, 64% of female inmates tested in the clinical range for mental health problems (Singer et al., 1995). Despite these remarkably high figures, women in some correctional systems tend to receive fewer services than male prisoners.

As an example, the Cook County Department of Corrections initiated a longitudinal study which examined what proportion of female and male detainees with mental disorders received treatment while in jail. The Cook County system actually does screen all detainees, although their treatment resources are very limited. Detainees were evaluated using standard instruments, the Brief Psychiatric Rating Scale and the Referral Decision Scale. They were classified as needing treatment if they had been previously diagnosed with schizophrenia or a major affective disorder and were symptomatic within 2 weeks of the interview, had severe cognitive impairment at the time of the interview, or if the subject reported a history of substance abuse and was disoriented at the time of the interview. According to these criteria, 10.7% of detainees needed mental health services. The study subjects were then followed for 6 months, or until their records were disposed of. It was determined that 23.5% of all female detainees received services, as opposed to 37% of all male inmates. The study concluded that in addition to gender, diagnosis had an effect on whether or not a detainee received treatment. Depression was the diagnosis least likely to be treated. In fact, only 3.5% of detainees suffering from depression received treatment. Women in jail have depression rates 4 times higher than men (Teplin, Abram, & McClelland, 1997).

Medical Problems

Access to health services is strained in our society in general, in prisons in particular, and in women's prisons most of all. Despite their rapidly growing numbers, women are still a small percentage of the prison population, and for that reason it has sometimes been considered less cost-effective to provide care for drug abuse and addiction, mental health issues, and counseling for trauma and posttraumatic stress disorder for incarcerated females (Teplin et al., 1997; Zaitzow, 2001).

One obvious significant and gender-specific health care issue is the need for adequate gynecological and obstetric services. At least 6% of female prisoners are pregnant when they are arrested. Since not all prisons and jails test all women, the prevalence of pregnancy is likely higher. For example, studies have found that about 18% of female inmates had given birth at some point during a past or present incarceration (Acoca, 1998; BJS, 1999b; National Institute of Justice, 2000; Women's and Children's Health Policy Center, 2000).

In the broadest terms, incarcerated women are less healthy than incarcerated men. Many women had poor health care prior to their arrest and incarceration. They are frequently survivors of sexual and physical abuse. Many are sex workers and are therefore exposed to both abuse and sexually transmitted diseases. Many have not received routine gynecological care and have not been treated for reproductive system disorders (Braithwaite, Treadwell, & Arriola, 2005). Many women have numerous health issues that are masked by drug dependency. Once sober, mental and physical health issues become apparent, ranging from dental problems to chronic infections.

Studies have demonstrated an extremely high prevalence of sexually transmitted diseases among female prison inmates. Not all those infected are diagnosed, because many facilities only test women who are symptomatic or who request testing. One study estimated that between 11 and 17% of women tested positive for chlamydia infection, while 9% tested positive for gonococcus infection. Juvenile facilities reported an even higher prevalence of infection. In Chicago, among female prisoners, the incidence of infection with chlamydia was 27% and that of gonococcus was 11%; the Birmingham rates were 22% and 17% (CDC, 1999). Annual data from the California Department of Corrections demonstrate an incidence among women of positive skin testing for tuberculosis of between 20 and 30%. In contrast, less than 0.5% of the general population demonstrate a positive skin test for tuberculosis. Another study from the California Department of Corrections showed that 54% of female prisoners tested positive for hepatitis C, as opposed to 39% of male prisoners (Acoca, 1998; CDC, 2005).

HIV/AIDS statistics are even more disturbing. Groups disproportionately affected by HIV/AIDS are the same socioeconomic and ethnic groups that are disproportionately represented in the prison population. Confirmed AIDS cases are three times higher in correction systems than in the United States as a whole.

The segment of society currently most affected by rising AIDS rates is that of adolescent and adult females (BJS, 2005a). There are a number of factors which account for the extremely high prevalence among females in the prison population. A large percentage of incarcerated women have a history of intravenous drug use, and studies have shown that many incarcerated women have shared needles. Incarcerated women have often traded sex for money or for drugs. Furthermore, the facts that women have poor health in general and high rates of sexually transmitted genital ulcer diseases in particular leave them vulnerable to infection with HIV.

Studies vary in their estimates of HIV prevalence but all demonstrate a higher percentage of HIV infection among female inmates than among males. One study reported that 2.2% of male offenders and 3.5% of female offenders are known to be HIV positive (Zaitzow, 2001; BJS 2005a). Many states do not test all entering inmates. Policies vary greatly from system to system but only 18 of 51 jurisdictions test all inmates on admission. The most common practice is to test inmates who exhibit symptoms or who ask to be tested. This is the case in 44 of 51 jurisdictions. Fifteen states test inmates who are in high-risk groups. Four jurisdictions and the Bureau of Prisons test inmates at release (Women and Children's Health Policy Center, 2000; Zaitzow, 2001). These cases are not distributed equally around the country. New York, Florida, and Texas have the largest number of identified HIV-positive inmates, accounting for 48% of confirmed AIDS cases. In New York, which does periodic blind testing, 14.6% of female inmates and 7.3% of male inmates were known to be HIV-positive (BJS, 2005a).

While many states provide state-of-the-art antiretroviral treatment to prisoners, the treatment of HIV requires specialist involvement. Most of the time, prison primary care doctors do not have the training and expertise to effectively treat infected women, and even if they do, they may lack the facilities and staff to do so, or a system to provide follow-up care (Farley et al., 2000; Zaitzow, 2001).

Theoretically, prison would seem to be an ideal situation for monitoring and treating disease, and for managing chronic conditions, from tuberculosis to HIV/AIDS. Instead, not only is there insufficient testing and limited treatment, there are often insufficient connections with health services outside the corrections system to provide further care. As a result, women may leave prison as sick as or sicker than when they arrived and in many cases they leave prison with insufficiently treated contagious diseases which can and will affect the community as a whole (Collica, 2002; Freudenberg, 2002, Braithwaite et al., 2005). Their health may deteriorate and they may wind up in emergency rooms, and in hospital beds, care which is significantly more expensive than treatment would have been within the prison system.

While these are issues for both men and women, they become gender specific, or perhaps more accurately gender critical, because without successful treatment and reentry programs women will have little choice but to return to a cycle of drug addiction, crime, and/or the sex trade.

Conceptual Challenges to Creating Effective Treatment and Reentry Programs for Women

Any attempt to design effective programs for women must take into account the statistical differences mentioned above, but they must also be responsive to the difference in gender roles and socioeconomic identity in contemporary society.

Female prisoners have unique needs because much of the time they are victims, not perpetrators, of crime. Programs that do not take into account the fact that so many women have histories of abuse and neglect and have witnessed and been the victim of domestic violence both as children and as adults are doomed to failure. A successful program intended to reintegrate women into society has to find ways to help women to have a sense of "agency." Women need, not as a luxury but as an essential need, a sense that they can alter their social environment (Bloome et al., 2002).

Women are more stigmatized by incarceration than men are. Their return to the world is therefore already more difficult. Over 80% have children, and they are often single parents. Men are far more likely to find that they can return to wives or girlfriends who have taken care of their children and kept family life functioning than are women (BJS, 2000).

Put another way, women prisoners tend to have a "social capital" deficit. That is, women, and especially women from low socioeconomic standing, and even more especially those with young children, are not tied into the information systems that help an individual acquire skills and knowledge, networks which help in finding employment, and contacts for financial assistance. All too often they return to the community with the same lack of resources they had before, but now they have a prison record (Reisig, Holtfreter, & Morash, 2002).

The successful reentry of female offenders is dependent on helping them to find and connect to networks that will provide them with structural resources. Any program that is going to work has to be holistic; for example, it is not enough to provide employment and education programs and substance abuse treatment, important as those needs are, without also considering these women in their social context, as part of communities and families, and as mothers. Many female prisoners strongly identify with their role as parents. They are motivated to succeed in treatment programs in order to regain or keep custody of their children (Mullings et al., 2003; Surratt, 2003).

To succeed, reentry programs must provide mental health counseling. Given the frequency of abuse and neglect, it is not surprising that so many female inmates suffer from low self-esteem, as well as depression and anxiety disorders (Singer et al., 1995; BJS, 2000). But the actual figures are staggering. A 2002 study of female juvenile offenders reported that 95.8% suffered from low self-esteem. In this study, 88.6% of the participants said they had been sexually abused, and 77.1% claimed to have been physically abused. On testing, 74.1% were found to have a developmental disability, and 73.5% were suffering from severe mental trauma as a result of abuse (Bloome et al., 2002).

Not surprisingly, outcome predictors for reentry programs seem to be different for men and for women. Inmates treated in residential treatment followed by outpatient treatment in the community have lower rates of drug relapse and rearrest. But in the case of women, more than with men, there was a distinct correlation with the length of the program. In the case of female inmates the length of time they spent in aftercare was a useful predictor of success. The outcome for women in extended treatment programs was better than the outcome for men (Hall, Prendergast, Hellish, Patten, & Cho, 2004; Messina et al., 2006). There is also a strong association between lower recidivism rates for women and having health insurance, as long as it includes treatment for mental illness and substance abuse, as well as treatment for chronic diseases, including but by no means limited to HIV/AIDS (Richie et al., 2001).

For women, other than the length of time in treatment the most important predictor for successful reentry is reducing the proportion of income that comes from illegal activity, which makes education and employment issues as critical as substance abuse treatment and mental health services. A second predictor is reducing homelessness. Without a job and a home, women will be back on the streets.

This supports the social capital argument in many ways. Education expands networks which increase the likelihood of stable employment. A settled home provides structure which makes emotional and social support possible. These can include traditional community based institutions like Twelve Step Programs (Reisig et al., 2002). Participating in these systems also counteracts the antisocial lifestyle that so often persists into adulthood for so many abused and neglected children, especially girls (National Institute of Justice, 2000).

It is reasonable to suggest that current methods for reducing rearrest figures are not successful. Many of the women who are in prison are the sole support of their families. Their children suffer while they are in jail, and when they get out they have fewer resources than they had when they were arrested. They haven't "learned a lesson"; they have little choice or incentive to do anything but return to the behavior for which they were arrested. The lesson they are passing on to their children is a continuing cycle of abandonment and hopelessness. Removing nonviolent offenders doesn't make the community safer, it weakens the community. These women need health care, drug treatment, and mental health treatment, as well as job training and parenting skills.

They are lonely and isolated and they have to be connected to productive communities. Family focused programs are essential as is effective discharge planning and follow-up care. These must be multifaceted and must address all of the relationships through which women tend to define themselves, including the family, social structure, employment, and childrearing practices.

Case Studies

There are programs designed to address the problem of female detainees within the criminal justice system. In 1992 the National Juvenile Justice and Delinquency Prevention Act of 1974 was reauthorized. The new language included directives specifically mandating the development of programs that addressed the needs of female juveniles. These programs were to focus on health and mental health services, education and vocational training, and parenting skills. Despite best intentions, a successful gender-specific program required a paradigm shift; without one the needs of women and girls cannot be met. For example, the criminal justice system is frequently organized so as to place juveniles as close to home as possible. While sensible and humane on the one hand, establishing that kind of procedure ignores the well-documented reality that many female juveniles have been sexually and/or physically abused, and in many cases the abuser was a member of the family or a close family friend. Proximity may not be a positive in those cases.

Many jurisdictions have moved to develop new programs and establish parity in terms of services for females. A best-practices study commissioned in 1997 found that while most of the programs they evaluated tried to provide counseling and skills training (though frequently they were underfunded and understaffed), health services were inadequate. There was very little emphasis on providing the young women with information about sexually transmitted diseases, family planning, or parenting skills. Substance abuse treatment was provided at about only half of the programs evaluated, and in many cases this primarily meant referrals to local Twelve Step Programs. Very few of these programs addressed the important issues of victimization and prior abuse, and without that component the needs of these young women would not be met (Bloome et al., 2002).

A study done by the Women's and Children's Health Policy Center at Johns Hopkins University School of Public Health recommended that providing ongoing integrated services that coordinated pre- and postrelease care was a critical component in reentry programs for women. They also found that programs for women generally fell into four main categories.

- Nursery programs which allow incarcerated women to keep their infants for a period of time and care for them while receiving child development education. There are several of these in New York State and Nebraska.
- Mentoring programs that stress self-esteem.
- Programs following self-help models, connecting women with networks of survivors, such as incest survivors, sexual and physical abuse survivors.
- A fourth group provide health and education services, which is clearly a broad description (Women's and Children's Health Policy Center, 2000).

Despite certain limitations there are certainly many programs which are innovative and sensitive to the needs of the populations they serve. The few briefly discussed below are examples chosen from among many others.

Healthlink, which began in 1992, is a program in New York City intended to reduce female recidivism through a comprehensive program to help women reintegrate into the community; it is also intended to help strengthen community institutions. The theoretical basis of the program is empowerment theory. The idea is to strengthen individuals and to make them realize that they can effect change both in their own lives and in their community. In turn, by providing services for inmates with their communities, the local networks are themselves strengthened. Community providers are empowered, and develop expertise which allows them to expand, and help more members of the community. As these provider organizations become stronger, they can begin to affect politics and social policy. This program creates the social networks so important to success, as well as repairing the social capital deficit that so often exists in lower socioeconomic communities. Healthlink focuses on two specific neighborhoods, which account for 15% of inmates in city jails, and in which the HIV/AIDS prevalence, and drug dependence, are more than twice as high as the rest of the city. The program stresses that its approach is client-centered, and services begin before release with discharge planning and counseling. The program includes residential treatment services as well as counseling and assistance with education, employment and housing. Counseling continues for 1 year after release, with the same counselor whenever possible. This coordinated and continuous care is critical to the success of the program. A 1-year postrelease study that compared women who had services only while in jail and women who had postrelease services found significant differences. The women who did not participate in the postrelease program had a rearrest rate of 59%, while the women who did participate had a 38% rearrest rate (Richie et al., 2001).

A Michigan program, Project PROVE (Post Release Opportunities for Vocational Education), operates on a different model of empowerment. The program was founded to address the issue that while education and training are supposed to be a critical part of rehabilitation, too often programs for women are limited, consisting primarily of training in cosmetology and clerical skills. Dead-end, poorly paid jobs weaken "workplace attachment," and increase the chance that women will be forced to obtain money illegally. The more a woman gets money illegally, the more likely she is to return to prison. Therefore, the goal of the program is to develop a model of reintegration that provides stability to former inmates and to the community through educational programs, housing assistance, and substance abuse counseling. In addition to mentoring, and assistance in finding employment, PROVE provides very practical help. They supply tutoring as well as counseling. They help women fill out applications. They can also pay off student loans, pay for licensing exam fees, and provide tuition assistance. This program, too, focuses on community networks and social capital though it does it rather differently.

Rhode Island programs are organized around a medical model (Farley et al., 2000). The state has only one prison, and a large number of HIV positive prisoners; 4% of males and 8% of females test positive during mandatory testing at admission. Rhode Island also has a high recidivism rate; 62% of women are reincarcerated between 2 and 10 times. The major source of HIV transmission seems to be use of intravenous drugs. The state developed a program intended to reduce both recidivism and the spread of HIV. The premise of the program is that multiple ongoing therapeutic relationships could help inmates plan for their discharges, prevent drug relapse, and encourage stability after release. Some of that counseling comes from peers and the contact continues after release. Another basic principle is that discharge planning is essential to remove women from situations that predispose them to drug use and sex work, because women are especially vulnerable immediately after release. In order to be eligible for the program, a woman has to be either an intravenous drug user, a commercial sex worker, or have a history of recidivism along with a poor educational background and poor work experience. While in prison the participants develop a relationship with a physician and a social worker. The program is focused on substance abuse issues, health care issues, and previous abuse. The same staff member remains in contact with the prisoner after discharge whenever possible. These combined services have proven successful; when compared to the general population discharged at the same time, these high-risk women have a lower recidivism rate. At 3 months the control group recidivism rate was 18.5% while the rate for women in the study was 5%. At 1 year after release, the recidivism rate for the general prison population was 45% while the rate for the women in the study was 33%. The women who stayed out of jail also reported a higher rate of condom use and a lower number of sexual partners.

While there are distinctions among these plans, all are holistic and integrate a wide variety of services, and all provide health care, education, and substance abuse treatment. All acknowledge social capital deficits and try to build new capital.

A Chain that Must Be Broken

An essential part of the "American" character is independence. Individuals are expected to pull themselves up by their bootstraps, and make something of themselves. As a society we believe that we are free to choose our own path, and are responsible for our behavior. But most of the women who are in prison were exposed as children to violence, abuse, drugs, and alcohol—all long before they were old enough to be making their own choices.

Most women in prison have children. Most of them understand that there is a connection between the trauma they suffered as children and their adult problems (Greene, Haney, & Hurtado, 2000). They say that they want to provide their children with something else, but the reality is that they are in prison. In 1997, 64% of the mothers in state prison, and 84% of the mothers in federal prison, had at least one of their children living with them at the time of their arrest (BJS, 2000). Even if they can maintain custody of their children, and many cannot, they have abandoned them for the length of their sentence. Their children will be placed in the foster care system, which statistically increases the risk of abuse for their children, as described above. Their children will grow up without the watchful eye of a parent and they are likely to run away, to turn to drugs and alcohol.

This isn't to suggest that these women should not be held responsible, but rather to suggest that the fact that so many of the women in prison were victims is relevant—and not just to them, but to society as a whole (Green et al., 2005).

In a California study, investigators interviewed female prisoners in three jails. All of them were mothers, with an average of 2.5 children. Most of them, 71%, lived with their children at the time of their arrest and expected to do so after their release. Seventy-one percent of the women said that they had been addicted to drugs and/or alcohol at one time. Seventy-nine percent had been arrested before. They had unstable upbringings; they had moved an average of seven times before they were 18. Eighty-six percent had either been abused or witnessed abuse at home. Sixty-two percent had parents or guardians involved with drugs or alcohol. Fifty-eight percent were involved in sexually abusive relationships as adults. They were raised without parents to protect them and they know that their children are being raised the same way. They reported that 83% of their children had been abused or had witnessed abuse at home. Their children, average age 10, had moved an average of three times (Greene et al., 2000).

Women place a high value on parenting and that including mothers in prison, and mothers who are dependent on drugs or alcohol. Perhaps there are better ways to make use of that desire. To protect their children we have passed laws that take them away from their parents, though as a society we do not have much to put in their place. The families of inmates may already be stretched to the limit. We have a severely stressed foster care system. Several decades of using the fear of losing their children to discipline mothers or as reminders of the value of self-reliance have not worked. Statistics suggest that they have not "learned their lesson." And they surely have not been "rehabilitated." We have to find an alternative because otherwise we are perpetuating a tragic cycle.

We all have a stake in finding better programs for female prisoners. The same things that make their situation unique have an impact on all of us. These women do not stay in jail forever and we don't want to see their children headed in that direction. Instead of making use of a moment for providing health care for an underserved population, and controlling chronic and infectious disease, we let the opportunity pass by. Over half of female inmates said that they had reported a condition requiring medical attention. About 28% got treatment within the prison system (BJS, 2001a). Without intervention these women will return to prison, but before they do, they will return to the streets, and many will return to sex work. They are part of our community, and they share their poor health with us. They pay. Their children pay. We all pay.

Things to consider:

- Female prisoners have different problems than male prisoners; treatment and reentry programs need to be tailored to their needs.
- To be effective, any reentry program for women must be holistic in nature. It must include substance treatment, psychological counseling, health care, education, and ongoing emotional support.
- The most successful programs include pre- and postrelease components. Continuity of staff is extremely valuable.
- Women who are mothers need to learn parenting skills for their own self-esteem and for the sake of their children, so that their children are not trapped in the same cycle.

References

Acoca, L. (1998). Defusing the time bomb: Understanding and meeting the growing health care needs of incarcerated women in America. *Crime and Delinquency, 44*, 49–69.

American Bar Association & National Bar Association. (2001). *Justice by gender: The lack of appropriate prevention, diversion and treatment alternatives for girls in the juvenile justice system.* Washington, DC.

Blank, S., Sternberg, M., Neylans, L.L., Rubin, S.R., Weisfuse, I.B., & Louis, M.E. (1999). Incident syphilis among women with multiple admissions to jail in New York City. *Journal of Infectious Diseases, 180,* 1159–1163.

Bloome, B., Owen, B., Deschenes, E.P., & Rosenbaum, J. (2002), Moving toward justice for female juvenile offenders in the new millennium: Modeling gender–specific policies and programs. *Journal of Contemporary Criminal Justice, 18,* 37–56.

Braithwaite, R.L., Treadwell, H.M., & Arriola, K.R.J. (2005). Health disparities and incarcerated women: A population ignored. *American Journal of Public Health, 95,* 1679–1681.

Bureau of Justice Statistics. (1999a). *Prior abuse reported by inmates and probationers.* Washington, DC: U.S. Department of Justice.

Bureau of Justice Statistics. (1999b). *Special report: Women offenders.* Washington, DC: U.S. Department of Justice.

Bureau of Justice Statistics. (2000). *Special report: Incarcerated parents and their children.* Washington, DC: U.S. Department of Justice.

Bureau of Justice Statistics. (2001a). *Special report: Medical problems of inmates, 1997.* Washington, DC: U.S. Department of Justice.

Bureau of Justice Statistics. (2001b). *Special report: Mental health treatment in state prisons, 2000.* Washington, DC: U.S. Department of Justice.

Bureau of Justice Statistics. (2004). *Special report: Profile of jail inmates, 2002.* Washington, DC: U.S. Department of Justice.

Bureau of Justice Statistics. (2005a). *Bulletin: HIV in prisons, 2003.* Washington, DC: U.S. Department of Justice.

Bureau of Justice Statistics. (2005b). *Special report: Substance dependence, abuse, and treatment of jail inmates, 2002.* Washington, DC: U.S. Department of Justice.

Bureau of Justice Statistics. (2006). *Special report: Prison and jail inmates at midyear 2005.* Washington, DC: U.S. Department of Justice.

Center for Disease Control, (1999) *High Prevalence of Chlamydial and Gonococcal Infection in Women Entering Jails and Juvenile Detention Centers.* Morbidity and Mortality Weekly Report, *48*(36), 793–776.

Center for Disease Control, (2006) *Trends in Tuberculosis, United States, 2005.* Morbidity and Mortality Weekly Report, *55*(11), 305–308.

Collica, K. (2002). Levels of knowledge and risk perceptions about HIV? AIDS among female inmates in New York State: Can prison-based HIV programs set the stage for behavior change? *The Prison Journal, 82,* 101–124.

Dalley, L. (2002). Policy implications relating to inmate mothers and their children: Will the past be prologue? *The Prison Journal, 82,* 243–268.

Farley, J.L., Mitty, J.A., Lally, M.A., Burzynski, J., Tashima, K., Rich, J.D., et.al. (2000). Comprehensive medical care among HIV-positive incarcerated women: The Rhode Island experience. *Journal of Women's Health & Gender-Based Medicine, 9,* 51–56.

Freudenberg, N. (2002). Adverse effects of US jail and prison policies on the health and well-being of women of color. *American Journal of Public Health, 92,* 1895–1900.

Green, B.L., Miranda, J., Daroowalla, A., & Siddique, J. (2005). Trauma exposure, mental health functioning, and program needs of women in jail. *Crime & Delinquency, 51,* 133–151.

Greene, S., Haney, C., & Hurtado, A.(2000). Cycles of pain: Risk factors in the lives of incarcerated mothers and their children. *The Prison Journal, 80,* 3–23.

Grella, C.E., & Greenwell, L. (2006). Correlates of parental status and attitudes toward parenting among substance-abusing women offenders. *The Prison Journal, 86,* 89–113.

Grey, T., Mays, G.L., & Stohr, M.K. (1995). Inmate needs and programming in exclusively women's jails. *The Prison Journal, 75*, 186–202.

Hall, E., Prendergast, M.L., Hellish, J., Patten, M., & Cao, Y. (2004). Treating drug-abusing women prisoners: An outcomes evaluation of the Forever Free Program. *The Prison Journal, 84*, 81–105.

Hogben, M., & Lawrence, J. (2000). HIV/STD risk reduction interventions in prison settings. *Journal of Women's Health & Gender-Based Medicine, 9*, 587–592.

McClellan, D.S., Farabee, D., & Crouch, B.M. (1997). Early victimization, drug use, and criminality: A comparison of male and female prisoners. *Criminal Justice and Behavior, 24*, 455–476.

Messina, N., Burdon,W., Hagopian, J.D., & Prendergast. (2006). Predictors of prison-based treatment outcomes: A comparison of men and women participants. *The American Journal of Drug and Alcohol Abuse, 32*, 7–28.

Mullings, J.L., Marquart, J.W., & Hartley, D.J. (2003). Exploring the effects of child-hood sexual abuse and its impact on HIV/AIDS risk-taking behavior among women prisoners. *The Prison Journal, 83*, 442–463.

National Institute of Justice. (2000). *Research on women and girls in the criminal justice system.* Washington, DC: U.S. Department of Justice.

Radosh, P.F. (2002). Reflections on women's crime and mothers in prison: A peace-making approach. *Crime & Delinquency, 48*, 300–315.

Reisig, M., Holtfreter, K., & Morash, M. (2002). Social capital among women offenders: Examining the distribution of social networks and resources. *Journal of Contemporary Criminal Justice, 18*, 167–187.

Richie, B.E., Freudenberg, N., & Page, J. (2001). Reintegrating women leaving jail into urban communities: A description of a model program. *Journal of Urban Health: Bulletin of the New York Academy of Medicine, 78*, 290–303.

Singer, M.I., Bussey, J., Song, L., & Lunghofer, L. (1995). The psychosocial issues of women serving time in jail. *Social Work, 40*, 103–113.

Staton, M., Leukefeld, C., & Webster, J.M. (2003). Substance use, health, and mental health: Problems and service utilization among incarcerated women. *International Journal of Offender Therapy and Comparative Criminology 47*, 224–239.

Surratt, H. (2003). Parenting attitudes of drug-involved women inmates. *The Prison Journal, 83*, 206–220.

Teplin, L.A., Abram, K.M., & McClelland,G.M. (1997). Mentally disordered women in jail: Who receives services? *American Journal of Public Health, 87*, 604–610.

Women's and Children's Health Policy Center. (2000). *Health issues specific to incarcerated women: Information for state maternal and child health programs.* Baltimore: Johns Hopkins University School of Public Health.

Zaitzow, B.H. (2001). Whose problem is it anyway? Women prisoners and HIVAIDS. *International Journal of Offender Therapy and Comparative Criminology, 45*, 673–690.

Chapter 20

Building the Case for Oral Health Care for Prisoners: Presenting the Evidence and Calling for Justice

Henrie M. Treadwell, Mary E. Northridge, and Traci N. Bethea

Note: Portions of this chapter were previously published in two papers written by the same lead author as for this chapter, Henrie M. Treadwell, and are incorporated into the text of this extended essay with the permission of the publishers who hold the corresponding copyrights. The two papers are:

Treadwell, H. M., & Formicola, A. J. (2005). Improving the oral health of prisoners to improve overall health and well-being. *American Journal of Public Health, 95*(10), 1677–1678.

Treadwell H. M., & Northridge, M. E. (2007). Oral health is the measure of a just society. *Journal of Health Care for the Poor and Underserved, 18*(1), 12–20.

Introduction

In various works of fiction and nonfiction written over time and place [see, e.g., the opening passage of *She Still Lives: A Novel of Tibet* (Magee, 2003)], missing teeth are universally distinguished as the physical markers of having been imprisoned. While few accurate data are available on nonlethal violence behind bars in the United States, missing front teeth in men are a sign of a much larger malignancy in U.S. prisons and jails: physical violence perpetrated by staff against prisoners as well as pervasive assaults among prisoners (Gibbons & Katzanbach, 2006).

There is no need to convince the editors of this volume of the importance of oral health and health care to the overall safety and well-being of incarcerated populations. By including this chapter, they have heeded the advice of former Surgeon General David Satcher in his landmark report *Oral Health in America* to reconnect the mouth to the rest of the body (U.S. Department of Health and Human Services, 2000).

What happens inside jails and prisons does not stay inside jails and prisons. It comes home with prisoners after they are released and with corrections officers at the end of each day's shift. When people live and work in facilities that are unsafe, unhealthy, unproductive, or inhumane, they carry the effects home with them. We must create safe and productive conditions of confinement not only because it is the right thing to do, but because it influences the safety, health, and prosperity of us all. (Gibbons & Katzanbach, 2006, p. 1)

The above quote introduces *Confronting Confinement*, a report on violence and abuse in U.S. jails and prisons, the broad impact of these conditions on public safety and public health, and the steps that correctional facilities can institute to help bring about needed reform (Gibbons & Katzanbach, 2006). Despite the report's stated focus on dangerous conditions of confinement that can also endanger corrections officers and the public, i.e., violence, poor health care, and inappropriate segregation, oral health care was never mentioned in the summary of findings and recommendations of this progressive report.

This omission did not shock or deter us. We have been here before. In October 2005, two of us (H.M.T. and M.E.N.) collaborated on a special issue of the *American Journal of Public Health* devoted to prisons and health. When a formal call for papers and personal solicitations failed to yield any papers on oral health in the prison system, we teamed up with our colleague Allan J. Formicola, D.D.S., former dean of the College of Dental Medicine at Columbia University, to fill this gap through writing and editing a front piece to the issue titled "Improving the Oral Health of Prisoners to Improve Overall Health and Well-Being" (Treadwell & Formicola, 2005).

In our ongoing work with the W. K. Kellogg funded initiative called *Community Voices: Health Care for the Underserved* (see www.communityvoices.org) we have come to appreciate that we cannot ensure overall health absent oral health nor can we secure respectful health care absent oral health care (Formicola et al., 2004). Moreover, when we realized that poor men in this country had become invisible and their health needs were being neglected (see, e.g., Treadwell & Ro, 2003), we began to link these unmet health and social needs to the soaring numbers of poor men in prison (Treadwell & Nottingham, 2005; Treadwell, Northridge, & Bethea, in press).

In the following section, "Why Oral Health Is a Public Health Priority," we introduce readers of this edited volume to the meaning of oral health as set forth in the Surgeon General's report *Oral Health in America* (U.S. Department of Health and Human Services, 2000). Next, in the section "Building the Case for Oral Health Care," we review the social patterning of oral health status and oral health care access in the United States and argue that people in prisons and jails suffer from egregious oral health and health care disparities compared to people in the United States overall. Then, given the sparse peer-reviewed literature on oral health care for incarcerated populations to date, we devote the bulk of the section "Presenting the Evidence" to a handful of thoughtful studies published on this topic and draw out essential methodological issues and take-home points. Finally, in the concluding section "Calling for Justice," we endorse a core set of recommendations for improving the oral health care of imprisoned populations in order to provide point-by-point, practical guidance for public policy makers and practitioners.

Why Oral Health is a Public Health Priority

Our hope for this chapter is to place the oral health and health care needs of incarcerated populations on the table as worthy of inclusion in efforts to improve public health and public safety. While there is a plethora of pressing issues for those behind bars, absent explicit attention to their mouths, it is unlikely that their oral health and health care needs will ever be met. A recent edited volume devoted to *Social Injustice and Public Health* (Levy & Sidel, 2006) included a particularly thoughtful and forward-thinking chapter on incarcerated people (Drucker, 2006). Unfortunately, oral health was totally absent from the section "The Health of Prisoners" and, indeed, all sections in this chapter. The omission of oral health from overall health and well-being is nearly universal in the public health literature. This lapse needs to be righted if we are to ever achieve equitable health and health care for all members of U.S. society.

On the other hand, the oral health community committed to social justice has often failed to include the critical needs of incarcerated populations as part of its agenda. The editors of the above-referenced volume *Social Injustice and Public Health*, Barry S. Levy and Victor W. Sidel (2006), are to be commended for commissioning a chapter on oral health from two leading public health dentists, Myron Allukian, Jr. and Alice M. Horowitz (2006). Nonetheless, if incarcerated populations were considered at all in this oral health chapter, it was only within a single mention of "institutionalized individuals" as part of a list of populations vulnerable to poor oral health due to social injustice (Allukian & Horowitz, 2006, p. 359).

Toward rectifying these oversights, we provide a primer on the meaning of oral health from the influential report *Oral Health in America* (U.S. Department of Health and Human Services, 2000). In addition to being an authoritative scientific work, it is also a well-written and accessible brief on oral health. Our overarching goal is to help redirect a significant portion of U.S. societal resources that are now expended in the criminal justice system—estimated at more than $100 billion annually (Drucker, 2006)—to respectful health care that includes oral health care, housing, education, and social supports in those communities most heavily affected by mass incarceration policies.

The Meaning of Oral Health

...The word oral, both in its Latin root and in common usage, refers to the mouth. The mouth includes not only the teeth and the gums (gingiva) and their supporting connective tissues, ligaments, and bone, but also the hard and soft palate, the soft mucosal tissue lining of the mouth and throat, the tongue, the lips, the salivary glands, the chewing muscles, and the upper and lower jaws, which are connected to the skull by the temporomandibular joints. Equally important are the branches of the nervous, immune, and vascular systems that animate, protect, and nourish the oral tissues, as well as provide the connections to the brain and the rest of the body. The genetic patterning of development in utero further reveals the intimate relationship of the oral tissues to the developing brain and to the tissues of the face and head that surround the mouth, structures whose location is captured in the word craniofacial.

...Oral health means much more than healthy teeth. It means being free of chronic oral-facial pain conditions, oral and pharyngeal (throat) cancers, oral soft tissue lesions, birth defects such as cleft lip and palate, and scores of other diseases and disorders that affect the oral, dental, and craniofacial tissues, collectively known as the craniofacial complex. These are tissues whose functions we often take for granted, yet they represent the very essence of our humanity. They allow us to speak and smile; sigh and kiss; smell, taste, touch, chew, and swallow; cry out in pain; and convey a world of feelings and emotions through facial expressions. They also provide protection against microbial infections and environmental insults.

The craniofacial tissues also provide a useful means to understanding organs and systems in less accessible parts of the body. The salivary glands are a model of other exocrine glands, and an analysis of saliva can provide telltale clues of overall health or disease. The jawbones are examples of other skeletal parts. The nervous system apparatus underlying facial pain has its counterpart in nerves elsewhere in the body. (U.S. Department of Health and Human Services, 2000, p. 17)

The Surgeon General's report on oral health excerpted above goes on to describe the mouth as a mirror of health or disease, as a sentinel or early warning system, as an accessible model for the study of other tissues and organs, and as a potential source of pathology affecting other systems and organs (U.S. Department of Health and Human Services, 2000). While improved nutrition and living standards after World War II have enabled certain population groups to enjoy far better oral health than their forebears did a century ago, not all Americans have achieved the same level of oral health and well-being. According to Allukian and Horowitz (2006), people are much more likely to have poor oral health if they are low-income, uninsured, developmentally disabled, homebound, homeless, medically compromised, and/or members of minority groups or other high-risk populations who do not have access to oral health services.

When an entire community suffers from a health concern, it becomes a social justice issue. As Allukian and Horowitz (2006, p. 370) argue, "Just as it takes a village to raise a child, it will take a village to resolve the neglected epidemic of oral diseases, especially for vulnerable populations."

Building the Case for Oral Health Care

The burden of oral diseases and conditions is disproportionately borne by those of lower versus higher social standing at each stage of life (Treadwell & Northridge, under review). Poor nutrition, lack of preventive oral health care, violence leading to facial trauma, and tobacco and alcohol use affect teeth and their supporting structures, leading to dental caries (beginning in early childhood and continuing throughout the life course), periodontal diseases and tooth loss (especially in adults), and oral and pharyngeal cancers (predominantly disorders of the elderly) (Northridge & Lamster, 2004). Furthermore, research is currently underway to understand the relationship between periodontal infections in mothers and preterm low birth weights of their babies (Mitchell-Lewis, Engebretson, Chen, Lamster, & Papapanou, 2001), which suggests that there may be intergenerational effects of oral diseases.

The Surgeon's General report *Oral Health in America* went beyond health to document the pervasive effects of oral diseases and conditions on the well-being of disadvantaged members of U.S. society (U.S. Department of Health and Human Services, 2000). That is, oral diseases and their treatments may undermine self-image and self-esteem, discourage family and other social interactions, and lead to chronic stress and depression—all at great emotional and financial costs. They also interfere with vital functions of daily living such as breathing, eating, swallowing, and speaking in assorted areas of activity, including work, school, play, and home (U.S. Department of Health and Human Services, 2000).

Poor oral health is not just a problem of individuals or families—entire communities are affected. Millions of U.S. residents succumb to unnecessary oral diseases and infections because proven, cost-effective, population-based primary prevention measures, such as community water fluoridation, have not been implemented (Allukian & Horowitz, 2006). Practices of the food and tobacco industries further contribute to oral health disparities between wealthy and impoverished populations. High-fat and high-sugar products are usually less expensive to purchase than healthy foods. The marketing practices of the tobacco industry, including the use of "giveaways" such as hats and lighters and the support of sporting events and other extracurricular activities in our nation's schools, are more successful in communities which lack other avenues for raising requisite funds (Allukian & Horowitz, 2006).

Furthermore, illicit methamphetamine use is reported widely by the U.S. news media and discussed increasingly among scholars, clinicians, and members of civic and law enforcement organizations and legislative bodies (Curtis, 2006). "Meth mouth" refers to a pattern of oral signs and symptoms of methamphetamine abuse, thought to include rampant caries and tooth fracture, leading to multiple tooth loss and edentulism (toothlessness) (Curtis, 2006). While population-based evidence is scant, meth mouth is considered to be especially prevalent among incarcerated populations.

Finally, regardless of location—rural or urban, within the United States or outside of its borders—impoverished communities are everywhere distinguished by crisis-oriented rather than preventive oral health care (Allukian & Horowitz, 2006). An in-person, community-based survey was conducted from 1992 to 1994 among 695 adults aged 18–65 in Central Harlem, a largely African-American community located in northern Manhattan, New York City (Fullilove et al., 1999). Of more than 50 health complaints that were part of the survey, problems with teeth or gums (30%) were the most frequently cited among respondents—greater than the percentage who recounted suffering from hypertension, asthma, or diabetes (Zabos et al., 2002). In contrast, only 10% of the participants surveyed in a 1989 special supplement on oral health in the National Health Interview Survey reported fair or poor oral health (Bloom, Gift, & Jack, 1992), meaning that three times as many Harlem adults (30%) as U.S. adults overall (10%) experience oral health problems.

How the Mouth Became Disconnected from the Rest of the Body

Beginning with the establishment of the first dental school in 1840, the medical and dental professions developed separately in the United States. Even today, U.S. medical schools teach very little, if anything, about oral health. Moreover, since medicine has played a dominant role in the development of health policy and practice in the United States, oral health is usually excluded or not considered part of primary health care (Allukian & Horowitz, 2006). As Allukian (2000, p.843) marveled, "It makes no sense that children, diabetic patients, or senior citizens with an abscess on their leg can receive care through their health insurance or a health program, but if the abscess is in their mouth, they may not be covered."

Only 4% of dental care is financed with public funds, compared with 32% of medical care (U.S. Department of Health and Human Services, 2000). But what does this coverage mean in terms of access to quality oral health care? Consider New York State, where Medicaid includes comprehensive primary oral health care coverage, Medicare has no dental component, and private insurance may or may not cover oral health services.

In the Central Harlem survey previously cited (Zabos et al., 2002), the oral health assessment consisted of the question, "During the past 12 months, have you had problems with your teeth or gums?" Those who answered yes to this question were then asked, "Did you see a dentist for problems with your teeth or gums?" Among participants reporting oral health complaints ($n = 209$), two thirds (66%) reported having seen a dentist for the complaint. Persons who had private insurance (87%) were more likely to have sought treatment from a dentist than those who had public insurance (62%) or were uninsured (48%). In the authors' view, "It is disturbing that a third of those who suffer from dental problems did not seek care. Among those who did, having insurance coverage was significantly associated with receipt of care. Those with private coverage were less likely to report having dental problems and more likely to report seeking treatment when problems existed than were those with public coverage or no coverage" (Zabos et al., 2002, p. 51).

Zabos et al. (2002, p. 51) then speculated: "Receipt of oral health services for people in need may be improved if those services can be integrated into comprehensive primary care programs. This problem is particularly vexing because the New York State Medicaid program has one of the most comprehensive dental benefit packages among the 50 states, providing coverage for people of all ages. This suggests that there are other barriers to care that need to be examined (e.g., geographic accessibility and availability of dentists who both accept Medicaid and provide culturally competent care).

Addressing Oral Health Disparities and Increasing Workforce Diversity

According to the Sullivan Commission (2004) report titled *Missing Persons: Minorities in the Health Professions*, African Americans, Hispanic Americans, and American Indians together make up more than 25% of the U.S. population, but only 9% of the nations' nurses, 6% of its physicians, and 5% of its dentists. Evidence of the direct link between poorer health outcomes for racial and ethnic minorities and the shortage of racial and ethnic minorities in the health care professions was compiled by the Institute of Medicine (2002) in its landmark report, *Unequal Treatment: Confronting Racial and Ethnic Disparities in Health Care*.

Mitchell and Lassiter (2006) recently reviewed the literature concerning health care disparities and workforce diversity issues, particularly within the oral health field. They then synthesized the recommendations intended to address identified needs, with a focus on the role of academic dental institutions (ADIs). They believe that, "First and foremost, ADIs need to develop a culture conducive to change and the implementation of diversity issues" (Mitchell & Lassiter, 2006, p. 2095). They further explain that developing such a culture will require consistent support from the leadership within ADIs, including a formal declaration of each institution's commitment to diversity, cultural competency, and the elimination of oral health care disparities (Mitchell & Lassiter, 2006).

In the coming decades, the racial and ethnic composition of the United States is expected to shift to include more people of color, particularly Hispanics (U.S. Census Bureau, 2004). The need for ADIs to enroll and support more applicants from underserved minority groups is crucial to the elimination of disparities in oral health care. In response to this impending crisis, 15 dental educators undertook a feasibility study with funding from the W. K. Kellogg Foundation which resulted in the publication of the report, *Bridging the Gap:*

Partnerships between Dental Schools and Colleges to Produce a Workforce to Fully Serve America's Diverse Communities (Community Voices: Health Care for the Underserved Study Committee, 2006). Findings suggest that "a collaborative model between colleges and dental schools can become a valuable way to enroll students of color but … the establishment of such programs would most likely depend on a demonstrated need for (1) new practitioners in a particular locale, and (2) an interested state legislature seeking to solve a dental workforce problem" (Community Voices: Health Care for the Underserved Study Committee, 2006, p. 7).

It is no wonder, then, given the striking economic and racial disparities in the application of incarceration [e.g., African Americans represent only 12% of the total U.S. population but comprise nearly 50% of the U.S. prison population (Drucker, 2006)] and the dearth of dentists of color in the oral health care workforce (Community Voices: Health Care for the Underserved Study Committee, 2006), that prisoners suffer from poor oral health and have unmet oral health care needs. The scant evidence on oral health care for prisoners that is available from government reports and the peer-reviewed literature is reviewed in the following section.

Presenting the Evidence

Dental care is listed as an essential health service by the National Commission on Correctional Health Care (Treadwell & Formicola, 2005). Nonetheless, the oral health status of prisoners is overridingly poor. As with other individuals of low social standing in the U.S. population, adults who are incarcerated in both federal and state prison systems are more likely to have extensive caries and periodontal disease, be missing teeth at every age, and endure a higher percentage of unmet dental needs than employed U.S. adults (Mixson, Eplee, Feil, Jones, & Rico, 1990; Salive, Carolla, & Brewer, 1989). Clare (1998) conducted a survey of dental decay, moderate periodontal pocket depth, and urgent treatment needs in a sample of adult felon admissions and found more unmet dental needs in the prison sample compared to those reported among participants in Phase One of the Third National Health and Nutrition Examination Survey (NHANES III). Clare (1998) hypothesized that a possible cause for the differences found between the adult felon survey results and the general adult U.S. population reference group results may be a higher representation of lower socioeconomic groups in the prison populations.

Even still, racial differences are evident. At the U.S. Penitentiary in Leavenworth, Kansas, white inmates had significantly fewer decayed teeth than did black inmates (Mixson et al., 1990).

The empirical evidence that exists to date indicates that prisoners deem oral health a priority and that access to oral health services improves the conditions of their mouths. For instance, among prisoners in Maine, smoking and dental health were the most commonly reported health problems after mental health and substance abuse (Maine Civil Liberties Union, 2003). A recent study of continuously incarcerated individuals in the North Carolina prison system found that the prison dental care system was able to markedly improve the oral health of a sample of inmates (Clare, 2002), affirming the idea that dental health improves when access to services is provided. Even still, despite improvement, the remaining dental needs of these felons were deemed to be substantial.

Limited surveys have documented the prevalence of oral health problems in both male and female inmates. Ormes, Carlyon, Thompson, and Brim (1997) examined a representative sample of 251 male inmates in the Michigan Department of Corrections. Results were that inmates aged 18–34 had a mean Decayed Missing Filled Teeth Index (DMFT) of 11.52 compared to a mean DMFT of 19.25 for inmates aged 35–44 and 24.70 for inmates aged 45 and older. Differences were also found in the number of decayed and filled teeth and the DMFT composite index with respect to the number of years a male inmate was incarcerated. When these results were compared to those of combined age categories in the NHANES and the Midwest Regional findings of the U.S. Employed Adults survey, the Ormes et al. (1997) inmate survey identified more decayed teeth than the general population surveys, but fewer missing and filled teeth.

Badner and Margolin (1994) investigated the oral health status and dental experience of 183 mostly African-American women detained by the New York City Department of Corrections at Riker's Island Correctional Facility. Almost one-third of the detainees complained of oral pain. Only 41.1 and 67.9% had received dental treatment within the past 12 and 24 months, respectively. One-third of the last treatments were for tooth extraction. The DMFT, time between appointments, need for emergency care, and utilization of extractions all indicated that New York female detainees have: (1) a large amount of unmet dental need, (2) a past dental history consisting of emergency dental care, and (3) limited utilization of preventive and restorative dental services (Badner & Margolin, 1994).

In 1998, the U.S. federal government spent $1.3 billion and the state governments spent $1.0 billion on dental care (U.S. Department of Health and Human Services, 2000). Dental care spending in prisons is paltry in comparison. For instance, in 2004 the North Dakota State Penitentiary spent $150,000 for dental work and supplies (Healthcare Mergers, Acquisitions & Ventures Week, 2004). This is almost three times the reported amount it spent in 2000 for dental care and supplies ($56,000), but likely still meager compared with the unmet dental needs of prisoners in this facility (Healthcare Mergers, Acquisitions & Ventures Week, 2004). There is no reliable information on what it would cost to bring prisoners who lack oral health care up to a reasonable level of oral health, but we provide below the information we could find on the current level of oral health care in state prisons.

Forty-five of 50 states and the District of Columbia (88% response rate) replied to a 1996 survey from the Department of Corrections (DOCs) that sought to examine the characteristics of dental care provided to state prisoners. Results indicated that there was substantial variation in the way that oral health care was provided to state inmate populations. For instance, 73% of respondents reported that they had dental directors who coordinated dental care in their state prisons, 72% described their DOCs as providing emergency dental care and some routine dental care, 52% required inmates to make a copayment for dental services, and 23% indicated that their states were providing dental care through managed care (Makrides & Schulman, 2002). Not unexpectedly, finances and staffing are major obstacles to the adequate provision of oral health care in prisons.

The recruitment of dentists to serve in the prison system is difficult, given the declining numbers of dentists in relation to population counts and the strong demand for dentists in private practice. Certain states are attempting to address this problem through their universities. The state dental schools of North Carolina and Florida have programs in which students or residents are rotated through prison facilities (Treadwell & Formicola, 2005). Further, we conducted a web search in August 2006 and found evidence that the University of Texas Medical Branch (see www.utmb. edu/cmc/Publications/dental/DentalProgramEffectiveness.asp), the Texas Tech University Health Sciences Center (see www.aamc.org/newsroom/ reporter/aug04/prisonhealth.htm), the University of Southern California (see www.usc.edu/schools/medicine/departments/family_medicine/education/ paetc/education/correctional/index.html and www.usc.edu/hsc/dental/update/ april02/admin_04.htm), and Ohio State University (see http://dent.osu.edu/ Outreach.php and http://outreach.osu.edu/database/record.php?dataid=368) all sponsor programs in which oral health care is provided to incarcerated populations. More such programs could help alleviate the shortage of dentists and hygienists in the prison system.

Loan forgiveness programs might also encourage dental school graduates to work in prisons. For instance, the National Health Services Corps is a federally funded program that offers a loan repayment program for dental students in return for placement and service in underprivileged areas (see www.dent. unc.edu/careers/career_options/uspubhlth.htm#cid10fbp).

Calling for Justice

The oral health status of inmates in the prison system is not routinely incorporated into data and reports that summarize the state of the nation's health. Yet the number of imprisoned citizens is already high and further increases are expected if current drug and incarceration policies remain in place (Drucker, 2006). Therefore, the health of prisoners is important to the overall health of the nation. The 630,000 people who migrate back and forth across the border between prisons and communities represent a public health opportunity that can be addressed if and when there is a safety net that serves these citizens both while they are detained and when they return to their communities (U.S. Department of Homeland Security, 2004).

To help people be all that they can be, we must pay attention to their entire well-being. Because oral health is inextricably linked to overall health, as well as to self-esteem, we have a responsibility to ensure that oral health services are available and accessible as part of our health care delivery systems both within and outside prison walls. If good oral health care is provided to prisoners, the benefits will extend to their families, their communities, and the nation as a whole. What can we do as a society to better ensure improved oral health and health care for incarcerated populations?

Recommendations and Conclusions

In closing, we have adapted the following core set of recommendations from the report titled, *Confronting Confinement: A Report of the Commission on Safety and Abuse in America's Prisons* (Gibbons & Katzanbach, 2006) to explicitly refer to improving the oral health care of imprisoned populations.

1. *Partner with oral health care providers from the community.* Departments of corrections and oral health providers from the community should join together in the common project of delivering high-quality oral health care.
2. *Build real partnerships within facilities.* Corrections administrators and officers must develop collaborative working relationships with individuals and organizations that provide oral health care to prisoners.
3. *Commit to caring for persons with oral health problems and providing them with culturally competent oral health care.* Legislators and executive branch officials, including corrections administrators, need to commit adequate resources to identify prisoners with oral health problems and provide them with culturally competent oral health care.
4. *Screen, test, and treat for oral disease.* Every U.S. prison and jail should screen, test, and treat for oral diseases under the oversight of public health authorities and in compliance with national guidelines and ensure continuity of oral health care on release.
5. *End copayments for oral health care.* State legislatures should revoke existing laws that authorize prisoner copayments for oral health care.
6. *Extend Medicaid to eligible prisoners.* Congress should change the Medicaid rules so that correctional facilities can receive federal funds to help cover the costs of providing oral health care to eligible prisoners. Until Congress acts, states should ensure that benefits are available to people immediately on release.

Our hope for this chapter is to provide public policy makers and practitioners with concrete guidance for improving the oral health and health care of incarcerated populations. By reuniting the mouth with the rest of the body and the body politic, we hope to improve the health and well-being of prisoners and thereby advance public health and public safety for their families, entire communities affected by mass incarceration, and U.S. society in the process.

References

Allukian, M. (2000). The neglected epidemic and the Surgeon General's report. A call to action for better oral health. *American Journal of Public Health, 90*, 843–845.

Allukian, M., & Horowitz, A. M. (2006). Oral health. In B. S. Levy & V. W. Sidel (Eds.), *Social injustice and public health* (pp. 357–377). New York: Oxford University Press.

Badner, V., & Margolin, R. (1994). Oral health status among women inmates at Rikers Island Correctional Facility. *Journal of Correctional Health Care, 1*, 55–72.

Bloom, B., Gift, H. C., & Jack, S. S. (1992). *Dental services and oral health: United States, 1989.* National Center for Health Statistics. DHHS Publication No. (PHS) 93–1511, Series 10, No. 183. Washington, DC: U.S. Government printing Office.

Clare, J. H. (1998). Survey, comparison, and analysis of caries, periodontal pocket depth, and urgent treatment needs in a sample of adult felon admissions, 1996. *Journal of Correctional Health Care, 5*, 89–101.

Clare, J. H. (2002). Dental health status, unmet needs, and utilization of services in a cohort of adult felons at admission and after three years incarceration. *Journal of Correctional Health Care, 9*, 65–75.

Community Voices: Health Care for the Underserved Study Committee. (2006). *Bridging the gap: Partnerships between dental schools and colleges to produce a workforce to fully serve America's diverse communities.* Retrieved August 25,

2006, from http://www.communityvoices.org/Uploads/DENTAL_PUBLICATION_00108_00139.pdf

Curtis, E. K. (2006). Meth mouth: A review of methamphetamine abuse and its oral manifestations. *General Dentistry, 54*, 125–129.

Drucker, E. M. (2006). Incarcerated people. In B. S. Levy & V. W. Sidel (Eds.), *Social injustice and public health* (pp. 161–175). New York: Oxford University Press.

Formicola, A. J., Ro, M., Marshall, S., Derksen, D., Powell, W., Hartsock, L., & Treadwell, H. M. (2004). Strengthening the oral health safety net: Delivery models that improve access to oral health care for uninsured and underserved populations. *American Journal of Public Health, 94,* 702–704.

Fullilove, R. E., Fullilove, M. T., Northridge, M. E., Ganz, M. L., Bassett, M. T., McLean, D. E., Aidala, A. A., Gemson, D. H., & McCord, C. (1999). Risk factors for excess mortality in Harlem: Findings from the Harlem Household Survey. *American Journal of Preventive Medicine, 16*(Suppl. 3), 22–28.

Gibbons, J. J., & Katzanbach, N. D. B. (2006). *Confronting confinement: A report of the Commission on Safety and Abuse in America's Prisons.* Washington, DC: Vera Institute of Justice.

Healthcare Mergers, Acquisitions & Ventures Week. (2004). *Correctional healthcare: Methamphetamine use takes major toll on inmates' dental health.* Retrieved August 30, 2006, from http://www.newsrx.com/article.php?articleID=134847

Institute of Medicine. (2002). *Unequal treatment: Confronting racial and ethnic disparities in health care.* Washington, DC: National Academy Press.

Levy, B. S., & Sidel, V. W. (Eds.). (2006). *Social injustice and public health.* New York: Oxford University Press.

Magee, B. (2003). *She still lives: A novel of Tibet.* Ithaca, NY: Snow Lion Publications.

Maine Civil Liberties Union. (2003). *The health status of Maine's prison population: Results of a survey of inmates incarcerated by the Maine Department of Corrections.* Portland: Author.

Makrides, J., & Schulman, J. (2002). Dental health care of prison populations. *Journal of Correctional Health Care, 9*, 291–303.

Mitchell, D. A., & Lassiter, S. L. (2006). Addressing health care disparities and increasing workforce diversity: The next step for the dental, medical and public health professions. *American Journal of Public Health, 96*, 2093–2097.

Mitchell-Lewis, D., Engebretson, S. P., Chen, J., Lamster, I. B., & Papapanou, P. A. (2001). Periodontal infections and pre-term birth: Early findings from a cohort of young minority women in New York. *European Journal of Oral Sciences, 109*, 34–39.

Mixson, J., Eplee, H., Feil, P., Jones, J., & Rico, M. (1990). Oral health status of a federal prison population. *Journal of Public Health Dentistry, 50*, 257–261.

Northridge, M. E., & Lamster, I. B. (2004). A lifecourse approach to preventing and treating oral disease. *Sozial- und Präventivmedizin, 49*, 299–300.

Ormes, W. S., Carlyon, D., Thompson, W. F., & Brim, M. (1997). The measurement of dental disease in a correctional setting and its importance to functional service delivery. *Journal of Correctional Health Care, 4*, 105–119.

Salive, M. E., Carolla, J. M., & Brewer, T. F. (1989). Dental health of male inmates in a state prison system. *Journal of Public Health Dentistry, 49*, 83–86.

Sullivan Commission. (2004). *Missing persons: Minorities in the health profession. A report of the Sullivan Commission on diversity in the healthcare workforce.* Retrieved May 30, 2006, from http://www.aacn.nche.edu/Media/pdf/SullivanReport.pdf.

Treadwell, H. M., & Formicola, A. J. (2005). Improving the oral health of prisoners to improve overall health and well-being. *American Journal of Public Health, 95*, 1677–1678.

Treadwell, H. M., & Northridge, M. E. (Forthcoming). Oral health is the measure of a just society. *Journal of Health Care for the Poor and Underserved.*

Treadwell, H. M., Northridge, M. E., & Bethea, T. N. (Forthcoming). Confronting racism and sexism to improve men's health. *American Journal of Men's Health.*

Treadwell, H. M., & Nottingham, J. H. (2005). Standing in the gap. *American Journal of Public Health, 95*, 1676.

Treadwell, H. M., & Ro, M. (2003). Poverty, race, and the invisible men. *American Journal of Public Health, 93*, 705–707.

U.S. Census Bureau. (2004). *Projected population of the United States, by race and Hispanic origin: 2000 to 2050*. U.S. Department of Commerce, Economics and Statistics Administration, U.S. Census Bureau. Retrieved May 31, 2006, from http://www.census.gov/ipc/www/usinterimproj/natprojtab01a.pdf.

U.S. Department of Health and Human Services. (2000). *Oral health in America: A report of the Surgeon General*. Rockville, MD: National Institute of Dental and Craniofacial Research, National Institutes of Health.

U.S. Department of Homeland Security. (2004). *2004 Yearbook of Immigration Statistics*. Retrieved June 27, 2005, from http://uscis.gov/graphics/shared/statistics/yearbook/index.html.

Zabos, G. P., Northridge, M. E., Ro, M. J., Trinh, C., Vaughan, R., Moon Howard, J., Lamster, I., Bassett, M. T., & Cohall, A. T. (2002). Lack of oral health care for adults in Harlem: A hidden crisis. *American Journal of Public Health*, *92*, 49–52.

Section 4

Tertiary Prevention

This fourth section of the book is about the treatment of established disease including rehabilitation. These three chapters each have to do with mental illness. Raymond Patterson, a forensic and correctional psychiatrist, and myself discuss the basic components of a psychiatric program behind bars, beginning with the intake assessment process and ending with discharge planning for reentry. The chapter emphasizes timely identification of mental illness and potential suicidality and the requirements for diagnosis, treatment planning, medication management, and discharge planning.

Roger Peters and colleague Nicole Bekman are academics who describe treatment and reentry specifically for inmates with co-occurring mental illness and substance abuse. This is a critical area, not only because of the high prevalence of this comorbidity in our institutions, but also because, historically, there has been such a high barrier between psychiatry and drug-abuse treatment behind bars. The authors underscore the need for step-by-step approaches to planning for discharge and the merits of diversion programs.

The chapter on pharmacologic treatment of substance abuse disorders is authored by medical school academics with correctional health care experience. Doug Bruce, Duncan Smith-Rohrberg, and Rick Altice provide a review of substance abuse in inmates, undertreatment with medication, and pharmacologic therapies, including both methadone and buprenorphine. They provide a scholarly and evidence-based argument for further development of pharmacologic treatments for substance abuse behind bars, programs which are currently in their infancy in the United States.

Chapter 21

Treatment of Mental Illness in Correctional Settings

Raymond F. Patterson and Robert B. Greifinger

Treatment for mental illness and other conditions related to mental functioning presents significant challenges to clinicians, administrators, and custody staff within correctional facilities. In this chapter, the term *correctional facility* refers to police lockups, jails, and prisons. The distinctions are important considerations in the provision of mental health care because of the varying lengths of stay.

In one way or another, the mission of all correctional facilities usually includes:

1. Custody
2. Maintenance of order, safety, and control
3. Punishment

"Rehabilitation" is found in some correctional mission statements, along with references to restoring an individual to function in the community. In even fewer mission statements is there a reference to medical care or "treatment." These functions are rarely considered part of the intent of confinement in a correctional setting.

The mission statements of health care providers and health care organizations are different. They usually include:

1. Focus on individuals and their health needs
2. Humane and responsive care and treatment
3. Confidentiality
4. Consent
5. Provision of treatment in the least restrictive environment

Ethical Guidelines

The American Medical Association promulgates principles of medical ethics, applicable generally and specifically to psychiatry. These principles are laudable. They form a backdrop for the development of an ethical and responsible mental health care program for inmates. Several sections of the principles are specifically relevant:

- "Because society has an obligation to make access to an adequate level of healthcare available to all of its members regardless of ability to pay, physicians should contribute their expertise at a policy-making level to achieve this goal."
- "To ensure justice, the process for determining the adequate level of healthcare should include the following considerations: (1) democratic decision-making with broad public input at both the developmental and final approval stages, (2) monitoring for variations in care that cannot be explained on medical grounds with special attention to evidence of discriminatory impact on historically disadvantaged groups, and (3) adjustment to the adequate level over time to ensure continued and broad public acceptance."
- Restraints "should not be punitive, nor should they be used for convenience or as an alternative to reasonable staffing." The principles specify that restraints should be used only in accordance with appropriate clinical indications (Council on Ethical & Judicial Affairs, 2006).
- "A physician shall be dedicated to providing competent medical service with compassion and respect for human dignity."
- "A physician shall respect the law and also recognize the responsibility to seek changes in those requirements which are contrary to the best interest of the patient."
- "A physician shall respect the rights of patients, of colleagues, and of other health professionals, and shall safeguard patient confidences within the constraints of the law." (Council on Ethical & Judicial Affairs, 2006)

Further, the American Academy of Psychiatry and the Law provides ethical guidelines for the practice of forensic psychiatry[1] (American Academy of Psychiatry and the Law, 2005). These require that confidentiality should be maintained to the extent possible given the legal context of the involvement of the psychiatrist, and specifically "special attention is paid to any limitations on the usual precepts of medical confidentiality." These guidelines require psychiatrists to assure that any limitations on confidentiality are communicated to patients. Each of these considerations with regard to medical ethics and the practice of psychiatry within a correctional context must be considered for any practitioners working within a correctional setting.

When the mission and purpose of corrections meets the mission and purpose of health care delivery systems, the combination is like "dancing with a bear," where the human partner understands that one must continue dancing in the manner dictated by the bear until the bear no longer wishes to dance.

The mental health problems encountered in prisons reflect the predictable issues that evolve when individuals with varying pathologies are contained in a crowded, stressful environment where the mission of the institution emphasizes containment, deterrence, and punishment, with limited concern and/or resources for rehabilitation. A relatively small number of seriously mentally ill individuals have been diverted from corrections through pretrial evaluations resulting in findings of insanity; however, many more individuals convicted

[1] A subspecialty of psychiatry in which scientific and clinical expertise is applied to legal issues and legal contexts embracing several criminal, correctional, civil, or legislative matters: forensic psychiatry should be practiced in accordance with guidelines and ethical principles enunciated by the profession of psychiatry."

and serving sentences do have serious mental disorders which were not identified or did not exist during the trial process or which did not meet the standard for legal insanity.

The incarcerated mentally ill, whether in lockups, jails, or prisons, require a broad range of psychiatric and other mental health services while in correctional facilities. What these services should be and how they should be provided in a correctional setting are described in detail in this chapter.

Developing a Mental Health Services Delivery System

How should we address the mental health needs of inmates and detainees housed in jails, lockups, and prisons given the historical, demographic, and public policy factors, such as sentencing structure and the deinstitutionalization of the mentally ill? The approach to addressing these needs begins with defining the six major areas essential for a comprehensive mental health services delivery system:

1. Initial intake screening and referral
2. Suicide assessment
3. Intake mental health screening
4. Mental health assessment
5. Treatment planning
6. Discharge planning

Step 1: Initial Intake Screening and Referral

At reception or intake, any detainee or inmate entering a correctional facility should receive an intake screening at the "front door," to identify those with acute medical or mental health needs. In lockups, such initial screening is frequently conducted by an arresting or receiving officer who has determined that someone in custody appears to have mental health, medical, and/or substance abuse issues that may require that they be transferred to the local hospital emergency room. Following clearance at the local hospital emergency room, the detainee/inmate is returned immediately to the lockup. If the inmate has an acute medical or mental illness or if the inmate is suffering from drug or alcohol withdrawal, the individual may require admission to the hospital. Again, given the very limited services available in most lockup environments, the police or sheriff deputies determine if there is a need and then transport the individual to an outside medical or mental health facility for evaluation.

The outcome of civil rights actions, including those by the U.S. Department of Justice under the Civil Rights of Institutionalized Persons Act (CRIPA), compel most jurisdictions to require staffing at jails that includes medical and mental health professionals, to determine when an individual in custody is in need of medical or mental health services. In small jails (less than 100 detainees), these services are frequently provided by the local hospital. In medium to large jails, there are staff and on-site programs for medical detoxification and mental health services for crisis intervention treatment. The reception or intake screening at jails is frequently conducted by correctional officers who should be trained in the proper administration of reception screens.

The screens are completed during intake processing (within minutes to a few hours of the prisoner's arrival). Frequently, the screening consists of a checklist of questions asked by the officer, inquiring for any history of mental health issues, medical/mental health treatment, suicide attempts, medication utilization, alcohol and/or drug use, and information as to whether the offense is considered high profile or shocking in nature. Typically, the reception/intake screening also includes documentation by the officer of his/her observations regarding the detainee's behavior, appearance, and apparent state of mind.

When the results of the reception/intake screening indicate the need for referral to a mental health professional, the detainee is to be evaluated within specified time frames. The specific time frames for evaluating referrals are:

1. "emergency" referrals are to be seen within minutes and the individual should be observed until seen;
2. "urgent" referrals are to be seen within 24 hours; and
3. "routine" referrals are to be seen within 3 to 5 days.

These criteria should be established through institutional policy so that the responses by mental health professionals to the referrals are timely. Adequate training for correctional officers at intake is essential to assure that the proper level of referral at the "front door" is generated.

In prisons, there is generally more information available to custody and mental health staffs than in lockups or jails. This is largely because there is usually more opportunity to accumulate information that should be available to custody and health care staffs, such as the results of evaluations that may have been conducted at a local hospital or at a jail. This information will often provide an inmate's history of treatment in a jail, whether medications were prescribed, self-injurious behaviors, and attempted suicide or self harm. Information on evaluations conducted prior to trial and conviction or during any previous incarcerations assists prison administrators, custody officers, and mental health practitioners to provide appropriate housing and timely services. Even though there may have been previous assessments conducted on a detainee/inmate, a reception/intake screening is still performed to determine the acute medical or mental health needs for the incoming population.

The purpose of reception/intake screening is to determine whether the arrestee, detainee, or inmate is in need of immediate medical or mental health services. The screening process does not presume that officers who conduct the screenings have extensive medical or mental health knowledge. The forms are designed to facilitate immediate referral for those in need of medical or mental health services on an acute basis.

The value of adequate training for staff who complete the screening tool and are responsible for notifying the appropriate personnel (custody, administrative, medical, and/or mental health) when positive responses are generated is obvious. Unless there are sufficient policies and procedures and post orders in place along with the training of correctional staff responsible for the reception/intake screening process, the process itself is subject to failure; and failures at the "front door" of any lockup, jail, or prison have been associated with an increased incidence of bad outcomes including medical and psychiatric complications and death, most notably suicide.

Step 2: Suicide Risk Assessment

As a result of numerous suicides, civil rights actions regarding these suicides, and standards for reducing risk of suicide (Hayes, 1995), there has been an increased emphasis on the importance of assessing the potential risk for suicide in correctional settings. The basic suicide risk assessment typically requires completion of a standardized form that identifies areas that are important for review and assessment. The risk assessment must be done face-to-face, with review of all pertinent records, including the medical records from prior incarcerations. Usually, the reasons for the suicide risk assessment include (1) statements made by a detainee or inmate indicating thoughts or intent to harm him- or herself, (2) behaviors that indicate the potential for self-harm, or (3) referral by facility staff for changes in behavior or exhibiting behavior that warrants referral for the suicide risk assessment. The reports of these behavior changes frequently result from training provided to correctional officers as well as other non-mental health staff who can then better recognize that an inmate's changes in behavior, demeanor, activity level, or relationship with other inmates or staff may be an indication of increased risk for suicide. These behavior changes may include giving away property, having disciplinary problems with staff or other inmates, or no longer taking part in previous activities.

Not infrequently, detainees and inmates send self-referrals (often called "sick slips" or "kites") to mental health or other staff with a request for an evaluation, "someone to talk to" or sometimes with overt statements of intent to commit suicide or otherwise harm him- or herself. Because there are often large numbers of sick call requests by inmates each day, a functional and responsive screening process is mandatory. This means that training is not only crucial for custody and health care staff, but also for any other staff who may actually handle sick call request slips.

After identifying the reason for completing the suicide risk assessment and the sources of information (including but not limited to the inmate, clinical and classification records, and collateral information in cases when the inmate is known to staff), a mental status examination should be done to clarify the patient's recent and historical functioning. The assessment then includes designation of static or historical risk factors, dynamic factors, and supportive factors, including:

• Age
• Race
• Length of sentence
• Number of times incarcerated
• History of suicidal behavior
• History of mental illness
• Current treatment for mental illness
• Other risk factors such as having new charges filed, getting a "third strike" or additional sentence in states with such provisions
• Changes in mental status
• Environmental support, family support, and compliance with treatment
• Religious and cultural factors support

Typically, mental health staff performs the suicide risk assessment, but it may also be done by non-mental health medical and nursing staff members who have received appropriate training in how to conduct a suicide risk assessment. In either case, it is essential that the facility have in place policies and procedures as well as post orders that require the detainee or inmate to be placed in a safe environment under observation until the risk assessment can take place in those instances where the referral suggests an emergency or urgent situation.

Segregated housing has been identified as a factor in 53% of suicides in the Federal Bureau of Prisons during a 15-year study (White, Shimmel, & Frickey, 2002) Based on a 6-year review of completed suicides in the California Department of Corrections, Patterson and Hughes (2006) determined that a number of additional factors should be considered both in the assessment of suicide risk as well as the management of inmates who present with potential suicide risks. Additional risk factors include:

- single-cell housing, particularly in administrative segregation or detention in which the inmate may be more isolated and at greater risk,
- changes in their dynamic risk factors, for example when the patients indicate by behavior or statements that they may believe they have run out of options or feel "backed into a corner," where they see suicide as the most immediate option,
- concomitant medical illnesses, particularly chronic and/or life-threatening illnesses,
- changes "from home" (i.e., dissolution of relationships, divorce),
- loss of visits,
- new charges that could result in a longer prison term, and
- fear of harm from other inmates.

The fear of harm from other inmates may be related to "prison politics," i.e., gang-related activities, "paperwork," i.e., inmates who may have been charged or convicted of particular offenses including child molestation or rape which may increase the risk of harm from other inmates, or social issues within the prison population including drug debts or other "favors" or obligations owed to other inmates.

Finally, the suicide risk is assessed, frequently described as "none," "low or minimal," "moderate," or "high." While there are a number of appropriate criticisms with regard to the ability or inability to predict future violence to self or others, the risk must be estimated and then interventions should be correlated with the risk assessment. Such interventions include but are not limited to placement on suicide watch (constant observation), placement on suicide precautions (usually meaning the inmate is physically observed by a correctional officer or health care professional every 5 to 15 minutes), transfer to a higher level of care (crisis bed care or hospital level of care), follow-up by a clinical case manager, psychiatrist, or other mental health professional within specific time frames, placement on a residential unit, or treatment as an outpatient. Some systems also require that an inmate have increased clinical and/or custody contacts after suicide watch or precautions are discontinued for a specified period of time, which may range from 1 to 5 days, to reduce the likelihood that they may harm themselves in the foreseeable future. It is also very helpful if the evaluating clinician notes specific comments including "statements made directly by the inmate" as well as their assessments and recommendations for continued follow-up care.

An obvious, but often faulty, component of suicide prevention is the emergency response process. The emergency response process includes not only assessment but also treatment activities and characteristically involves both custody and clinical staffs. Given that the great majority of individuals who are attempting suicide are discovered by custody staff, the policies and procedures and post orders on custody responses are crucial. The activation of medical and custody alarms to indicate an emergency situation is frequently the very first step taken by a custody officer after determining that an inmate may be unresponsive or behaving in a bizarre manner.

However, once that occurs there may be some ambiguity as to the custody officer's responsibility to enter the cell, which depends largely on post orders, and may vary depending on the security level of the inmate. Often, segregated inmates may not have their cells entered (by policy) until a supervisor, other officers, or a cell extraction team has been assembled. This means that valuable time may elapse from the moment of discovery until the actual emergency clinical response process is put into place. There are obvious risks to staff in entering cells housing inmates who have already been determined to represent a threat to the staff or the facilities' safety. Therefore, the facilities must have operational policies and procedures and post orders to allow for the safety of its staff as well as the immediate response to an inmate who may be hanging, bleeding, or unconscious.

Greater than 90% of completed suicides within correctional facilities are by hanging. The use of a cut-down tool is imperative. Cut-down tools must be readily available and supplied to trained custody staff for use prior to resuscitation. Even the use of cardiopulmonary resuscitation is debated in some systems. In a few jurisdictions, custody staff believes it is inappropriate for them to perform emergency procedures, because they are not medical personnel and not trained to determine whether CPR is indicated.

In addition to custody staff, all medical and mental health staff should be trained to respond to an emergency code and implement CPR on anyone who is without pulse or respiration. There have been some cases where medical or mental health staff have declared CPR unnecessary and have even pronounced the inmate deceased, which in most states is typically the responsibility of a physician. In a study of suicides in California prisons, the one component that contributed the most to foreseeable or preventable suicides was failure of staff to follow established policies and procedures when responding to an emergency in which an inmate was attempting suicide (Patterson & Hughes, 2006).

Step 3: Intake Health Screening and Referral

The mental health and medical screening is a more comprehensive process conducted after the reception/intake screening done by custody staff. The task force report on Psychiatric Services in Jails and Prisons (2000) indicates that a brief mental health assessment should be conducted within 72 hours of the time of a positive screening and referral, with provision for more immediate assessment if there is a determination that the referral should be completed on an urgent basis. This screening may be completed by medical or mental health personnel within a relatively short period of time (during intake processing) for every newly admitted detainee/inmate. The screening is structured to include: review of the intake screening done by custody on arrival; any past medical records and mental health history; information on the individual's adjustment to the correctional environment since admission; and suicide risk. The intake health screening form is typically 31 questions, approximately half of which may focus on mental health issues.

It is essential that the intake health screening be consistently administered to newly arriving prisoners within a short, specified time period, and that the information obtained be documented on a standardized form (handwritten or electronically). The form must include "trigger questions," so that immediate emergency referral for further mental health assessment is accomplished, with safe housing placement until the emergency assessment is completed. The health screening process also identifies those in need of referrals that are not "emergent," for example, "urgent," with a need for the inmate to be seen within 24 hours, or "routine," which allows for typically 3 to 5 days for inmates to be seen for further mental health assessments.

Performance on meeting time-standards for referrals should be monitored to assure that the screening and referral process is being followed according to existing policies and procedures. This monitoring should be conducted by trained correctional and health care personnel.

Based on the results of the initial intake screening or the intake health screening, when emergency mental health services are indicated, staff must be available on an emergency basis, 24 hours per day. This may be very difficult in lockups where there may be no mental health staff on the premises for extended periods of time, resulting in transportation of the arrestee to a local hospital emergency room. In jail programs, depending on the size and complexity of the program, there may be mental health staff on the premises of the facility. The detainee must be maintained in a safe environment, typically on one-to-one direct observation by a correctional officer, until the referral has been completed.

Some jails use video monitoring of prisoners on suicide watch or suicide precautions instead of one-to-one observation. In our experience, this is an extremely risky procedure, if video monitoring is the sole mechanism used for observation of a prisoner who is awaiting a more intensive mental health evaluation. Video monitoring should be used only as a supplement to direct human observation, if at all. Although there may be cost-efficiencies of video monitoring of multiple inmates, there are a number of potential pitfalls:

1. the arrangement of the cameras inside a cell, as cells frequently have blind spots;
2. the resolution on the monitors may be quite poor, obscuring sufficient detail to detect and prevent self-harm;
3. the officer may not be located proximate to the cell, leading to slow response time;
4. the officer may be in a control booth, with additional responsibilities that can lead to distractions;
5. post orders may require officers to wait for additional correctional staff to arrive before the cell can be opened, delaying attempts to intervene with a suicidal patient. Potential harm to the inmate and danger to the staff must be carefully considered and reflected in policies, post orders, and training.

Step 4: Mental Health Assessment

The mental health assessment is a formal assessment and includes initial plans for treatment and management. The task force (Psychiatric Services in Jails and Prisons, 2000) recommended that the assessment should be conducted by a trained mental health professional, within a time frame appropriate to the level of urgency, with a face-to-face interview with the patient and review of available health care records and collateral information (Psychiatric Services in Jails and Prisons, 2000). Last, a comprehensive mental health evaluation should include additional assessment tools such as psychological testing, laboratory testing, and neuroimaging procedures, where clinically appropriate.

The task force report defines the role of the psychiatrist in developing policies and procedures, conducting training and supervision, and providing direct services, when indicated. They recommend that the psychiatrist provide direct service and take responsibility for supervision of mental health staff.

The National Commission on Correctional Health Care (NCCHC, 2003) requires a comprehensive documented mental health evaluation within 14 days of intake.

Step 5: Treatment and Treatment Planning

In providing mental health services to incarcerated individuals with serious mental illness, a primary issue is the balance between security and treatment needs. While there is no inherent contradiction between the provision of appropriate security and the provision of quality treatment, they often appear to have competing goals. In practice, security usually takes precedence over treatment, except in emergency or urgent situations in which security and treatment processes share equal importance. High-quality treatment programs encourage a patient's participation and assumption of responsibility for his/her behavior.

Security requirements typically reduce the individual's responsibility and substitute a *parens patriae* authority which includes the practice of assuming decision-making for the inmate, as a matter of course.

Barriers

Many traditional correctional practices can negatively impact individuals with serious mental disorders. For example, accumulating "good time" (shorter sentence) can be difficult or impossible for an inmate living on a psychiatric unit in prison since participation in work assignments, education, or recreation activities can be limited or prohibited. In jails and prisons, the practice of isolating prisoners who have been disruptive to the environment or threatening to the safety of the institution is a longstanding practice. Only in the last two decades have there been serious efforts to ensure that prisoners in isolation are not seriously mentally ill or if they have a serious mental illness are appropriately screened and managed by mental health staff. They should be removed from isolation if their condition requires more intensive mental health services.

In lockups, individuals who are "fresh off the street" may have mental health, other medical or substance abuse histories and/or current behaviors or symptoms that can be very difficult to distinguish by correctional personnel. The historical use of the "drunk tank" to allow new arrestees to "dry out" has also resulted in bad and even fatal outcomes when those individuals had medical and/or mental health issues that were unrecognized and untreated, not the least of which were consequences of intoxication or withdrawal.

In any correctional environment, behaviors caused by hallucinations or delusional thinking can result in "tickets" or lead to violations that may result in punishment including isolation, restriction of visitors, or transfer to a more secure setting. Tickets may be given for rule infractions that range from not getting up on time to verbal or other confrontations with security staff, including, in some jurisdictions, "attempting suicide." In all correctional settings, detainees/inmates who exhibit behaviors that result in the accumulation of infractions cannot amass "good time," and consequently are more likely to serve their maximum sentence. The mentally ill in prisons may not be eligible for transfer to halfway houses because of the exhibition of behaviors that may very well be related directly to their mental disorders.

Treatment in jails and prisons should cover a broader range of services including crisis services, residential services, outpatient services, and access to hospital services when necessary.

Levels of Care

Mental health crisis services usually consist of short-term (10 days or less) stays in designated areas that, in some states, are licensed by the State Mental Health Authority or other licensing body. These cells are typically part of an infirmary-like setting in which there may be medical as well as mental health cells specifically used for crisis management. The distinction between medical and mental health cells is important because cells used for mental health crisis management require special security provisions within the cells. For example, the cells need to have sinks and toilets without sharp edges or protrusions by which a detainee/inmate can hang or cut him- or herself, the absence of clothing hooks, bed frames with no holes in them, no bunk beds as they have ladders that can be used for hanging, security air vents to reduce the likelihood of threading sheets or other materials used for ligatures through the air vents, modified window screens, and other physical plant enhancements. These cells may also include cameras for video monitoring of inmates who are on suicide observation and/or observation for psychiatric decompensation. Policies and procedures typically specify that inmates who have not improved to the extent that they can be transferred to a lower level of care within a specified time frame, for example, 10 days, should be considered for transfer to a hospital level of care because of the need for more intensive services. More often than not, these crisis bed cells are managed from a custodial point of view in much the same way as administrative segregation or detention cells are managed with meals provided to the inmate through a food-port in modified food trays; limited yard and out-of-cell time and showers, and "limited issue" materials such as paper gowns, suicide-proof blankets, and "sporks" (plastic spoons/forks). These crisis bed infirmary-like cells require 24-hour nursing and custody support for inmate movement in and out of cells for whatever reasons.

The next less intensive level of services in most jails and prisons that have a comprehensive mental health services delivery system is residential services. Residential services programs are for inmates who have been determined, as a result of the assessment process, to have a serious mental illness or severe personality disorder with self-harming or other behaviors that may require housing with other inmates similarly diagnosed. These inmates require a range of services not available to outpatients. These services are typically provided on a self-contained unit with food service available on that unit, individual and group therapies, and at times a separate yard for outside activities. The services on residential units are provided by trained mental health staff, including 24-hour nursing. These units usually have individual and group treatment space in rooms or cubicles that allow correctional staff to visually observe interactions between clinical staff and inmates but limit the correctional staff's ability to hear what is being discussed providing for a "sound confidential" treatment process. This compromise within many correctional facilities is intended to allow for some degree of confidentiality in the treatment process, while having safety of staff and inmates reinforced by visual observation by correctional officers.

Residential units, depending on the size of the prison and the size of the unit, may be designed for inmates who are "higher functioning" and it is anticipated they will be returning to the general population at some point in the reasonably near future, i.e., weeks to months versus units where inmates are felt to be "low functioning" and would require housing on a separate and specialized unit for an extended period of time, in some cases the full lengths of their sentences. The distinction between "higher functioning" and "low functioning" allows for consideration of other factors that may contribute to the inmate's overall functioning including co-occurring mental retardation or developmental disability, medical illnesses including brain damage, and chronic substance abuse which may also have contributed to an inmate being at a lower functioning level than would be solely explained by their mental illness.

Outpatient services for inmates in prison are provided within the facilities or halfway houses in which they are confined. Outpatient services typically consist of scheduled appointments with a clinical case manager or other clinician, as well as scheduled appointments with a psychiatrist for inmates who may be prescribed psychotropic medications or who are in need of a medication evaluation. The achievement of sound confidentiality for outpatients can be more problematic than on residential or crisis management units because of custody reasons including an inmate not being able to come to an appointment or who may be required to remain in their cell, such as in a lockdown. This means the patient may need to be seen at cell-side or cell–front; other inmates would most likely be able to overhear at least some of the conversation between the clinician and the patient. This reduces the likelihood of legitimate information being provided to the clinician. All efforts to achieve a sound confidential setting for interviews should be undertaken.

A special circumstance for outpatient services occurs in administrative segregation and detention units, as well as protective custody. These units are typically not mental health units but are part of the general population. However, the movement of inmates within these units is strictly limited and compromises sound confidentiality even further should inmates not be able to leave their cells. In cases such as these, a few systems have developed "therapeutic holding cells," "therapeutic modules," or "individualized treatment cells" which are essentially wire-meshed enclosures that may be 2 by 3 feet and 7 feet tall in which an inmate who is under special custody conditions can be removed from their cell, placed in such individual treatment modules, and interviewed by clinicians in a semi-sound confidential setting. There have been attempts also for those inmates who require more intensive mental health services than outpatient services to arrange for several of these individual treatment modules to be in the same space or proximity to promote a group therapy experience with the inmates within the modules and the therapist in the center of a semicircle of the modules where various clinical activities can be instituted. These are some of the most difficult challenges in providing treatment in a correctional setting in which an inmate has demonstrated the need for such interventions that would ordinarily be provided on a residential or hospital unit, but are of such concerns from a security and safety prospective that they are housed in the most limit-setting environments within correctional facilities.

Access to hospital-level services must be provided either within the correctional facility or by agreement with a hospital. In the great majority of instances, hospital-level services, when outside of the correctional environment, are provided in the local or closest forensic hospital in which security concerns and measures are in place and staff include the usual mental health staff, i.e., psychiatrists, psychologists, social workers, nurses, psychiatric technicians, activities and creative arts therapists, and medical personnel, but also include custody staff to provide security and overall management of the units. The process for referral to a hospital level of care is typically instituted by clinical staff within the correctional facility with an agreed upon approval process for transfer. Once transport is arranged, it should be accomplished within a short time frame, because the process is intended to provide the appropriate level of care to inmates in need of acute or intermediate hospital-level services. The hospital services typically consist of services that are similar to crisis bed and residential services including more out-of-cell time, participation in verbal psychotherapies, access to a greater range of diagnostic tests including psychological testing, neuroimaging, other medical procedures, and medication management.

Medication Management

An area of concern in many systems is medication management and the administration of medications on a "watch take" or direct observation basis for inmates receiving psychotropic medications that can be used as contraband and traded within a prison environment, or where compliance may be an issue for specific inmates. Another issue of concern may be the differences between the formulary in the hospital versus the correctional formulary. The same medications that are available at the hospital should be available at the prison. The waiver process for nonformulary medications should be a rapid process without excessive requirements for approval that delays timely access to medically necessary medication. Medical, mental health, and nursing staff must be made aware of when inmates are moved from one area of a prison to another to avoid disruptions to the continuity of treatment services and medication.

Treatment Planning

A basic requirement for all of the services that have been described in this chapter is the requirement for a comprehensive treatment plan. The initial treatment plan formulated during the intake process or after initial referral of a patient is by the clinician completing the assessment. This is a short-term plan. Later, multidisciplinary treatment planning for ongoing treatment is imperative. This treatment plan should be timely and well-documented with diagnoses, staff participants, planned interventions, updates, and discharge plans. Correctional staff should be involved in psychiatric treatment planning for inmate patients.

Correctional staff includes officers and supervisors, but also classification personnel who have access to classified records and information regarding what restrictions or enhancements are applicable for the specific inmate during treatment planning. There may be policies and procedures that limit the participation of correctional staff in the actual treatment planning process. Given that correctional officers are within the facilities 24 hours a day, 7 days a week, their observations and information shared between them are extremely important for the appropriate development of a quality and comprehensive treatment plan.

The treatment plan should be based on the assessment process, but also should take into consideration the inmate's security status and housing. This will allow development of objectives for the treatment team including goals for the inmate to achieve or address for optimal functioning and milestones to demonstrate when the inmate is ready for transfer to a less restrictive level of care or for a modification in services. Conversely, when those goals are not being reached, the reasons should be documented, such as nonparticipation in treatment activities, nonadherence with medication, changes in correctional status, or other factors. The patient should have the treatment plan discussed with him or her, and he or she should sign the treatment plan and be allowed to comment on any areas where there may be disagreement with the treatment team.

Effective and quality treatment planning begins long before the detainee or inmate enters a facility or is identified as a potential patient. It begins with the creation and implementation of policies and procedures designed to govern the treatment planning process. There are a number of basic requirements for this process to be effective and meet the mental health needs of specific detainees and inmates:

1. Policies and procedures that define the appropriate content of treatment plans including:
   A. Identification of presenting symptoms as reported by the inmate
   B. Inclusion of collateral information from past records, transfer documents from previous facilities, and observations of officers or others who had access to the detainee/inmate
   C. A complete and appropriate mental status examination including not only the detainee/inmate's self-report, but the observations and evaluation of the clinician conducting the mental status examination
   D. The diagnostic impressions of the examining clinician including the accepted diagnostic categories including Axis I through V, as follows:
      1) Axis I—the major mental disorders, substance abuse/dependencies, and other potential areas of focus including diagnosis of malingering, when appropriate
      2) Axis II—identification of personality disorders and developmental disabilities, particularly with regard to their impact on the potential adjustment and behavior issues related to correctional confinement

3) Axis III—medical conditions, disorders, or diagnoses, whether or not they have direct impact on mental health care
4) Axis IV—the stressors that the detainee/inmate is experiencing that include reasons for the inmate currently being a focus of treatment
5) Axis V—Global Adaptive Function (GAF), a percentage estimate of the detainee/inmate's current level of functioning in the areas of social, occupational, or other important functional categories and capacities

While these basic categories are very much in concert with the *Diagnostic and Statistical Manual of Mental Disorders*, *4th Edition*, they must be applied with particular care in a correctional environment. The absolute necessity to identify Axis I and Axis II disorders and to then apply the treatment process to addressing those disorders is essentially the same as it would be in the community, with the exception that there may be particular limitations on what interventions may be available within a correctional environment. This applies not only to what are often considered the talking therapies such as individual and group therapy, but also to creative arts therapies, and other therapeutic interventions. All of these interventions are influenced by custodial practice and may prove challenging in areas such as confidentiality, the clinician–patient relationship, and the inclusion of nonclinicians in the treatment planning process, to be addressed later in this chapter.

Axis III conditions including any medical diagnoses, disorders, or problems the detainee/inmate may be experiencing or may have historical risk for developing conditions must also be incorporated, not only because of the potential impact on mental health functioning, but also because of the very real consequences of medication interactions when the mental health clinicians are unaware of what other clinicians may be prescribing and vice versa. The risk of metabolic syndrome in inmates who may be prescribed second-generation or atypical antipsychotic medications, as a prime example, is an area for necessary collaboration that is frequently absent. With regard to Axis IV, it is standard correctional practice for clinicians to identify the stressor bringing the inmate or detainee into mental health treatment at the time of the preparation of the treatment plan. Terms such as "criminal justice issues" or "incarceration" are woefully inadequate descriptions of what the inmate may be suffering; simply limiting the Axis IV descriptors to these categories implies that every "incarcerated" individual should be in mental health treatment based on that stressor alone. In reading the actual descriptions of inmate behavior and inmate reporting of symptoms, it becomes very clear that incarceration may certainly be a concomitant factor, but there is need for much more comprehensive identification of the specific stressors for an inmate to be a focus of treatment at any given time. With regard to Axis V, the Global Adaptive Functioning obviously must be modified for those issues relative to functioning in a correctional environment. The "occupation" of an inmate may very well be "inmate," although certainly many inmates are working in shops, as porters, in food service, and other job activities and/or training activities. Educational pursuits vary by facility and the availability of educational opportunities may be limited to obtaining a GED or may include formal classes at some facilities in some systems; inmates with serious and persistent mental illness may be excluded from work and/or educational activities such that they may not be able to participate based on the errant assumption that their mental illness precludes such participation. Very careful consideration of the inmate's overall functioning in a correctional environment should drive the identification of the level of functioning and the GAF score, which ranges from 0 to 100. Currently, inmates with GAF scores of 30 or below need crisis intervention services and may require hospitalization. Inmates with GAF scores between 30 and 50 frequently need residential level services, and accompanying special housing and activities to address their level of functioning. Inmates with GAF scores above 50 are most frequently outpatients; however, there are certainly inmates whose GAF score fluctuates based on other factors, including where and how they are housed and with whom they are housed. These factors underscore the need for participation in the treatment planning process of clinician *and* custodial and classification personnel to address not only the clinical needs but also the housing and other placement supports.

All treatment planning must be based on proper and timely assessment by a professional and qualified clinician. The use of the terms "professional" and "qualified" are included, because in community and hospital practice outside of corrections, states and the federal systems recognize licensure or certification as requirements for clinicians to make independent clinical decisions with regard to diagnosis. Unfortunately, in correctional settings, there are sometimes waivers of such qualifications, and a clinician who is identified as "mental health clinician" without further definition may be placed in a position of assigning diagnoses and developing treatment plans without proper qualification and training. It is essential that qualified and professional personnel be assigned this task and be provided in adequate numbers to appropriately assess the mental health needs of detainees and inmates and make diagnoses. Qualifications, privileges, and policies and procedures for clinical personnel must be well defined.

This does not mean that basic licensure or certification can substitute for appropriate training and experience. For example, physicians are licensed to practice medicine and surgery in most states; however, they may have not practiced in a particular area of expertise for many years. Psychiatrists, for example, are not typically asked to perform general surgery in a prison hospital because they have not engaged in surgical practice since their internships and/or residencies which may have been many years before. Similarly, surgeons should not be in the business of making psychiatric diagnoses when their latest experiences with psychiatric patients may have been during their training years.

While policies and procedures describe the information that should be provided in the treatment plan, the timeliness of the treatment plan becomes the next important factor. Treatment plans should always be based on assessments. Initial treatment plans, which are usually done at the time of the first thorough mental health assessment, may be authored by one clinician as a short-term management strategy until a full, comprehensive treatment plan can be completed. This is usually within the first 3 to 5 days of the inmate's admission to a facility after the need was determined through the screening or assessment process. A mental health assessment may determine that the detainee or inmate does not require mental health treatment. In this case, a treatment plan would not be necessary. However, if the assessment determines the detainee or inmate is in need of mental health treatment, there should be: (1) diagnoses, (2) an assigned level of care, e.g., outpatient, residential, crisis bed, or hospital, and (3) a management plan to be in effect until the full comprehensive treatment plan has been completed, usually within 14 days.

The comprehensive treatment plan is, indeed, a multidisciplinary treatment plan that requires input from several disciplines including psychiatry, psychology, social work, nursing, and activity/creative arts therapies, plus the presence and participation of custody staff including day-to-day management staff such as correctional officers, and classification staff who should be keenly aware of the inmate's custody status, "points" (number of custody case factors that establish that an inmate should be placed at minimum, medium, or maximum security), and medical staff, as needed. It is unusual for non-mental health medical staff to be present at treatment plans, and it is a waste of their time to be present through the course of all mental health treatment planning. However, it is essential for medical staff to be present in specific cases when inmate medical care is involved, such as inmates with chronic pain, seizure disorders, or risk factors for the development of complications related to psychotropic medications, such as metabolic syndrome.

Metabolic syndrome is a constellation of symptoms that has been associated with the use of atypical antipsychotics and includes elevations in glucose, hemoglobin A1c, lipids, and associated weight gain and a variety of symptoms that are preventable. Unless the mental health staff, particularly the psychiatrist, is keenly aware of the inmate's medical status, and monitors these parameters via laboratory analysis on a periodic (3 to 6 month) basis, the development of metabolic syndrome is a serious consequence for patients taking second-generation antipsychotic medication. There are similar risks for inmates on antidepressants and other medications, particularly when used in combination with medications prescribed by nonpsychiatric physicians.

The Joint Commission on Accreditation of Healthcare Organizations (JCAHO), the Center for Medical Services (CMS), and the National Commission on Correctional Healthcare (NCCHC) indicate that treatment planning should be timed to the level of care provided to the specific inmate or patient. The frequency of mental health treatment planning should be as follows:

- inmates in crisis care: every 3 to 7 days
- inmates in residential or transitional care units: every 3 months
- inmates who are outpatients: from 6 to 12 months

All of these treatment planning time frames include the development of a comprehensive treatment plan at the first meeting of the treatment team with treatment plan revisions or updates at no longer than the stated frequency, or sooner when there are any significant changes in the inmate's mental status and/or functioning. All accrediting, certifying, and reviewing bodies indicate the need for timely treatment planning based on the inmate's needs, with the frequency for treatment plan review to also be based on those needs but no longer than the stated time periods.

The next most important area is the composition of the treatment team. As previously stated, it should be a multidisciplinary team that includes various clinical staff but in a correctional system should also include custody representatives. There was a time when there were concerns regarding confidentiality of issues discussed in a treatment team meeting and whether correctional officers and other custody staff could be included in those discussions. This issue has been approached at a number of facilities in various ways, such as:

1. Custody staff members are required to sign confidentiality statements;
2. Custody staff are invited for portions of treatment team meetings where they can provide their input relative to the inmate's adjustment or observed behaviors, custody points score and security status, limits on possible transfers to other facilities that may have particular treatment programs or may be "closer to home" to facilitate visiting by family members; or
3. No participation of custody staff in the treatment planning process.

In these authors' experience, the first two options have been very beneficial for the overall treatment and management of inmates, as custody staff spends much more time with the inmates than clinical staff; and without an understanding of the custodial requirements for housing, security, and placement imposed by the jail or prison system, mental health staff could make plans that will never be realized. Facilities that do not allow the participation of custody staff, and "hide behind" the concept of not violating confidentiality, are missing an important source of information for effective treatment planning.

The treatment plan itself consists of not only descriptions of symptoms reported by the inmate and signs of mental illness as determined by clinical assessment, but also diagnoses and specific criteria for addressing the symptoms and signs of mental illness. The process includes the development of a "problem list" that describes in behavioral terms the kinds of signs and symptoms the inmate is exhibiting. For example, auditory hallucinations, suicidal thoughts, lack of socialization with other inmates, and nonadherence with medication are all important behavioral signs and symptoms. Invalid descriptor signs or symptoms include "schizophrenia" or "bipolar disorder" or "personality disorder," because the manifestations of each of these diagnoses may differ from inmate to inmate. The behaviors are the focus of the treatment interventions. True interventions should describe the plan of action, including the assignment of responsibility for executing the plan. Interventions may include: (1) medication, which in most facilities, is prescribed by a psychiatrist and administered by nursing staff, and (2) talking therapies, such as individual and/or group sessions that should be focused on the inmate's mental health signs and symptoms rather than simply being "round robin" groups comprised of whichever inmates feel like participating that day. This is an unacceptable way of conducting group therapy, but is often used to demonstrate "the numbers" for reviewers monitoring how many inmates are involved in group therapy, without the specificity that the particular inmates in the group are benefiting from the group and whether the group addresses their issues. The treatment planning process not only should assign patients to specific groups, but also should review whether or not group participation has been meaningful and effective in addressing the patient's mental health needs. Other interventions include suicide watch or suicide precautions, placement in a crisis or residential bed, or placement in outpatient services.

The intensity of services decreases with the lessening of the level of care from hospital through outpatient level of care, and the level of responsibility and access to other activities within a prison increases with decreases in the level of care. Inmates who are in hospital crisis beds experience the least involvement with other prison activities; inmates in outpatient are in "general population" and, therefore, may have recreational and other activities with inmates who do not have mental illness. These factors should be very seriously considered in determining not only the level of care, but more specifically what interventions are available and at what frequency the interventions will be provided at each level of care. The frequency of clinical contacts for inmates in hospital or crisis beds is usually daily because these inmates have been evaluated as in need of the most intensive level of care. The frequency of seeing outpatients may vary from once a month to once every 3 months because the outpatient in general population is seen as most stable and has the least need for mental health interventions and is housed in the least restrictive environment.

The interventions should be provided to address specific objectives. For example, if the problem "hearing voices telling him to harm himself" is addressed by interventions including medication, verbal therapy, and housing in a crisis bed unit to prevent harm to himself, including suicide precautions, the objective should be to reduce the impact of the voices and reduce the likelihood of harm to self. When these objectives have been met, based on the interventions provided, then the problem may indeed be resolved or improved to the extent that a crisis bed is no longer necessary. When the treatment plan identifies a specific problem with specific interventions and objectives, the discharge plan from crisis bed is also being developed. Therefore, the discharge plan should include where the inmate is to go next, which may be to a residential treatment unit or to outpatient services, as a less restrictive environment than hospital or crisis bed services.

Conversely, if the objective of reducing the impact of the voices and reducing the likelihood of harm to self is not met in a crisis bed, then transfer to a higher level of care (hospital) may be the most appropriate intervention. If the inmate is already in a hospital, maintaining the inmate may be the appropriate intervention if the objective of reducing the impact of voices and harm to self has not been achieved. This is just one example of an identified problem with associated interventions to address that problem and the specified objectives to be met by that intervention. Overall, the short- and long-term goals should also be identified in the treatment plan, which is a compilation of all of the objectives. In the short term, the objectives, if achieved, may result in a decrease in the level of care; and, if not achieved, may result in a change to either a higher level of care or maintenance of the inmate at the same level of care. The long-term goals may be to (1) maintain the inmate in a residential housing unit if he or she has a serious or persistent mental illness that prevents the inmate from functioning in general population; (2) return the inmate to general population if the interventions successfully satisfy the objectives and short-term goals such that the inmate can be housed in a less restrictive environment; or (3) provide planning for discharge, which may include community-based services as a condition of parole or the determination that no further mental health services are necessary when the inmate is returned to the community.

In the treatment planning process, it is not infrequent to read in medical records the impressions by clinical staff that an inmate is "manipulative" or "malingering." Unfortunately, this frequently occurs with the suggestion that because an inmate is manipulative or malingering they are excluded from having legitimate mental illness. Manipulation and mental illness are not mutually exclusive.

In prison environments, our experience is that some inmates attempt to control or otherwise influence their environment by reporting they have mental illness, particularly suicidality, or by disruptive/offensive behaviors, such as smearing feces or "gassing" (throwing bodily fluids on staff). One of the crucial questions to be asked by any clinician evaluating an inmate for the presence or absence of mental illness or the presence or absence of malingering or manipulative behavior is to ask the inmate "what do you want?" or "what are you trying to achieve by this behavior?" Although these may seem to be fairly simple questions, they frequently are not asked of the inmate (lest the inmate "control" the situation) and a struggle between the inmate and facility staff including clinicians and custody staff can occur. This kind of "struggle" may result in "upping the ante" with accelerated disruptive or self-destructive behavior to achieve unexpressed goals.

With careful interviewing, inmates tend to acknowledge that they are attempting to influence their conditions of confinement for reasons other than true suicidality or even serious symptoms of mental illness, such as hallucinations and delusions. For such a dialogue to occur, there must be an effective and useful relationship between clinical and custody staff. Unfortunately, to return an inmate to the very same conditions that they are attempting to avoid by manipulating staff or malingering illness, can result in more serious attempts to change that environment or change their placement in it and greater morbidity and mortality and/or increased risks to staff.

Clinicians and correctional administrators need to be keenly aware of the following issues relative to mental health treatment in correctional systems:

1. In a closed environment, with at times competing or seemingly incompatible missions, the success of any mental health services delivery system depends on collaboration, communication, and mutual respect.
2. Clinicians must understand that when working in corrections, they are working in "somebody else's house." To effectively coexist and achieve reasonable success, both guest and host must appreciate the expertise and limitations of the other.
3. For detainees and inmates who "don't fit" and staff struggle with whether they are "mad" or "bad," consider they may be either or both. Our approach, therefore, requires working together to address their issues, manage their behaviors, and treat illness where it exists. It may also require, at times, "checking one's ego at the door" lest we get into unproductive power struggles with the inmate and/or each other.
4. Cultural awareness and sensitivity includes not only "where we come from" but "where we are," in this case behind bars. Correctional institutions have a culture of their own, determined and influenced by history, and reality and belief systems. Effective and quality mental health services not only assist the inmate, but support the delivery of quality correctional practices and safety.

Step 6: Discharge Planning and Aftercare

Inmates who have been identified as having serious and persistent mental illnesses should have a discharge plan that provides for community-based services on their return to the community, where feasible. The community-based services should include an evaluation and assessment of the inmate's mental health needs at the time of discharge, and monitoring should continue for several months while the discharged individual attempts to become reintegrated into society in his or her local community, which may or may not be a well-supported and reasonable transition.

As part of the treatment planning process, discharge planning is essential. The timeliness of discharge planning is very frequently related to an inmate's length of sentence or anticipated length of incarceration. In lockups, treatment plans typically do not occur because inmates are released or transferred to the jail within hours to days.

In jails, while initial treatment planning may occur when the inmate is assessed, with "bridge orders" of medication, the assessment process may not be fully realized until up to 14 days into the incarceration. A high proportion of jail inmates will have bonded out or been released prior to the development of a treatment plan or an appropriate discharge plan. When detainees in the jail are in treatment, a comprehensive multidisciplinary treatment plan should be completed and a discharge plan should be initiated on the supposition that the detainee will require treatment for a year or possibly 2 years when released to a prison or to the community. The collaboration between correctional practitioners and community providers is a critical component of successful treatment.

In prisons, discharge planning is frequently based on level-of-care determinations and length of incarcerations. For inmates who are on a higher level of care, the treatment planning generally focuses on what interventions are necessary to meet objectives for particular inmates to move to a lower level of care or remain stable. When those objectives are met and, in the instances when inmates are transferred to other facilities where services may be different, the discharge plan should be updated by the sending facility staff and reviewed in detail and incorporated into the treatment planning process by the receiving staff. In those instances where inmates are serving long sentences, it is important to remember that these sentences do come to term. For condemned inmates who will most probably die in prison, treatment services should address their changing mental health needs.

The provision of discharge summaries to identified clinicians in the community, with scheduled appointments and adequate medications to bridge the period between release and the appointment, is vital for continuity of mental health care for inmates to have a reasonable chance of successful reentry to the community.

In his chapter on transition to community outpatient services for the mentally ill released from correctional institutions, Dr. Steven Hoge provides an excellent description of some of the challenges and mechanisms for success in providing appropriate discharge and transition planning. These two chapters should be seen as a continuum discussing those issues relative to detainees and inmates who may be incarcerated, as well as services and issues to promote their successful reintegration into the community.

References

American Academy of Psychiatry and the Law, Membership Director, 2005 , American Academy of Psychiatry and the Law.

Beck, A., Karberg, J. & Harrison, P (2002). *Prisons and jail inmates at midyear 2001.* Bureau of Justice Statistics Bulletin. Washington, DC.

Council on Ethical & Judicial Affairs (2006). Code of Medical Ethics, Current Opinions with Annotations 2006–2007. Chicago: American Medical Association.

Greenfield, L.A. (1994). *Women in prison*. Bureau of Justice Statistics Special Report. Washington, DC.

Hayes, L. (1989). National study of jail suicides. Seven years later. *Psychiatric Quarterly*, *60*, 7–29.

Hayes, L. (1995). Prison suicide: An overview and guide to prevention. *The Prison Journal*, *75*, 431–456.

Maddow, R. (2002). *Pushing for progress: HIV/AIDS in prisons*. Washington, DC: National Minority AIDS Council.

Metzner, J.L. (1993). Guidelines for psychiatric services in prisons. *Criminal Behavior and Mental Health*, *3*, 252–267.

National Center on Addiction and Substance Abuse at Columbia University (1998). *Behind bars: Substance abuse and America's prison population*. New York.

National Commission on Correctional Healthcare. (2003). *Standards for health services in jails*. Chicago: Author.

Patterson, R., & Greifinger, R. (2004). Insiders as outsiders: Race, gender, and cultural considerations affecting health outcome after release to the community. *Journal of Correctional Health Care*, *10*, 437–455.

Patterson, R., & Hughes, K. (2006). Six year review of completed suicides in the California Department of Corrections and Rehabilitation.

Psychiatric Services in Jails and Prisons: Report of a Task Force on Psychiatric Services in Jails and Prisons. (1989 and 2000). American Psychiatric Association.

U.S. Department of Justice (2004). *Prison and jail inmates at Midyear 2003*. Bureau of Justice Statistics Bulletin.

U.S. Department of Justice. (2005). *Suicide and homicide in State prisons and local jails*. Bureau of Justice Statistics Bulletin.

Vitek v Jones, 445 US 480, 100 S.C. + 1254 (1980).

White, T., Shimmel, D., & Frickey, R.I. (2002). A comprehensive analysis of suicide in federal prisons: A fifteen-year review. *Journal of Correctional Health Care*, *9*, 321–343.

Chapter 22

Treatment and Reentry Approaches for Offenders with Co-occurring Disorders

Roger H. Peters and Nicole M. Bekman

Introduction

An increasing number of offenders in jail, prison, and community corrections settings have mental health and substance abuse problems. In a recent survey conducted within state prisons, 24% of inmates reported a recent history of mental health problems (Bureau of Justice Statistics, 2006), and prevalence estimates of mental disorders in jails and prisons range from 10 to 15% (Lamb, Weinberger, & Gross, 2004; National GAINS Center, 2004; Teplin, Abram, & McClelland, 1996, 1997). Approximately three-quarters of prisoners have had a diagnosable substance abuse or dependence disorder in their lifetime (Peters, Greenbaum, Edens, Carter, & Ortiz, 1998). Rates of both mental health and substance use disorders among offenders far surpass those found in the general population (Robins & Regier, 1991).

A significant proportion of offenders have co-occurring mental health and substance use disorders (National GAINS Center, 2004), including 80% of probationers sentenced to participate in substance abuse treatment (Hiller, Knight, & Simpson, 1996) and as many as half of female offenders and juvenile detainees (Jordan, Schlenger, Fairbank, & Caddell, 1996; Teplin, Abram, McClelland, Dulcan, & Mericle, 2002). Research indicates that from 72 to 87% of offenders with severe mental disorders have co-occurring substance use disorders (Abram & Teplin, 1991; Abram, Teplin, & McClelland, 2003; Chiles, Cleve, Jemelka, & Trupin, 1990; Bureau of Justice Statistics, 2006).

A number of factors explain the influx of inmates with co-occurring disorders to jails and prisons. These include the closing and "downsizing" of state mental hospitals, adoption of restrictive civil commitment criteria, inadequate access to community support services, widespread availability of relatively cheap and rapidly addicting street drugs, and law enforcement efforts to eliminate drug use and drug-related street crime. Studies examining persons with mental disorders in community settings indicate that having co-occurring disorders increases the risk for community violence and for arrest (Monahan et al., 2001, 2005). Once arrested, persons with co-occurring disorders are more likely to be incarcerated, and once incarcerated, these persons remain in jail significantly longer than other inmates, and are more likely to receive a sentence that involves a period of custody (Bureau of Justice Statistics, 2006; Peters, Sherman, & Osher, in press).

The increasing numbers of offenders with co-occurring mental and substance use disorders has been of great concern to correctional and health care administrators. One significant challenge is that these offenders tend to rapidly cycle between various parts of the criminal justice and social service systems, and are frequently unemployed, homeless, and without financial or social supports (Peters et al., in press). Offenders with co-occurring disorders who are released from correctional settings are not easily placed in traditional residential or other intensive treatment services, and frequently experience difficulty engaging in these services (Chandler, Peters, Field, & Juliano-Bult, 2004). Other potential problems following release include access to medications and psychiatric consultation, affordable housing, transportation, and reinstatement of income supports and entitlements (Osher, Steadman, & Barr, 2002; Weisman, Lamberti, & Price, 2004).

Given the high rates of co-occurring disorders, available treatment services in most correctional settings are inadequate to meet the needs of the vast majority of offenders (National GAINS Center, 2004; Peters, LeVasseur, & Chandler, 2004; Peters & Wexler, 2005). For example, correctional mental health services have grown only nominally in the past decade, despite the tremendous increase in offenders with mental illness who were incarcerated during this period. Moreover, there are few existing specialized co-occurring disorders treatment programs that have been developed in correctional settings (Peters et al., 2004). In recent years, however, several new offender treatment programs have been developed that provide an integrated approach, consistent with evidence-based practices developed in nonjustice settings (Sacks & Ries, 2005). Research indicates that well-coordinated and integrated services provided in custody and postcustody settings can significantly reduce recidivism among offenders with co-occurring disorders (Sacks, Sacks, McKendrick, Banks, & Stommel, 2004).

This chapter explores emerging and innovative approaches for treatment and reentry of offenders who have co-occurring disorders in jails, prisons, and diversion settings. Key areas highlighted in this chapter include evidence-based models of treatment, program features and principles, reentry approaches, and program outcomes. Several challenges to correctional program implementation and funding are also explored, and implications are discussed for policy development and future research.

Correctional Treatment and Reentry Services for Co-occurring Disorders

Prison Services for Co-occurring Disorders

In the past, treatment for offenders with co-occurring disorders has been fragmented and typically provided within the constraints of traditional mental health or substance abuse programs. These programs have been characterized by diverse theoretical orientations and approaches toward treatment, variable levels of staff training in co-occurring disorders, and relatively few attempts to provide integrated services (Wexler, 2003). Correctional mental health and substance abuse programs are often housed in separate units, funded through different channels, independently staffed, and typically do not provide specialized services for co-occurring disorders. In many correctional settings, offenders with co-occurring disorders have been excluded from either mental health or substance abuse services because the programs and affiliated staff are only equipped to deal with single disorders. However, there is a growing recognition that this population requires specialized services using an integrated approach, building on evidence-based approaches that have been developed in community settings (Chandler et al., 2004).

Prison-Based Treatment Programs

In a recent national survey (Peters et al., 2004), 20 co-occurring disorders treatment (CDT) programs were identified within 13 state prison systems across the country, as well as 6 additional programs that were being developed. Most of these programs were housed in freestanding treatment units and many were located in prisons designed specifically for inmates who are in need of treatment. The CDT programs surveyed ranged in size from 12 to 320 inmates, and almost all were operating at capacity and had waiting lists. About half of the programs admitted inmates voluntarily, and the length of stay varied from 3 to 24 months. The most common mental disorders treated in these programs included major depression (26%), posttraumatic stress disorder (PTSD) (19%), bipolar disorder (15%), schizophrenia (15%), anxiety disorders (13%) and schizoaffective disorder (6%). Prison inmates treated in CDT programs are often diagnosed with one or more Axis II (personality) and Axis III (medical) disorders, reflecting the need for a structured treatment approach and a comprehensive array of services.

Prison CDT programs generally provide an integrated set of mental health and substance abuse services, an approach that is supported by the research literature (Hills, 2000; Sacks et al., 2004). Most programs provide a structured and intensive treatment environment and use a range of interventions that are based on cognitive–behavioral and social learning models. For example, many of the programs are provided within therapeutic community (TC) settings. Key interventions include psychoeducational skills groups, criminal thinking groups, peer support groups (e.g., AA and NA groups), regular behavioral feedback from peers and staff, individual assignments, behavioral contracts, and role playing and modeling of behaviors.

Prison Reentry Programs

Activities designed to prepare for reentry and transition to the community are particularly important for offenders with co-occurring disorders, and include development of reentry plans, relapse prevention, engagement with ongoing mental health and substance abuse services, and review of housing, transportation, and employment/vocational needs. Most prison CDT programs feature designated staff (e.g., case managers, transition counselors, outreach workers) who are responsible for linking inmates to community services. These staff often make arrangements for housing, transportation, and employment, and make initial appointments for medical, psychiatric, psychological, and substance abuse services. Some prison CDT programs continue to track offenders once they enter the community, and monitor treatment outcomes. For example, the Community Orientation and Reintegration Program operated by the Pennsylvania Department of Corrections provides supervised prison reentry services for special needs offenders in community corrections centers (Couturier, Maue, & McVey, 2005).

Principles of Prison-Based Programs

Key principles of CDT programs in prisons include the following (Hills, 2000; Peters & Hills, 1997; Peters et al., 2004): (1) early interventions focused on engagement, motivation, and readiness for treatment, (2) a comprehensive approach that addresses mental illness, substance abuse, and criminal thinking and behaviors, (3) tailoring treatment through ongoing assessment of offenders' needs, and (4) continuity of treatment while in custody and postcustody settings. Several treatment modalities have proven effective for this population, including TCs, which have been adapted to provide additional peer and staff support, cognitive–behavioral interventions, relapse prevention, and case management services (Hills, 2000; Sacks et al., 2004).

Several *structural modifications* to prison CDT programs (Peters et al., 2004) include the following:

- Extending the duration of treatment to allow for coverage of new material, and for repetition and overlap of material.
- Developing a highly structured daily treatment schedule.
- Shortening the length of group sessions and other treatment activities.
- Providing an early focus on motivation and treatment engagement.
- Cross-training of treatment staff, program administrators, case managers, security staff, and probation and parole staff in approaches for CDT treatment, supervision, and management.
- Addition of outreach and case management staff who provide prerelease/transition planning and who track and assist program participants as they return to the community.
- Identification of community treatment agencies/vendors that provide services that are similar and complementary to those offered in prison CDT programs.

Clinical modifications to prison CDT programs include the following:

- Decreasing the amount and intensity of confrontation. Confrontation initiated by staff and peers is used less frequently, and is often replaced by supportive feedback in both individual and group settings.
- Treatment modules and interventions related to medication management, symptom management, and affect regulation.
- Twelve-step groups with a specialized focus on co-occurring disorders, such as Dual Diagnosis Anonymous and Double Trouble groups.
- Treatment groups that address criminal thinking.
- Greater use of supervised study groups, peer mentors, and peer support groups.
- More frequent reinforcement provided for positive behaviors.
- Training staff in techniques to work with participants who have memory problems or cognitive impairment, such as repetition of material and instructions and monitoring to ensure participants' comprehension.
- Review of factors related to co-occurring disorders that may precipitate relapse.

Outcomes of Prison-Based Programs

Several studies have explored outcomes associated with prison-based CDT programs. Sacks et al. (2004) examined the effectiveness of a modified therapeutic community (MTC) in comparison to traditional prison mental health treatment services (MH) for inmates with co-occurring disorders. In this rigorous controlled study conducted within the Colorado prison system, inmates with co-occurring disorders were assigned to one of three levels of treatment: MTC, MH, and MTC plus involvement in postcustody aftercare treatment services, consisting of a 6-month residential TC program in the community. Twelve-month follow-up results indicated that offenders assigned to receive MTC plus aftercare treatment had the lowest rate of reincarceration (5%), followed by those in the MTC group (16%) and the MH group (33%). The MTC plus aftercare group also experienced the lowest rate of arrest for drug-related offenses (30%), in comparison to the MTC group (44%) and the MH group (67%). These findings reveal the cumulative positive effect of specialized CDT treatment received in prison and in the community, following release from prison.

Similar findings were reported from a study of Wisconsin prison inmates with co-occurring disorders, who were either assigned to a specialized TC program or who did not receive the specialized treatment services (Van Stelle & Moberg, 2004). At 3 months following release from prison, the TC participants were significantly more likely to remain abstinent than the comparison sample (63% versus 49%), and were more likely to routinely take their prescribed medications and to be rated as having stable mental health functioning, in comparison to untreated inmates. These outcomes from prison CDT programs are likely to translate into significant cost savings related to criminal processing and incarceration.

Jail Services for Co-occurring Disorders

As in prisons, there are few specialized treatment programs for inmates with co-occurring disorders in jails, and program services are traditionally provided in either mental health or substance abuse treatment units within the jails. Although all jails are required to provide basic mental health services, most jail programs are frequently understaffed to provide more than screening, stabilization on medications, and routine monitoring (e.g., for suicidal and aggressive behavior, and acute mental health symptoms). Although standards developed by professional correctional and mental health organizations indicate the need for other jail services such as short-term treatment and discharge/release planning, due to the overwhelming numbers of jail inmates with mental and other co-occurring disorders, many do not receive comprehensive services to address these problems (Peters et al., in press; Veysey, Steadman, Morrissey, & Johnsen, 1997).

Jail-Based Treatment Programs

Jail-based treatment programs operate quite differently from those in prison, primarily because of the brevity of incarceration. Rather than providing long-term residential treatment, jail programs for co-occurring disorders often focus on screening and assessment, psychoeducational interventions, linkage with community services, and reentry planning (Hills, 2000). Accurate assessment of co-occurring disorders can provide valuable information regarding the need for treatment, readiness for treatment, and appropriate types of community services that may be mandated by the courts at the time of presentence hearings or at sentencing. Other key services include court liaison, reentry planning, and linkage to community services. Jail programs that are designed for sentenced inmates tend to be longer in duration (typically up to 1 year), and include psychoeducational and peer support groups, interventions designed to increase motivation and engagement in treatment, and transition planning with community agencies. Joint reentry planning with community treatment and supervision agencies can help inmates to meet their legal obligations and to maintain sobriety and involvement in mental health and substance abuse services. Jail inmates with co-occurring disorders also frequently need support to identify sober and safe housing, transportation, employment/vocational services, and to restore eligibility for SSI/SSDI and other benefits.

Principles of Jail-Based Programs

Jail-based treatment programs for inmates with co-occurring disorders are generally organized around four key principles, as described in the following section. These principles tend to guide the process of implementing services across several sequential jail-based program components, including identification, screening, stabilization, assessment and treatment, and reentry.

Focus on Meeting Immediate and Basic Needs: Jail inmates with co-occurring disorders have a variety of acute needs, including stabilization of acute psychological symptoms (e.g., through use of psychotropic medications), detoxification from alcohol and drugs, and suicide screening, prevention, and monitoring. Other urgent needs include treatment of physical illness and injuries, and dental care.

Integrated Delivery of Mental Health and Substance Abuse Services: As indicated previously, integrated or blended treatment for co-occurring disorders is the preferred approach in jails and other correctional settings. These services are most effectively provided in an isolated treatment unit that is geographically separate from other general population housing units. Treatment staff typically include those with experience in both the mental health and substance abuse fields. Staff are frequently cross-trained in techniques for assessment, use of specialized engagement and motivation approaches, and stage-specific treatment interventions for co-occurring disorders.

Preparation for Release: Reentry and transition planning begin following screening and enrollment in jail services, and continue throughout the course of treatment and incarceration.

Collaboration with Community Agencies to Enhance Continuity of Care: In-reach programs are designed to involve community treatment providers and supervision officers in reentry planning activities. Efforts are also made to ensure continuity of benefits and entitlements (e.g., SSI, SSDI, and Medicaid).

Components of Jail-Based Programs

A number of sequential components are included in most jail treatment programs for inmates with co-occurring disorders, and these are described in this section.

Identification and Screening: Jails often provide the initial point of contact and opportunity for assessment and triage following arrest. This creates a unique opportunity to identify co-occurring disorders and needs for specialized services both within and outside the institution. Effective jail systems provide multiple points for identifying co-occurring disorders, including at booking, classification, within mental health and substance abuse treatment units, and through referral by health care staff, correctional officers, or other service providers. In Rensselaer County, New York (Walsh, 2000), a range of jail personnel are tasked with identifying inmates with co-occurring disorders and provide referrals to a Forensic Coordinator. The Forensic Coordinator then reviews the referral information and arranges for a comprehensive assessment by a "MICA coordinator" within the jail.

Stabilization: Jail inmates with co-occurring disorders are often in crisis due to destabilization of their mental disorders, acute intoxication, and related behavioral problems that brought them into contact with law enforcement officers. As a result, these inmates often require emergency services and placement in specialized housing units that allow for close monitoring, ongoing observation, isolation from other inmates, and access to general medical and mental health services. At admission to jail, the focus of interventions is on stabilizing an inmate's physical and psychological condition by providing medication, adequate nutrition, and attending to emergency medical needs. For inmates with co-occurring disorders, both mental health stabilization and detoxification are primary areas of concern. Treatment must be coordinated to ensure that there are no adverse effects of combining certain medications with recently ingested alcohol or other drugs, and to monitor detoxification from these substances. Several jails have developed freestanding crisis response teams that serve the entire jail facility by assessing emergency needs for mental health treatment, substance abuse treatment, and close management services, and that provide triage to these services (Steadman & Veysey, 1997).

Assessment: Comprehensive medical and psychosocial assessments are essential elements of jail-based programs for co-occurring disorders, and provide the capability for developing individualized treatment plans based on the offender's unique needs for in-jail and reentry services. Both short- and long-term goals should be considered, with an emphasis on locating services that address needs for housing, transportation, financial support, and treatment following release from jail. For example, in the MISA (Mentally Ill Substance Abuse) treatment program in Beaver County, Pennsylvania (Bell, Jaquette, Sanner, Steele-Smith, & Wald, 2005), assessments help to determine whether inmates will be placed in jail treatment tracks that focus on either drug and alcohol rehabilitation, mental health needs, or co-occurring disorders (through the MISA program).

Integrated Treatment: Effective treatment of co-occurring disorders in jails and other correctional settings requires an integrated approach that addresses both mental and substance use disorders (Osher, 2006). This usually requires staff involvement from both disciplines, and who have experience and training related to both disorders. A phased treatment approach is generally used (Peters et al., 2004; Peters & Wexler, 2005; Sacks & Pearson, 2003) that provides an initial focus on stabilization of acute symptoms, medication consultation, assessment, and enhancing motivation and engagement in treatment. Secondary treatment phases focus on skills development, relapse prevention, involvement with peer supports, and interventions to restructure "criminal thinking." Final treatment phases focus on development of a reentry/transition plan and linkages to community services. In-jail treatment services for inmates with co-occurring disorders include psychiatric consultation and use of psychotropic medications, individual counseling, psychoeducational groups, peer support groups, and other specialized groups that focus on co-occurring disorders. Other specialized individual or group counseling services may be offered, such as those provided by the TAMAR Project in Maryland for female victims of trauma (Russell, 1999) or by the WINGS Program in the Riker's Island jail in New York City that provides support groups and parenting skills classes for female inmates (Sacks & Pearson, 2003).

Unlike prison-based programs, jail programs do not typically feature a lengthy course of treatment, and focus on preparing inmates to effectively engage in services upon their release. One means to encourage rapid engagement in community services is through in-reach of community treatment providers to the jails (Steadman, Fallon, Mireles, Williams, & Aronson, 2005). In-reach activities frequently involve participation in treatment planning, reentry planning, and assessment of eligibility for enrollment in various community treatment programs (e.g., specialized intensive outpatient or residential programs for co-occurring disorders). For example, in Beaver County, Pennsylvania, the MISA program hosts weekly treatment team meetings with community treatment providers, forensic case managers, probation officers, and other community service providers to provide case consultation and to assist in reentry planning (Bell et al., 2005). Cross-training between jail treatment staff, jail correctional staff and administrators, and community treatment and supervision staff also helps to facilitate better communication and problem-solving within jail treatment programs, and to develop consensus regarding reentry needs of inmates who have co-occurring disorders.

Accessing and Restoring Benefits: Individuals with co-occurring disorders who are placed in jails and prisons will generally need to access public assistance and health care benefits (e.g., through SSI and SSDI) once they are released to the community. However, access to these benefits is limited by federal regulations, and these are often suspended or discontinued once an individual is incarcerated. Several state and local initiatives have been implemented to streamline the process of restoring benefits prior to release, and to help encourage rapid engagement in mental health, substance abuse, and other health care services in the community. Key strategies employed by these initiatives are summarized by the Bazelon Center for Mental Health Law (Koyanagi & Blasingame, 2006), and include the following activities:

- Screening for mental illness and prior benefits on entry to prison or jail.
- Suspending rather than terminating inmates' Supplemental Security Income (SSI), Social Security Disability Income (SSDI) and Medicaid benefits.
- Helping inmates to complete applications for enrollment in these programs or for restoration of benefits, and expediting the review and processing of these applications.
- Using Web-based applications.
- Ensuring that inmates have valid IDs prior to release.
- Providing coverage for services and medication after release while applications for benefits are pending.
- Sharing information across correctional and community service agencies.
- Working with the Social Security Administration to coordinate prerelease applications for benefits.

Some jail-based initiatives have led to significant improvements in accessing and restoring benefits, such as the NYC Link program at Riker's Island, in which case workers help file benefit applications on behalf of inmates. One of the first programs designed to facilitate continuity of benefits for jail inmates was developed in Lane County, Oregon, in which SSI/SSDI and Medicaid applications are processed in 1–2 days. Medicaid benefits are sustained for 14 days after placement in jail, and are suspended rather than terminated after this time, to ease the process of reinstatement of benefits upon release (Lipton, 2001; National GAINS Center, 2002).

Reentry/Prerelease Planning: Unlike prison-based programs, reentry planning in jails begins as soon as an inmate is enrolled in treatment services. Reentry services anticipate offenders' needs for basic services and for specialized services related to co-occurring disorders. One key concern following release from jail is providing continuity of mental health services, including ongoing psychiatric monitoring and a supply of medication that will last until follow-up psychiatric consultation can be arranged. To address this issue, jail programs such as the one in Hampden County, Massachusetts, provide inmates with a 30-day prescription and 5-day supply of medications on release (Koyanagi & Blasingame, 2006).

Coordination with community service providers in reentry planning is of vital importance in preventing relapse and recidivism. For inmates with co-occurring disorders, transition services are often instrumental in providing a single point of contact to help with crisis management, appointments with mental health providers, liaison and advocacy with service providers, courts, and community supervision; and to provide monitoring and surveillance for early warning signs of relapse and criminal behavior. One effective model for managing offenders with co-occurring disorders is Assertive Community Treatment (ACT) teams, which provide an interdisciplinary set of staff, case management services, and single point of contact and support for high-risk clients (Lurigio, Fallon, & Dincin, 2000).

In order to effectively facilitate reentry and transition from jail, Osher et al. (2003) have introduced the "APIC" model for planning reentry services. This model provides a practical framework for reentry planning with jail inmates who have co-occurring disorders and multiple service needs, and can be implemented in jails of all sizes, and in settings that feature varying lengths of incarceration and program duration. The APIC model provides a structured approach to accomplish the following key activities:

- **A**ssess the inmate's clinical and social needs, and public safety risks
- **P**lan for treatment and services required to address these needs
- **I**dentify required community and correctional programs responsible
- **C**oordinate the transition plan to ensure execution and avoid gaps in care

The APIC approach is particularly useful for inmates who are incarcerated for brief periods of time (i.e., less than 72 hours), who are eligible for placement in noncustody settings, and who require rapid assessment and triage. The APIC and other reentry planning approaches are most effective if inmates are encouraged to actively participate in the assessment process, identification of services, and implementation of the reentry plan. A reentry "checklist" has been developed to help facilitate implementation of the APIC model (Osher, Steadman, & Barr, 2003), and can assist jail and community treatment and supervision staff to prepare for different components of the transition/reentry plan. The checklist format provides quadruplicate copies to allow dissemination of the reentry plan to jail treatment/medical staff, community service providers, the courts, and the inmate. Key areas addressed in the APIC reentry checklist include:

- Mental health services
- Psychotropic medications
- Housing
- Substance abuse services
- Health care services and benefits
- Income support/benefits
- Food/clothing
- Transportation

Diversion Programs for Co-occurring Disorders

A variety of pre- and postbooking programs have been developed to divert offenders with co-occurring disorders from incarceration, and to expedite access to community treatment and housing (Peters & Matthews, 2002; Steadman, Morris, & Dennis, 1995; Steadman & Naples, 2005). Prebooking diversion programs include specially training law enforcement crisis interventions teams (CIT); postbooking diversion programs include drug courts, mental health courts, and specialized jail-based case management services to provide early identification, court liaison, and triage to community services. The number of diversion programs has increased in recent years (Steadman & Naples, 2005) due in part to assumptions that offenders with mental health and substance abuse problems are more effectively and economically treated and supervised in community settings, and that diversion programs can reduce the pattern of rapid cycling within the treatment, health care, and criminal justice systems.

Several common elements of postbooking diversion programs include: (a) identification of arrestees with co-occurring disorders, (b) screening and assessment for mental and substance use disorders, (c) counseling and discharge planning, (d) use of "boundary-spanning" staff who are versatile in working with the mental health treatment, substance abuse treatment, and criminal justice systems, and (e) referral to community services and/or monitoring following release (Conly, 1999). These programs differ significantly in the location of diversion activities (e.g., in jails, courts, community treatment agencies) and the types of services provided (Broner, Lattimore, Cowell, & Schlenger, 2004).

A wide range of court-based diversion programs have emerged in the past decade, including drug courts, mental health courts, domestic violence courts, community courts, and reentry courts. In the past, many of these programs have been reluctant to admit offenders with co-occurring disorders, due to anticipated high rates of recidivism and to difficulties in treating and managing this population (Peters & Osher, 2004). However, a number of specialized court diversion programs have now emerged to address the needs of offenders with co-occurring disorders. For example, the Treatment Alternatives to the Dually Diagnosed (TADD) program in Brooklyn, New York, provides court-supervised diversion services including identification, screening and assessment, deferred sentencing arrangements, case management, supervision, and court monitoring (Broner, Nguyen, Swern, & Goldfinger, 2003). In some jurisdictions such as Lane County, Oregon, and in Butler County, Ohio, specialized court dockets have been established for offenders with co-occurring disorders, and operate in a similar fashion to drug courts (Ohio Substance Abuse and Mental Illness Coordinating Center of Excellence, 2002; Peters & Osher, 2004). These programs provide integrated assessment, intensive case management and judicial oversight, specialized dual disorders groups, psychiatric consultation, family involvement, and participation in peer support groups such as "Dual Recovery Anonymous."

Implementing and Sustaining Correctional Services for Co-occurring Disorders

There are several challenges to developing and sustaining co-occurring disorders treatment services in correctional settings (Chandler et al., 2004). As noted previously, mental health and substance abuse services in jails and prisons are often situated in separate programs, provided by different sets of staff or contract vendors, and are typically supported by different funding sources. As a result, it is difficult to generate blended sources of funding, and to promote collaboration between program staff who may not have previously worked together. The emphasis of correctional institutions and programs has traditionally been on punishment and protection of public safety, and rehabilitative programs are often the first to be eliminated in times of budget cuts. Another major challenge is in providing advanced skills training for clinical and supervision staff to work effectively with offenders who have co-occurring disorders. Finally, the absence of reentry services in many jails and prisons prevents effective linkage to the community, and contributes to the risk for relapse and recidivism.

Several resources are available to support the development of correctional programs, services, and research related to co-occurring disorders (Chandler et al., 2004). The National GAINS Center for People with Co-Occurring Disorders in the Justice System provides technical assistance through the TAPA Center for Jail Diversion and the Center for Evidence-Based Programs in the Justice System, and assists in disseminating information related to effective screening, assessment, treatment, supervision, and management of offenders with co-occurring disorders. Diversionary and corrections-based programs for offenders with co-occurring disorders have also been supported in the past through the Center for Mental Health Services (CMHS) Targeted Capacity Expansion (TCE) program (National GAINS Center, 2006), and the Justice and Mental Health Collaboration Program (JMHCP), created by the Mentally Ill Offender Treatment and Crime Reduction Act of 2004 (U.S. Department of Justice, 2006). Both the National Institute of Mental Health (NIMH) and the National Institute on Drug Abuse (NIDA) support research examining treatment approaches for use with offenders who have co-occurring disorders. NIDA's current portfolio of research projects includes the Criminal Justice Drug Abuse Treatment Studies (CJ-DATS) network, which has encouraged exploratory and developmental studies of services and interventions for co-occurring disorders in correctional settings (Fletcher, 2005).

Conclusions and Implications for Policy and Research

Offenders with co-occurring mental health and substance use disorders are being placed in jails, prisons, and other correctional settings in increasing numbers. These individuals are at high risk for recidivism, reincarceration, premature dropout from treatment, homelessness, and a range of other poor outcomes following release from correctional systems (Osher, 2006). Offenders with co-occurring disorders have not fared well in traditional treatment programs or in regular supervision caseloads. Poor outcomes obtained using these approaches are often misattributed to poor motivation, lack of engagement in treatment, skills deficits, and behavioral problems, rather than to the absence of specialized interventions to address both sets of disorders, and the failure to make accommodations for cognitive impairment, motivation level, and effects of mental disorders and medication on problematic behaviors.

Specialized co-occurring disorders treatment programs and supervision caseloads have only recently been developed for correctional populations (Peters et al., 2004). Despite the implementation of several innovative programs in jails, prisons, and diversion settings, there is still a tremendous gap between the need for co-occurring disorders treatment and available services. This gap has been fueled in part by the demand over the past decade for new jail and prison construction, with relatively few resources reserved to upgrade and expand the scope of treatment, reentry, and supervision services. The parallel structure and funding of correctional mental health and substance abuse treatment systems has also discouraged collaborative efforts to develop specialized services for offenders with co-occurring disorders (Chandler et al., 2004). Moreover, staff have not been adequately trained in the past to provide effective interventions for both disorders, and treatment programs have generally reflected a primary focus on one or the other disorder. Finally, management information and data systems in correctional systems are often segmented to capture either mental health or substance abuse information. As a result, correctional administrators are sometimes unaware of the number of offenders who have co-occurring disorders, and may be unable to quantify or justify the need for specialized services.

Specialized co-occurring disorders treatment programs have been successfully implemented in both jails and prisons (Peters et al., 2004, in press). In-custody programs feature a number of structural and clinical modifications. For example, these programs are highly structured, provide an emphasis on motivation and engagement to treatment, follow a phased structure of graduated intensity, and include a significant focus on prerelease planning to address transitional needs for housing, employment, and ongoing treatment. Specialized prison treatment programs are quite comprehensive in scope and are generally of longer duration than those provided in jails. Prison programs provide a range of integrated treatment and peer support activities, and are often situated in long-term residential therapeutic communities. Jail programs are typically less intensive, and focus on stabilization, assessment, access and restoration of benefits, and prerelease planning and reentry needs. In-reach of community treatment and supervision agencies is used by most specialized jail programs to facilitate continuity of services for offenders with co-occurring disorders.

A number of innovative jail-based and court-based diversion programs for offenders with co-occurring disorders have also emerged in recent years (Broner, Lattimore, Cowell, & Schlenger, 2004; Peters & Osher, 2004). Key elements of jail-based diversion programs include early identification or case finding, assessment, court liaison, and triage and referral to community services. Court-based diversion programs include those located in drug courts, mental health courts, and other alternatives to incarceration programs. In addition, dedicated court dockets and affiliated treatment services have been developed in some jurisdictions for offenders with co-occurring disorders, using some of the same principles and structures that have been operationalized in drug court programs. These programs offer a range of incentives for participation, sanctions for infractions and noncompliance, and involvement in treatment over a sustained period of time.

Based on the current discussion and findings, several recommendations may help guide development of effective programs and policies related to co-occurring disorders in correctional settings:

- Planning to develop new correctional services related to co-occurring disorders should be conducted with broad multidisciplinary participation, and using a community systems perspective. Clearly, this population moves rapidly between a number of public health systems (e.g., mental health, substance abuse, emergency health) and the criminal justice system, and consumes vast financial resources in each system. Narrowly crafted programmatic solutions in one setting may temporarily address the needs of this population, but are unlikely to reduce the pattern of relapse, recidivism, and rapid cycling between systems. As a result, communitywide and statewide task forces are needed to address the needs of offenders with co-occurring disorders. These groups should develop strategies for collaborative and interagency funding of specialized services, sharing of information between agencies, identifying and resolving barriers related to service eligibility and access (e.g., changing policies and procedures related to reimbursement for specialized co-occurring disorders services), and implementing long-term and multidisciplinary programmatic interventions, such as Assertive Community Treatment (ACT) teams for offenders with co-occurring disorders.
- Organizations at the state and national/federal level should be tasked with disseminating information regarding evidenced-based and innovative approaches for treatment and reentry of offenders who have co-occurring disorders. These organizations should work closely with courts, local jails, and state correctional authorities to develop strategic planning related to specialized interventions for co-occurring disorders, and to provide incentives for collaboration in this process. These organizations should also work closely with existing groups such as the National GAINS Center for People with Co-Occurring Disorders in the Justice System, the Co-Occurring Center for Excellence (COCE Center), and the Addiction Technology Transfer Centers (ATTCs) to promote training, sharing of key resources (e.g., training curricula, treatment manuals, descriptions of program models, program contact information), identification of programmatic and practice approaches, and prioritization of these approaches for implementation in correctional settings.
- Management information systems (MIS) within treatment and correctional agencies and within state social service and correctional agencies should be modified to capture information regarding offenders with co-occurring

disorders. These MIS systems should have the capacity for identifying current and yearly totals of offenders who have co-occurring disorders, diagnoses, living arrangements, medication use, utilization and outcomes of treatment services, use of sanctions and administrative confinement, length of incarceration, reentry needs, placement in reentry or other community services, and outcomes following release from custody.

- Statewide efforts should be developed to track offenders with co-occurring disorders who are released from correctional settings, and to describe their engagement in services, response to services, and rates of hospitalization and criminal recidivism. From these tracking efforts, cost models should be constructed to examine the economic benefits of providing specialized services in jails and prisons, and of specialized reentry services; and the relative costs associated with offenders who are not engaged in institutional or reentry services.

Research examining effective interventions for offenders with co-occurring disorders is in the early stages of development, and much of our knowledge regarding these interventions is drawn from community-based samples involving nonoffenders (Chandler et al., 2004). As such, additional research is needed to identify outcomes in adapting evidence-based community treatment approaches within correctional settings. Preliminary research indicates that specialized institutional and postcustody services independently produce reductions in recidivism and substance abuse among offenders with co-occurring disorders (Sacks et al., 2004). Further work is needed to clarify the contribution of treatment components such as prerelease planning and reentry services, case management, and specialized interdisciplinary treatment teams (e.g., ACT teams) to outcomes obtained with this population.

Existing research examining outcomes related to diversion programs has been equivocal, and has not provided definitive answers regarding program interventions and components that contribute to positive outcomes. Research with offenders who have co-occurring disorders should also examine a wider range of outcomes, including those related to mental health functioning, substance abuse, utilization of services, criminal behavior, incarceration, and costs associated with these outcomes. Controlled studies of treatment interventions are needed that include both male and female offenders, employ large samples, and feature different types of comparison groups (e.g., no treatment, mental health or substance use treatment "as usual," and either custody-based treatment or reentry treatment versus a combined approach).

References

Abram, K.M., & Teplin, L.A. (1991). Co-occurring disorders among mentally ill jail detainees: Implications for public policy. *American Psychologist, 46*, 1036–1045.

Abram, K.M., Teplin, L.A., & McClelland, G.M. (2003). Comorbidity of severe psychiatric disorders and substance use disorders among women in jail. *American Journal of Psychiatry, 160*, 1007–1010.

Bell, A., Jaquette, N., Sanner, D., Steele-Smith, C., & Wald, H. (2005). Treatment of individuals with co-occurring disorders in county jails: The Beaver County, Pennsylvania experience. *Corrections Today, 67*(3), 86–90.

Broner, N., Lattimore, P.K., Cowell, A.J., & Schlenger, W.E. (2004). Effects of diversion on adults with co-occurring mental illness and substance use: Outcomes from a national multi-site study. *Behavioral Sciences and the Law, 22*, 519–542.

Broner, N., Nyugen, H., Swern, A., & Goldfinger, S. (2003). Adapting a substance abuse court diversion model for felony offenders with co-occurring disorders: Initial implementation. *Psychiatric Quarterly, 74*, 361–385.

Bureau of Justice Statistics. (2006). *Special report: Mental health problems of prison and jail inmates.* Washington, DC: U.S. Department of Justice.

Chandler, R.K., Peters, R.H., Field, G., & Juliano-Bult. (2004). Challenges in implementing evidence-based treatment practices for co-occurring disorders in the criminal justice system. *Behavioral Sciences and the Law, 22*, 431–448.

Chiles, J.A., Von Cleve, E., Jemelka, R.P., & Trupin, E.W. (1990). Substance abuse and psychiatric disorders in prison inmates. *Hospital and Community Psychiatry, 41*, 1132–1134.

Conly, C. (1999). *Coordinating community services for mentally ill offenders: Maryland's Community Criminal Justice Treatment Program.* Washington, DC: National Institute of Justice.

Couturier, L., Maue, F., & McVey, C. (2005). Releasing inmates with mental illness and co-occurring disorders into the community. *Corrections Today*, (April), 82–85.

Fletcher, B.W. (2005). National Criminal Justice Drug Abuse Treatment Studies (CJ-DATS): Update and progress. Justice Research and Statistics Association: *The Forum, 23*(3), 5–7.

Hiller, M.L., Knight, K., & Simpson, D. D. (1996). An assessment of comorbid psychological problems in a residential criminal justice drug treatment program. *Psychology of Addictive Behaviors, 10*, 181–189.

Hills, H.A. (2000). *Creating effective treatment programs for persons with co-occurring disorders in the justice system.* Delmar, NY: The National GAINS Center for People with Co-Occurring Disorders in the Justice System.

Jordan, K., Schlenger, W.E., Fairbank, J.A., & Caddell, J. M. (1996). Prevalence of psychiatric disorders among incarcerated women. *Archives of General Psychiatry, 53*, 513–519.

Koyanagi, C., & Blasingame, K. (2006). *Best practices: Access to benefits for prisoners with mental illnesses.* A Bazelon Center Issue Brief. Washington, DC: Bazelon Center for Mental Health Law.

Lamb, H.R., Weinberger, L.E., & Gross, B.H. (2004). Mentally ill persons in the criminal justice system: Some perspectives. *Psychiatric Quarterly, 75*, 107–126.

Lipton, L. (2001). Jail program helps inmates avoid health care gap. *Psychiatric News, 36*(16), 9.

Lurigio, A.J., Fallon, J.R., & Dincin, J. (2000). Helping the mentally ill in jails adjust to community life: A description of a post-release ACT program and its clients. *International Journal of Offender Therapy and Comparative Criminology, 44*, 532–548.

Monahan, J., Steadman, H., Robbins, P., Appelbaum, P., Banks, S., Grisso, T., Heilbrun, K., Mulvey, E., Roth, L., & Silver, E. (2005). An actuarial model of violence risk assessment for persons with mental disorders. *Psychiatric Services, 56*, 810–815.

Monahan, J., Steadman, H., Silver, E., Appelbaum, P., Robbins, P., Mulvey, E., Roth, L., Grisso, T., & Banks, S. (2001). *Rethinking risk assessment: The MacArthur study of mental disorder and violence.* New York: Oxford University Press.

National GAINS Center for People with Co-Occurring Disorders in the Justice System (2002). *Maintaining Medicaid benefits for jail detainees with co-occurring mental health and substance use disorders.* Fact Sheet Series. Delmar, NY.

National GAINS Center for People with Co-Occurring Disorders in the Justice System. (2004). *The prevalence of co-occurring mental illness and substance use disorders in jails.* Fact Sheet Series. Delmar, NY.

National GAINS Center for People with Co-Occurring Disorders in the Justice System. (2006). *Targeted Capacity Expansion initiative for jail diversion programs.* The

National GAINS Center for People with Co-Occurring Disorders in the Justice System: http://gainscenter.samhsa.gov/html/tapa/cmhs/overview.asp.

Ohio Substance Abuse and Mental Illness Coordinating Center of Excellence. (2002). *SAMI Matters Newsletter, 1*(2), 1–2. Northfield, Ohio.

Osher, F., Steadman, H.J., & Barr, H. (2002). *A best practice approach to community re-entry from jails for inmates with co-occurring disorders: The APIC model.* Delmar, NY: The National GAINS Center for People with Co-Occurring Disorders in the Justice System.

Osher, F., Steadman, H.J., & Barr, H. (2003). A best practice approach to community reentry from jails for inmates with co-occurring disorders: The APIC Model. *Crime and Delinquency, 49*, 79–96.

Osher, F.C. (2006). *Integrating mental health and substance abuse services for justice-involved persons with co-occurring disorders.* Delmar, New York: The National GAINS Center for Systemic Change for Justice-Involved People with Mental Illness.

Peters, R.H., Greenbaum, P.E., Edens, J.F., Carter, C.R., & Ortiz, M.M. (1998). Prevalence of DSM-IV substance abuse and dependence disorders among prison inmates. *American Journal of Drug and Alcohol Abuse, 24*, 573–587.

Peters, R.H., & Hills, H.A. (1997). *Intervention strategies for offenders with co-occurring disorders: What works?* Delmar, NY: The National GAINS Center for People with Co-Occurring Disorders in the Justice System.

Peters, R.H., LeVasseur, M.E., & Chandler, R.K. (2004). Correctional treatment for co-occurring disorders: Results of a national survey. *Behavioral Sciences and the Law, 22*, 563–584.

Peters, R.H., & Matthews, C.O. (2002). Substance abuse treatment programs in prisons and jails. In T.J. Fagan & R.K. Ax (Eds.), *Correctional mental health handbook* (pp. 73–99). Laurel, MD: Sage Publications.

Peters, R.H., Matthews, C.O., & Dvoskin, J.A. (2005*).* Treatment in prisons and jails. In J.H. Lowinson, P. Ruiz, R.B. Millman, & J.G. Langrod (Eds.), *Substance abuse: A comprehensive textbook* 4th ed., (pp. 707–722). Baltimore: Williams & Wilkins.

Peters, R.H., & Osher, F. (2004). *Co-occurring disorders and specialty courts.* Delmar, NY: National GAINS Center for People with Co-Occurring Disorders in the Justice System and the TAPA Center for Jail Diversion.

Peters, R.H., Sherman, P.B., & Osher, F.C. (in press). Treatment in jails and prison. In K.T. Mueser & D.V. Jeste (Eds.), *Clinical handbook of schizophrenia.* New York: Guilford Press.

Peters, R.H., & Wexler, H.K. (Eds.). (2005). *Substance abuse treatment for adults in the criminal justice system.* Center for Substance Abuse Treatment, Treatment Improvement Protocol (TIP) Series 44. DHHS Publication No. (SMA) 05-4056. Rockville, MD: Substance Abuse and Mental Health Services Administration.

Robins, L.N., & Regier, D.A. (1991). *Psychiatric disorders in America: The Epidemiologic Catchment Area study.* New York: Free Press.

Russell, B. (1999). New approaches to the treatment of women with co-occurring disorders in jails. *American Jails*, March/April, 21–25.

Sacks, S., & Pearson, F.S. (2003). Co-occurring substance use and mental disorders in offenders: Approaches, findings and recommendations. *Federal Probation, 67*(2), 32–39.

Sacks, S., & Ries, R.K. (2005) (Eds). *Substance abuse treatment for persons with co-occurring disorders.* Center for Substance Abuse Treatment, Treatment Improvement Protocol (TIP) Series 42. DHHS Publication No. (SMA) 05-3922. Rockville, MD: Substance Abuse and Mental Health Services Administration.

Sacks, S., Sacks, J.Y., McKendrick, K., Banks, S., & Stommel, J. (2004). Modified TC for MICA offenders: Crime outcomes. *Behavioral Sciences and the Law, 22*, 477–501.

Steadman, H. J., Fallon, J., Mireles, P., Williams, K., & Aronson, L. (2005). *Establishing collaborations with local jails: An edited transcript of the PATH national teleconference sponsored by the Substance Abuse and Mental Health Services Administration (SAMSHA)*. Retrieved on November 15, 2006, from PATH: Projects for Assistance in Transition from Homelessness: http://www.pathprogram.samhsa.gov/tech_assist/default.asp.

Steadman, H.J., Morris, S.M., & Dennis, D.L. (1995). The diversion of mentally ill persons from jails to community-based services: A profile of programs. *American Journal of Public Health, 85*, 1630–1635.

Steadman, H.J., & Naples, M. (2005). Assessing the effectiveness of jail diversion programs for persons with serious mental illness and co-occurring substance use disorders. *Behavioral Sciences and the Law, 23*, 163–170.

Steadman, H.J., & Veysey, B.M. (1997). Providing services for jail inmates with mental disorders. *National Institute of Justice: Research in Brief*, NCJ 162207, 1–10.

Teplin, L.A., Abram, K.M., & McClelland, G.M. (1996). Prevalence of psychiatric disorders among incarcerated women—I. Pretrial jail detainees. *Archives of General Psychiatry, 53*, 505–512.

Teplin, L.A., Abram, K.M., & McClelland, G.M. (1997), Mentally disordered women in jail: Who receives services? *American Journal of Public Health, 87*(4), 604–609.

Teplin, L.A., Abram, K.M., McClelland, G.M., Dulcan, M.D., & Mericle, A.A. (2002). Psychiatric disorders in youth in juvenile detention. *Archives of General Psychiatry, 59*, 1133–1143.

U.S. Department of Justice (2006). *Justice and Mental Health Collaboration Program: FY 2006 competitive grant announcement # BJA-2006-1381*. Retrieved on November 15, 2006, from Bureau of Justice Assistance Programs: http://www.ojp.usdoj.gov/BJA/grant/06MIOsol.pdf.

Van Stelle, K.R., & Moberg, D.P. (2004). Outcome data for MICA clients after participation in an institutional therapeutic community. *Journal of Offender Rehabilitation, 39*, 37–62.

Veysey, B.M., Steadman, H.J., Morrissey, J.P., & Johnsen, M. (1997). In search of the missing linkages: Continuity of care in the U.S. jails. *Behavioral Sciences and the Law, 15*, 383–397.

Walsh, A. (2000). Should jails be messing with mental health or substance abuse? *American Jails, 14*, 60–66.

Weisman, R.L., Lamberti, J.S., & Price, N. (2004). Integrating criminal justice, community healthcare, and support services for adults with severe mental disorders. *Psychiatric Quarterly, 75*, 71–85.

Wexler, H.K. (2003). The promise of prison-based treatment for dually diagnosed inmates. *Journal of Substance Abuse Treatment, 25*, 223–231.

Chapter 23

Pharmacological Treatment of Substance Abuse in Correctional Facilities: Prospects and Barriers to Expanding Access to Evidence-Based Therapy

R. Douglas Bruce, Duncan Smith-Rohrberg, and Frederick L. Altice

Introduction: Untreated Substance Abuse among Incarcerated Populations

The individual and societal costs of untreated substance abuse are enormous. These costs include overuse of hospital emergency departments, death due to overdose, high unemployment, illegal activity, and incarceration (Mark, Woody, Juday, & Kleber, 2001; Wall et al., 2000). Substance users, especially injection drug users, tend to be among society's most disease-burdened individuals, with a high prevalence of infectious diseases—HIV, hepatitis B and C, and tuberculosis (Edlin, 2002; Hagan et al., 2002; Kapadia et al., 2002; Martin, Cayla, Bolea, & Castilla, 2000; Spaulding, Greene, Davidson, Schneidermann, & Rich, 1999)—and comorbid psychiatric conditions (Milby et al., 1996).

Throughout the 1980s, in an effort to combat the increasing prevalence of substance misuse, many state and federal governments enacted stringent antidrug laws. Largely as a result of these measures, incarceration rates in the United States have dramatically increased and have imposed pressures on a system ill-prepared to address the medical and social consequences of substance abuse (Pollack, Khoshnood, & Altice, 1999). According to the Bureau of Justice, 82% of jail inmates and 83% of state prisoners have a history of substance abuse; 64% and 70%, respectively, used drugs "regularly" (at least once a week for at least a month) in the period immediately preceding incarceration (Dunkle et al., 2004; Hammett, Harmon, & Rhodes, 2002). While the high rates of drug-related arrests, recidivism, and the large numbers of substance abusers within the correctional system are alarming, they also represent an important public health opportunity (Glaser & Greifinger, 1993) Due to the large number of substance users who enter and reenter the nation's prisons and jails, the correctional system is one setting where access to necessary psychological and pharmacological therapies for substance dependence can be greatly expanded. In fact, the structured environment of the correctional setting can be an ideal place to initiate such treatment.

Despite the serious need for evidence-based pharmacological treatment for substance abuse, such interventions have not been implemented or evaluated sufficiently among incarcerated and soon-to-be released prisoners. Currently only 32% of state prisoners and 36% of federal prisoners with substance abuse problems receive any form of treatment while in prison, and almost none receive medically indicated pharmacotherapy (Mumola, 1999). Interview-based data suggest that a large population of inmates desire treatment in prison but are unable to access it (Brooke, Taylor, Gunn, & Maden, 1998). Among the federally approved medications to treat substance abuse, only methadone has been used in a correctional setting, and this has occurred only in a few model programs (Tomasino, Swanson, Nolan, & Shuman, 2001). This is despite over 40 years of accumulated evidence demonstrating its effectiveness at reducing drug-related harms. On the outside, only 15 to 20% of opiate-dependent patients presently receive medically indicated pharmacological treatment (Fiellin & O'Connor, 2002; Kreek & Vocci, 2002; Sporer, 2003).

The lack of providing effective evidence-based pharmacotherapies to treat substance abuse is counter productive for society and the criminal justice system. In the absence of prison-based treatment and linkage to community care following release, rates of drug abuse and recidivism will remain high (Langan & Levin, 2002). Interventions initiated in corrections, and continued into the community, could reduce recidivism and the many psychosocial and medical problems that result from untreated opiate use and dependence.

The aim of this chapter is to review a much-neglected area of correctional health care: the pharmacological treatment of substance abuse. The particular focus of this review will be on the evidence, prospects, and barriers to implementation among the five federally approved and currently available medications for the pharmacological treatment of substance abuse: methadone, naltrexone, buprenorphine, disulfiram, and acamprosate. We will discuss each of these, as well as provide additional insights into the prospects for treatment of cocaine and methamphetamine abuse. These two additional conditions are also serious public health concerns and are highly prevalent among incarcerated populations (Cartier, Farabee, & Prendergast, 2006; Miura, Fujiki, Shibata, & Ishikawa, 2006). It is likely that over the next decades we will see the advent of several new drugs to adequately treat these chemical dependencies, and when that time comes, it will be important to build from a successful foundation of correctional experiences with other pharmacotherapies of substance abuse.

The Pharmacological-Free Approach to Substance Abuse: Not Enough

Multiple therapeutic modalities have demonstrated effectiveness for the treatment of substance dependence. These modalities can be classified into two broad classes: drug-free therapeutic communities (TCs) and pharmacological interventional therapies. Hybrid models are also possible, although the basic philosophies of these two types of programs often conflict. It is beyond the scope of this review to discuss in-depth the TC approach in the prison setting, which has been subject to extensive study. TCs are typically more favored and understood by correctional officials (Butzin, Martin, & Inciardi, 2002; Hiller, Knight, & Simpson, 1999; Hofmann et al., 1996; Knight, Simpson, & Hiller, 1999; Wexler, Melnick, Lowe, & Peters, 1999), and indeed are the dominant mode of treatment in correctional facilities. It is thus worth providing a concise overview of TCs, even if they, in the authors' opinions, represent only a partial solution to the problem.

Briefly, traditional TCs are residential, long-term (6–12 months and longer) programs that provide the behavioral and psychosocial skills necessary to remain abstinent from drugs. Central to this philosophy, pharmacological treatments are discouraged and often viewed as enabling. TCs primarily focus on the teaching of "living right" and emphasize responsibility for self and others (De Leon, 1996) in an attempt to achieve "lasting life-style changes" (Hofmann et al., 1996). Perhaps the single greatest value of TCs is that they work toward getting the client off *all* drugs, and for this reason can treat comorbid cocaine and alcohol misuse and can avoid medication dependence that can develop in pharmacological programs.

A few generalizations can be made regarding situations that might be beneficial for prison-based TCs: (1) inmates with prolonged sentences who therefore have time to spend in an intensive program; (2) correctional systems with resources to fund comprehensive TC-based services linked to adequate aftercare programs; (3) individuals who are highly motivated (De Leon, Melnick, Kressel, & Jainchill, 1994; Wexler et al., 1999); (4) individuals with a history of severe drug abuse (Hiller et al., 1999; Hofmann et al., 1996; Knight et al., 1999); and (5) those without co-occurring mental illness or those whose mental illness is adequately treated (Brambilla et al., 1999; Milby et al., 1996). Motivation of the staff, cooperation of prison authorities, increasing levels of client responsibility, consensus-based decision-making, and provision of aftercare are all also central to success of TC-based programs (Jones, 1980; Rouse, 1991). Additionally, in terms of both recidivism and relapse rates, and cost-effectiveness, linkage to community programs on release is central to the success of such prison-based TCs (Chanhatasilpa, MacKenzie, & Hickman, 2000; Friedland et al., 1999; Hiller et al., 1999; Hofmann et al., 1996; Knight et al., 1999).

It is clear that TCs benefit many patients. The problem with the TC approach has not been strategy but rather the rhetoric surrounding them. They are typically presented as the only option for the treatment of substance abuse, and indeed, the current situation in U.S. correctional facilities is one where, if any treatment at all is available, TCs predominate. As such, there is generally little experience with or utilization of pharmacological treatments for substance-dependent correctional inmates. This is related to the logistical failures of such programs in the 1970s and the increased societal demands to reduce "coddling" of criminal offenders. Correctional administrators, the majority of whom are not familiar with chemical dependency as a medical and psychiatric disease, tend to favor drug-free options such as TC-based programs rather than more medically relevant options for patients with severe substance use disorders. The provision of medical treatments is especially vital for opioid-dependent patients who are at high risk for relapse, overdose, and death on release. Despite prior participation in TC-based programs, overdose continues to threaten the opioid-dependent user, especially on release from a correctional setting where tolerance has declined (Bird & Hutchinson, 2003; Brugal et al., 2005; Verger, Rotily, Prudhomme, & Bird, 2003). The goal of the remainder of this chapter is to present the available information on evidence-based medical treatment with pharmacotherapies for substance abuse as medically relevant and necessary aspects of complete substance abuse treatment.

Current Pharmacological Options for the Treatment of Opioid Dependence

It is estimated that almost 900,000 Americans are currently opiate dependent, with heroin dependence being the most common reported (Kreek & Vocci, 2002). Over 146,000 new individuals began using heroin in 2000, a number that continues to increase (SAMHSA, 2004). Mortality rates among heroin injectors are between 6 and 20 times higher than their drug-free peers (Sporer, 2003). Furthermore, the medical consequences of opiate use—infectious diseases, mortality, and emergency department use—have increased in recent years (National Consensus Development Panel on Effective Medical Treatment of Opiate Addiction, 1998). The overall economic costs of opiate dependence, especially to poor urban communities, are tremendous. Annual losses due to medical care, lost productivity, crime, and social welfare of heroin abuse alone cost the United States $21.9 billion (Mark et al., 2001). To combat these individual and societal problems, three pharmacological treatment strategies have been demonstrated to be effective in the treatment of opioid-dependent patients.

Naltrexone

Naltrexone, a long-acting, pure opiate antagonist that competitively inhibits the euphoric effects of opiates, has been in use for the treatment of opioid dependence for decades (Farren, O'Malley, & Rounsaville, 1997). A typical naltrexone regimen is 100 mg Monday and Wednesday and 150 mg on Friday, although 50 mg daily and twice weekly 100/150 mg have also been studied (Kirchmayer, Davoli, & Verster, 2002). Treatment initiation generally requires an effective supervised medical withdrawal from opioids for at least 5–7 days prior to treatment initiation to prevent the precipitation of severe withdrawal. The efficacy and safety of naltrexone for the treatment of opiate dependence have been demonstrated in several randomized, controlled clinical trials (J. P. Gonzalez & Brogden, 1988).

The major strength of this medication is that there are no opiate-related side effects, no overdose risk, no negative consequences on cessation (e.g., withdrawal), and no possibility for diversion. Additionally, naltrexone has some beneficial effects in the treatment of moderate alcoholism (Aditya et al., 2004; Marmot, Siegrist, Theorell, & Feeney, 1999), a common comorbid condition among opiate users. Naltrexone's effectiveness has been hampered by decreased adherence because, unlike methadone, there is no negative reinforcement for discontinuation (i.e., opioid withdrawal). Hence, the effectiveness of naltrexone heavily depends on the motivation and social support system of the patient (Greenstein, Evans, McLellan, & O'Brien, 1983). Indeed, the drug is most effective among "white-collar" opiate users, such as dependent health care professionals, and has achieved its best results when treatment was contingent on continued employment (Roth, Hogan, & Farren, 1997; Washton, Gold, & Pottash, 1984).

Systematic meta-analysis indicates that naltrexone is no better than placebo except when used in combination with behavioral therapy; and this effect was explained primarily by subject motivation (Kirchmayer, Davoli, Verster, et al., 2002). Recently, Schottenfeld and colleagues reported on the first comparison of naltrexone to an opioid agonist (in this case buprenorphine) treatment in a double-blinded placebo-controlled study of 126 patients in Malaysia. After complete withdrawal from opiates, subjects were randomized to one of three arms: standardized counseling, buprenorphine with standardized counseling, or naltrexone with standardized counseling. Buprenorphine with standardized counseling was associated with a longer duration of abstinence compared with drug counseling alone or drug counseling with naltrexone, suggesting that, where feasible, agonists such as buprenoprhine should be preferred over antagonists such as naltrexone (Mazlan, Schottenfeld, & Chawarski, 2006; Schottenfeld, Mazlan, & Chawarski, 2006).

The lack of effect of naltrexone, as discussed above, has been attributed to a lack of motivation on the part of subjects. Correctional settings offer a location where motivation can be affected by concerns of punishment. Naltrexone was first used in the United States among incarcerated populations as part of a work-release program, involving 691 work-release inmates in Nassau County, New York (Brahen, Henderson, Capone, & Kordal, 1984). While the program was not a controlled experiment and had no outcomes described for the subjects, the involved correctional officials, clients, and physicians viewed naltrexone favorably. Subsequently, a pilot study was conducted among 51 federal parolees in whom naltrexone therapy was stipulated as a condition for parole (Cornish et al., 1997). Parole officers directly observed naltrexone administration and tested the urine weekly for opiates. Using historical controls, both retention in treatment (52% in treatment versus 33% in control) and mean opiate positive urine test (8% versus 30%) were improved. Notwithstanding these preliminary results, randomized controlled trials with appropriate controls and longer follow-up beyond the period of parole are necessary to determine long-term effectiveness. The effectiveness of such programs depends on prisoners who have probation or parole stipulations which act as enhancers of motivation and adherence, the duration of the stipulation, and the degree to which parole or probation officers are co-trained in the area of drug treatment. Still, especially for highly motivated subjects under a structured environment, naltrexone remains a viable option.

A 1-month injectable depo-naltrexone formulation was recently approved by the Food and Drug Administration for the treatment of alcohol dependence. Although approved for alcohol dependence, naltrexone's ability to block exogenous opiates such as heroin may expand naltrexone's applicability in both community and correctional settings. For example, it might be administered soon after incarceration for unsentenced inmates and immediately prior to release for sentenced prisoners. As such, it may allow for a reprieve from immediate recidivism to opiate use and prevent overdose (especially in the week following release from custody) while social factors are stabilized. Such clinical applications, however, await carefully designed research trials to demonstrate effectiveness in correctional settings.

Methadone

Methadone is a full opiate agonist with a long half-life of 12–36 hours that can be administered once daily because of its relatively constant plasma levels over a 24-hour period. Daily dosing regimens are variable and patient-specific. Higher doses, on the order of 80–100 mg, are overall more effective than lower doses (e.g., 40–50 mg) in reducing illicit opiate use (Strain, Bigelow, Liebson, & Stitzer, 1999). This may be because while lower doses suppress heroin withdrawal symptoms, higher doses block the opiate receptor, thereby limiting both craving and blocking the effect of exogenous heroin (Donny, Walsh, Bigelow, Eissenberg, & Stitzer, 2002). Since methadone takes 2 to 6 hours to attain peak levels, it does not provide a euphoric sensation when properly dosed in stabilized patients. Dependency develops rapidly, and missed doses result in severe opiate withdrawal symptoms (Liu & Wang, 1984).

Over 40 years of experience and extensive research in the United States have demonstrated the cost-effectiveness of methadone at increasing retention in treatment, decreasing heroin use, and reducing crime and HIV risk behaviors (Barnett, Zaric, & Brandeau, 2001; Marsch, 1998; Mattick, Breen, Kimber, & Davoli, 2002; Yoast, Williams, Deitchman, & Champion, 2001). Nevertheless, in the United States and many countries, community-based methadone treatment clinics are strictly regulated and rarely able to meet treatment demand (Rettig & Yarmolinsky, 1995). Regulation is central in reducing diversion to illicit use, but this practice severely limits access to treatment because of the resultant small number of funded treatment slots. Recently, attempts to expand access, by transitioning stable methadone-maintained patients from methadone clinics to physician-prescribed treatment, have demonstrated considerable clinical success (Fiellin et al., 2001). Despite these findings, transition programs to office-based methadone treatment that would be exempt from strict federal regulations in the United States (as in buprenorphine) have not been implemented outside of research settings due to federal licensure requirements. It is still unclear where the balance between limiting diversion and increasing access might lie. One recent report from the United Kingdom, where methadone is made available through prescription by general practitioners, demonstrated that fewer deaths result from methadone than from heroin (Hickman et al., 2003). This suggests that the U.S. system has placed a greater emphasis on preventing methadone-related deaths at the expense of preventing heroin-related deaths.

There have been several experiments worldwide in which methadone maintenance treatment is provided to prison populations. In Canada, early success in the reduction of illicit drug use among methadone-maintained participants in provincial prison (Rothon, 1997) was followed in 1998 by a Correctional Service of Canada sponsored program to provide methadone maintenance for opiate-dependent federal prisoners (Sibbald, 2002). Initially, incarcerated individuals who were enrolled in community-based methadone maintenance were allowed to continue their treatment while in prison. The success of the program and the lack of diversion resulted in a significant policy change in May 2002, such that all opioid-dependent prisoners are now provided methadone treatment. In 1987, New South Wales, Australia, initiated a prison-based methadone treatment program that has since gained widespread acceptance by correctional officers, medical staff, and inmates (Elliott et al., 1998), in part because it has been shown to reduce injection drug use practices in prison (Dolan, Hall, & Wodak, 1996). Unfortunately, none of these programs have been rigorously evaluated for effectiveness in reducing crime and illicit use.

While there has been relatively little experience with a prison-based Methadone Maintenance Treatment Program (MMTP) in the United States, one model program, New York's Riker's Island, Key Extended Entry Program (Project KEEP), has been implemented and evaluated since 1987 (Tomasino et al., 2001). In order to address the concerns of correctional officials regarding diversion to illicit use, Project KEEP used community-based strategies such as directly observed therapy (DOT) using a public health nurse and correctional officer. This has minimized diversion in this setting (Tomasino et al., 2001). The lack of diversion and reduction of "difficult" behaviors of inmates experiencing opioid withdrawal have resulted in the acceptance, and even encouragement, of methadone maintenance by correctional officers and administrators.

Project KEEP's success is dependent on the linkage between the prison- and community-based MMTPs that provides a continuum of care between the community and prison. As such, patients entering the prison already on methadone are maintained. The program also offers methadone initiation or supervised opioid withdrawal for opioid dependent patients who are not already on pharmacological treatment. On release, patients may continue to receive methadone in the community-based programs.

Successful outcomes for this program include linkage to continued MMTP in the community (74–80%) (Tomasino et al., 2001), a higher linkage to community-based drug treatment programs than those who underwent supervised opiate withdrawal (85% versus 37%), and a decrease in injection drug behaviors at 6 months postrelease (70% versus 44%) (Magura, Rosenblum, Lewis, & Joseph, 1993). Despite success of Project KEEP in linking more patients to community drug treatment, the 6-month retention was modest; 27% of KEEP versus 9% of patients who underwent supervised opioid withdrawal remained in treatment (Magura et al., 1993). Successful linkage to and retention in drug treatment after prison release varied among individuals within KEEP. Participants who were on methadone prior to incarceration and methadone-naive participants who were placed on higher methadone doses (>30 mg/day) fared best (Tomasino et al., 2001). This latter finding is in keeping with the several studies that have demonstrated that patients on higher dose methadone do better than those on a lower dose (Dole, Nyswander, & Kreek, 1966; Donny et al., 2002; Strain et al., 1999).

In sum, methadone maintenance is gradually gaining acceptance in several countries as a viable option for treatment among opiate-dependent inmates. Perhaps the most important rationale for expanded methadone programs in the correctional system is to continue therapy for inmates already on methadone in the community prior to incarceration. A major risk factor for the use of illicit drugs within prison is related to a failure to continue methadone maintenance treatment that the inmate had been receiving in the community prior to incarceration (Gore & Bird, 1995; Vormfelde & Poser, 2001). Withdrawal symptoms due to forced abstinence from methadone following incarceration are a major source of negative attitudes toward methadone among injection drug users (Zule & Desmond, 1998). Expanded access to MMTPs for methadone participants in the correctional setting could help to resolve this problem. The system-level political obstacles that have hindered methadone acceptance in U.S. correctional facilities are important to remember in analyzing the feasibility of other pharmacotherapies, including buprenorphine.

Buprenorphine

Buprenorphine has been studied since 1978 as a synthetic partial opioid for the treatment of pain (Jasinski, Pevnick, & Griffith, 1978). Unlike full opioid agonists (e.g., methadone), buprenorphine is a partial agonist at the mu-opioid receptor. As a partial agonist, there is a plateau of its agonist effects at higher doses that enhances its safety profile compared to full agonists and tempers its likelihood for street diversion (Fiellin & O'Connor, 2002; Ling & Smith, 2002). This "ceiling effect" includes an upper limit on the severity of side effects associated with overdose, such as respiratory depression (Liguori, Morse, & Bergman, 1996; Walsh, Preston, Stitzer, Cone, & Bigelow, 1994).

As with all opioids, a potential for abuse exists (Seet & Lim, 2006; Tzschentke, 2002). To combat this potential for abuse, buprenorphine is primarily marketed in combination with naloxone (Suboxone®), though buprenorphine alone (Subutex®) is also available. In Suboxone, the naloxone (NTX) has limited bioavailability when administered sublingually. However, when crushed and injected, NTX has the potential to precipitate opioid withdrawal in buprenorphine-maintained subjects (Comer & Collins, 2002; G. M. Robinson, Dukes, Robinson, Cooke, & Mahoney, 1993). In addition, buprenorphine can precipitate opioid withdrawal in opioid-maintained (e.g., heroin or methadone) subjects because it binds to the μ-receptor with greater affinity than heroin, thus dislodging the heroin (Clark, Lintzeris, & Muhleisen, 2002; Greenwald, Schuh, Hopper, Schuster, & Johanson, 2002). Finally, buprenorphine dissociates slowly from the μ-receptor; therefore, its effects at the receptor site are long acting and can allow for alternate-day dosing (Fudala, Jaffe, Dax, & Johnson, 1990; Johnson et al., 1995).

Several randomized, controlled trials have demonstrated buprenorphine's efficacy in managing opiate withdrawal(Gowing, Ali, & White, 2002; Mattick, Kimber, Breen, & Davoli, 2002) and opiate dependence (Doran et al., 2003; Johnson et al., 2000). These studies led to U.S. FDA approval of Suboxone® and Subutex® in October 2002. Additionally, buprenorphine's pharmacological properties compelled the U.S. DEA to classify it as a Class III controlled substance, thereby allowing its prescription by properly trained generalist practitioners under the Drug Addiction Treatment Act of 2000. The goal was to expand access to pharmacological treatments by avoiding the need for the tightly regulated, specialist clinics that have hampered the expansion of MMTPs. France approved physician prescription of buprenorphine in 1996, and the Australian government has also begun implementing a national buprenorphine program (Caplehorn & Deeks, 2006).

Since a continuity-of-care program following incarceration will require community-based treatment on release, an examination of studies in community settings is informative for the development of future correctional-to-community interventions. While buprenorphine's efficacy has been proven through numerous clinical trials, it has been subject to fewer tests of effectiveness in real-world settings. France has had the most experience with community-based buprenorphine treatment; within a few years after its approval in 1996, the number of buprenorphine maintenance patients exceeded that of methadone by a factor of 10 (Auriacombe, Franques, & Tignol, 2001). Remarkably, approximately 20% of French physicians are using buprenorphine to treat the estimated 150,000 problem heroin users in France (Auriacombe, Fatseas, Dubernet, Daulouede, & Tignol, 2004). One prospective study of 105 community-based French physicians and 909 opioid-dependent patients showed improvements in housing, employment, social status, and self-reported heroin and other illicit drug intake; low HIV, HBV, and HCV seroconversion was also demonstrated (Fhima, Henrion, Lowenstein, & Charpak, 2001).

There were several problems, however, with the widespread introduction of buprenorphine in France. Buprenorphine was used illicitly, primarily by injection in combination with benzodiazepines, resulting in unanticipated morbidity and mortality (Claudon-Charpentier, Hoibian, Glasser, Lalanne, & Pasquali, 2000). Overdose and death occurred in some individuals when buprenorphine was coadministered intravenously with benzodiazepines; despite these occurrences, the overall overdose rate has declined in France since the start of buprenorphine treatment (Auriacombe et al., 2004). These anecdotal reports, however, did lead the manufacturer to caution the use of buprenorphine in patients abusing benzodiazepines (Obadia, Perrin, Feroni, Vlahov, & Moatti, 2001). Still, the problem of overdose appears to be less than with full opioid agonists; in a review of all cases from 1994 to 1998 in France reported to a centralized illicit drug use agency, methadone use had a mortality that was three times greater than buprenorphine (Auriacombe et al., 2001).

Compared with France, the U.S. experience has been more limited. One pilot study of 46 subjects compared buprenorphine administered thrice weekly in a primary care clinic to methadone administered at a specialized MMTP. Buprenorphine resulted in higher levels of retention and opiate-free urine toxicology than methadone (O'Connor et al., 1998). One speculation from this study is that primary care clinics have less stigma than traditional drug treatment settings and provide more comprehensive services that are often required for a population with multiple comorbid medical and social problems. This pilot is small and its findings remain to be established in a larger sample, however. In Australia, a comparison of methadone and buprenorphine found methadone superior largely due to improved cost-effectiveness, but also in treatment outcomes (Caplehorn & Deeks, 2006). Importantly, one recent smaller study involving 14 patients in a 13-week clinical trial demonstrated that, in combination with a brief counseling intervention, buprenorphine was effective in the ambulatory primary care setting; 11 patients were retained through the maintenance phase (Fiellin et al., 2002). Another series of pilot studies have been conducted among HIV-infected patients, suggesting the feasibility of treating patients with comorbid medical conditions (Sullivan et al., 2006). These preliminary studies suggest that buprenorphine may prove effective as it is implemented in community settings, especially in sites such as correctional settings which have been traditionally resistant to methadone.

While corrections-based programs have yet to be implemented in the United States, the French Ministry of Health has provided buprenorphine to incarcerated injection drug users since 1996 (Berson et al., 2001). This represents the longest and largest program internationally. A retrospective cohort study of over 3600 medical files of French prisoners analyzed the comparative effectiveness of methadone, buprenorphine, and abstinence treatment following the legalization of prison-administered buprenorphine. Compared to abstinence-based treatment, both buprenorphine and MMTP within prison resulted in reduced recidivism rates (Peters, LeVasseur, & Chandler, 2004). The early successes of the French experience with buprenorphine in correctional settings highlights the need to utilize and evaluate buprenorphine treatment within the U.S. correctional system. Recent work is being conducted within Project KEEP at Riker's Island to introduce buprenorphine for incoming opioid dependent inmates. This protocol is in its early stages and no data are available. In addition, the Connecticut Department of Corrections has started using buprenorphine for supervised clinical withdrawal of opioid dependent inmates who present to Connecticut jails in objective opiate withdrawal as assessed by the Clinical Opiate Withdrawal Scale (COWS). This program is in its early phases and has not been evaluated to date.

Pharmacological Treatment Options for Alcohol Dependence

Compared to opiate dependence, the neurobiology of alcohol dependence does not lend itself well to a substitution strategy. As such, treatment for alcohol dependence centers on reducing problematic drinking and relapse prevention through the pharmacological attenuation of relapse in the case of acamprosate or naltrexone, and the aversive response with relapse in the case of disulfiram. Although all three medications have been studied in the general population, the only published studies to date in a postcorrectional setting are with disulfiram. Therefore, many of the recommendations on the pharmacological use in correctional settings or on release are therefore extrapolations from existing studies in nonincarcerated settings.

Disulfiram

Disulfiram was first discovered as a possible treatment for alcoholism in 1937 by E.E. Williams and was FDA approved for the treatment of alcohol dependence in 1951 (Suh, Pettinati, Kampman, & O'Brien, 2006). Disulfiram works by blocking the oxidation of alcohol, resulting in 5- to 10-fold increased levels of acetaldehyde. The accumulation of acetaldehyde produces many unpleasant symptoms that include flushing, headache, nausea, vomiting, sweating, chest pain, palpitations, and tachycardia. In rare cases, life-threatening reactions can occur including hypotension, cardiovascular collapse, convulsions, and death ("Disulfiram," 2006). The psychopharmacological principle was aversive conditioning. This was achieved by titrating the exact dose of disulfiram to the minimum dose required to experience aversion when administered ethanol. The goal is for the patient to experience the aversive effect of ethanol with disulfiram with the hope that the patient would avoid future ethanol administration. Over time physicians stopped having patients purposefully experience the disulfiram–ethanol interaction. Instead, physicians described the interaction, hoping the fear of an adverse effect rather than aversive conditioning itself would be sufficient to reduce ethanol consumption.

Achieving optimal adherence, a challenge for all pharmacological treatments, is particularly difficult in the case of disulfiram, which only provides negative reinforcement. In an attempt to improve adherence that would not depend on patient motivation or legal requirements (e.g., parole), an implantable formulation was developed. This formulation, however, is not available in the United States. Because the principal benefit of disulfiram appears to be the fear of an adverse experience, rather than a receptor mediated agonist effect such as methadone for opioid dependence, it appears the treatment is currently more a psychological rather than physiological treatment. As a result, in the few well controlled studies that have been conducted, it appears to be of similar benefit to placebo (Kranzler & Rounsaville, 1998). Therefore, individuals often discontinue treatment because there is no aversive effect of stopping the medication (as opposed to discontinuing methadone). Hence, the individual taking the disulfiram either must be highly motivated internally due to a desire to remain abstinent from alcohol or must be externally motivated such as in the coercive nature of linkage of treatment with parole/probation.

Indeed, some of the greatest successes with disulfiram have been in settings where adherence was coercive or subjects were otherwise highly motivated to remain in treatment. Several studies have examined disulfiram among recently released inmates. In an uncontrolled observational study with inmates released from an Atlanta correctional facility who had daily disulfiram therapy directly observed by either a family member or a probation officer, 64 (48%) of 132 subjects remained abstinent from alcohol at 3 months (Bourne, Alford, & Bowcock, 1966). In another, uncontrolled study among 141 inmates released on parole who were given disulfiram on alternate days with supervised dosing, 46% demonstrated a beneficial response by the end of 1 year (Haynes, 1973). In a study using thrice-weekly observed dosing of disulfiram in 68 patients, 58% remained abstinent over 6 months (Sereny, Sharma, Holt, & Gordis, 1986). Gallant and colleagues, however, were unable to replicate these results in offenders, finding only a 10% improvement in drinking (Gallant et al., 1968).

While the data are limited, there is some evidence to suggest that disulfiram may be beneficial in certain circumstances. Any "pure" effect of disulfiram, however, is amplified by the legal sanctions associated with being on parole/probation.

Naltrexone and Acamprosate

In addition to its use for the treatment of opioid dependence, naltrexone is an FDA-approved medication for the treatment of alcohol dependence. It is believed that naltrexone works to prevent relapse by attenuating the pleasure response associated with a return to drinking, thereby decreasing the reinforcement associated with that behavior (O'Malley, 1996; O'Malley & Froehlich, 2003). Specifically, ethanol appears to activate the endogenous opioid system that results in an activation of various neurotransmitters, such as dopamine. This pleasurable cycle constitutes the reinforcing effects of ethanol (Gianoulakis, Krishnan, & Thavundayil, 1996; O'Brien, 2005). Interruption of this cycle with naltrexone results in a decrease in heavy drinking as well as a prolongation of abstinence (Balldin et al., 2003; Monterosso et al., 2001; Petrakis et al., 2005). As with disulfiram, poor adherence increases treatment ineffectiveness, however. To address adherence, an injectable formulation was recently developed which provides therapeutic doses of naltrexone over a 30-day period. The injectable formulation has not been evaluated in correctional settings, but its potential to decrease relapse to both alcohol and opiates when administered prior to release from correctional settings is an important area for future research.

Acamprosate, a structural analogue of the GABA neurotransmitter whose mechanism of action is not completely understood, was FDA-approved in 2004 for the treatment of alcohol dependence ("Acamprosate," 2006). Studies have suggested that acamprosate facilitates the function of GABA receptors and/or may attenuate the effect of glutamate at NMDA-type receptors. The cumulative effect results in restoration of a balance between neuronal excitation and inhibition in the central nervous system that is hypothesized to be altered in chronic alcoholics and plays a role in relapse ("Acamprosate," 2006; Littleton, 1995; Mason et al., 2002). Sixteen trials with a total of more than 4500 patients have demonstrated a modest advantage over placebo in maintaining abstinence from alcohol (Mason, 2001). On the other hand, a large multicenter trial comparing naltrexone, acamprosate, or a combined behavioral intervention did not demonstrate a benefit of acamprosate over placebo (Krupitsky et al., 2006).

Adherence is also a major challenge with acamprosate. Dosing requires two capsules three times a day, and this increased pill burden, compared to naltrexone and disulfiram, adversely impacts adherence. Methods to improve adherence in this population will be necessary to improve clinical outcomes.

Although no studies have been conducted to date with naltrexone and acamprosate within correctional settings, the previous case studies with disulfiram suggest that acamprosate or naltrexone may have similar benefits. Well-designed clinical trials which evaluate pharmacological treatments as interventions to prevent relapse on release from correctional settings are urgently needed to more appropriately inform clinical practice.

Implementing Pharmacological Therapies for Substance Dependence in the Correctional System

The recent expansion of pharmacological treatments for substance dependence in the primary care setting provides a potentially exciting opportunity to revisit the use of these therapies within the correctional setting as well as in transitioning inmates with a history of substance dependence to community-based programs. Pharmacological treatments for alcohol dependence do not pose the risk of diversion that methadone and buprenorphine may pose and may be more easily incorporated into the correctional setting. Because the pharmacological treatments of alcohol dependence are for the purposes of relapse prevention only and do not treat the symptoms of withdrawal, these pharmacological therapies could be instituted prior to release and do not need to be offered immediately on incarceration.

Methadone maintenance as relapse prevention for opiate-dependent prisoners transitioning to the community has been fraught with the following problems: (1) the logistical and regulatory impediments of providing methadone within the correctional setting; (2) the lack of available methadone treatment slots after release to the community; (3) the lack of financial resources of impoverished correctional inmates as they leave prison or jail; and (4) the relatively slow dose escalation to therapeutic doses of methadone (Fiellin & O'Connor, 2002; Fudala et al., 2003). The more recent availability of buprenorphine now promises compelling reasons to consider this as an alternative transitional treatment for inmates transitioning to the community. Buprenorphine offers the following advantages: (1) it can be safely started and can achieve a therapeutic dose faster than methadone prior to release; (2) it does not require stringent regulations to administer both within and outside the correctional setting; (3) it has a lower risk of overdose than methadone. However, as with methadone, it will require the availability of financial resources to cover the costs of the medication and any additional drug treatment (e.g., counseling). Notwithstanding these exciting possibilities, there are several obstacles that will hinder the use of buprenorphine, and other medications for the treatment of addiction, in both corrections and the community. These will be discussed, with some analysis of previous practical attempts at surmounting these obstacles.

Structural Obstacles

Perhaps the most important obstacles, certainly those that have paralyzed expansion of MMTPs, are structural ones relating to acceptability, availability, and access of services for the treatment of substance dependence (Khoshnood, Blankenship, Pollack, Roan, & Altice, 2000). First, physicians may not fully embrace and gain the necessary skills to prescribe a pharmacological agent such as buprenorphine or naltrexone. This may be particularly true for correctional physicians who often lag behind the community with regard to "best practices" (Skolnick, 1998). Second, some correctional settings are often ill-equipped to provide psychosocial and medical services necessary for an effective chemical dependency treatment program (see below). Third, the lack of access to and desire to see primary care clinicians among some drug-dependent patients released from correctional institutions will hinder linkage-to-care programs. While linkage-to-care is essential for the success of both buprenorphine and methadone, it is particularly critical for the treatments of alcohol dependence that rely solely on relapse prevention. Finally, current federal law limits access to opioid substitution therapy (OST) on release by requiring methadone maintenance through federally licensed MMTP sites and by requiring a patient limit for each physician willing to prescribe buprenorphine for OST (currently at 100 patients per physician).

Reduction in the illicit use of prescribed buprenorphine is important in gaining political acceptance among the public and correctional officers—and therefore in gaining the support necessary to fight these structural obstacles. This is a very real concern, especially globally. For example, the decline in heroin availability and the clinical practice of prescribing injectable (intramuscular) buprenorphine to heroin users led to widespread illicit buprenorphine use in parts of India (Ball, Rana, & Dehne, 1998). As discussed previously, Suboxone® (buprenorphine/naloxone) may reduce diversion; a New Zealand study presented evidence of diminished, though not eliminated, abuse of a co-formulated tablet (buprenorphine/naloxone) following its introduction in 1991 (Stoller, 2003; G. M. Robinson, Dukes, Robinson, Cooke, & Mahoney, 1993). Often diversion is secondary to limited treatment availability and, while diversion and abuse are concerns that require appropriate attention and funding, they should not be used as an argument to restrict access to this important medication (Fudala & Johnson, 2006; S. E. Robinson, 2006).

The Need for Psychosocial Services

Substance-dependent patients have multiple unmet psychosocial needs that place them at high risk for recidivism, relapse, and overdose following release from incarceration (Nurco, Hanlon, & Kinlock, 1991). These same unmet needs increase risk for transmission of HIV, viral hepatitis, and sexually transmitted diseases (Sheu et al., 2002; Thompson et al., 1998). Additionally, pharmacological treatment for one specific illness (e.g., opioid dependence) may fall short due to use of other illicit drugs (e.g., cocaine abuse). For example, in the KEEP study, 25% of the participants were also cocaine users (Magura et al., 1993; Tomasino et al., 2001); national samples indicate that as many as 40% of heroin users also use cocaine (Hser, Anglin, & Fletcher, 1998). Opioid substitution therapy will substantially reduce opioid-associated behavior that puts the user at risk for infectious disease. OST alone, however, will not ensure safe sex, abstinence from other drugs, involvement in primary care, and improved social habits—activities that would improve infectious- and non-infectious-associated morbidity and mortality. Pharmacological therapies should thus be viewed as a part of the larger promotion for public health and the improved health and psychosocial status of chemically dependent inmates.

The extent and nature of ancillary psychosocial services are thus essential for successful outcomes, regardless of which treatment is selected for the patient. For example, provision of transportation (Friedmann, Lemon, & Stein, 2001) and contact with state social services (Desland & Batey, 1991) have been shown to play a role in retention in community-based clinics. Additionally, psychiatric care, involvement by family members, employment, and medical services are predictive of positive outcomes across a wide range of treatment modalities (McLellan et al., 1994). Given the high rates of incarceration of people of color in the U.S. correctional system (Blankenship, Smoyer, Bray, & Mattocks, 2005), cultural considerations (i.e., bilingual and bicultural services) are important (Osemene, Essien, & Egbunike, 2001). Case management services both within and outside correctional facilities are a central component to the treatment of drug abuse and dependence, since treatment is oftentimes hindered by the individuals' inability to meet basic needs such as shelter and food (Hasson, Grella, Rawson, & Anglin, 1994). These linkage services have been shown in retrospective cohort studies to be effective and inexpensive interventions that promote short-term retention in treatment and prevent relapse in patients discharged from various treatment programs (Shwartz, Baker, Mulvey, & Plough, 1997).

The Need for Health Care Services

In a population with serious medical needs, access to health care on release from correctional settings is an integral part of an effective transitional treatment intervention (Osemene et al., 2001). Traditional methods to improve access to primary care services, such as community health centers and mobile health care units, for chemically dependent inmates (Altice, Springer,

Buitrago, Hunt, & Friedland, 2003; Kuo, Sherman, Thomas, & Strathdee, 2004; Liebman, Pat Lamberti, & Altice, 2002) will need to be explored as options in maintaining the prison-to-community care continuum for pharmacotherapies of substance dependence (e.g., buprenorphine and naltrexone). Once patients are within the health care system, it is critical that community clinicians are prepared to decide which patients would benefit from outpatient pharmacotherapy in the primary care setting and which ones would need a specialized drug treatment clinic. A staging system using admission questions, similar to those used in cancer prognosis, has been developed to achieve this objective (Favrat, Rao, O'Connor, & Schottenfeld, 2002).

Despite the clear need for access to ancillary social services among chemically dependent inmates, such services are often unavailable or ineffective, leading to underutilization of these effective components of successful treatment (Widman, Platt, Lidz, Mathis, & Metzger, 1997). There is extensive variability in the delivery of these ancillary interventions, depending on site, staff, and patient characteristics (Widman et al., 1997), complicating policy and health care decision-making. This is due in part to the paucity of randomized controlled trials looking at how provision of these services impacts pharmacological treatments.

The need for such trials is demonstrated by the few good controlled trials that have been done. One such trial involving MMTP alone, MMTP plus counseling, and MMTP plus medical services, employment, and family counseling, showed a clear gradation of effectiveness depending on the level of social services provided (McLellan, Arndt, Metzger, Woody, & O'Brien, 1993). Although these are effective components of a successful treatment program, a cost-effectiveness analysis, however, suggested that money could be better spent expanding access to traditional MMTPs (which are limited in number compared to the large need) as opposed to enhancing existing ones through added social services (Kraft, Rothbard, Hadley, McLellan, & Asch, 1997).

A Team Approach to Pharmacological Therapies—Communication between Community and Corrections

Because of the complex needs of opiate-dependent patients, especially those within the correctional system, communication among the different providers both inside and outside of the correctional system is vital. In addressing this problem, the Glasgow "shared care" methadone system is instructive. This program consisted of general practitioners who agreed to maintain common treatment standards and attend monthly educational sessions, and who were compensated for their extra efforts. Drug counselors and pharmacists were involved to reduce the clinician responsibility and to provide the social and psychological support necessary to maintain proper adherence to treatment. Finally, as mentioned above, pharmacy-based supervised self-administration of the methadone helped reduce diversion. This program showed excellent participation and retention of physicians and pharmacists (Gruer et al., 1997) The program resulted in reduced injection practices, opiate use and overdose, crime, and money spent on drugs. This was especially true for individuals who remained in the program for at least 12 months (Hutchinson, Corbie-Smith, Thomas, Mohanan, & del Rio, 2004).

In addition to working toward integration of services among community-based pharmacists, counselors, and physicians, a model of communication between the correctional and community physicians is essential for a program's success. This will require the establishment of a network of community physicians who can accept referrals for treatment with little or no notice as jail detainees and prisoners are released from the correctional setting secondary to commuted sentences, payment of bond, or unanticipated release from court.

A Team Approach to Pharmacological Therapies—Structure within Corrections

A "one treatment fits all" approach in correctional settings is not compatible with community standards and will significantly diminish the benefit to the public's health. Therefore, careful attention to the specific correctional environment and assessment of the individual inmate is required to prescribe appropriate and clinically meaningful pharmacological treatment within correctional settings. The evaluation of the inmate should begin with appropriate intake assessments which should be utilized to develop a meaningful and effective treatment plan. The following are central to an initial evaluation of the inmate: (1) likelihood of release for jail detainees; (2) duration of sentence for prisoners; (3) primary substance to which the inmate is dependent (e.g., heroin); (4) severity and duration of dependence; (5) dependence on other drugs; (6) comorbid medical conditions such as HIV or viral hepatitis which may complicate treatment (e.g., methadone and HIV therapy interactions); (7) comorbid mental illness which may be addressed concurrently with pharmacological treatment for chemical dependence or may need to precede this treatment; (8) levels of social support including employment; and (9) living circumstances after release to the community.

In order to address drug treatment needs throughout the correctional system, it will be essential to examine the conditions and infrastructure of both jails and prisons. The approaches are likely to be different given the differing populations and time constraints. Jails house pretrial detainees and sometimes prisoners sentenced to less than 2 years. Thus, the majority of unsentenced detainees will be released from jail within days to weeks while those who are sentenced serve a median time of 9 months (Dunkle et al., 2004). Policy changes for jails are likely to be more erratic because they are usually under the jurisdiction of local communities. In a jail setting, brief structural interventions such as pharmacotherapy for chemical dependence might be initiated with the plan to transition to a community-based program or practitioner on release. Jail inmates are also likely to be younger and to have used psychoactive substances just prior to incarceration than those who reside within the prison system. For these individuals, there is a critical moment where drug treatment opportunities exist before release to the community. This is especially true in the case of new opiate users who enter the jail system briefly and have yet to make the transition to injecting heroin use. The possibility for preventing hepatitis C and HIV rests on the ability to reach these opiate abusers early, before they have made the transition to injection drug use and seroconverted (Altice et al., 1998).

The landscape is different for prison inmates. The longer sentences imposed on prisoners provide an optimal time to address multiple social, psychological, and criminal problems that would otherwise confound drug treatment. Interventions among longer-sentenced prisoners can be less immediate, but need to be substantial and long term to be effective. Prison-based TCs may be highly effective with some of these prisoners, but such an approach requires high investment in infrastructure to promote the drug-free environment. This infrastructure must incorporate this goal within the prison, throughout the transitional period, and must plan for aftercare on release in order to be effective. In the absence of this commitment, pharmacological therapy initiated in prison may serve as an effective conduit to treatment after release for individuals with a high likelihood of relapse.

Depending on the assessment gleaned and the treatment plan developed (which must take into consideration the length of incarceration and location as discussed above), decisions can be made regarding the optimal course of action for the patient. For example, buprenorphine may well find its niche where prison- or community-based methadone specialty clinics are not feasible and where methadone is not suitable (e.g., short-term opioid dependent patients and adolescents). It may also be of use when correctional systems are unwilling or unable to comply with the strict regulations required for methadone maintenance. Additionally, pharmacotherapies for alcohol will lend themselves to discharge planning and these medications especially, because they lack the reenforcing properties of the opiates, will require good correction-to-community communication and discharge planning. In this setting, depo-formulations of medications may be especially helpful in assisting inmates to maintain adherence to pharmacotherapy between the time of release and their first postdischarge medical visit. Finally, all pharmacotherapies for chemical dependence should also be considered as part of alternative to incarceration strategies that seek to reform young and first-time offenders by providing drug treatment and community service in lieu of incarceration.

New Pharmacological Therapies and Old Barriers to Access

It is time to reexamine the realm of possibilities of pharmacological treatment for chemical dependence within the correctional system. Correctional health care provides a unique opportunity to engage some of society's most marginalized individuals by screening for chemical dependence and initiating effective treatment. Both the World Health Organization and the Institute of Medicine have written that pharmacological maintenance programs should be developed where practical in prisons as a means to reduce drug use and its severe consequences, and to control the spread of HIV/AIDS among injection drug users (Rettig & Yarmolinsky, 1995; WHO, 1993). Despite the pressing needs for chemical dependency treatment in this country and internationally, treatment expansion has been slow. While therapeutic communities have made great strides in corrections, MMTP implementation in prisons remains noticeably absent, due to a lack of acceptance by politicians, the public, and correctional officers, and the logistical difficulties of developing effective and safe programs in correctional facilities.

Buprenorphine opens a new avenue for the treatment of opiate dependence in a correctional-to-community program. By reducing diversion for illicit use, increasing availability and acceptance, and reducing stigma, buprenorphine may prove a highly effective tool in reducing crime, infectious disease, and recidivism rates among opiate-dependent inmates. Yet many of the barriers and potential problems that have hindered other treatments are likely to plague buprenorphine.

Similarly, the three FDA-approved treatments for alcohol dependence—disulfiram, naltrexone, and acamprosate—have yet to take much hold among correctional health care systems. Pilot and observational studies have suggested that these treatments may offer some benefit, particularly in situations where they are used in conjunction with law enforcement tactics to promote adherence.

Extensive work is under way to find new pharmacological treatment options in addiction medicine. For example, therapeutic vaccines for the treatment of methamphetamine and cocaine dependence are currently in development or under investigation in clinical trials (Kosten & Biegel, 2002; Kosten et al., 2002; Martell, Mitchell, Poling, Gonsai, & Kosten, 2005). However, these vaccines are years from moving into clinical treatment. Recently, promising data with disulfiram (Carroll et al., 2004), topiramate (Kampman et al., 2004), tiagabine (G. Gonzalez et al., 2003), modafinil (Dackis, Kampman, Lynch, Pettinati, & O'Brien, 2005), and baclofen (Brebner, Childress, & Roberts, 2002; Brebner, Phelan, & Roberts, 2000) for the treatment of cocaine dependence have emerged. All of these therapeutic modalities remain investigational and require extensive research to demonstrate efficacy prior to use in clinical care, however. Although lagging behind the advances in research discussed above, NIDA is actively working on the development of pharmacotherapies to reduce the serious problem of methamphetamine use (Vocci & Ling, 2005).

While the benefits of these treatments remain to be seen, it is clear that over the next several decades, more and more options will become available for the treatment of chemical dependence in correctional settings. Lessons learned from expanding access to already-approved medications will allow correctional health systems to more rapidly and effectively incorporate new treatments. This makes the study of methadone, buprenorphine, disulfiram, naltrexone, and acamprosate all the more fruitful and important.

Rigorous controlled clinical effectiveness trials should be pursued to determine the contextual factors that affect pharmacological treatment programs in correctional settings and in the community, as well as interventions that impact continuity of care from prison to community. Research is also needed into ways to expand access to pharmacological therapies through nontraditional avenues to care among drug users. Medical, psychological, drug treatment, and social service professionals will have to lead this dialogue, together with community groups, to educate the public and reduce barriers to effective implementation. The hope is that newer and effective treatment modalities will gain acceptance as important public health interventions in both correctional and community settings.

A Prescription for the Future

Pharmacological treatment for chemical dependency is evidence-based and the keystone for much of effective drug treatment. Such approaches are in their infancy in correctional settings and will continue to paint the future landscape of treatment. It is now time to unshackle the constraints for providing evidence-based pharmacological treatments in correctional settings and develop a continuum of care model that follows the individual from the community through the correctional system and back to the community. Such approaches will require collaboration and coordination from a number of stakeholders, all of whom should be devoted to improving the health status of the inmate and their community. Ineffective approaches, similar to the ones witnessed over the past few decades, that view chemical dependence in moral rather than medical terms, will not reduce recidivism to prison and cannot reduce ongoing drug abuse in our communities.

References

Acamprosate Publication. (2006). Retrieved November 29, 2006, from Thomson MICROMEDEX: http://mdx.med.yale.edu:81/hcs/librarian/ND_PR/Main/PFPUI/ vC3skXa1ChBW79/ND_PG/PRIH/CS/88A250/ND_T/HCS/ND_P/Main/ DUPLICATIONSHIELDSYNC/ACFCFB/ND_B/HCS/PFDefaultActionId/hcs. main.KeywordSearch.Search.

Aditya, G. S., Mahadevan, A., Santosh, V., Chickabasaviah, Y. T., Ashwathnarayanarao, C. B., & Krishna, S. S. (2004). Cysticercal chronic basal arachnoiditis with infarcts, mimicking tuberculous pathology in endemic areas. *Neuropathology: Official Journal of the Japanese Society of Neuropathology, 24*, 320325.

Altice, F. L., Mostashari, F., Selwyn, P. A., Checko, P. J., Singh, R., Tanguay, S., et al. (1998). Predictors of HIV infection among newly sentenced male prisoners. *J Acquir Immune Defic Syndr Hum Retrovirol, 18*, 444453.

Altice, F. L., Springer, S., Buitrago, M., Hunt, D. P., & Friedland, G. H. (2003). Pilot study to enhance HIV care using needle exchange-based health services for out-of-treatment injecting drug users. *J Urban Health, 80*, 416427.

Auriacombe, M., Fatseas, M., Dubernet, J., Daulouede, J. P., & Tignol, J. (2004). French field experience with buprenorphine. *American Journal on Addictions, 13*(Suppl. 1), S17S28.

Auriacombe, M., Franques, P., & Tignol, J. (2001). Deaths attributable to methadone vs buprenorphine in France. *JAMA, 285*, 45.

Ball, A. L., Rana, S., & Dehne, K. L. (1998). HIV prevention among injecting drug users: Responses in developing and transitional countries. *Public Health Reports, 113*(Suppl. 1), 170181.

Balldin, J., Berglund, M., Borg, S., Mansson, M., Bendtsen, P., Franck, J., et al. (2003). A 6-month controlled naltrexone study: Combined effect with cognitive behavioral therapy in outpatient treatment of alcohol dependence. *Alcoholism: Clinical & Experimental Research, 27*, 1142–1149.

Barnett, P. G., Zaric, G. S., & Brandeau, M. L. (2001). The cost-effectiveness of buprenorphine maintenance therapy for opiate addiction in the United States. *Addiction, 96*, 1267–1278.

Berson, A., Gervais, A., Cazals, D., Boyer, N., Durand, F., Bernuau, J., et al. (2001). Hepatitis after intravenous buprenorphine misuse in heroin addicts. *Journal of Hepatology, 34*, 346–350.

Bird, S. M., & Hutchinson, S. J. (2003). Male drugs-related deaths in the fortnight after release from prison: Scotland, 1996–99. *Addiction, 98*, 185–190.

Blankenship, K. M., Smoyer, A. B., Bray, S. J., & Mattocks, K. (2005). Black–white disparities in HIV/AIDS: The role of drug policy and the corrections system. *Journal of Health Care for the Poor & Underserved, 16*(4 Suppl. B), 140–156.

Bourne, P. G., Alford, J. A., & Bowcock, J. Z. (1966). Treatment of skid-row alcoholics with disulfiram. *Quarterly Journal of Studies on Alcohol, 27*, 42–48.

Brahen, L. S., Henderson, R. K., Capone, T., & Kordal, N. (1984). Naltrexone treatment in a jail work-release program. *J Clin Psychiatry, 45*(9 Pt 2), 49–52.

Brambilla, D., Reichelderfer, P. S., Bremer, J. W., Shapiro, D. E., Hershow, R. C., Katzenstein, D. A., et al. (1999). The contribution of assay variation and biological variation to the total variability of plasma HIV-1 RNA measurements. The Women

Infant Transmission Study Clinics. Virology Quality Assurance Program. *AIDS, 13*, 2269–2279.

Brebner, K., Childress, A. R., & Roberts, D. C. (2002). A potential role for GABA(B) agonists in the treatment of psychostimulant addiction. *Alcohol & Alcoholism, 37*(5), 478–484.

Brebner, K., Phelan, R., & Roberts, D. C. (2000). Effect of baclofen on cocaine self-administration in rats reinforced under fixed-ratio 1 and progressive-ratio schedules. *Psychopharmacology, 148*, 314–321.

Brooke, D., Taylor, C., Gunn, J., & Maden, A. (1998). Substance misusers remanded to prison—A treatment opportunity? *Addiction, 93*, 1851–1856.

Brugal, M. T., Domingo-Salvany, A., Puig, R., Barrio, G., Garcia de Olalla, P., & de la Fuente, L. (2005). Evaluating the impact of methadone maintenance programmes on mortality due to overdose and AIDS in a cohort of heroin users in Spain. *Addiction, 100*, 981–989.

Butzin, C. A., Martin, S. S., & Inciardi, J. A. (2002). Evaluating component effects of a prison-based treatment continuum. *J Subst Abuse Treat, 22*, 63–69.

Caplehorn, J., & Deeks, J. J. (2006). A critical appraisal of the Australian comparative trial of methadone and buprenorphine maintenance. *Drug & Alcohol Review, 25*, 157–160.

Carroll, K. M., Fenton, L. R., Ball, S. A., Nich, C., Frankforter, T. L., Shi, J., et al. (2004). Efficacy of disulfiram and cognitive behavior therapy in cocaine-dependent outpatients: A randomized placebo-controlled trial. *Archives of General Psychiatry, 61*, 264–272.

Cartier, J., Farabee, D., & Prendergast, M. L. (2006). Methamphetamine use, self-reported violent crime, and recidivism among offenders in California who abuse substances. *J Interpers Violence, 21*, 435–445.

Chanhatasilpa, C., MacKenzie, D. L., & Hickman, L. J. (2000). The effectiveness of community-based programs for chemically dependent offenders: A review and assessment of the research. *J Subst Abuse Treat, 19*, 383–393.

Clark, N. C., Lintzeris, N., & Muhleisen, P. J. (2002). Severe opiate withdrawal in a heroin user precipitated by a massive buprenorphine dose. *Med J Aust, 176*, 166–167.

Claudon-Charpentier, A., Hoibian, M., Glasser, P., Lalanne, H., & Pasquali, J. L. (2000). Drug-addicted prisoners: Seroprevalence of human immunodeficiency virus and hepatitis B and C virus soon after the marketing of buprenorphine. *Rev Med Interne, 21*, 505–509.

Comer, S. D., & Collins, E. D. (2002). Self-administration of intravenous buprenorphine and the buprenorphine/naloxone combination by recently detoxified heroin abusers. *Journal of Pharmacology & Experimental Therapeutics, 303*, 695–703.

Cornish, J. W., Metzger, D., Woody, G. E., Wilson, D., McLellan, A. T., Vandergrift, B., et al. (1997). Naltrexone pharmacotherapy for opioid dependent federal probationers. *J Subst Abuse Treat, 14*, 529–534.

Dackis, C. A., Kampman, K. M., Lynch, K. G., Pettinati, H. M., & O'Brien, C. P. (2005). A double-blind, placebo-controlled trial of modafinil for cocaine dependence. *Neuropsychopharmacology, 30*, 205–211.

De Leon, G. (1996). Therapeutic communities: AIDS/HIV risk and harm reduction. *J Subst Abuse Treat, 13*, 411–420.

De Leon, G., Melnick, G., Kressel, D., & Jainchill, N. (1994). Circumstances, motivation, readiness, and suitability (the CMRS scales): Predicting retention in therapeutic community treatment. *Am J Drug Alcohol Abuse, 20*, 495–515.

Desland, M., & Batey, R. (1991). High retention rates within a prospective study of heroin users. *Br J Addict, 86*, 859–865.

Disulfiram Publication. (2006). Retrieved November 29, 2006, from Thomson MICROMEDEX: http://mdx.med.yale.edu:81/hcs/librarian/ND_PR/Main/

SBK/1/PFPUI/vC3skXa1ChuIHW/ND_PG/PRIH/CS/3FC297/ND_T/HCS/
ND_P/Main/DUPLICATIONSHIELDSYNC/588F76/ND_B/HCS/PFActionId/
hcs.common.RetrieveDocumentCommon/DocId/184770/ContentSetId/42/
SearchTerm/disulfiram/SearchOption/BeginWith.

Dolan, K., Hall, W., & Wodak, A. (1996). Methadone maintenance reduces injecting in prison. *BMJ, 312*, 1162.

Dole, V. P., Nyswander, M. E., & Kreek, M. J. (1966). Narcotic blockade. *Arch Intern Med, 118*, 304–309.

Donny, E. C., Walsh, S. L., Bigelow, G. E., Eissenberg, T., & Stitzer, M. L. (2002). High-dose methadone produces superior opioid blockade and comparable withdrawal suppression to lower doses in opioid-dependent humans. *Psychopharmacology (Berl), 161*, 202–212.

Doran, C. M., Shanahan, M., Mattick, R. P., Ali, R., White, J., & Bell, J. (2003). Buprenorphine versus methadone maintenance: A cost-effectiveness analysis. *Drug Alcohol Depend, 71*, 295–302.

Dunkle, K. L., Jewkes, R. K., Brown, H. C., Gray, G. E., McIntryre, J. A., & Harlow, S. D. (2004). Gender-based violence, relationship power, and risk of HIV infection in women attending antenatal clinics in South Africa. *Lancet, 363*, 1415–1421.

Edlin, B. R. (2002). Prevention and treatment of hepatitis C in injection drug users. *Hepatology, 36*(5 Suppl. 1), S210–S219.

Elliott, A. J., Uldall, K. K., Bergam, K., Russo, J., Claypoole, K., & Roy-Byrne, P. P. (1998). Randomized, placebo-controlled trial of paroxetine versus imipramine in depressed HIV-positive outpatients. *The American Journal of Psychiatry, 155*, 367–372.

Farren, C. K., O'Malley, S., & Rounsaville, B. (1997). Naltrexone and opiate abuse. In S.M. Stine & T. R. Kosten (Eds.), *New treatments for opiate dependence* (pp. 104–123). New York: Guilford Press.

Favrat, B., Rao, S., O'Connor, P. G., & Schottenfeld, R. (2002). A staging system to predict prognosis among methadone maintenance patients, based on admission characteristics. *Subst Abus, 23*, 233–244.

Fhima, A., Henrion, R., Lowenstein, W., & Charpak, Y. (2001). Two-year follow-up of an opioid-user cohort treated with high-dose buprenorphine (Subutex). *Ann Med Interne (Paris), 152*(Suppl. 3), IS26–36.

Fiellin, D. A., & O'Connor, P. G. (2002). Clinical practice. Office-based treatment of opioid-dependent patients. *N Engl J Med, 347*, 817–823.

Fiellin, D. A., O'Connor, P. G., Chawarski, M., Pakes, J. P., Pantalon, M. V., & Schottenfeld, R. S. (2001). Methadone maintenance in primary care: A randomized controlled trial. *JAMA, 286*, 1724–1731.

Fiellin, D. A., Pantalon, M. V., Pakes, J. P., O'Connor, P. G., Chawarski, M., & Schottenfeld, R. S. (2002). Treatment of heroin dependence with buprenorphine in primary care. *Am J Drug Alcohol Abuse, 28*, 231–241.

Friedland, G. H., Pollard, R., Griffith, B., Hughes, M., Morse, G., Bassett, R., et al. (1999). Efficacy and safety of delavirdine mesylate with zidovudine and didanosine compared with two-drug combinations of these agents in persons with HIV disease with CD4 counts of 100 to 500 cells/mm^3 (ACTG 261). ACTG 261 Team. *J Acquir Immune Defic Syndr, 21*, 281–292.

Friedmann, P. D., Lemon, S. C., & Stein, M. D. (2001). Transportation and retention in outpatient drug abuse treatment programs. *J Subst Abuse Treat, 21*, 97–103.

Fudala, P. J., Bridge, T. P., Herbert, S., Williford, W. O., Chiang, C. N., Jones, K., et al. (2003). Office-based treatment of opiate addiction with a sublingual-tablet formulation of buprenorphine and naloxone. *N Engl J Med, 349*, 949–958.

Fudala, P. J., Jaffe, J. H., Dax, E. M., & Johnson, R. E. (1990). Use of buprenorphine in the treatment of opioid addiction. II. Physiologic and behavioral effects of daily and alternate-day administration and abrupt withdrawal. *Clin Pharmacol Ther, 47*, 525–534.

Fudala, P. J., & Johnson, R. E. (2006). Development of opioid formulations with limited diversion and abuse potential. *Drug Alcohol Depend, 83* (Suppl. 1), S40–S47.

Gallant, D. M., Bishop, M. P., Faulkner, M. A., Simpson, L., Cooper, A., Lathrop, D., et al. (1968). A comparative evaluation of compulsory (group therapy and-or antabuse) and voluntary treatment of the chronic alcoholic municipal court offender. *Psychosomatics, 9*, 306–310.

Gianoulakis, C., Krishnan, B., & Thavundayil, J. (1996). Enhanced sensitivity of pituitary beta-endorphin to ethanol in subjects at high risk of alcoholism. [erratum appears in Arch Gen Psychiatry 1996 Jun;53(6):555]. *Archives of General Psychiatry, 53*, 250–257.

Glaser, J. B., & Greifinger, R. B. (1993). Correctional health care: A public health opportunity. *Ann Intern Med, 118*, 139–145.

Gonzalez, G., Sevarino, K., Sofuoglu, M., Poling, J., Oliveto, A., Gonsai, K., et al. (2003). Tiagabine increases cocaine-free urines in cocaine-dependent methadone-treated patients: Results of a randomized pilot study. *Addiction, 98*, 1625–1632.

Gonzalez, J. P., & Brogden, R. N. (1988). Naltrexone. A review of its pharmacodynamic and pharmacokinetic properties and therapeutic efficacy in the management of opioid dependence. *Drugs, 35*, 192–213.

Gore, S. M., & Bird, A. G. (1995). Mandatory drug tests in prisons. *BMJ, 310*, 595.

Gowing, L., Ali, R., & White, J. (2002). Buprenorphine for the management of opioid withdrawal. *Cochrane Database Syst Rev*(2), CD002025.

Greenstein, R. A., Evans, B. D., McLellan, A. T., & O'Brien, C. P. (1983). Predictors of favorable outcome following naltrexone treatment. *Drug Alcohol Depend, 12*, 173–180.

Greenwald, M. K., Schuh, K. J., Hopper, J. A., Schuster, C. R., & Johanson, C. E. (2002). Effects of buprenorphine sublingual tablet maintenance on opioid drug-seeking behavior by humans. *Psychopharmacology (Berl), 160*, 344–352.

Gruer, L., Wilson, P., Scott, R., Elliott, L., Macleod, J., Harden, K., et al. (1997). General practitioner centred scheme for treatment of opiate dependent drug injectors in Glasgow. *BMJ, 314*, 1730–1735.

Hagan, H., Snyder, N., Hough, E., Yu, T., McKeirnan, S., Boase, J., et al. (2002). Case-reporting of acute hepatitis B and C among injection drug users. *J Urban Health, 79*, 579–585.

Hammett, T. M., Harmon, M. P., & Rhodes, W. (2002). The burden of infectious disease among inmates of and releasees from US correctional facilities, 1997. *Am J Public Health, 92*, 1789–1794.

Hasson, A. L., Grella, C. E., Rawson, R., & Anglin, M. D. (1994). Case management within a methadone maintenance program. A research demonstration project for HIV risk reduction. *J Case Manag, 3*, 167–172.

Haynes, S. N. (1973). Contingency management in a municipally-administered antabuse program for alcoholics. *Journal of Behavior Therapy and Experimental Psychiatry, 4*, 31.

Hickman, M., Madden, P., Henry, J., Baker, A., Wallace, C., Wakefield, J., et al. (2003). Trends in drug overdose deaths in England and Wales 1993–98: Methadone does not kill more people than heroin. *Addiction, 98*, 419–425.

Hiller, M. L., Knight, K., & Simpson, D. D. (1999). Prison-based substance abuse treatment, residential aftercare and recidivism. *Addiction, 94*, 833–842.

Hofmann, B., Afzelius, P., Iversen, J., Kronborg, G., Aabech, P., Benfield, T., et al. (1996). Buspirone, a serotonin receptor agonist, increases CD4 T-cell counts and modulates the immune system in HIV-seropositive subjects. *AIDS (London, England), 10*, 1339–1347.

Hser, Y.-I., Anglin, M. D., & Fletcher, B. (1998). Comparative treatment effectiveness: Effects of program modality and client drug dependence history on drug use reduction. *Journal of Substance Abuse Treatment, 15*, 513–523.

Hutchinson, A. B., Corbie-Smith, G., Thomas, S. B., Mohanan, S., & del Rio, C. (2004). Understanding the patient's perspective on rapid and routine HIV testing in an inner-city urgent care center. *AIDS Education and Prevention: Official Publication of the International Society for AIDS Education, 16*, 101–114.

Jasinski, D. R., Pevnick, J. S., & Griffith, J. D. (1978). Human pharmacology and abuse potential of the analgesic buprenorphine: A potential agent for treating narcotic addiction. *Arch Gen Psychiatry, 35*, 501–516.

Johnson, R. E., Chutuape, M. A., Strain, E. C., Walsh, S. L., Stitzer, M. L., & Bigelow, G. E. (2000). A comparison of levomethadyl acetate, buprenorphine, and methadone for opioid dependence. *N Engl J Med, 343*, 1290–1297.

Johnson, R. E., Eissenberg, T., Stitzer, M. L., Strain, E. C., Liebson, I. A., & Bigelow, G. E. (1995). Buprenorphine treatment of opioid dependence: Clinical trial of daily versus alternate-day dosing. *Drug Alcohol Depend, 40*, 27–35.

Jones, M. (1980). Desirable features of a therapeutic community in a prison. In H. Toch (Ed.), *Therapeutic communities in corrections*. New York: Praeger.

Kampman, K. M., Pettinati, H., Lynch, K. G., Dackis, C., Sparkman, T., Weigley, C., et al. (2004). A pilot trial of topiramate for the treatment of cocaine dependence. *Drug & Alcohol Dependence, 75*, 233–240.

Kapadia, F., Vlahov, D., Des Jarlais, D. C., Strathdee, S. A., Ouellet, L., Kerndt, P., et al. (2002). Does bleach disinfection of syringes protect against hepatitis C infection among young adult injection drug users? *Epidemiology, 13*, 738–741.

Khoshnood, K., Blankenship, K. M., Pollack, H. A., Roan, C. T., & Altice, F. L. (2000). Syringe source, use, and discard among injection-drug users in New Haven, Connecticut. *AIDS Public Policy J, 15*, 88–94.

Kirchmayer, U., Davoli, M., & Verster, A. (2002). Naltrexone maintenance treatment for opioid dependence. *Cochrane Database Syst Rev*(2), CD001333.

Kirchmayer, U., Davoli, M., Verster, A. D., Amato, L., Ferri, A., & Perucci, C. A. (2002). A systematic review on the efficacy of naltrexone maintenance treatment in opioid dependence. *Addiction, 97*, 1241–1249.

Knight, K., Simpson, D. D., & Hiller, M. L. (1999). Three-year reincarceration outcomes for in-prison therapeutic community treatment in Texas. *The Prison Journal, 79*, 337–351.

Kosten, T. R., & Biegel, D. (2002). Therapeutic vaccines for substance dependence. *Expert Review of Vaccines, 1*, 363–371.

Kosten, T. R., Rosen, M., Bond, J., Settles, M., Roberts, J. S., Shields, J., et al. (2002). Human therapeutic cocaine vaccine: Safety and immunogenicity. *Vaccine, 20*, 1196–1204.

Kraft, M. K., Rothbard, A. B., Hadley, T. R., McLellan, A. T., & Asch, D. A. (1997). Are supplementary services provided during methadone maintenance really cost-effective? *Am J Psychiatry, 154*, 1214–1219.

Kranzler, H. R., & Rounsaville, B. J. (1998). *Dual diagnosis and treatment: Substance abuse and comorbid medical and psychiatric disorders*. New York: Dekker.

Kreek, M. J., & Vocci, F. J. (2002). History and current status of opioid maintenance treatments: Blending conference session. *J Subst Abuse Treat, 23*, 93–105.

Krupitsky, E. M., Zvartau, E. E., Lioznov, D. A., Tsoy, M. V., Egorova, V. Y., Belyaeva, T. V., et al. (2006). Co-morbidity of infectious and addictive diseases in St. Petersburg and the Leningrad region, Russia. *Eur Addict Res, 12*, 12–19.

Kuo, I., Sherman, S. G., Thomas, D. L., & Strathdee, S. A. (2004). Hepatitis B virus infection and vaccination among young injection and non-injection drug users: Missed opportunities to prevent infection. *Drug Alcohol Depend, 73*, 69–78.

Langan, P. A., & Levin, D. J. (2002). *Recidivism of prisoners released in 1994* (No. NCJ 193427). U.S. Department of Justice.

Liebman, J., Pat Lamberti, M., & Altice, F. (2002). Effectiveness of a mobile medical van in providing screening services for STDs and HIV. *Public Health Nurs, 19*, 345–353.

Liguori, A., Morse, W. H., & Bergman, J. (1996). Respiratory effects of opioid full and partial agonists in rhesus monkeys. *J Pharmacol Exp Ther, 277*, 462–472.

Ling, W., & Smith, D. (2002). Buprenorphine: Blending practice and research. *J Subst Abuse Treat, 23*, 87–92.

Littleton, J. (1995). Acamprosate in alcohol dependence: How does it work? *Addiction, 90*, 1179–1188.

Liu, S. J., & Wang, R. I. (1984). Relationship of plasma level and pharmacological activity of methadone. *NIDA Res Monogr, 49*, 128–135.

Magura, S., Rosenblum, A., Lewis, C., & Joseph, H. (1993). The effectiveness of in-jail methadone maintenance. *Journal of Drug Issues, 23*, 75–99.

Mark, T. L., Woody, G. E., Juday, T., & Kleber, H. D. (2001). The economic costs of heroin addiction in the United States. *Drug Alcohol Depend, 61*, 195–206.

Marmot, M. G., Siegrist, J., Theorell, T., & Feeney, A. (1999). Health and the psychosocial environment of work. In M. G. Marmot & R. Wilkinson (Eds.), *Social determinants of health* (pp. 106–133). Oxford: Oxford University Press.

Marsch, L. A. (1998). The efficacy of methadone maintenance interventions in reducing illicit opiate use, HIV risk behavior and criminality: A meta-analysis. *Addiction, 93*, 515–532.

Martell, B. A., Mitchell, E., Poling, J., Gonsai, K., & Kosten, T. R. (2005). Vaccine pharmacotherapy for the treatment of cocaine dependence. *Biological Psychiatry, 58*, 158–164.

Martin, V., Cayla, J. A., Bolea, A., & Castilla, J. (2000). Mycobacterium tuberculosis and human immunodeficiency virus co-infection in intravenous drug users on admission to prison. *Int J Tuberc Lung Dis, 4*, 41–46.

Mason, B. J. (2001). Treatment of alcohol-dependent outpatients with acamprosate: A clinical review. *Journal of Clinical Psychiatry, 62*(Suppl. 20), 42–48.

Mason, B. J., Goodman, A. M., Dixon, R. M., Hameed, M. H., Hulot, T., Wesnes, K., et al. (2002). A pharmacokinetic and pharmacodynamic drug interaction study of acamprosate and naltrexone. *Neuropsychopharmacology, 27*, 596–606.

Mattick, R. P., Breen, C., Kimber, J., & Davoli, M. (2002). Methadone maintenance therapy versus no opioid replacement therapy for opioid dependence (Cochrane Review). *Cochrane Database Syst Rev*(4), CD002209.

Mattick, R. P., Kimber, J., Breen, C., & Davoli, M. (2002). Buprenorphine maintenance versus placebo or methadone maintenance for opioid dependence (Cochrane Review). *Cochrane Database Syst Rev*(4), CD002207.

Mazlan, M., Schottenfeld, R. S., & Chawarski, M. C. (2006). New challenges and opportunities in managing substance abuse in Malaysia. *Drug Alcohol Rev, 25*, 473–478.

McLellan, A. T., Alterman, A. I., Metzger, D. S., Grissom, G. R., Woody, G. E., Luborsky, L., et al. (1994). Similarity of outcome predictors across opiate, cocaine, and alcohol treatments: Role of treatment services. *J Consult Clin Psychol, 62*, 1141–1158.

McLellan, A. T., Arndt, I. O., Metzger, D. S., Woody, G. E., & O'Brien, C. P. (1993). The effects of psychosocial services in substance abuse treatment. *JAMA, 269*, 1953–1959.

Milby, J. B., Sims, M. K., Khuder, S., Schumacher, J. E., Huggins, N., McLellan, A. T., et al. (1996). Psychiatric comorbidity: Prevalence in methadone maintenance treatment. *Am J Drug Alcohol Abuse, 22*, 95–107.

Miura, H., Fujiki, M., Shibata, A., & Ishikawa, K. (2006). Prevalence and profile of methamphetamine users in adolescents at a juvenile classification home. *Psychiatry Clin Neurosci, 60*, 352–357.

Monterosso, J. R., Flannery, B. A., Pettinati, H. M., Oslin, D. W., Rukstalis, M., O'Brien, C. P., et al. (2001). Predicting treatment response to naltrexone: The influence of craving and family history. *American Journal on Addictions, 10*, 258–268.

Mumola, C. (1999). *Substance abuse and treatment, state and federal prisoners, 1997* (No. NCJ 172871). U.S. Department of Justice.

National Consensus Development Panel on Effective Medical Treatment of Opiate Addiction. (1998). Effective medical treatment of opiate addiction. *JAMA, 280*, 1936–1943.

Nurco, D. N., Hanlon, T. E., & Kinlock, T. W. (1991). Recent research on the relationship between illicit drug use and crime. *Behav Sci Law, 9*, 221–242.

Obadia, Y., Perrin, V., Feroni, I., Vlahov, D., & Moatti, J. P. (2001). Injecting misuse of buprenorphine among French drug users. *Addiction, 96*, 267–272.

O'Brien, C. P. (2005). Anticraving medications for relapse prevention: A possible new class of psychoactive medications. *American Journal of Psychiatry, 162*, 1423–1431.

O'Connor, P. G., Oliveto, A. H., Shi, J. M., Triffleman, E. G., Carroll, K. M., Kosten, T. R., et al. (1998). A randomized trial of buprenorphine maintenance for heroin dependence in a primary care clinic for substance users versus a methadone clinic. *Am J Med, 105*, 100–105.

O'Malley, S. S. (1996). Opioid antagonists in the treatment of alcohol dependence: Clinical efficacy and prevention of relapse. *Alcohol & Alcoholism, 31*(Suppl. 1), 77–81.

O'Malley, S. S., & Froehlich, J. C. (2003). Advances in the use of naltrexone: An integration of preclinical and clinical findings. *Recent Developments in Alcoholism, 16*, 217–245.

Osemene, N. I., Essien, E. J., & Egbunike, I. G. (2001). HIV/AIDS behind bars: An avenue for culturally sensitive interventions. *J Natl Med Assoc, 93*, 481–486.

Peters, R. H., LeVasseur, M. E., & Chandler, R. K. (2004). Correctional treatment for co-occurring disorders: Results of a national survey. *Behav Sci Law, 22*, 563–584.

Petrakis, I. L., Poling, J., Levinson, C., Nich, C., Carroll, K., Rounsaville, B., et al. (2005). Naltrexone and disulfiram in patients with alcohol dependence and comorbid psychiatric disorders. *Biological Psychiatry, 57*, 1128–1137.

Pollack, H., Khoshnood, K., & Altice, F. (1999). Health care delivery strategies for criminal offenders. *J Health Care Finance, 26*, 63–77.

Rettig, R. A., & Yarmolinsky, A. (1995). *Federal regulation of methadone treatment.* Washington, DC: Institute of Medicine.

Robinson, G. M., Dukes, P. D., Robinson, B. J., Cooke, R. R., & Mahoney, G. N. (1993). The misuse of buprenorphine and a buprenorphine–naloxone combination in Wellington, New Zealand. *Drug & Alcohol Dependence, 33*, 81–86.

Robinson, S. E. (2006). Buprenorphine-containing treatments: Place in the management of opioid addiction. *CNS Drugs, 20*, 697–712.

Roth, A., Hogan, I., & Farren, C. (1997). Naltrexone plus group therapy for the treatment of opiate-abusing health-care professionals. *J Subst Abuse Treat, 14*, 19–22.

Rothon, D. A. (1997). Methadone in provincial prisons in British Columbia. *Can HIV AIDS Policy Law Newsl, 3–4*(4–1), 27–31.

Rouse, J. J. (1991). Evaluation research on prison-based drug treatment programs and some policy implications. *Int J Addict, 26*, 29–44.

SAMHSA. (2004). *Results from the 2003 National Survey on Drug Use and Health: National findings* (No. NSDUH Series H-25, DHHS Publication No. SMA 04-3964). Rockville, MD: Author.

Schottenfeld, R. S., Mazlan, M., & Chawarski, M.C. (2006). *Randomized, double blind comparison of drug counseling combined with buprenorphine, naltrexone or placebo for treating opioid dependence and reducing HIV risk in Malaysia.* Paper presented at the College on Problems of Drug Dependence. From http://biopsych. com/cpdd/CPDD06_PDFs/CPDD06_442931517333.pdf.

Seet, R. C., & Lim, E. C. (2006). Intravenous use of buprenorphine tablets associated with rhabdomyolysis and compressive sciatic neuropathy. *Annals of Emergency Medicine, 47*, 396–397.

Sereny, G., Sharma, V., Holt, J., & Gordis, E. (1986). Mandatory supervised antabuse therapy in an outpatient alcoholism program: A pilot study. *Alcoholism: Clinical & Experimental Research, 10*, 290–292.

Sheu, M., Hogan, J., Allsworth, J., Stein, M., Vlahov, D., Schoenbaum, E. E., et al. (2002). Continuity of medical care and risk of incarceration in HIV-positive and high-risk HIV-negative women. *J Womens Health (Larchmt), 11*, 743–750.

Shwartz, M., Baker, G., Mulvey, K. P., & Plough, A. (1997). Improving publicly funded substance abuse treatment: The value of case management. *Am J Public Health, 87*, 1659–1664.

Sibbald, B. (2002). Methadone maintenance expands inside federal prisons. *CMAJ, 167*, 1154.

Skolnick, A. A. (1998). Correctional and community health care collaborations. *JAMA, 279*, 98–99.

Spaulding, A., Greene, C., Davidson, K., Schneidermann, M., & Rich, J. (1999). Hepatitis C in state correctional facilities. *Prev Med, 28*, 92–100.

Sporer, K. A. (2003). Strategies for preventing heroin overdose. *BMJ, 326*, 442–444.

Stoller, N. (2003). Space, place and movement as aspects of health care in three women's prisons. *Soc Sci Med, 56*, 2263–2275.

Strain, E. C., Bigelow, G. E., Liebson, I. A., & Stitzer, M. L. (1999). Moderate- vs high-dose methadone in the treatment of opioid dependence: A randomized trial. *JAMA, 281*, 1000–1005.

Suh, J. J., Pettinati, H. M., Kampman, K. M., & O'Brien, C. P. (2006). The status of disulfiram: A half of a century later. *Journal of Clinical Psychopharmacology, 26*, 290–302.

Sullivan, L.E., Bruce, R., Haltiwanger, D., Lucas, G.E., Eldred, L., Finkelstein, R., & Fiellin, D.A. (2006). Initial strategies for integrating buprenorphine into HIV care settings in the United States. *Clinical Infectious Diseases, 43*, S191–S196.

Thompson, A. S., Blankenship, K. M., Selwyn, P. A., Khoshnood, K., Lopez, M., Balacos, K., et al. (1998). Evaluation of an innovative program to address the health and social service needs of drug-using women with or at risk for HIV infection. *J Community Health, 23*, 419–440.

Tomasino, V., Swanson, A. J., Nolan, J., & Shuman, H. I. (2001). The Key Extended Entry Program (KEEP): A methadone treatment program for opiate-dependent inmates. *Mt Sinai J Med, 68*, 14–20.

Tzschentke, T. M. (2002). Behavioral pharmacology of buprenorphine, with a focus on preclinical models of reward and addiction. *Psychopharmacology (Berl), 161*, 1–16.

Verger, P., Rotily, M., Prudhomme, J., & Bird, S. (2003). High mortality rates among inmates during the year following their discharge from a French prison. *Journal of Forensic Sciences, 48*, 614–616.

Vocci, F., & Ling, W. (2005). Medications development: Successes and challenges. *Pharmacology & Therapeutics, 108*, 94–108.

Vormfelde, S. V., & Poser, W. (2001). Death attributed to methadone. *Pharmacopsychiatry, 34*, 217–222.

Wall, R., Rehm, J., Fischer, B., Brands, B., Gliksman, L., Stewart, J., et al. (2000). Social costs of untreated opioid dependence. *J Urban Health, 77*, 688–722.

Walsh, S. L., Preston, K. L., Stitzer, M. L., Cone, E. J., & Bigelow, G. E. (1994). Clinical pharmacology of buprenorphine: Ceiling effects at high doses. *Clin Pharmacol Ther, 55*, 569–580.

Washton, A. M., Gold, M. S., & Pottash, A. (1984). Successful use of naltrexone in addicted physicians and business executives. *Advances in Alcohol & Substance Abuse, 4*, 89–96.

Wexler, H. K., Melnick, G., Lowe, L., & Peters, J. (1999). Three-year reincarceration outcomes for Amity in-prison therapeutic community and aftercare in California. *The Prison Journal, 79*, 321–336.

WHO. (1993). *WHO guidelines on HIV infection and AIDS in prisons.* Geneva: Author.

Widman, M., Platt, J. J., Lidz, V., Mathis, D. A., & Metzger, D. S. (1997). Patterns of service use and treatment involvement of methadone maintenance patients. *J Subst Abuse Treat, 14*, 29–35.

Yoast, R., Williams, M. A., Deitchman, S. D., & Champion, H. C. (2001). Report of the Council on Scientific Affairs: Methadone maintenance and needle-exchange programs to reduce the medical and public health consequences of drug abuse. *J Addict Dis, 20*, 15–40.

Zule, W. A., & Desmond, D. P. (1998). Attitudes toward methadone maintenance: Implications for HIV prevention. *J Psychoactive Drugs, 30*, 89–97.

Section 5

Thinking Forward to Reentry—Reducing Barriers and Building Community Linkages

The final section of *Public Health Behind Bars* is about reentry, a much discussed topic in the past few years. With all the talk, though, there has not been nearly as much action, for a variety of reasons, not the least of which are the categorical and separate funding streams for criminal justice, public health, and community health care. Nick Freudenberg, a professor and researcher, leads the section with a chapter on the state of correctional health care research including a discussion of the barriers and challenges to meaningful scholarship in this field.

Christy Visher and Kamala Mallik-Kane, public policy researchers, provide us with interesting and provocative information derived from studies of men reentering their home communities. They offer a detailed look at health, family, and community issues for returning state prison inmates.

Steven K. Hoge, a forensic and correctional psychiatrist, details the historical background for incarceration of the mentally ill and a description of the mentally ill in prisons and jails today. Further, Dr. Hoge writes a prescription for effective reentry services for the mentally ill who are incarcerated.

Karen Terry is a social scientist with expertise in sexual violence. In her chapter, Professor Terry gives us valuable definitions and the history of public policy regarding sex offenders. She outlines issues of community supervision, civil commitment, and describes the challenges and opportunities for community reintegration of sex offenders.

In this book, we address a wide variety of challenges. High on the list is improving communication, particularly through medical records. Ralph Woodward, a physician executive in corrections, has written a primer on the value of electronic medical records and the need for correctional authorities to carefully consider keeping pace with the development of electronic medical records in the community. He emphasizes the necessity to develop platforms that can easily communicate with community health care providers. Dr. Woodward artfully describes what can be achieved today with electronic information systems and what could be achieved with effective leadership and persistence.

Tom Lincoln is a correctional physician working in the jail that pioneered a public health/community health model of care. Along with Steve Scheibel, a correctional health physician working on reentry, and John Miles, a public servant with a long-time commitment to correctional health care, Dr. Lincoln describes the essential elements of public health and community health collaborations. The authors carefully detail the rationale and components for an effective health care program that reaches into correctional facilities and out to the community.

The final chapter of the book is written by Sandra Springer and Rick Altice, academic physicians with expertise in corrections, HIV, and drug abuse treatment. Drs. Springer and Altice review the essentials of planning for release of HIV-infected inmates, including antiretroviral treatment and attention to substance abuse treatment and mental illness.

Chapter 24

Health Research Behind Bars: A Brief Guide to Research in Jails and Prisons

Nicholas Freudenberg

While most people make staying out of jail and prison a priority, a growing number of researchers are eager to get into correctional facilities in order to study the criminal justice system, the causes and consequences of incarceration, and the role of corrections in our society.

For health researchers and their collaborators, the audience for this chapter, correctional facilities offer several unique advantages: a population at high risk of many health problems including infectious and chronic diseases, substance abuse, and mental health problems; social and physical environments that can enhance or impede well-being; a setting that is a focal point for the class, racial/ethnic, and gender differences that divide the United States; a site where health and mental health services and prevention programs are offered and can be evaluated; a controlled environment for administration of treatments such as directly observed therapy for tuberculosis; and a stopping point in the cycle of incarceration and reentry that so profoundly affects community well-being.

In this chapter, I consider the benefits and perils of doing health research in jails and prisons. The chapter begins with a brief overview of the different types of health research conducted within correctional facilities and among those leaving jail or prison. I then describe some of the unique obstacles that correctional health researchers encounter and assess some of the methods they have used to overcome these obstacles. Since researchers in correctional settings face significant ethical dilemmas, I next consider recent frameworks for making ethical decisions about this research. Finally, I suggest an agenda for future health research in correctional settings.

Scope of Health Research in Correctional Settings

In recent decades, researchers from a variety of disciplines including health services research, public health, medicine, criminal justice studies, sociology, psychology, anthropology, organizational studies, and others have initiated studies on health in the correctional system. A brief typology of the different categories of questions these investigators have asked will help to set the stage for our consideration of approaches to correctional research.

1. What are the health and social characteristics of people in jail and prison?

   Numerous studies have examined the health and demographic profile of incarcerated populations. These vary from large studies based on national samples and using multiple health outcomes such as the reports of the National Correctional Health Care Commission on the health status of soon-to-released inmates (2002a, 2002b) or of the health status of inmates in Texas prisons (Baillargeon, Black, Pulvino, & Dunn, 2000) to studies of a single outcome such as hepatitis C among California inmates (Fox et al., 2005). The various reports of the Bureau of Justice Statistics on mental health, substance use, and other health conditions (e.g., James & Glaze, 2006, Karberg & James, 2005) summarize data across U.S. jurisdictions, providing an opportunity for correctional and health officials to identify incarcerated populations in higher need. Other studies describe patterns of health care utilization among inmate populations (Leukefeld et al., 2006). Investigators often compare the health status of different subpopulations, e.g., men to women (Peters, Strozier, Murrin, & Kearns, 1997), or African-Americans and Latinos to whites (Rounds-Bryant, Motivaus, & Pelissier, 2003).
   These descriptive studies are used to identify the needs of various segments of the incarcerated populations, to compare changing incidence or prevalence of conditions over time, or to serve as a baseline for the subsequent evaluation of interventions. Research imperatives in these studies are consistent definitions of dependent and independent variables, uniformity in data collection methods in multisystem studies, and sampling strategies that enable generalizations to other settings.

2. How does the health of inmates differ from that of nonincarcerated populations?

   A second group of studies compare the health of incarcerated populations with the health of the general population or with samples of nonincarcerated people. For example, Teplin and colleagues' studies of the prevalence of mental health conditions among women and juveniles in Chicago jails found higher rates of some psychiatric conditions in incarcerated populations than in similar populations living in the same catchment area from which inmates had been arrested (Teplin, 1990; Teplin et al., 1996). These studies set the stage for the next group of studies. Methodological issues in this type of study include selecting an appropriate comparison group.

3. How does incarceration itself affect the health of incarcerated populastions?

   Both correctional and public health authorities want to know whether observed differences between incarcerated and nonincarcerated populations are due to differences in the composition of the populations or to the experience of incarceration, a variant of the classic epidemiological task of distinguishing between compositional (i.e., characteristics of the population) and contextual effects (i.e., characteristics of an environment). For example, numerous investigators have sought to determine whether the higher prevalence of HIV infection among U.S. prison populations was due to intraprison transmission or to criminal justice policies that led to incarceration for people already HIV infected (Hammett, 2006; Krebs & Simmons, 2002). Most studies suggest the latter route is more important, reassuring correctional authorities that within-prison transmission, while it does occur, is not a major factor in higher rates. On the other hand, studies in the early 1990s established that TB transmission did occur within the facility, leading to substantial efforts to prevent such transmission (Bellin Fletcher, & Safyer, 1993). Others have investigated whether incarceration is associated with homelessness and mental illness (McNeil, Binder, & Robinson, 2005). The main analytic task in these studies is to distinguish between causal and noncausal associations between incarceration and selected health outcomes.

4. What are the health effects of criminal justice policies and practices on the health of inmates?

    Criminal justice policies often have unintended effects on incarcerated populations. Documenting the positive and negative impact of these policies can serve as a starting point for policy change. For example, a study in a large public hospital in New York City found that many admissions for diabetic ketoacidosis were related to the court practice of denying inmates access to insulin medications in court pens (Keller et al., 1993). Health impact assessment, an analytic method developed to assess the health effects of both health and non-health-related policies, offers a promising approach to consider the health consequences of various prison and criminal justice policies (Davenport, Mathers, & Parry, 2006; Kemm, 2001, Veerman, Barendregt, & Mackenbach, 2005). To date, however, this approach does not seem to have been used to assess the impact of U.S. correctional policies on inmate or community health.

5. What is the impact of interventions designed to care for or improve the health of incarcerated populations?

    A key practical question for correctional, public health, and correctional health officials is the effect of the programs they run on the well-being of the populations in custody. Evaluation studies seek to document the utilization of health services (Lindquist & Lindquist, 1999); assess their impact on health or health care utilization (e.g., Chan, Vilke, Smith, Sparrow, & Dunford, 2003; Edens, Peters, & Hills, 1997); analyze the cost-benefits of an intervention (NCCHC, 2002a); or compare the cost-effectiveness of various approaches to a specified health problem, e.g., screening for HIV or other infectious diseases within correctional settings (Resch, Altice, & Paltiel, 2005; Kraut-Becher, Gift, Haddix, Irwin, & Greifinger, 2004). In these studies, methodological issues include the specification of clearly defined outcomes, the use of standard accepted measures for assessing costs and benefits of various interventions, and the design of evaluation studies that are both methodologically sound and operationally feasible.

6. How does reentry affect the health of incarcerated populations?

In the last decade, correctional health researchers have begun to follow their research participants back into the community, examining their success in finding health services or drug treatment (Jarrett, Adeyemi, & Huggins, 2006; Lincoln et al., 2006), maintaining control of a mental health condition (Wilson & Draine 2006), or in improving HIV care or reducing HIV risk behavior (Bauserman et al., 2003; Rich et al., 2001; Myers et al., 2005). These studies can be part of an evaluation of a reentry program (e.g., Needels, James-Burdumy, & Burghardt, 2005) or a descriptive study of the outcomes of the reentry process (e.g., Freudenberg et al., 2005).

7. What is the impact of incarceration rates on the well-being of communities and populations?

Finally, a growing number of researchers are studying the impact of incarceration and correctional policies on the health of families, communities, and populations. For example, some research looks at the impact of incarceration on children and other family members (Murray & Farrington, 2005; Barreras, Drucker, & Rosenthal, 2005). Researchers have asked whether incarceration policies have contributed to the community transmission of HIV infection (Leh, 1999; Johnson & Raphael, 2006) or other sexually transmitted infections (Thomas & Sampson, 2005), community rates of violence (Rose & Clear, 2003), or disparities in health between black and white U.S. populations (Taxman, Byrne, & Pattav, 2005; Johnson & Raphael, 2006; Iguchi, Bell, Ramchand, & Fain, 2005). These studies can help policy makers consider the impact of various incarceration policy choices.

This brief summary of the types of questions that correctional health researchers have sought to answer illustrates the scope of the field. For neophyte investigators, becoming familiar with the findings and methodological challenges in the extant literature relevant to their question of interest can save years of trial and error in this difficult setting and avoid duplication of effort. For more experienced researchers, a familiarity with the scope of prior research can help them move from descriptive to analytic and intervention studies. Several recent reviews provide a good starting place for becoming familiar with recent correctional health research (Edens et al., 1997; Freudenberg, 2001; Magaletta, Diamond, Dietz, & Jahnke, 2006, Morris, 2001; Pollack, Khoshnood, & Altice, 1999).

Stakeholders in Correctional Health Research

Successful health research in correctional settings requires familiarity with the existing literature described in the previous section, a knowledge of the research methods applicable to the correctional setting, discussed in the next section, and an understanding of the various stakeholders in correctional health, discussed here. Without a map of this organizational landscape, even skilled researchers can lose their way.

Key participants in developing and implementing research studies in correctional settings include correctional officials, correctional health providers, public health authorities, other researchers and research institutions, elected officials, funders, prison and reentry advocacy groups and inmates and their families. Each of these constituencies has the potential both to improve research and to stop studies before they get off the ground. Thus, the practical researcher will want to understand how to enlist each of these groups in supporting the research process.

Correctional officials need to approve and at least not oppose any research study conducted in their facility. Their main concerns are the extent to which research may pose a threat to safety and regular prison routines, fear of bad publicity, cost and liability concerns, or additional demands on their staff. Researchers who can reassure correctional officials on these matters will have an easier time pursuing their studies. Investigators who are unable (or unwilling) to provide these assurances may need to consider other approaches to their research, such as interviewing participants after their release from jail or prison.

In most situations, research studies will need the tacit support of at least three levels of correctional authorities: senior departmental managers (e.g., commissioners/directors or sheriffs); wardens of the facility(ies) where the study takes place; and frontline correctional staff. Each level brings different concerns and requires different assurances in order to allow the research to proceed. For example, frontline correctional officers who may be required to bring participants to the researcher for interviews or medical examinations want to make sure these procedures do not interfere with their routines or increase staff workloads. Wardens often need to be assured that no research procedure will jeopardize security. In another example, a jail security warden was concerned that a stylus for a handheld computer device used for interviews with inmates could be used as a weapon. It took several meetings between a warden and a research team to agree on a type of stylus and interview procedures. Senior officials of corrections departments are sometimes ambivalent about studying illegal behavior such as drug use or voluntary or coercive sexual behavior. If they know that a problem exists, they may have an obligation to address it so that agreeing to research on these topics can have significant administrative, legal, and cost implications. Researchers will need to be prepared to address these concerns.

Correctional health providers have a constitutional mandate to provide health care to people in custody, offering a theoretical rationale for research that helps to improve care or make it more efficient or economical. In practice, however, since the types and quality of these services are often the subject of litigation (Nathan, 2004), health providers often filter requests for participation in research projects through their potential impact on current or future litigation. In addition, similarly to corrections officials, correctional health authorities often believe that if they know about a problem they will be required to take action to address it. This has made some officials reluctant to support research on difficult—and expensive—conditions such as hepatitis C (Spaulding et al., 2004). Researchers who want to study such topics will need to be able to address these concerns.

Correctional health providers operate under a variety of auspices, including public departments of corrections or health, universities, voluntary hospitals, or for-profit companies (Mellow & Greifinger, 2006). These differing organizational sponsorships influence a unit's openness to research and their motivation to participate in research studies. As with other potential stakeholders, researchers need to initiate a straightforward discussion to identify areas of common interest and potential conflict before beginning a study.

In some cases, correctional health providers have themselves initiated evaluation studies to guide practice. For example, the University of Texas, which has a contract to provide health services for inmates in Texas prisons, commissioned an independent evaluation of its services. The report generally lauded the Texas program and made several suggestions for more systematic quality assessment (Texas Medical Foundation, 2005).

Public health authorities often have a legal mandate to provide oversight of correctional health services and always have responsibility for providing core public health services to people returning to their communities. These obligations provide an incentive for research that can identify unmet needs, improve the effectiveness or quality of care or reduce its costs, or demonstrate the impact of interventions. In practice, some state and municipal health departments have close and positive relationships with correctional health researchers and enlist their help in identifying and solving problems. Others, either as a result of fears of litigation, new mandates for service, or unfavorable media attention, may be reluctant to establish partnerships with researchers.

Other researchers and research institutions can provide an important resource for both experienced and neophyte correctional health investigators. They can share their frontline experiences doing research in specific correctional systems or facilities, the study designs and instruments they have used, their solutions to issues of confidentiality and informed consent, or their findings from their previous research. In the last decade or so, a number of research centers focused on correctional health or reentry have been established, gaining valuable experience and producing a body of work that can inform future studies. Some of these are listed in Table 24.1. Since some federal funding agencies prefer multijurisdiction research projects in order to increase generalizability, establishing partnerships with experienced centers can help to design such studies and win funding for them.

Elected officials in both the executive and legislative branches are sometimes needed to approve funding for research studies (e.g., evaluation of publicly funded health or reentry interventions) or to pose questions that need study to correctional or health officials (e.g., how best to provide substance abuse treatment services to people in and returning from correctional facilities). In order to help these officials take on these roles, researchers can provide them with information documenting the problem, cost arguments on the potential savings from new approaches, and the public health benefits of correctional health services. Many elected officials worry that supporting health services or even research on the health needs of people in jail or prison might lead to charges that they are "soft on crime" or coddling criminals. Research evidence that can reframe the issues as public health, public safety, or economic concerns may help to provide a rationale for interest.

Funders provide the financial support for correctional and reentry health research and thus for this research to develop they must be willing to provide the level and continuity of funding needed to develop the field. Given that both private and public funders always have more requests for support than resources, that prison health is always a less popular choice than, say, children's health or education, and that many funders change their priorities

Table 24.1 Selected research centers on issues related to incarceration and health.

Research center	Research areas projects	Selected references	For more information
Abt Associates, Inc.	Research on social, economic, and health policy; criminal justice, HIV/AIDS, public health research	Hammett (2006), Hammett et al. (2002)	www.abtassociates.com (see Research, Criminal Justice or Publications)
Brown University, *Infectious Diseases in Corrections Report*	National forum for research and discussion of HIV/AIDS and hepatitis issues in corrections	Arriola et al. (2006), Jürgens (2006)	www.idcronline.org/index.html
Rutgers University, Center for Mental Health Services and Criminal Justice Research	Research and evaluation of mental health services, prevalence of mental illness, reentry and mental illness	Draine et al. (2005), Wolff et al. (2005)	www.cmhs-cjr.rutgers.edu/
University of California San Francisco, Center for AIDS Prevention Studies (CAPS)	Centerforce project: HIV prevention education and evaluation research	Comfort et al. (2000), Grinstead et al. (2001)	www.caps.ucsf.edu/projects/ Centerforce/
University of Connecticut Health Center	Research on ethical issues in correctional research, psychiatric illness, substance abuse	Lazzarini & Altice (2000), Lewis (2006)	www.connecticuthealth.org/ projects/index.html
University of Texas Medical Branch, Galveston, Program on Legal and Ethical Issues in Correctional Health	Training for NIH researchers, needs assessment of health issues for correctional health care workers; research on sex offenders, aging offenders, access to clinical trials	Stone et al. (2000), Stone & Winslade (1998)	www.utmb.edu/imh/ CorrectionalHealth/
Urban Institute, The Reentry Roundtable	Forum for research and discussion of policy, social, and health issues affecting formerly incarcerated individuals	Freudenberg (2006), Roberts et al. (2004)	www.urban.org/projects/reentry-roundtable/
Yale University, HIV in Prisons Program, Center for Interdisciplinary Research on AIDS	Consultation and management for HIV/ AIDS, TB, hepatitis, STDs; research on HIV/AIDS and antiretroviral therapy	Altice et al. (2005), Springer et al. (2004)	http://cira.med.yale.edu/

regularly, researchers face an uphill battle in winning the resources they need to pursue a comprehensive research agenda on correctional health.

Funders who have provided significant support to correctional health research include public agencies such as the National Institutes of Drug Abuse, Alcohol Abuse and Alcoholism, Mental Health, and Allergy and Infectious Diseases, the Centers for Disease Control and Prevention, the National Institute of Justice, and some state and local governments. Private funders include the Robert Wood Johnson Foundation, the Kellogg Foundation, the Open Society Institute, and the Jeht Foundation, among others.

To ensure long-term support, correctional health researchers will need to educate public and private funders about the connections between correctional health and public safety, public health, and social justice as well as to find ways to integrate correctional health issues into research on a variety of health and social problems.

Prison and reentry advocacy groups serve as important bridge between inmates and their families and the wider community. They also have the potential to influence policy makers, elected officials, and the media. Their opposition to unsafe or unhealthy prison conditions, inadequate medical care, or violations of civil liberties have contributed to the development of standards for correctional health care and greater public attention to these issues (Nathan, 2004).

The mission, scope, and activities of these groups vary widely, from national organizations such as the National Prison Project of the American Civil Liberties Union, which brings legal action against correctional systems alleged to violate inmate rights, and Critical Resistance, an alliance of regional groups dedicated to radical reform of the criminal justice system, to local groups that seek to coordinate reentry programs or organize prison visiting programs.

For researchers, these groups can provide detailed knowledge about prison conditions, inmate perceptions of problems, and the local political climate on correctional issues including health. Establishing relationships of mutual trust and respect, even when the two parties may disagree on the causes or solution to a problem of interest, can deepen investigators' understanding of the context in which their research is carried out.

Finally, *inmates and their families* can provide the insider knowledge that can determine the success or failure of a research project. Their understanding of the real-world intersection of policy and practice, the actual living conditions of inmates, and the problems that people leaving jail and prison face when they return home can help researchers to design their studies, develop their research instruments, and interpret their findings. Many researchers have noted the benefits of participatory research—deeper knowledge of the problem under study, greater engagement of research participants in the process, and more meaningful interpretation of results (Israel, Schulz, Parker, & Becker, 1998; Metzler et al., 2003).

In summary, correctional health researchers interact with a variety of stakeholders. At worst, these interactions can appear as a gauntlet of opponents, each with contradictory perceptions and demands that threaten the integrity of the research process and have the potential to disrupt or even halt any study. At best, however, each stakeholder can offer unique insights into the research problem, contribute distinct resources to the research process, and assist in making findings lead to improvements in practice, policy, and health. Thus, developing skills in successfully negotiating these interactions is an essential prerequisite for the correctional health researcher.

Methods of Research

Researchers in correctional facilities have used a wide variety of data sources to study inmate health. These include surveys of inmates or correctional authorities, clinical studies of inmate health, secondary analyses of national datasets, ethnographies, and reviews of existing prison health or criminal justice records. Each of these sources of data has unique advantages and disadvantages. Increasingly, researchers combine different types of data in order to gain deeper insights into the question of interest. For example, many correctional health studies will integrate survey data from participants, medical records from a correctional health service, and official criminal justice records in order to assess the impact of intervention programs.

In general, the methodological questions in correctional health are similar to those in other settings: e.g., how to define variables of interest consistently, how to ensure that the data collected are reliable and valid, and how to select appropriate samples and comparison groups. A variety of standard research texts can help investigators to become familiar with these issues (e.g., Boruch, 2005; Datzker, 1999; Noaks & Wincup, 2004; Patton, 2001).

Research in correctional settings does pose some particular methodological challenges. For example, longitudinal studies that follow inmates into the postrelease period face the problem of locating participants after release. Since people leaving jail or prison often lack residential stability and may not want further contact with those associated with the incarceration experience, achieving acceptable follow-up rates can be difficult. Strategies that have been used to increase follow-up rates include collection of multiple contact names at study entry; frequent interim contacts in order to maintain updated locators, use of both service and financial incentives, and use of public records (e.g., "rap sheets" and criminal records) in lieu of face-to-face contacts.

Correctional health researchers, like other investigators, often struggle to design and implement multilevel studies that seek to understand the cumulative impact of more than one level of organization on inmate or community health. They may collect data on individuals, social networks such as family and peers, communities, correctional facilities, and jurisdictions, then seek to analyze the contribution each level makes to a specified outcome. For example, a study of women and male adolescents leaving New York City jails examined the impact of individual characteristics, the jail and reentry experience, conditions in the returning community, and changing municipal policies on crime, welfare, and housing on returning inmates' drug use, HIV risk behavior, and reincarceration (Freudenberg et al., 2005). Multilevel analyses consider the contributions of variables at multiple levels to the variability in a particular individual-level dependent variable, e.g., drug use. In public health, multilevel research is increasingly used to assess the relative influence of neighborhood and individual-level variables on health (Diez-Roux, 2001). By comparing these two influences within different jurisdictions, a third level of organization (i.e., city or state policies or services) can be studied.

Health research in correctional settings also faces organizational and logistical issues. These include finding space for confidential interviews (an extremely challenging task in overcrowded jails and prisons), negotiating use of technology such as computer-assisted interviewing devices with prison security officials, providing clearance and escorts for researchers, and gaining consistent and reliable access to research participants within the security confines of the facility.

Solving these logistical problems requires a close and collaborative relationship between researchers and correctional officials. Defining common objectives at the inception of research, developing procedures for resolving conflicts before they emerge, and maintaining open communications with all levels of correctional authorities—from frontline correctional officers to wardens and commissioners—can help to reduce logistical problems. Most importantly, researchers who choose to work in correctional settings must be willing to act as guests in someone else's house, rather than expect to develop their own rules of conduct. Researchers who are unable or unwilling to accept this reality will face difficulty in working in prisons or jails.

Ethical Issues in Correctional Health Research

Perhaps the most challenging aspect of health research in correctional settings is meeting the competing demands for ethical research practice as mandated by various bodies as well as the researcher's own ethical standards. Prisoners pose ethical dilemmas for researchers not only because they lack the freedom to make the choices that most individuals in the free world take for granted, but also because so many prisoners experience other problems that make them vulnerable as research subjects: low levels of literacy, HIV infection, mental illness, victims or perpetrators of violence, as well as being adolescents. Ethical questions correctional health researchers must address include:

- What procedures ensure that all incarcerated people involved in studies have been given the opportunity to give informed and voluntary consent to participate in the research?
- What research practices can guarantee that inmates have as much right to choose to participate in research as any other population?
- How do correctional health researchers balance their ethical responsibilities to the correctional officials who commission their work or provide access to inmates with their responsibility to inmates?
- What level of individual or population benefits in correctional health research balances potential risks?
- How can researchers ensure that participation in correctional health research studies will not lead to harm through disclosure of confidential medical or criminal justice information to third parties?
- What ethical responsibility do researchers have to bring the findings of their research in correctional settings to policy makers or others who can act on these finding?

A brief review of the recent history of ethical issues in prison research helps to illustrate the competing forces and changing policy priorities. More in-depth discussion of this history can be found elsewhere (Gostin, Vanchieri, & Pope, 2006;

Kalmbach & Lyons, 2003; DeGroot, Bick, Thomas, & Stubblefield, 2001; Haney & Zimbardo, 1998; Hornblum, 1998).

In 1997, Hornblum observed that "from the early years of this century, the use of prison inmates as raw materials became an increasingly valuable component of American scientific research" (Hornblum, 1997). For example, in the 1960s, major pharmaceutical companies, Dow Chemical, and the U.S. Army tested 153 experimental drugs at the Holmesburg Prison in Pennsylvania (Hornblum, 1998). In 1976, based in part on disclosures of research abuses in prisons, the National Commission for the Protection of Human Subjects of Biomedical and Behavioral Research (1976) issued a report that set the framework for subsequent federal involvement in setting ethical standards for human experimentation. Their report called for additional protection for certain "vulnerable" populations, including children, neonates, pregnant women, and prisoners. In 1978, the Commission issued a report titled "Additional Protections Pertaining to Biomedical and Behavioral Research Involving Prisoners as Subjects" (U.S. DHHS, 2005). The main goal of these early guidelines was to protect incarcerated individuals from serving as involuntary or coerced "guinea pigs" in research that offered no direct benefits and had the potential for harm.

In the 1980s and early 1990s, the AIDS epidemic raised new ethical concerns for correctional health researchers. In some cases, prisoners with HIV infection or AIDS were not permitted to join clinical trials for new AIDS medications, based on various beliefs including their inability to give truly voluntary consent and their perceived unwillingness to comply with prescribed regimens. Some health researchers and prisoners rights advocates argued that such a ban violated ethical principles and that prisoners should have the same access to experimental treatments and clinical trials as other sectors of the population. From this perspective, ethical guidelines should place a priority on ensuring access to potential beneficial treatments (Dubler and Sidel, 1989) — a priority that may conflict with the previous emphasis on protecting inmates from researchers.

In 2006, the Institute of Medicine commissioned another review of ethical issues involved in prisoner research (Gostin, Vanchieri, & Pope, 2006). Based on several reviews of the more recent literature and testimony from dozens of witnesses including researchers, inmates, and correctional officials, the Committee on Ethical Considerations for Protection of Prisoners Involved in Research made fourteen recommendations in five broad categories (Table 24.2). These recommendations strive to find an appropriate and updated balance between the protection and access imperatives embodied in previous ethical standards. Whether these Institute of Medicine recommendations lead to changes in federal guidelines for prison research or in practice remains to be seen.

In practice, among the vexing problems correctional health researchers face are obtaining voluntary consent in jails or prisons, informing research participants about the benefits and risks of research, getting consent for randomized trials in which some participants receive no potential benefit, protecting the privacy of research participants, and negotiating with IRBs that may lack expertise in the realities of prison research.

Defining "voluntary" consent in the coerced environment of a correctional facility is sometimes difficult. Among the practices that can compromise free choice are promises of services not ordinarily available to inmates (e.g., certain

Table 24.2 Institute of Medicine committee recommendations for revisions to DHHS regulations for protection of prisoners involved in research.

1. Expand the definition of prisoner to include all those involuntarily confined in a penal institution, including detainees, parole violators, and those in alternatives to incarceration programs.

2. Ensure Universal, Consistent Ethical Protection
   * Establish uniform guidelines for all human subjects research involving prisoners, not just those funded by NIH or other federal agencies.
   * Maintain a public database of all research involving prisoners in order to make it easier to provide ethical oversight on this research.
   * Ensure transparency and accountability in the research enterprise.

3. Shift from a Category-Based to a Risk Benefit Approach to Research Review
   * Apply a risk–benefit framework to research review, shifting from the current model based on categories of excluded work to a system based on weighing of risk and benefits for the individual research participant.

4. Update the Ethical Framework to Include Collaborative Responsibility
   * Use a collaborative research approach that obtains input on research design and conduct from prisoners and other relevant stakeholders.
   * Ensure adequate standards of care such that prisoners are not encouraged to participate in research simply to get care that should be available to all.
   * Support critical areas of correctional research.

5. Enhance Systematic Oversight of Research Involving Prisoners
   * Strengthen monitoring of research involving prisoners.
   * Strengthen local IRBs abilities to reach independent decisions on prison research.
   * Enhance the Office of Human Research Protections capacity to provide systematic oversight of research involving prisoners.
   * Ensure voluntary informed consent for all prisoners involved in research.
   * Protect the privacy of prisoner involved in research.

Source: Gostin et al. (2006).

types of health services), the presence of correctional officers in the area where consent is being solicited, the unavailability of the independent advice on participation that is normally available to research participants in the free world, or the implied offer to use participation in research in exchange for a shorter sentence or favorable consideration by a judge or parole board. Since no set of rules can govern all the situations that can jeopardize voluntary consent, for any particular study the ethical researcher ought to consult experienced correctional researchers, correctional officials at the study site, prisoners rights advocates, and current and former inmates in order to obtain a variety of perspectives on the best procedures to insure voluntary consent.

Similarly, the process of informing research participants in correctional settings of the risks and benefits of a study can be challenging. Many inmates have low levels of literacy; many distrust correctional and health authorities, sometimes based on their own past experiences; and, unlike most research in medical settings, an added risk is disclosure of information that can cause harm to participants from other inmates, correctional staff, legal authorities, or the wider public. Research on stigmatized conditions such as HIV infection, mental illness, and substance use almost always poses such risks. Methods that researchers have used to overcome these obstacles are to engage current and former inmates in the design of informed consent materials and as members of

IRBs, to hire independent advisors who are not part of the research team to help inmates make decisions about participation, and to obtain federal certificates of confidentiality to minimize risk of disclosure of confidential information.

While some inmates and ethicists express concerns about the coercion implicit in any research in the correctional setting, the recent IOM report(Gostin et al., 2006) also noted that other inmates strongly oppose restrictions on inmate participation in research. Some are concerned about lack of access to cutting-edge treatments for HIV or cancer; others object to the loss of opportunities for compensation or enhanced living situations.

A specific problem facing researchers involved in clinical trails in which some forms of treatment are withheld from some participants is convincing both staff and participants of the rationale for a randomized trial. From a researcher's point of view, the lack of definitive evidence of the benefits of an intervention is sufficient rationale for such a trial but for staff and participants, withholding services perceived to be beneficial may seem unethical. When staff are not convinced of the morality of a research study, they may intentionally or unintentionally undermine the study, either by providing services to the "control" group or by communicating their discomfort to research participants, thus discouraging enrollment in a study. For this reason, it is important for researchers to address this issue forthrightly.

Strategies to minimize this problem include offering all research participants some level of services above the standard care in the correctional facility, comparing different interventions to each other rather than to no special services, educating research staff about the ethics of offering unevaluated services to all participants, and, as the Institute of Medicine report on correctional research suggests (Gostin et al., 2006), joining advocacy efforts to improve the basic standard of care in all correctional facilities.

In my experience, many correctional health researchers complain about the extensive and lengthy process required to get IRB approval for their research study and suggest that it can discourage them from pursuing worthy projects. In some cases, several different IRBs need to approve a single study and occasionally offer conflicting guidance on how to proceed. These complaints have a variety of sources: some investigators prefer the old way of business where researchers alone decided on the conduct of their studies. But even researchers who support the importance of protecting prisoners note that IRB members often lack expertise in the day-to-day realities of correctional institutions and the nonresearch risks inmates encounter daily. They also report that IRB committees often reflect the wider tension between protecting participants from research harm and ensuring access to beneficial services and in their effort to maximize both of these aims impose unreasonable demands on researchers.

A possible solution is to assist IRBs to find a member who is experienced in correctional settings and correctional research—not only to meet the DHHS regulatory requirement to include such a person but also to obtain practical advice on devising realistic and ethical resolution of problems. For example, one state prison system IRB included an attorney who specialized in inmate litigation. Another solution, as recommended by the IOM report (Gostin et al., 2006), is to develop universal national standards for review of prison research so that all research is reviewed using uniform criteria.

Developing a Research Agenda on Correctional Health

At present, correctional health researchers respond to a variety of heterogeneous influences — other criminal justice, medical, public health, and public policy researchers; local, state, and federal correctional and health officials; correctional health providers; a variety of professional organizations; elected policy makers; and various criminal justice and health advocacy organizations, among others. It is therefore not surprising that in this anarchic and complex environment correctional health researchers have yet to develop a coherent and comprehensive research agenda driven by existing scientific knowledge and public policy imperatives. However, the fact that it may be difficult to envision and articulate such an agenda should not stop the effort. In fact, as health and correctional officials and researchers request additional support for correctional health research, it is inevitable that they will be asked to set priorities. And if researchers themselves fail to take the lead in this process, others will impose an agenda on them.

While the development of a comprehensive research agenda for correctional health is beyond the scope of this chapter, I conclude by suggesting some steps that might move the field in this direction.

First, we need to begin a national dialogue on research needs that include researchers, correctional and health officials, policy makers, and advocates. Questions to discuss include: what are the most promising avenues of research to lead to short- and middle-term improvements in the health of incarcerated populations? What are potential stable funding streams for this research? How best can we develop consistent frameworks for research so that clinical, practice, and policy decisions can be more evidence-based? Who are the constituencies that will support a national research agenda on correctional health and how can these constituencies be organized into a coherent force? What correctional research might be particularly beneficial both to the health of the incarcerated and to the larger health of the public?

Organizations that can play a role in this national discussion include the National Institute of Justice, NIH Institutes and the Centers for Disease Control and Prevention, the National Commission on Correctional Health Care, various health professional organizations, and the Reentry Policy Council.

Second, researchers need to synthesize the existing and disparate literature on correctional health to identify common findings, gaps in the literature, and future priorities. This literature is dispersed in several different disciplines and among the peer-reviewed and "gray" literatures, i.e., public and voluntary organization reports and studies. One possible sponsor for such a critical review would be the Institute of Medicine.

Third, as recommended by the recent IOM report on correctional health research (Gostin et al., 2006), the United States should establish more consistent and uniform guidelines for ethical health research among incarcerated populations. Such guidelines will protect researchers and inmates and help to resolve the continuing debate between protection from researchers and full access to the benefits of research.

Fourth, any agenda should consider the range of settings in which correctional health plays out, including courts, jails, prisons, parole and probation services, alternatives to incarceration, and reentry programs. Too often, each setting has been its own silo with a cadre of researchers and officials. The evidence of the past decades suggests that in fact these settings constitute a single if sometimes disorganized system in which changes in one component affect all others. Thus, health research needs to examine these systemic interactions in order to avoid shifting problems for one sector to another.

Finally, correctional health research has to be considered a branch of population health research and therefore address the broadest questions that affect the health of the public. In the past, some correctional health researchers have limited their attention to those individuals served in correctional health settings—the patients who walked through their clinic doors. While these concerns will continue to be important and warrant focused investigation, they are not sufficient to realize the full opportunity for correctional health researchers to improve health.

Research questions that need to be addressed in the coming decade include: How does incarceration influence socioeconomic, racial, and gender disparities in health in the United States? How does incarceration affect the health of the families and communities of incarcerated individuals? What role can correctional health services play in reducing community incidence, prevalence, severity, or costs of conditions such as HIV infection, hepatitis C, diabetes, asthma, addiction, violence, depression, or lack of health insurance? By expanding their focus to these questions, correctional health researchers have the potential to contribute to solving our nation's most pressing health problems.

References

Altice, F.L., Marinovich, A., Khoshnood, K., Blankenship, K.M., Springer, S.A., & Selwyn, P.A. (2005). Correlates of HIV infection among incarcerated women: Implications for improving detection of HIV infection. *J Urban Health*, *82*, 312–326.

Arriola, K.J., Braithwaite, R.L., & Newkirk, C.F. (2006). At the intersection between poverty, race, and HIV infection: HIV-related services for incarcerated women. *Infectious Diseases in Corrections Report*, *9*.

Baillargeon, J., Black, S.A., Pulvino, J., & Dunn, K. (2000). The disease profile of Texas prison inmates. *Ann Epidemiol*, *10*, 74–80.

Barreras, R.E., Drucker, E.M., & Rosenthal, D. (2005). The concentration of substance use, criminal justice involvement, and HIV/AIDS in the families of drug offenders. *J Urban Health*, *82*, 162–170.

Bauserman, R.L., Richardson, D., Ward, M., Shea, M., Bowlin, C., Tomoyasu, N., & Solomon, L. (2003). HIV prevention with jail and prison inmates: Maryland's Prevention Case Management program. *AIDS Educ Prev*, *15*, 465–480.

Bellin, E.Y., Fletcher, D.D., & Safyer, S.M. (1993). Association of tuberculosis infection with increased time in or admission to the New York City jail system. *JAMA*, *269*, 2228–2231.

Boruch, R.F. (2005). *Randomized experiments for planning and evaluation: A practical guide* (Applied Social Research Methods). Beverly Hills: Sage Publications.

Chan, T.C., Vilke, G.M., Smith, S., Sparrow, W., & Dunford, J.V. (2003). Impact of an after-hours on-call emergency physician on ambulance transports from a county jail. *Prehosp Emerg Care*, *7*, 327–331.

Comfort, M., Grinstead, O.A., Faigeles, B., & Zack, B. (2000). Reducing HIV risk among women visiting their incarcerated male partners. *Criminal Justice and Behavior*, *21*, 57–71.

Datzker, M.L. (Ed.). (1999). *Readings for research methods in criminology and criminal justice.* Butterworth–Heinemann.

Davenport, C., Mathers, J., & Parry, J. (2006). Use of health impact assessment in incorporating health considerations in decision making. *J Epidemiol Community Health, 60,* 196–201.

De Groot, A., Bick, J., Thomas, D., & Stubblefield, B. (2001). Clinical trials in correctional settings: Right or regression? *The AIDS Reader, 11,* 34–40.

Diez Roux, A.V. (2001). Investigating neighborhood and area effects on health. *Am J Public Health, 91,* 1783–1789.

Draine, J., Wolff, N., Jacoby, J., Hartwell, S., & Duclos, C. (2005). Understanding community re-entry among former prisoners with mental illness: A conceptual model to move new research. *Behav Sci Law, 23,* 689–707.

Dubler, N.N., & Sidel, V.W. (1989). On research on HIV infection and AIDS in correctional institutions. *Milbank Q, 67,* 171–207.

Edens, J.F., Peters, R.H., & Hills, H.A. (1997). Treating prison inmates with co-occurring disorders: An integrative review of existing programs. *Behav Sci Law, 15,* 439–457.

Fox, R.K., Currie, S.L., Evans, J., Wright, T.L., Tobler, L., Phelps, B., Busch, M.P., & Page-Shafer, K.A. (2005). Hepatitis C virus infection among prisoners in the California state correctional system. *Clin Infect Dis, 41,* 177–186.

Freudenberg, N. (2001). Jails, prisons, and the health of urban populations: A review of the impact of the correctional system on community health. *J Urban Health, 78,* 214–235.

Freudenberg, N., Daniels, J., Crum, M., Perkins, T., Richie, B.E. (2005). Coming home from jail: the social and health consequences of community reentry for women, male adolescents, and their families and communities. *Am J Public Health, 95,* 1725–1736.

Freudenberg, N. (2006). *Coming home from jail*: A *review of health and social problems facing US jail populations and of opportunities for reentry interventions.* Washington, DC: Jail Reentry Roundtable Initiative, Urban Institute.

Gostin, L.O., Vanchieri, C., & Pope, A. (Eds.). (2006). *Ethical considerations for research involving prisoners.* Washington, DC: National Academy Press.

Grinstead, O., Zack, B., & Faigeles, B. (2001). Reducing postrelease risk behavior among HIV seropositive prison inmates: The health promotion program. *AIDS Educ Prev, 13,* 109–119.

Hammett, T.M. (2006). HIV/AIDS and other infectious diseases among correctional inmates: Transmission, burden, and an appropriate response. *Am J Public Health, 96,* 974–978.

Hammett, T.M., Harmon, M.P., & Rhodes, W. (2002). The burden of infectious disease among inmates of and releasees from US correctional facilities, 1997. *Am J Public Health, 92,* 1789–1794.

Haney, C., & Zimbardo, P. (1998). The past and future of U.S. prison policy: Twenty-five years after the Stanford Prison Experiment. *Am Psychol, 53,* 709–727.

Hoofnagle, J.H. (2006). A framework for management of hepatitis C in prisons. *Ann Intern Med, 144,* 762–769.

Hornblum, A. (1997). They were cheap and available: Prisoners as research subjects in twentieth century America. *Br Med J, 315,* 1437–1441.

Hornblum, A.M. (1998). *Acres of skin: Human experiments in Holmesberg Prison.* New York: Routledge.

Iguchi, M.Y., Bell, J., Ramchand, R.N., & Fain, T. (2005). How criminal system racial disparities may translate into health disparities. *J Health Care Poor Underserved, 16*(4 Suppl. B), 48–56.

Israel, B.A., Schulz, A.J., Parker, E.A., & Becker, A.B. (1998). Review of community-based research: Assessing partnership approaches to improve public health. *Annu Rev Public Health, 19,* 173–202.

James, D.J., & Glaze, L.E. (2006). *Mental health problems of prison and jail inmates.* Bureau of Justice Statistics Special Report. NCJ 213600; 1–12.

Jarrett, N.C., Adeyemi, S.A., & Huggins, T. (2006). Bridging the gap: Providing health care to newly released men. *J Health Care Poor Underserved, 17*(1 Suppl.), 70–80.

Johnson, R.C., & Raphael, S. (2006). *The effects of male incarceration dynamics on AIDS infection rates among African-American women and men.* National Poverty Center Working Paper Series. Available at http://www.npc.umich.edu/publications/working_papers/.

Jürgens, R. (2006). From evidence to action on HIV/AIDS in prisons: A report from the XVI International AIDS Conference. *Infectious Diseases in Corrections Report.*

Kalmbach, K.C., & Lyons, P.M. (2003). Ethical and legal standards for research in prison. *Behav Sci Law, 21*, 671–686.

Karberg, J.C., & James, D.J. (2005). *Substance dependence, abuse and treatment of jail inmates, 2002.* Bureau of Justice Statistics Special Report NCJ 209588: 1–12.

Keller, A.S., Link, R.N., Bickell, N.A., Charap, M.H., Kalet, A.L., & Schwartz, M.D. (1993). Diabetic ketoacidosis in prisoners without access to insulin. *JAMA, 269*, 619–621.

Kemm, J. (2001). Health impact assessment: A tool for healthy public policy. *Health Promotion International, 16*, 79–85.

Kraut-Becher, J.R., Gift, T.L., Haddix, A.C., Irwin, K.L., & Greifinger, R.B. (2004). Cost-effectiveness of universal screening for chlamydia and gonorrhea in US jails. *J Urban Health, 81*, 453–471.

Krebs, C.P., & Simmons, M. (2004). Intraprison HIV transmission: An assessment of whether it occurs, how it occurs, and who is at risk. *AIDS Educ Prev, 14*(5 Suppl. B), 53–64.

Lazzarini, Z., & Altice, F.L. (2000). A review of the legal and ethical issues for the conduct of HIV-related research in prisons. *AIDS Public Policy J, 15*(3–4), 105–135.

Leh, S.K. (1999). HIV infection in U.S. correctional systems: Its effect on the community. *J Community Health Nurs, 16*, 53–63.

Leukefeld, C.G., Hiller, M.L., Webster, J.M., Tindall, M.S., Martin, S.S., Duvall, J., Tolbert, V.E., & Garrity, T.F. (2006). A prospective examination of high-cost health services utilization among drug using prisoners reentering the community. *J Behav Health Serv Res, 33*, 73–85.

Lewis, C. (2006). Treating incarcerated women: Gender matters. *Psychiatr Clin North Am, 29*, 773–789.

Lincoln, T., Kennedy, S., Tuthill, R., Roberts, C., Conklin, T.J., & Hammett, T.M. (2006). Facilitators and barriers to continuing healthcare after jail: A community-integrated program. *J Ambul Care Manage, 29*, 2–16.

Lindquist, C.H., & Lindquist, C.A. (1999). Health behind bars: Utilization and evaluation of medical care among jail inmates. *J Community Health, 24*, 285–303.

Magaletta, P.R., Diamond, P.M., Dietz, E., & Jahnke, S. (2006). The mental health of federal offenders: A summative review of the prevalence literature. *Adm Policy Ment Health, 33*, 253–263.

McNiel, D.E., Binder, R.L., & Robinson, J.C. (2005). Incarceration associated with homelessness, mental disorder, and co-occurring substance abuse. *Psychiatric Serv, 56*, 840–846.

Mellow, J., & Greifinger, R. (2006). Successful reentry: The perspective of private correctional health care providers. *J Urban Health, 84*, 85–98.

Metzler, M.M., Higgins, D.L., Beeker, C.G., Freudenberg, N., Lantz, P.M., Senturia, K.D., Eisinger, A.A., Viruell-Fuentes, E.A., Gheisar, B., Palermo, A.G., & Softley, D. (2003). Addressing urban health in Detroit, New York City, and Seattle through community-based participatory research partnerships. *Am J Public Health, 93*, 803–811.

Morris, R.E. (2001). The health of youth in the juvenile justice systems. *Adolesc Med, 12*, 471–483.

Murray, J., & Farrington, D.P. (2005). Parental imprisonment: Effects on boys' antisocial behaviour and delinquency through the life-course. *J Child Psychol Psychiatry, 46,* 1269–1278.

Myers, J., Zack, B., Kramer, K., Gardner, M., Rucobo, G., & Costa-Taylor, S. (2005). Get Connected: An HIV prevention case management program for men and women leaving California prisons. *Am J Public Health, 95,* 1682–1684.

Nathan, V.M. (2004). Taking stock of the accomplishments and failures of prison reform litigation: Have the courts made a difference in the quality of prison conditions? What have we accomplished to date? *Pace Law Rev, 24,* 419–425.

National Commission for the Protection of Human Subjects of Biomedical and Behavioral Research. (1976). *Report and recommendations research involving prisoners.* Washington, DC.

National Commission on Correctional Health Care. (2002a). *The health status of soon-to-be-released inmates: A report to Congress.* Vol. 1. Chicago: Author.

National Commission on Correctional Health Care. (2002b). *The health status of soon-to-be-released inmates: A report to Congress.* Vol. 2. Chicago: Author. (Cost-Effectiveness Studies, pp. 81–166.)

Needels, K., James-Burdumy, S., & Burghardt, J. (2005). Community case management for former jail inmates: Its impacts on rearrest, drug use, and HIV risk. *J Urban Health, 82,* 420–433.

Noaks, L., & Wincup, E. (2004). *Criminological research: Understanding qualitative methods.* Beverly Hills: Sage.

Patton, M.Q. (2001). *Qualitative research and evaluation methods* (3rd ed.). Beverly Hills: Sage.

Peters, R.H., Strozier, A.L., Murrin, M.R., & Kearns, W.D. (1997). Treatment of substance-abusing jail inmates Examination of gender differences. *J Substance Abuse Treatment, 4,* 339–349.

Pollack, H., Khoshnood, K., & Altice, F. (1999). Health care delivery strategies for criminal offenders. *J Health Care Finance, 26,* 63–77.

Resch, S., Altice, F.L., & Paltiel, A.D. (2005). Cost-effectiveness of HIV screening for incarcerated pregnant women. *J Acquir Immune Defic Syndr, 38,* 163–173.

Rich, J.D., Holmes, L., Salas, C., Macalino, G., Davis, D., Ryczek, J., & Flanigan, T. (2001). Successful linkage of medical care and community services for HIV-positive offenders being released from prison. *J Urban Health, 78,* 279–289.

Roberts, C., Kennedy, S., & Hammett, T.M. (2004). Linkages between in-prison and community-based health services. *Correctional Health Care, 10,* 333–368.

Rose, D., & Clear, T. (2003). Incarceration, reentry, and social capital: Social networks in the balance. In J. Travis & M. Waul (Eds.), *Prisoners once removed: The impact of incarceration and reentry on children, families, and communities* (pp. 313–342). Washington, DC: Urban Institute Press.

Rounds-Bryant, J.L., Motivans, M.A., & Pelissier, B. (2003). Comparison of background characteristics and behaviors of African-American, Hispanic, and white substance abusers treated in federal prison: Results from the TRIAD Study. *J Psychoactive Drugs, 35,* 333–341.

Spaulding, A.C., Weinbaum, C.M., Lau, D.T., Sterling, R., Seeff, L.B., Margolis, H.S., Springer, S.A., Pesanti, E., Hodges, J., Macura, T., Doros, G., & Altice, F.L. (2004). Effectiveness of antiretroviral therapy among HIV-infected prisoners: Reincarceration and the lack of sustained benefit after release to the community. *Clin Infect Dis, 38,* 1754–1760.

Springer, S.A., Pesanti, E., Hodges, J., Macura, T., Doros, G., Altice, F.L. (2004). Effectiveness of antiretroviral therapy among HIV-infected prisoners: reincarceration and the lack of sustained benefit after release to the community. *Clin Infect Dis. 38,* 1754–1760.

Stone, T.H., & Winslade, W.I. (1998). Report on a national survey of correctional health facilities: A needs assessment of health issues. *J Correctional Health Care, 5,* 5–49.

Stone, T.H., Winslade, W.J., & Klugman, C.M. (2000). Sex offenders, sentencing laws and pharmaceutical treatment: A prescription for failure. *Behav Sci Law, 18*, 83–110.

Taxman, F.S., Byrne, J.M., & Pattavina, A. (2005). Racial disparity and the legitimacy of the criminal justice system: Exploring consequences for deterrence. *J Health Care Poor Underserved, 16*(4 Suppl. B), 57–77.

Teplin, L.A. (1990). The prevalence of severe mental disorder among male urban jail detainees: comparison with the Epidemiologic Catchment Area Program. *Am J Public Health, 80*, 663–9.

Teplin, L.A., Abram, K.M., McClelland, G.M. (1996). Prevalence of psychiatric disorders among incarcerated women. I. Pretrial jail detainees. *Arch Gen Psychiatry, 53*, 505–12. Erratum in: *Arch Gen Psychiatry, 1996, 53*, 664.

Texas Medical Foundation. (2005). An evaluation of correctional health care services provided by University of Texas Medical Branch Correctional Managed Care to the Texas Department of Criminal Justice: An assessment of managed care service delivery systems, adherence to correctional health care standards and clinical outcomes. Available at http://www.utsystem.edu/news/2005/BORMar2005-Presentations/PrisonHealthCare-TMFExecSummary031005.pdf

Thomas, J.C., & Sampson, L.A. (2005). High rates of incarceration as a social force associated with community rates of sexually transmitted infection. *J Infect Dis, 191* (Suppl. 1):S55–S60.

U.S. Department of Health and Human Services. (2005). *Code of Federal Regulations: Title 45. Public Welfare. Part 46: Protection of Human Subjects*. Washington, DC: U.S. DHHS.

Veerman, J.L., Barendregt, J.J., & Mackenbach, J.P. (2005). Quantitative health impact assessment: Current practice and future directions. *J Epidemiol Community Health, 59*, 361–370.

Wilson, A.B., & Draine, J. (2006). Collaborations between criminal justice and mental health systems for prisoner reentry. *Psychiatr Serv, 57*, 875–878.

Wolff, N., Maschi, T., & Bjerklie, J.R. (2005). Reentry planning for mentally disordered inmates: A social investment approach. *J Offender Rehabil, 41*, 21–42.

Chapter 25

Reentry Experiences of Men with Health Problems

Christy A. Visher and Kamala Mallik-Kane

One of the most profound challenges facing American society is the reintegration of more than 650,000 individuals who leave state and federal prisons and return home each year. The fourfold increase in incarceration rates over the past 25 years has had far-reaching consequences. Four million citizens have lost their right to vote. One and a half million children have a parent in prison. Men and women leave correctional facilities with little preparation for life on the outside, insufficient assistance with reintegration, and a high likelihood of return to prison for new crimes or parole violations. Nationwide, over half of released prisoners are expected to return to prison within 3 years (Langan & Levin, 2002), and some states experience even higher rates of recidivism. This cycle of incarceration and return of large numbers of adults, mostly men between the ages of 18 and 35, creates specific health needs and risks for returning prisoners, their families, and the community at large. The challenges to improve the health profile of the prison population and protect the health of their families and communities to which they return are numerous. Persons released from prison are disproportionately afflicted with illness and tend to be sicker, on average, than the U.S. general population (Davis & Pacchiana, 2003). The prevalence of chronic, communicable, and mental illnesses is often higher among prisoners than in the general population due, in part, to higher levels of socioeconomic disadvantage and substance use compared to the average American (National Commission on Correctional Health Care [NCCHC], 2002). It is also common for many in the prisoner population to have multiple, co-occurring health conditions (Davis & Pacchiana, 2003).

Released prisoners are returning in relatively high concentrations to a small number of communities in America's urban centers (Lynch & Sabol, 2001), thereby having a profound and disproportionate impact on community life, family networks, and social capital in these neighborhoods. The Urban Institute has found that large numbers of prisoners return to a relatively small number of cities, and returning prisoners are often clustered in a few neighborhoods within those cities. For example, in 2001, Chicago and Baltimore received more than half of the prisoners returning to Illinois and Maryland, respectively (La Vigne & Kachnowski, 2003; La Vigne and Mamalian, 2003).

Moreover, 8% of Chicago communities (6 of 77) accounted for 34% of all prisoners returning to Chicago (La Vigne & Mamalian, 2003) and 11% of Baltimore communities (6 of 55) accounted for 36% of the prisoners returning to Baltimore (La Vigne & Kachnowski, 2003). Houston received a quarter of all prisoners returning to Texas, and 25% of those returned to just seven Houston communities (Watson, Solomon, La Vigne, & Travis, 2004).

Social and economic disadvantage often characterize these communities with high concentrations of returning prisoners, compounding the challenges and burdens that this population brings with it. The Chicago, Baltimore, Cleveland, and Houston communities that are home to the greatest concentrations of released prisoners have above-average rates of unemployment, female-headed households, and families living below the federal poverty level (La Vigne & Kachnowski, 2003; La Vigne & Mamalian, 2003; La Vigne & Thomson, 2003; Watson et al., 2004). These communities are often already deprived of resources and ill equipped to meet the health needs and other difficulties that characterize this population. Research also suggests that high rates of incarceration and reentry of community residents cycling in and out of the criminal justice system may further destabilize these communities (Clear, Rose, & Ryder, 2001).

Addressing prisoner health would not only benefit individual prisoners, but could also improve the overall public health in these communities of return. Given the extent to which many individuals cycle in and out of correctional facilities, prisoners and former prisoners comprise a respectable share of the population in certain communities. The concentration of prisoners and former prisoners in some of the most disadvantaged urban areas has created a public health opportunity whereby attending to the health needs of prisoners may affect the course of a number of epidemics. Research has shown that sizable portions of the total number of Americans with HIV, tuberculosis, and hepatitis, for example, serve time in correctional facilities each year (NCCHC, 2002). The time spent in prison can be used to engage individuals in treatment, thereby reducing the burden of illness and potentially preventing the further transmission of disease.

Attending to prisoner health needs also has the potential to influence reentry outcomes. A successful reentry, defined as establishing a drug-free and crime-free life with a job and sufficient income, represents a great challenge for returning prisoners, many of whom have limited educational and vocational skill sets as well as troubled personal histories (Gaes & Kendig, 2002). Returning prisoners face multiple, often simultaneous tasks as they embark on the process of reestablishing their lives outside of prison. One of their immediate challenges is to obtain housing. Over time, other things become important as well: getting a job, having enough money to live on, reconnecting with children and family, and staying healthy and sober. The ability to live a drug-free and crime-free life depends on many of these intermediary steps.

Anecdotal evidence suggests that prisoners with health problems may have a more difficult reentry process than others (Travis, 2005). Unresolved health and substance use problems may further complicate an already challenging transition. Returning prisoners with health problems are additionally confronted with the tasks of managing their health problems, such as accessing health care and keeping up with medications or appointments. They may be unable to engage in work or other activities because of pain or sickness, and their families may be unwilling or unable to serve as a fallback support. Those with severe or unmanaged health problems face an increased risk of adverse outcomes, including physical illness, relapse into drug use, or, particularly in the case of mental illness, inappropriate behavior that provokes a police response. Previous Urban Institute work in Illinois showed that returning prisoners with mental illness experienced more postrelease unemployment and used drugs more often than returning prisoners without mental illness (Mallik-Kane, 2005). It stands to reason that successful treatment of returning prisoners' health conditions could improve their chances of reentry success by improving their ability to work, support themselves, and abstain from substance use, all of which have been shown to contribute to desistance from criminal activity.

The work presented here is an empirical examination of how the reentry experiences of prisoners with health problems differ from those without. Although there are many reasons to believe that prisoners with health problems would have a different reintegration process than the "average" returning prisoner, there has been little work done to quantify the specific differences. This study takes a wide view of health and includes physical health, mental health, and substance abuse in the analysis. The high level of substance use in correctional populations is indeed a health concern. Substance use at the level of addiction is an illness in its own right, an Axis II disorder according to the *Diagnostic and Statistical Manual of Mental Disorders* (DSM-IV). Moreover, regardless of addiction, the physiological effects of drugs and alcohol are damaging to overall physical health. In addition to the risk of overdose, substance use increases the likelihood of developing other chronic conditions, including cardiovascular disease and cirrhosis of the liver (National Institute on Drug Abuse [NIDA], 2004). Substance use also contributes to the transmission of other diseases, most notably HIV.

The data for this analysis come from Returning Home: Understanding the Challenges of Prisoner Reentry, a multistate, longitudinal study of prisoner reentry being conducted by the Urban Institute. Following an overview of the data collection methodology and sample characteristics, this chapter presents a description of the health status of returning prisoners and the extent to which they received treatment for their health problems. The reentry experiences of those with and without physical, mental, and substance abuse problems are then compared and contrasted in order to identify the ways in which they differ from the average reentry experience. We then offer empirically based recommendations for improving the reentry outcomes of prisoners with health problems.

Overview of Returning Home Study

In 2001, the Urban Institute launched a multistate, longitudinal study to document the transition from prison to home and understand the pathways of reintegration for men and women released from state prisons. This project, Returning Home: Understanding the Challenges of Prisoner Reentry, examines the factors that contribute to a successful or unsuccessful reentry experience, and identifies how those factors can inform policy and practice. The Returning Home study conducted interviews with individual prisoners once before and up to three times after their release from state correctional facilities. Through these interviews, returning prisoners shared their thoughts and experiences related to a number of important reentry challenges, such as finding housing, gaining employment, and remaining crime-free. The interviews also addressed factors that are hypothesized to influence reentry success, including attitudes and expectations, physical and mental health, substance use and treatment, family and peer relationships, and programmatic interventions. In addition to these interviews, the study conducted focus groups in the neighborhoods to which many prisoners return, interviewed reentry policymakers and practitioners, and reviewed state laws and policies relevant to reentry.

This chapter reports on the reentry experiences of men returning from Ohio and Texas prisons during 2004 and 2005. Because prison populations are largely comprised of individuals from urban areas, the study focuses on the reentry process within an urban context. In Ohio the study surveyed a representative sample of 424 men returning from state prisons to Cuyahoga County (metropolitan Cleveland), and in Texas the study surveyed a representative sample of 414 men returning to Harris County (metropolitan Houston). In both states, individuals completed a self-administered survey in the month before their release from prison and participated in a series of one-on-one interviews after their release. This chapter focuses on early outcomes reported at the first postrelease interview that was conducted, on average, 2 months after release.

The men in our sample were representative of released prisoners in their states who had been sentenced to at least 1 year in prison and planned to return to the Cleveland or Houston areas. Respondents were 36 years old, on average, at the time of release. Most were from minority racial groups, with 81% describing themselves as being black or of another (nonwhite) race. About 1 in 10 respondents reported Hispanic ethnicity and almost all were U.S. citizens. Roughly one half were parents of minor children when they entered prison and one-quarter had been married. (Table 25.1 displays these and other selected characteristics of study respondents.)

The typical respondent had been incarcerated for 18 months during this term, though about one-fifth of respondents were being released after terms of 5 or more years. Most respondents served their time in state prisons, but one-quarter had been in state jails intended for prisoners convicted of somewhat less serious felony offenses and serving shorter sentences. (These state jails, located in Texas, are distinct from local jails; they are meant for low-level convicted felons with sentences of 2 years or less.) One-third served this term for a drug offense and one-fifth each were in prison this time for violent and property offenses. Nearly two-thirds (62%) were being released to a term of parole supervision, with the remainder being released from custody with no supervision requirements.

The men in our sample would need to overcome several hurdles to establish a stable, drug-free and crime-free life in the community. Finding and maintaining employment would be challenging, as 3 out of 10 were leaving prison without having completed a high school education. Many had spotty employment histories with over one-quarter having been unemployed in the 6 months preceding this prison term.

Maintaining sobriety would not come easily either, with many reporting past troubles with substance use. About two-thirds came from a family in which someone had a drug or alcohol problem, and the vast majority (84%) reported using drugs or drinking to intoxication in the 6 months preceding their prison term. Levels of use commensurate with abuse and addiction were

Table 25.1 Selected characteristics of *Returning Home* respondents ($n = 838$).

Demographics	
Age (median)	36 years
Black or African American race	67.2%
White or Caucasian race	19.5%
Other race	13.3%
Hispanic ethnicity	12.2%
U.S. citizenship	98.4%
Education and employment	
High school diploma or GED at release	69.7%
Employed at any time in the 6 months before prison	72.5%
Family relationships	
Married or living together as married before prison	24.0%
Had children under age 18	52.6%
Number of close family relationships before prison (median)	3
Number of close family relationships during prison (median)	3
Criminal history	
Age at first arrest (median)	17 years
Served time in a juvenile correctional facility	36.0%
Previously convicted of a crime	82.3%
Served time in prison before	66.0%
Had parole or probation revoked before	48.9%
Current prison sentence	
Time served in prison (median)	18 months
Violent offense conviction	22.8%
Property offense conviction	20.5%
Drug dealing conviction	11.1%
Drug possession conviction	24.7%
Other offense conviction	20.9%
Current term resulted from probation or parole violation	35.6%
Will be released to parole supervision	62.2%

common. Before their incarceration, two-thirds of all respondents used drugs or drank to intoxication more than once a week and nearly one-half (45%) did so daily.

A cessation of criminal activity would also require many to make a break from the past, as most respondents had extensive familial and personal criminal histories. Close to two-thirds reported that a family member had served time in prison before and many had their own first encounter with the criminal justice system at a young age. Half of the men were first arrested by age 17 and over one-third had served time in a juvenile facility. Overall, 8 out of 10 respondents had been convicted of a crime before and over half had served time in prison. Nearly one-half reported having had their parole revoked in the past.

Health Status of Returning Prisoners

When we interviewed men during the month before their release from prison, most had positive feelings about their health, with 8 out of 10 describing their overall physical health as excellent or good. Despite feeling healthy, however, the majority of respondents also reported having been diagnosed with a chronic physical or mental health condition. One half of men reported that a doctor or nurse had told them they had a chronic physical health condition and 15% reported a history of mental illness. Table 25.2 shows the full range of conditions respondents were asked about and their self-reported rates of illness; for comparison purposes, these are displayed alongside national prevalence estimates for correctional populations developed by the National

Table 25.2 Health conditions reported by *Returning Home* respondents (*n* = 838).

	Returning Home respondents	U.S. correctional population[1]
Any physical health condition	49.8%	–
Arthritis	7.3%	–
Asthma	10.3%	8.5%
Back pain	6.3%	–
Cancer	2.0%	–
Chronic lung disease	2.8%	–
Diabetes	5.4%	4.8%
Heart disease	5.5%	–
Hepatitis B or C	11.2%	Hepatitis B, 2.0% Hepatitis C, 17.0–18.6%
High blood pressure	20.1%	18.3%
High cholesterol	8.1%	–
HIV or AIDS	2.0%	HIV, 2.3–2.98% AIDS, 0.5%
Stroke	1.3%	–
Tuberculosis	4.7%	Latent infection, 7.4% Active disease, 0.04%
Any mental health condition	14.9%	–
Depression	12.8%	Major depression, 7.9–15.2% Dysthymia, 2.7–4.2%
Other condition	7.0%	Schizophrenia/psychosis, 1.0–1.1% Bipolar disorder, 1.5–2.6% Posttraumatic stress disorder, 4.0–8.3% Anxiety, 14.1–20.0%
Preprison substance use		
Any alcohol intoxication or drug use	84.2%	83.2%[2]
More than once a week	66.0%	69.2%[2]
Daily	45.1%	–

Note: Dashes indicate that data are not available.

[1] Prevalence estimates of physical and mental health conditions in the U.S. correctional population are from Chapter 3 of *The Health Status of Soon-to-Be-Released Prisoners, Volume 1*, by the National Commission on Correctional Health Care, 2002.

[2] Prevalence estimates of preprison substance use are from Table 1 of *Drug Use and Dependence, State and Federal Prisoners, 2004* by Christopher J. Mumola and Jennifer C. Karberg, 2006. The numbers presented here represent, respectively, the percentage of state prisoners reporting any past drug use and weekly drug use for at least 1 month.

Commission on Correctional Health Care (2002). The men we surveyed most often reported having had high blood pressure (20%), depression (13%), hepatitis (11%), and asthma (10%). For the most part, the rates of illness reported by respondents were comparable to national estimates, though it is important to note that respondent self-reports often underestimate the true prevalence of disease since many conditions remain undetected without proper screening and medical care. For some serious and communicable diseases, notably hepatitis and tuberculosis, respondents' reported rates were lower than the national estimates; these differences may reflect regional variation in the prevalence of these diseases.

Chronic communicable diseases are of particular importance to the public health since, without intervention, they can be transmitted to other prisoners, correctional staff, and the families and communities to which prisoners return. Chronic communicable diseases (i.e., HIV, active TB, and hepatitis) were reported by 17% of the men in our sample. Men reported hepatitis most often (11%), followed by tuberculosis infection (5%) and HIV (2%). Fifteen percent of the men we surveyed reported having a mental health condition; this was assessed by asking respondents whether a doctor or another health care provider had told them they had such a condition. This is somewhat lower but comparable to the results from a recent Bureau of Justice Statistics (BJS) study, which found that 22% of men in state prisons reported a recent history of mental illness (James & Glaze, 2006). The actual prevalence of mental illness, however, is likely to be double the self-reported rate. James and Glaze (2006) found that while 22% of male state prisoners reported receiving a diagnosis or treatment for mental illness, 48% reported symptoms consistent with the DSM-IV criteria for depression, mania, and psychotic disorders.

A history of substance use was particularly common among returning prisoners. Most of the men surveyed, roughly four out of five, had used illegal drugs or gotten intoxicated at least once in the 6 months leading up to their prison term. A large share reported levels of use consistent with substance abuse or dependence. Overall, two-thirds reported drinking to intoxication (i.e., "getting drunk") or using drugs more than once a week in the 6 months leading up to their prison term. One-third used marijuana and one-quarter used cocaine at this frequency, while another one-quarter reported drinking to intoxication more than once a week (see Figure 25.1). Substance use more than once a week was significantly correlated with adverse consequences resulting from use, such as problems at work, arguments with family, and driving while impaired. Substance use at this frequency was also significantly correlated with signs of addiction (e.g., increased tolerance, greater than intended use, and inability to stop use).

Using a definition of health problem that includes preprison substance abuse shows that there are very few returning prisoners without a health problem. Over 8 out of 10 respondents reported at least one of the following: a chronic physical health condition, a mental health condition, or a substance abuse problem (defined as preprison drug use or alcohol intoxication more often than once a week). Four out of 10 men had multiple health concerns. Figures 25.2 and 25.3 provide different views of the interplay between physical health, mental health, and substance abuse in our sample of returning prisoners. Figure 25.2 displays the relative share of each of these conditions and

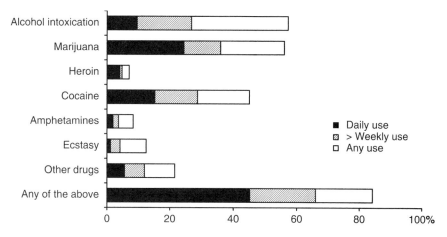

Figure 25.1 Substance use in the 6 months before incarceration. Substance use more than once a week was significantly correlated with problems resulting from use and signs of addiction.

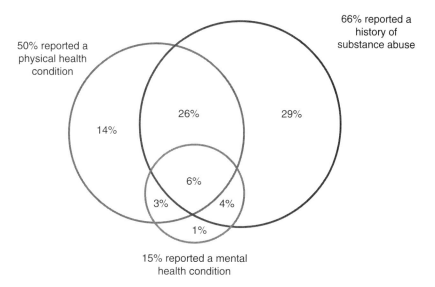

Figure 25.2 Interplay of physical health, mental health, and substance abuse. Eighty-five percent of men reported having at least one of these health conditions and 40% reported two or more.

overlap among them and Figure 25.3 illustrates the extent to which individuals with one type of health condition are affected by others. Among men with physical health conditions, two-thirds also reported a history of substance abuse and one-fifth had a history of mental illness. Among men with mental health conditions, nearly all had co-occurring physical and substance abuse problems. (Of particular interest to practitioners are individuals dually diagnosed with co-occurring substance use and mental health disorders; by our estimation, 11% of male returning prisoners fit this description.) Among men with substance abuse histories, one-half also had physical health problems and 16% reported mental health conditions. Furthermore, we found that 6% had coexistent physical, mental health, and substance abuse issues. The prevalence

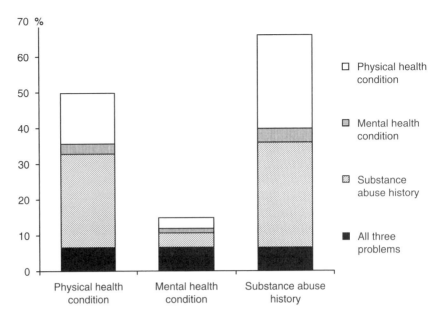

Figure 25.3 Prevalence of co-occurring health conditions. More often than not, men with any given health condition reported a second, co-occurring condition.

of multiple, coexisting health conditions is important for practitioners and policymakers to bear in mind. Prisoners seeking treatment for one type of health concern are likely to have others and, as clinical experience with co-occurring substance use and mental health disorders has shown (Quello, Brady, & Sonne, 2005), incomplete attention to one type of health condition may decrease the likelihood of successfully treating the others.

Health Care Received During Prison

Shortly before release, respondents were asked whether they were under medical care or receiving treatment for the health conditions they reported having (Table 25.3). Among those with a chronic physical health condition, the majority (63%) reported receiving treatment in prison; however, about one-third of those with health problems did not receive treatment. Among those with a history of mental illness, the rates are similar, albeit a little lower; 61% reported receiving mental health treatment in prison, and 4 out of 10 who had had a mental health diagnosis were without treatment. Among those with a substance abuse problem, defined as preprison drug use or alcohol intoxication more than once a week, approximately one-half (52%) received some type of drug or alcohol treatment services. When asked specifically about prescription medicines, about one-quarter (27%) of all respondents reported they were taking medication on a regular basis in the month before their release.

The treatment rates reported were highly variable across different physical health conditions. On the high end, treatment rates were above 70%. Most (89%) of those with diabetes, 82% of those with HIV, and 71% with high blood pressure reported being treated for those conditions. Other conditions,

Table 25.3 Treatment received by *Returning Home* respondents with health conditions, before and after prison release.

	During prison (*n* = 838)	2 months postrelease (*n* = 665)
Treatment of any physical health condition	63.0%	45.8%
Arthritis	50.8%	40.0%
Asthma	58.8%	36.3%
Back pain	46.2%	39.1%
Cancer	52.9%	37.5%
Chronic lung disease	47.8%	30.0%
Diabetes	88.9%	89.2%
Heart disease	60.9%	53.5%
Hepatitis B or C	37.6%	18.5%
High blood pressure	71.1%	60.3%
High cholesterol	50.7%	49.2%
HIV or AIDS	82.4%	100.0%[1]
Stroke	27.3%	53.8%[1]
Tuberculosis	23.1%	13.8%
Treatment of any mental health condition	60.5%	46.3%
Depression	59.4%	44.6%
Other mental health condition	60.3%	53.7%
Treatment of substance abuse[2]	51.9%	30.6%
Alcoholics or Narcotics Anonymous	47.7%	27.5%
Inpatient or outpatient treatment	29.4%	8.3%

[1] The treatment rate is based on the fewer than 10 respondents reporting this condition.
[2] Substance abuse is defined as preprison drug use or alcohol intoxication more often than once a week.

however, had treatment rates below 50%, such as back pain (46%), hepatitis B or C (38%), and tuberculosis infection (23%).

Of particular concern is the treatment of prisoners with chronic communicable diseases because of its impact on the well-being of the affected individuals as well as its implications for disease transmission to others within the prison setting and the larger community. Public health experts advocate in-prison screening, diagnosis, and treatment as a means of reaching typically hard-to-serve populations. Given the high proportion of individuals with hepatitis, HIV, and sexually transmitted infections who pass through correctional facilities, prisons may be a cost-effective point of contact for intervention (NCCHC, 2002). Although prisoners with HIV had treatment rates exceeding 80%, those infected with tuberculosis and hepatitis reported considerably lower treatment rates, between 20 and 40%. It is hard to determine whether this is an accurate reflection of actual treatment rates because these infections often have long periods of latency and treatment decisions are sometimes subjective. For example, tuberculosis infection is treated for 9 months, if at all, depending on the patient's age, when he became infected, and other clinical factors (Centers for Disease Control and Prevention, 2006). Similarly, viral hepatitis has a lengthy incubation period (20 to 40 years) and clinical guidelines recommend treatment during a specific window period (Centers for Disease Control and Prevention,

2003). Given the seriousness of these health problems, this issue bears further investigation; a targeted study of tuberculosis and hepatitis treatment in prison would be needed to evaluate whether these treatment rates are medically appropriate. Examining substance abuse treatment services, we found that the majority of respondents did not receive any treatment services in prison. Overall, 47% of all men participated in some type of substance abuse recovery program during prison. Typically, this meant attending self-help groups like Alcoholics Anonymous (AA) or Narcotics Anonymous (NA), which 43% reported having done. About one-quarter (26%) reported participating in a drug or alcohol treatment program, many of whom also attended AA or NA meetings.

Additionally, drug and alcohol treatment services in prison did not seem well matched to the level of need. Among those who reported preprison drug use, only one-half reported receiving any substance abuse treatment services (defined as participation in substance abuse treatment programs or self-help groups like AA and NA). However, the proportion receiving such services in prison did not seem to differ by the extent of preprison use. The participation rate for those with any substance use (50%) was similar to the participation rate of those reporting frequent or even daily substance use before prison (52% for each). Previous research involving Returning Home participants in Illinois showed a similar mismatch between prisoners' level of need and receipt of treatment services (Winterfield & Castro, 2005). This raises questions about whether scarce prison resources are being targeted toward the prisoners with the greatest need or likelihood of recidivism.

Health Care Received After Prison

Even when individuals have received adequate health and substance abuse treatment services while in prison, they often face limited access and insufficient linkages to community-based health care on release (Hammett, Roberts, & Kennedy, 2001). Service providers have identified the lack of available resources for services and the competition for funding as significant problems in delivering services to former prisoners, especially those with the most serious health needs (Visher, Naser, Baer, & Janetta, 2005). In addition, Medicaid benefits are suspended during incarceration. Restoring eligibility can take several months, interrupting access to prescription drugs and putting individuals at high risk of adverse outcomes.

We assessed the extent to which Returning Home participants were able to access health care in the community within their first 2 months out of prison. Overall, one-third of respondents had visited a doctor in the community within 2 months of release. Nearly one-tenth (9%) sought care in the emergency room and 4% were hospitalized. Understandably, respondents with physical and mental health problems were more likely to access health care than the average respondent. Men with mental health problems appeared to use health services more than those with physical problems: 54% visited a doctor (compared to 42%), 19% went to the emergency room (compared to 12%), and 12% were hospitalized (compared to 5%). Men with substance abuse problems were not any more likely than others to use such health services.

We found that the proportion receiving treatment for their health conditions fell by one-fifth, on average. Table 25.3 displays the range of health conditions we asked about and shows a comparison of treatment rates before and after release. Treatment rates for physical health conditions fell by over one-quarter, but there was considerable variation across conditions. Treatment for asthma, for example, fell by nearly 40%, whereas treatment for HIV seemed to remain constant. Disturbingly, treatment for other communicable diseases fell sharply: hepatitis treatment fell by half and tuberculosis treatment fell by 40%. Mental health treatment rates declined also. Treatment for depression fell by about one-quarter, whereas treatment for other mental health conditions remained more consistent, falling by about 10%. Perhaps the worst drop-off in care was for those with substance abuse problems. Participation in AA and NA decreased by about 40% and participation in a substance abuse treatment program fell by over 70%. Some of this reduction in care likely reflects the lack of insurance coverage among this population. Two months after release, 78% had no health insurance after prison. Just 6% had Medicaid coverage; the remainder reported private insurance (6%), Medicare (2%), Veterans' benefits (3%), and other sources (6%).

Focusing on prescription medications, we found that the majority of those who had been taking medication in prison were continuing to do so 2 months after release. Of those who had taken medications in prison, most (82%) said they had received a supply of medication from the prison at release and about two-thirds (64%) were still using the same medication (though it was unclear whether it came from the same supply). It is important to note, however, that one-third stopped taking the medications they used in prison within 2 months of release. Among those who stopped, the primary reason given for stopping was that the respondent had decided that he no longer needed it, pointing to a need for improved patient education before release. Other common reasons were that the medication cost too much and that the respondent's doctor in the community determined it was no longer needed.

Reentry Experiences of Former Prisoners with Health Problems

All prisoners, regardless of their health status, face numerous challenges when they are released from prison. Prisoners with health problems are thought to have more difficulties, partly because their health conditions diminish their capacity to meet reentry challenges, and partly because accessing and maintaining treatment creates an added burden. To explore this issue empirically, we analyzed Returning Home data gathered 2 months after release in order to compare and contrast the early reentry experiences of those with and without health problems. Bivariate analyses were conducted to compare those with and without three specific types of health problems—physical illness, mental illness, and substance abuse (defined as preprison drug use or alcohol intoxication more often than once a week)—with regard to a range of reentry outcomes. We examined three intermediate outcomes—housing, family relationships, and employment—as well as postprison substance use and involvement in criminal activity. Table 25.4 presents a summary of these findings. The following sections address each of these five reentry outcomes individually. In each, we describe men's reentry experiences in general, followed by a discussion of the ways in which men with physical health, mental health, and substance abuse problems had significantly different experiences ($p < 0.10$) from those without such conditions.

Table 25.4 Reentry outcomes reported by *Returning Home* respondents 2 months after prison release, by type of health condition.

	All (n=665)	Type of health condition		
		Physical (n=414)	Mental (n=124)	Substance abuse (n=552)
Housing				
Stayed with family the first night out	54%	54%	45%*	54%
Lived with family	63%	62%	52%***	66%**
Lived on one's own	24%	24%	23%	21%**
Lived with former prisoners	20%	22%	27%*	23%**
Lived with drug users	9%	10%	16%**	11%*
Experienced any homelessness	6%	6%	9%	5%
Number of residences since release (mean)	1.35	1.42*	1.38	1.40
Expected to live in current residence	77%	74%*	66%**	76%
Hope to live elsewhere in a year	63%	64%	64%	63%
Family—relationships with minor children				
Had minor children	49%	49%	42%	47%
Lived with minor children	13%	12%	8%**	11%**
Financially supported minor children	33%	31%	24%**	31%
Contact with minor children (0=none to 3=daily)	2.24	2.21	2.09	2.27
Level of involvement in raising minor children (0=low to 2=high)	1.13	1.05***	0.91**	1.08*
Family—other relationships and support received				
Number of close family relationships (mean)	6.2	5.9	6.3	5.7**
Family relationship quality (1=weak to 4=strong)	3.28	3.28	3.05**	3.28
Emotional support from family (1=low to 4=high)	3.33	3.34	3.11**	3.33
Tangible support from family (1=low to 4=high)	3.21	3.20	2.99**	3.21
Financial support from family	81%	81%	73%**	81%
Family helpfulness relative to expectations (1=less to 3=more helpful than expected)	2.20	2.20	2.03**	2.17
Family member threatened or hurt respondent	1.4%	1.2%	2.8%	1.6%

Respondent threatened or hurt family member	0.5%	0.6%	0.9%	0.7%*
Employment and income				
Employed since release	53%	51%	36%**	54%
Employed "under the table" since release	37%	34%	40%	39%*
Employed at the time of interview	37%	34%**	26%**	37%
Received public assistance (e.g., food stamps)	19%	25%**	28%**	17%***
Received SSI/SSDI payments	3%	5%**	8%*	3%
Illegal activities were a source of income	4%	4%	8%	5%***
Monthly income from all sources (mean)	$1092	$870	$1049	$1110
Worried about surviving financially	0.79	0.83	0.95**	0.83
Barely had enough money to get by	0.77	0.80	0.96**	0.79
Had trouble paying bills	0.70	0.75*	0.82*	0.72
Had trouble keeping housing	0.45	0.52*	0.57	0.48
Had trouble getting food	0.45	0.49	0.59**	0.45
Conflicts with friends/family over money	0.47	0.54**	0.67**	0.50
Substance use				
Any drug use or alcohol intoxication	27%	23%**	29%	34%**
Any drug use	18%	16%	19%	23%**
Any alcohol intoxication	17%	14%**	22%	22%**
Any marijuana use	13%	11%	10%	17%**
Any heroin use	1%	2%	2%	2%
Any cocaine use	8%	8%	13%*	10%**
Any amphetamine use	1%	1%	1%	1%
Number of problems due to drinking (mean)	0.68	0.82**	0.96*	0.73**
Number of problems due to drug use (mean)	0.37	0.41	0.67	0.46**
Sought help for drug/alcohol problem	8%	10%	15%**	10%
Participated in any treatment, including AA or NA	26%	33%**	31%	31%**
Participated in inpatient or outpatient treatment	6%	8%	10%	8%***
Recidivism				
Committed crime since release	11%	10%	20%**	14%**
Arrested since release	11%	10%	13%	13%**
Of those on parole, violated supervision conditions	21%	18%*	22%	26%**
Any of the above	25%	22%*	32%*	29%**

Note: *T* tests were conducted to compare respondents who reported a physical health problem with those who did not; respondents who reported a mental health condition with those who did not; and respondents who reported substance abuse (defined as preprison drug use or alcohol intoxication more often than once per week) with those who did not. Participants with multiple health conditions appear in more than one column.
*$p \leq 0.10$. **$p \leq 0.05$.

Housing

Finding housing is perhaps the most immediate challenge that returning prisoners face on release, and 3 out of 10 respondents did not have a place to live lined up when we surveyed them in the month before release. While many returning prisoners plan to stay with family, as 77% of the men in our sample did, those who do not confront limited housing options. Potential housing options for former prisoners include the private market; federally subsidized and administered housing; and homeless assistance supportive housing, service-enhanced housing, and special needs housing supported by the U.S. Department of Housing and Urban Development (HUD). However, the process of obtaining housing is often complicated by a host of factors: the scarcity of affordable and available housing; legal barriers, regulations, and prejudices that restrict tenancy for this population; and strict eligibility requirements for federally subsidized housing (Roman & Travis, 2004).

The majority of the men we surveyed believed that having a place to live would be important to avoid a return to prison. This belief is supported by research findings that released prisoners who do not have stable housing arrangements are more likely to return to prison (Metreaux & Culhane, 2004), suggesting that the obstacles to securing both temporary and permanent housing warrant the attention of policymakers, practitioners, and researchers. The men we surveyed most often spent the first night out of prison with a family member (54%) and over the course of the first 2 postrelease months, 6 out of 10 lived with family members for at least some of the time. About one-quarter of respondents lived in their own houses or apartments. The remainder reported other arrangements, like living with friends or in transitional housing such as a halfway house. A relatively small share of respondents (about 6%) experienced periods of homelessness during these first 2 months, and 5% reported having been homeless on their first night out of prison. For the most part, men's housing situations in the first 2 months after release matched what they had expected during prison: 77% said the place they were currently living in was where they had expected to be living. At the same time, many considered these to be temporary housing situations. Over one-fifth (23%) had already moved at least once and the majority (63%) hoped to be living somewhere else in a year's time.

Men with health problems were significantly more likely to face challenges with regard to housing (Table 25.4). Those with physical, mental, and substance abuse problems were all less likely to have had a place to live lined up before release and, once released, they were more likely to experience housing instability. Their specific housing experiences differed somewhat by the type of health condition. Men with physical health problems were more likely than men without to have changed residences during the first 2 months after prison. They were also more likely to report that their current residence was not someplace they had expected to be living while they were still incarcerated. Men with mental health conditions had more housing difficulties relative to men without mental illness. They were significantly less likely to have lived with family members since their release, even on the first night out of prison, and they were more likely to report living in a place they had not expected to be in while still incarcerated. Additionally, men with mental health conditions were more likely to report having lived with substance users and other former prisoners. Men with substance abuse histories were more likely than others to have lived with family members since their release, but they also reported changing residences more often in the first 2 months. They were more likely to report having lived with other substance users and former prisoners since release. Despite this instability, 2 months out of prison, men with these different types of health concerns did not report rates of homelessness that were significantly different than others (about 6%), even though those with mental illness and those with a history of substance abuse were significantly more likely to have been homeless before their incarceration.

Family Relationships and Support

The impact of incarceration and reentry on families is significant and, in many respects, difficult to measure. More than half of U.S. prisoners are parents of children under 18 years old (Harrison & Beck, 2002) and this was mirrored in our sample. When a parent is sent to prison, the family structure, financial responsibilities, emotional support systems, and living arrangements are all affected. These changes can drastically disrupt spousal relationships, parent–child relationships, and family networks (Travis, Cincotta, & Solomon, 2003). Restoring these relationships, reunifying with family members, and undertaking familial roles and responsibilities on return also pose a unique set of challenges. Recent research has found that strengthening the family network and maintaining supportive family contact can improve outcomes for both family members and prisoners (Sullivan, Mino, Nelson, & Pope, 2002).

Two months after release, men typically reported having four close family members. (This was the median.) This was similar to the number of close family relationships they had reported having before and during prison. After release, respondents rated their family relationships as relatively strong and reported receiving both emotional and tangible support from their family members. Families provided much practical support to returning prisoners. As noted previously, about two-thirds lived with family members for at least some time during the first 2 months out of prison. Eight out of 10 also reported receiving financial support from their families. Overall, men felt that the support they received from their families exceeded their expectations.

Examining men with health concerns, we found that the level of family support varied with the type of health issue (Table 25.4). Across the board, men with physical health problems and men with substance abuse histories experienced similarly high levels of family support as men without such problems. However, those with mental health conditions experienced somewhat lower levels of support. While respondents with mental health conditions generally received emotional and tangible support from their families, they rated the level of support as significantly lower than what men without mental illness reported. Although men with mental illness felt that their families' support exceeded their expectations, it was not by as much as others reported; moreover, their prerelease expectations of support tended to be lower compared to men without mental illness.

Looking conversely at men's support of their families, we found that many provided financial support for their minor children and were involved in the upbringing of those children (as measured by how often they did things like supervise homework or set limits) although they generally did not live with their children. Two months after release, only about one-third of fathers lived with their minor children, but about two-thirds were in contact with them at least weekly and provided some financial support. Fathers with health problems (physical, mental, or substance abuse-related) were significantly less likely to be involved in the raising of their children. Additionally, men with mental health and substance abuse problems were significantly less likely to live with or provide financial support for their children.

Employment

Finding and maintaining a job is a critical dimension of successful prisoner reentry. The majority of the men we surveyed felt that employment would be important to helping them stay out of prison. Research has shown that both employment and higher wages are associated with lower rates of criminal activity (Bernstein & Houston, 2000; Western & Pettit, 2000). An evaluation of the Opportunity to Succeed program, a comprehensive reentry program that included employment services, found that an increase in levels of employment was a predictor of reductions in drug dealing, violent crime, and property crime (Rossman & Roman, 2003).

However, former prisoners face tremendous challenges in finding and maintaining legitimate job opportunities, including low levels of education, limited work experience, and limited vocational skills (Harlow, 2003). This is further compounded by the incarceration period, during which they both forfeit the opportunity to gain marketable work experience and sever the professional connections and social contacts that could lead to legal employment on release (Western, Kling, & Weiman, 2001). In addition, the general reluctance of employers to hire former prisoners serves as a barrier to job placement (Holzer, Raphael, & Stoll, 2004). Nearly three-quarters of the men we surveyed had been employed in the 6 months before prison, but just over half reported being employed in the 2 months since their release from prison. Not all retained these jobs, though, as only about one-third (37%) were employed at the time of the interview. Regardless of employment, respondents did not have much money to live on. Overall, the median monthly income was just $600, while those with a job reported $900. Nearly two-thirds cited family and friends as being the most common source of financial support. The majority of respondents worried about surviving financially, and over one-quarter reported specific worries about getting food or keeping their housing. Employment outcomes for men with health concerns varied according to the type of the health condition (Table 25.4). About half of the men with physical health conditions had worked for some time since release (a rate similar to others) yet they were significantly less likely to have still been employed at the time of their study interview. They reported a significantly lower level of income and were more likely to receive support through public assistance programs, like food stamps, and disability payments through the Social Security Disability Insurance (SSDI) and Supplemental Security Income (SSI) programs. Men with physical health problems were more likely to report having trouble paying their bills and keeping housing than those without. They also were more apt to report conflicts with family and friends over money.

Men with mental health conditions had a different experience in that they were less likely to have worked at all since release (36%) and less likely to have a job at the time of the interview (26%). Despite their higher levels of unemployment, men with mental health problems did not have a significant difference in their monthly income compared to other returning prisoners. They were, however, more likely to receive public assistance and disability payments through SSI or SSDI and, at the same time, more likely to report worries about getting food and surviving financially.

Interestingly, men with a history of substance abuse were no different from other returning prisoners in terms of having been employed after release and having a job at the time of the interview. Their monthly income was also similar to other returning prisoners, but their sources of income differed: those with substance abuse histories were more likely to report income from illegal activities and were less likely to receive support from public assistance or disability programs.

Substance Use

Substance use presents a range of challenges to the reentry process. The very act of possessing or using many common drugs of abuse is illegal and places individuals at risk for arrest or parole revocation. Beyond that, substance abuse, legal or otherwise, can hinder the ability to find and keep a job, interfere with family relationships, and encourage antisocial peer relationships (NIDA, 2004). Additionally, the cost of purchasing drugs leads some users to commit income-generating crimes, such as drug dealing and theft (Wish, 1990–1991). Although the majority of state prisoners have a history of drug use, only a small fraction receive treatment while incarcerated (Mumola & Karberg, 2006). At the same time, prison-based drug treatment has been shown to reduce drug use and criminal activity, especially when coupled with aftercare treatment in the community (Gaes, Flanagan, Motiuk, & Stewart, 1999; Harrison, 2000).

Nearly one-fifth (18%) of respondents reported using drugs within the first 2 months after prison. The proportion reporting any postprison substance use comes to over one-quarter (27%) when alcohol intoxication is included with drug use. Perhaps not surprisingly, men with histories of substance abuse before prison were significantly more likely than others to report using again after prison (Table 25.4). Close to one-quarter (23%) reported postprison drug use, particularly marijuana and cocaine use, and the proportion reporting any postprison substance use reached about one-third (34%) when alcohol intoxication is included with drug use. Among all the respondents who reported substance use after prison (i.e., any drug use or alcohol intoxication), those who had reported preprison abuse were significantly more likely to report problems (e.g., with work or family) resulting from their postprison use. Those with histories of substance abuse were significantly more likely to seek help for drug problems and be involved in recovery programs, with 31% having participated in some type of recovery program (including AA or NA) and 8% having participated specifically in an inpatient or outpatient treatment program.

Men with physical health problems were significantly less likely to report any substance use after prison, even though about two-thirds had been frequent users before this most recent term in prison. Still, it is worth noting that nearly one-quarter (23%) had been intoxicated or used drugs in the first 2 months out of prison, and men with physical health concerns were more likely than healthier men to have experienced alcohol-related problems postrelease. Finally, men with physical health problems were more likely to have taken part in a recovery program (including AA and NA) after prison, with one-third reporting they had done so. Men with mental health conditions reported rates of postprison substance use that were similar to others. However, cocaine use was more common among mentally ill men, with 13% reporting any use since release. Also, alcohol use seemed to cause more problems for mentally ill men than others (though their rates of drinking to intoxication were not significantly higher) with a significantly greater share reporting problems due to their drinking. Men with mental health concerns were more likely to report seeking help for their substance use after prison; however, they were no more or less likely to have received such help, as their rate of participation in recovery programs was similar to others.

Criminal Activity

Considering the high rates of recidivism, prisoner reentry presents a tremendous public safety dilemma. The Bureau of Justice Statistics estimates that within 3 years of release, more than two-thirds of prisoners are rearrested for a new crime—most within the first year out of prison. Forty-seven percent of all released prisoners are reconvicted for a new crime and more than half are reincarcerated for a new crime or parole violation (Langan & Levin, 2002). Released prisoners make a substantial contribution to new crime; one study estimates that recent prison releasees account for about one-fifth of all adult arrests made by police (Rosenfeld, Wallman, & Fornango, 2005).

The Returning Home data on recidivism were gathered from respondent self-reports 2 months after their release from prison. One-quarter of men reported having committed a new crime, having been arrested, or violating a parole condition. Eleven percent reported committing a new crime, with the most common offenses being, in order, drug possession, drug dealing, theft, burglary, and assault. Eleven percent also reported having been arrested at least once. Among those on parole, one-fifth reported violating their supervision conditions. Additionally, 4% reported that part of their income came from illegal activities.

Men's reported criminal involvement after prison varied depending on their health status (Table 25.4). Those with physical health problems were less likely to recidivate, using a combined measure of self-reported criminal activity, arrests, and parole violations, whereas men with mental illness or a history of substance abuse were more likely to recidivate. Mental illness and substance abuse were correlated with committing a new crime, but physical health status was not. One-fifth (19%) of those with mental illness reported committing a new crime (compared to 10% of those without mental illness) and 14% of those with a history of substance abuse reported committing a new crime (compared to 6% of those without such a history). Among those on parole, men with a substance abuse history were more likely to report violating their conditions, whereas men with physical health problems were less likely to do so; men's mental health status did not affect parole violation rates in the first 2 months after prison. Despite these patterns of variation in criminal activity and parole violations, only substance abusers experienced significantly different and higher rates of arrest, with 14% having been arrested within 2 months of prison release.

Discussion

This examination of data from the Returning Home study corroborates previous findings on the prevalence of health problems among returning prisoners. Overall, one-half of men reported a physical health condition, 15% reported mental illness, and two-thirds reported preprison substance use at levels consistent with abuse and addiction (i.e., more than once a week). Looking at the interplay between these health conditions showed that over 4 out of 5 returning prisoners had at least one of these conditions and 2 out of 5 had multiple conditions. However, available services did not appear to meet this population's needs. Among men with physical or mental health conditions, roughly 3 in 5 received treatment in prison; 2 months after release this figure was closer to 2 in 5. Among men with a history of substance abuse, about one-half participated in recovery programs (including AA or NA) in prison; 2 months after release, less than one-third did.

By comparing the early reentry experiences of those with and without physical health, mental health, and substance abuse problems, this research demonstrates the ways in which returning prisoners with health problems face unique challenges that set them apart from the average returning prisoner. Our findings add support to the idea that a "one size fits all" approach to improving reentry outcomes is ill-advised. Men with health concerns had significantly different reentry experiences in the first 2 months after prison. Through the identification of statistically significant differences across a number of domains—housing, family support, employment, substance use, and criminal activity—this work lends itself to the development of empirically based interventions to improve outcomes for different subpopulations of returning prisoners.

Looking separately at men with physical health conditions, men with mental illnesses, and men with substance abuse histories—while recognizing that there is substantial crossover between these groups—we found that each of these groups' experiences in the first 2 months after prison release set them apart from the others. In general, those with physical health conditions had the fewest differences from those without such conditions, as well as the most positive outcomes with regard to substance use and recidivism 2 months postrelease. Men with mental health conditions tended to experience the most reentry challenges across a variety of domains, and their recidivism outcomes 2 months postrelease were worse than those without mental illness. Men with histories of substance abuse had a somewhat different experience from both the others. Although they tended to experience fewer challenges with regard to intermediate outcomes of housing, family, and employment, their rates of substance use relapse and recidivism 2 months postrelease were worse than those without a history of substance abuse.

For men with physical health conditions, the greatest challenges 2 months after release appeared to be housing and employment. They were less likely to have arranged their housing before release and, after release, they moved around more often compared to men without physical health problems. They were also more likely to worry about keeping the housing they were in at the time of the interview. This housing instability is likely related to employment difficulties after release. Although men with physical problems were just as likely as others to have worked for some time after prison, they were more likely to have lost those jobs by the time of the study interview, 2 months after release. Over one quarter reported that their health problems limited their ability to work or engage in other ordinary activities. As a result, men with physical health problems reported significantly less income and more reliance on public assistance and SSI/SSDI payments than others. At the same time, men with physical health problems reported being supported by their families, and the types and levels of support they reported were similar to those without health problems: the majority lived with family members and received some financial support from them. Despite housing and employment challenges, men with physical health problems reported better outcomes with regard to substance use and criminal activity. They were significantly less likely to report using drugs or alcohol 2 months after prison and more likely to be in a self-help recovery group like AA or NA. Those who were on parole supervision were less likely to report violating conditions of their release, though overall reports of committing new crimes and being arrested were similar to others.

Men with mental health conditions experienced unique reentry challenges in every domain we examined. Perhaps the most striking difference was in their family relationships. Men with mental health conditions reported weaker family relationships and lower levels of both emotional and tangible support when compared to others, even those with physical health problems or substance abuse histories. Men with mental health conditions were significantly less likely to receive financial support from family members or live with them (even on the first night out of prison); in fact, they were more likely to have lived with other former prisoners and substance users. They experienced particular challenges with regard to housing in that they were less likely to have made housing arrangements before release and, 2 months after release, were less likely to be living someplace they had expected to beforehand. Their rate of homelessness, at 9%, was somewhat higher than those without mental illness; though this difference was not statistically significant ($p = 0.14$), it is consistent with their significantly greater history of homelessness before prison. Men with mental health conditions also experienced poorer employment outcomes after release. Significantly fewer worked at all after release, with 2 in 5 reporting that their health problems interfered with their ability to work. Compared to others, they often relied on public assistance programs and SSI/SSDI payments, and worried more about surviving financially and having enough money for food. With regard to substance use, men with mental illness were similar to others in terms of reporting any substance use 2 months after prison, but they were more likely to specifically report cocaine use. Disturbingly, they reported seeking help for a substance use problem more often, but were no more or less likely to have participated in AA, NA, or substance abuse treatment after release. Furthermore, men with mental health conditions were more likely to report having committed a new crime in the 2 months since release, though they did not report violating parole or being arrested at greater rates.

Men with substance abuse histories had a different reentry pathway in the first 2 months after release. In some ways, they appear to have encountered fewer barriers with respect to housing, family support, and employment—for example, they were more likely to report living with family and getting financial support from family and friends—and yet, they experienced poorer substance use and recidivism outcomes, suggesting that issues related to substance use (or deviance more generally) might influence these outcomes. While men with substance abuse histories were more likely to have lived with family members after release, the benefit of this is somewhat unclear, as their families were more likely than others to have problems with drugs and crime. After release, men with substance abuse histories reported changing residences more often than others and were more likely to have lived with other former prisoners and substance users. This suggests two possibilities: first, that respondents initially lived with family members, but then moved on to more unstable living arrangements, or, second, that the family members they lived with were themselves destabilizing influences. Regarding employment, men with substance abuse histories were as likely as others to have a job, but formal employment was more likely to be supplemented with "under the table" employment and illegal activity. Ultimately, men with substance abuse histories were significantly more likely to report using again in the first 2 months after prison (though they were also more likely to seek and receive help, including AA, NA, and substance abuse treatment programs). They were also significantly more likely to report that they had committed new crimes, violated parole conditions, and been arrested.

Implications for Policy and Practice

This research has identified ways in which the transition from prison to the community differs for individuals with health problems; knowledge of these differences can and should facilitate the development of specific interventions for returning prisoners with health needs. However, to implement such policies, practitioners must know which prisoners have health needs and what those specific needs are. It is not sufficient to rely on prison medical records, as our findings indicate that roughly 40 to 50% of men with health needs did not receive care while incarcerated. A logical first step is for practitioners to conduct a prerelease health assessment with each prisoner in order to identify current or ongoing problems. This assessment could be as simple as a self-reported checklist to screen for potential health problems (including substance abuse) requiring follow-up. (Table 25.5 presents our recommendations.)

All prisoners with health needs need care after release. However, on average, one-fifth of those who had been receiving health services in prison were no longer being treated 2 months after release. A comprehensive strategy to address the drop in health treatment would include assessing each prisoner's eligibility for Medicaid before release and applying for or reinstating benefits

Table 25.5 Recommendations for practitioners and policymakers.

• Recognize that nearly all men in prison (85%) have physical health, mental health, or substance abuse-related needs.

• Expand access to health and substance abuse treatment services in prison. Nearly 4 out of 10 men with physical health problems, 4 out of 10 men with mental health problems, and nearly half of men with a substance abuse history did not report receiving treatment services in prison.

• Recognize that male prisoners presenting with one health problem often have others. Two out of five returning prisoners we surveyed reported overlapping physical, mental, or substance abuse problems.

• Assess each returning prisoner's health needs (including substance abuse treatment needs) shortly before release. This could be as simple as a self-administered checklist.

• Develop a reentry health plan for each returning prisoner with physical health, mental health, or substance abuse concerns with an emphasis on continuity of care:
  – Refer prisoners to specific community treatment providers. For those with serious health needs, schedule appointments with community treatment providers in advance of their release.
  – Provide prisoners with a supply of current medications, a prescription for obtaining more medication, and information about any community providers offering free or reduced price medications.
  – Educate prisoners about their current medications and explain the risks of stopping medication without medical supervision.
  – Assess Medicaid eligibility and help those who are eligible apply for or reinstate benefits before release.

• Facilitate continuity of care and information sharing with community health providers by asking prisoners to sign a release form authorizing in-prison providers to share medical and substance use treatment records with community providers.

• Offer housing assistance to returning prisoners with physical and mental health problems, as well as those with substance abuse histories. Evaluate family members' willingness, capacity, and fitness to house returning prisoners for up to 1 year after release.

• Help returning prisoners with physical health problems apply for or reinstate SSI/SSDI payments and other public assistance.

• Offer intensive case management services and/or criminal justice supervision to men with mental health conditions, as they reported multiple needs (housing instability, lower employment, food insecurity, lower family support, more postrelease cocaine use, and more postrelease criminal activity).

• Help returning prisoners with substance abuse histories access community treatment services, as they were more likely than others to recidivate.

as indicated; fostering relationships between correctional health services and community health care so that referrals to specific community service providers (or appointments for especially serious health conditions) could be made before release; and developing a reentry health plan for each prisoner emphasizing continuity of care and specifying medication management and adherence.

One promising approach is the Hampden County, Massachusetts, public health model of correctional health care, in which physicians and case managers are dually based both at the correctional facility and at community health care centers (Hammett et al., 2004). There are also less sweeping changes that correctional and community providers can take to improve outcomes. Coordination between the prison and community providers can be improved by making prison health records easily available to community health care providers; as part of the discharge planning process, prisoners could be asked to sign a release form authorizing the release of their health information to other medical or substance abuse treatment providers. This would result in community practitioners spending less time retracing medical histories and fewer interruptions in the course of treatment (Anno, 2003). Finally, prerelease health education is also important in light of the finding that many of the returning prisoners who stopped taking prescription medications did so because they decided they no longer needed them.

With regard to other reentry outcomes, our research has shown that all respondents with health concerns, be they physical, mental health, or substance abuse-related, were significantly less likely than others to firm up housing arrangements before being released from prison. They were also more likely to experience housing instability after release. Discharge planning for men with health problems, particularly those with mental health conditions, should emphasize locating stable housing (and, ideally, stable people to live with) before release.

Given that returning prisoners with different types of health problems had different reentry pathways, other interventions should be more problem-specific. In the case of men with physical health problems, this research has shown that in addition to housing instability, these men had particular difficulties with employment and income during the first 2 months out, reporting more unemployment, less income, and greater reliance on public safety net programs. Discharge planning for such prisoners should include beginning the application process for food stamps, SSI or SSDI benefits, and other public assistance before release to minimize the amount of time between prison release and receipt of services. Moreover, the finding that men with physical health problems had found jobs but were unable to keep them points to a need to effectively manage health problems so that individuals can continue working and, hopefully, be less dependent on public safety net programs.

The early reentry experiences of men with mental health conditions demonstrate a need for assistance in navigating several reentry challenges. They reported higher rates of housing instability, unemployment, postrelease cocaine use, and criminal involvement compared to other returning prisoners, and had lower levels of family support in dealing with these challenges. They also need access to health care, and the strategies outlined above for improving continuity of care are equally applicable to improving the outcomes of mentally ill returning prisoners. Given their multitude of needs, returning prisoners with mental health conditions would likely benefit the most from an intensive case management approach to their reentry.

The postrelease experience of men with substance abuse histories suggests that their greatest challenges in the first 2 months, relative to other prisoners, are stable housing and substance abuse treatment. They also experienced significantly higher rates of recidivism in the first 2 months. With respect to housing, these men were more likely to have lived with family, but were also more likely to have lived with other former prisoners and drug users, and more likely to have changed residences in the first 2 months. The implication for discharge planning is that placement with family is not necessarily a positive stable situation. Returning prisoners either lived with family for only a short time, or lived with family members for whom drugs and crime were also problematic; additional research using Returning Home data with longer follow-up periods is planned to investigate this issue. In either case, this finding points to a need to evaluate the willingness and capacity of the family members with whom returning prisoners plan to live. Substance abuse treatment is also a pressing need, given that participation in recovery programs dropped substantially after release and one-third reported using again within 2 months of release. Our findings showed less continuity of care with substance abuse treatment compared to other health problems. This is perhaps because substance abuse treatment is not widely regarded as being health care; for example, substance abuse treatment was not a distinct component of Hampden County's correctional health care model (Hammett et al., 2004). Bringing substance abuse treatment under the rubric of health care, and applying the same principles and standards of continuity of care may help to improve outcomes for returning prisoners.

We must state one important caveat. These typologies of reentry experiences and service needs are intended to inform policymakers and practitioners about the types of problems that men with specific health conditions face, but they cannot take the place of client-centered discharge planning. While this analysis examined distinct categories of men with physical health problems, men with mental health problems, and men with substance abuse histories, it is important to remember the extent to which returning prisoners reported overlapping health problems. Among men with physical health and substance abuse problems, about one-half reported having a second type of problem. Among men with mental health problems, the vast majority reported having a second type of problem. This is to say that individual returning prisoners with one type of health problem may also have needs related to other health issues. The actual services provided to individual returning prisoners must be targeted to their particular needs.

This analysis has established that men with health problems faced different reentry challenges and often poorer outcomes in the first 2 months after prison. This begs the question of whether health treatment (including substance abuse treatment) would contribute to improved outcomes. Future research will examine this issue over a longer follow-up period and will include multivariate analyses to test whether health status and health treatment are causally related to reentry outcomes. Improved care for returning prisoners has many potential benefits, including reduced transmission of infectious disease, lower health care costs through the reduced use of emergency rooms and hospitalization, and improved public safety. Ideally, the improvement of individual health and well-being would be enough motivation to improve health care treatment and linkages between correctional and community health care systems, but there is little political will to invest in improvements solely for the sake of the well-being of returning prisoners. A deeper understanding of the societal benefits of improving prisoner health care will be necessary to effect improvements in correctional health.

References

Anno, B. J. (2003). Prison health services: An overview. *Journal of Correctional Health Care, 10*, 287–301.

Bernstein, J., & Houston, E. (2000). *Crime and work: What we can learn from the low-wage labor market.* Washington, DC: Economic Policy Institute.

Centers for Disease Control and Prevention. (2003). Prevention and control of infections with hepatitis viruses in correctional settings [Recommendations and Reports]. *Morbidity and Mortality Weekly Report, 52*(RR-1).

Centers for Disease Control and Prevention. (2006). Prevention and control of tuberculosis in correctional and detention facilities: Recommendations from CDC [Recommendations and Reports]. *Morbidity and Mortality Weekly Report, 55*(RR-09), 1–44.

Clear, T. R., Rose, D. R., & Ryder, J. A. (2001). Incarceration and the community: The problem of removing and returning offenders. *Crime and Delinquency, 47,* 335–351.

Davis, L. M., & Pacchiana, S. (2003). Health profile of the state prison population and returning offenders: Public health challenges. *Journal of Correctional Health Care, 10,* 303–331.

Gaes, G. G., Flanagan, T. F., Motiuk, L. L., & Stewart, L. (1999). Adult correctional treatment. In M. Tonry & J. Petersilia (Eds.), *Prisons.* Chicago: University of Chicago Press.

Gaes, G., & Kendig, N. (2002, January 30–31). *The skill sets and health care needs of released offenders.* Presented at the "From Prison to Home" Conference. U.S. Department of Health and Human Services.

Hammett, T. M., Roberts, S., & Kennedy, S. (2001). Health-related issues in prisoner reentry to the community. *Crime and Delinquency, 47,* 390–409.

Hammett, T. M., Roberts, C., Kennedy, S., Rhodes, W., Conklin, T., Lincoln, T., et al. (2004). *Evaluation of the Hampden County Public Health Model of Correctional Health Care: Final Report to the National Institute of Justice* (Grant #1999-IJ-CX-0047). Cambridge, MA: Abt Associates.

Harlow, C. W. (2003). *Education and correctional populations* (Bureau of Justice Statistics Special Report No. NCJ 195670). Washington, DC: U.S. Department of Justice.

Harrison, L. D. (2000, October). *The challenge of reintegrating drug offenders in the community.* Presented at the Urban Institute Reentry Roundtable, Washington, DC

Harrison, P. M., & Beck, A. J. (2002). *Prisoners in 2001* (Bureau of Justice Statistics Bulletin No. NCJ 195189). Washington, DC: U.S. Department of Justice.

Holzer, H., Raphael, S., & Stoll, M. (2004). Will employers hire former offenders? Employer preferences, background checks, and their determinants. In B. Western, M. Patillo, & D. Weiman (Eds.), *Imprisoning America: The social effects of mass incarceration.* New York: The Russell Sage Foundation.

James, D. J., & Glaze, L. E. (2006). *Mental health problems of prison and jail inmates* (Bureau of Justice Statistics Special Report No. NCJ 213600). Washington, DC: U.S. Department of Justice.

Langan, P. A., & Levin, D. J. (2002). *Recidivism of prisoners released in 1994* (Bureau of Justice Statistics Special Report No. NCJ 193427). Washington, DC: U.S. Department of Justice.

La Vigne, N. G., & Kachnowski, V. (2003). *A portrait of prisoner reentry in Maryland.* Washington, DC: The Urban Institute.

La Vigne, N. G., & Mamalian, C. A. (2003). *A portrait of prisoner reentry in Illinois.* Washington, DC: The Urban Institute.

La Vigne, N., & Thomson, G. L. (2003). *A portrait of prisoner reentry in Ohio.* Washington, DC: The Urban Institute.

Lynch, J. P., & Sabol, W. J. (2001). *Prisoner reentry in perspective.* Washington, DC: The Urban Institute.

Mallik-Kane, K. (2005). *Returning Home Illinois policy brief: Health and prisoner reentry.* Washington, DC: The Urban Institute.

Metreaux, S., & Culhane, D. P. (2004). Homeless shelter use and reincarceration following prison release. *Criminology and Public Policy, 3*, 139–160.

Mumola, C. J., & Karberg, J. C. (2006). *Drug use and dependence, state and federal prisoners, 2004* (Bureau of Justice Statistics Special Report No. NCJ 213530). Washington, DC: U.S. Department of Justice.

National Commission on Correctional Health Care. (2002). *The health status of soon-to-be released prisoners* (Volume 1). Retrieved August 19, 2004, from http://www.ncchc.org/stbr/Volume1/Health%20Status%20(vol%201).pdf

National Institute on Drug Abuse. (2004). *Cocaine abuse and addiction* (NIDA Research Report Series No. 99-4342). Washington, DC: National Institutes of Health.

Quello, S. B., Brady, K. T., & Sonne, S. C. (2005). Mood disorders and substance use disorder: A complex comorbidity. *NIDA Science and Practice Perspectives, 3*(1).

Roman, C. G., & Travis, J. (2004). *Taking stock: Housing, homelessness, and prisoner reentry.* Washington, DC: The Urban Institute.

Rosenfeld, R., Wallman, J., & Fornango, R. J. (2005). The contribution of ex-prisoners to crime rates. In J. Travis & C. A. Visher (Eds.), *Prisoner reentry and public safety in America.* New York: Cambridge University Press.

Rossman, S. B., & Roman, C. G. (2003). Case-managed reentry and employment: Lessons from the opportunity to succeed program. *Justice Research and Policy, 5*(2).

Sullivan, E., Mino, M., Nelson, K., & Pope, J. (2002). *Families as a resource in recovery from drug abuse: An evaluation of La Bodega de la Familia.* New York: Vera Institute of Justice.

Travis, J. (2005). *But they all come back: Facing the challenges of prisoner reentry.* Washington, DC: The Urban Institute.

Travis, J., Cincotta, E. M., & Solomon, A. L. (2003). *Families left behind: The hidden costs of incarceration and reentry.* Washington, DC: The Urban Institute.

Visher, C., La Vigne, N. G., & Travis, J. (2004). *Returning Home: Understanding the challenges of prisoner reentry* (Maryland Pilot Study: Findings from Baltimore). Washington, DC: The Urban Institute.

Visher, C. A., Naser, R. L., Baer, D., & Janetta, J. (2005). *In need of help: Experiences of seriously ill prisoners returning to Cincinnati.* Washington, DC: The Urban Institute.

Watson, J., Solomon, A. L., La Vigne, N. G., & Travis, J. (2004). *A portrait of prisoner reentry in Texas.* Washington, DC: The Urban Institute.

Western, B., Kling, J. R., & Weiman, D. F. (2001). The labor market consequences of incarceration. *Crime and Delinquency, 47*, 410–427.

Western, B., & Pettit, B. (2000). Incarceration and racial inequality in men's employment. *Industrial and Labor Relations Review, 54*, 3–16.

Winterfield, L., & Castro, J. (2005). *Returning Home Illinois policy brief: Treatment matching.* Washington, DC: The Urban Institute.

Wish, E. D. (1990–91). U.S. drug policy in the 1990s: Insights from new data from arrestees. *The International Journal of the Addictions, 25*(3a), 377–409.

Chapter 26

Providing Transition and Outpatient Services to the Mentally Ill Released from Correctional Institutions

Steven K. Hoge

Introduction

More than a generation ago, the mentally ill began to flood our jails and prisons. Correctional institutions were not prepared for the influx of mentally disordered offenders and numerous reports have graphically detailed deficiencies in the provision of needed services (Center for Mental Health Services, 1995; National Commission on Correctional Health Care, 2002a,b; The Correctional Association of New York, 2004). However, little attention has been focused on the problems related to transitioning this population to the community and the provision of outpatient-based mental health services. Though the quality of institutional care remains woefully inadequate in many jurisdictions, it has become increasingly apparent that community-based care is an urgent necessity.

Parallels between the current state of correctional mental health services and the civil public psychiatric system can be drawn. For many years, the public sector struggled with the problem of the "revolving door": following discharge from inpatient care, many mentally ill individuals were unable to function in the community, relapsed, and were readmitted. In most jurisdictions, efforts to address this problem have relied on an increased emphasis on discharge planning for patients transitioning from state civil hospitals to community-based treatment and, once in the community, aggressive support services. There is now universal recognition that these measures are essential ingredients to maintaining many of the seriously mentally ill in the community. At present, correctional care systems have not broadly adopted such services, with predictable results. A study from the state of Washington illustrates the consequences. A cohort of mentally ill individuals convicted of felonies was followed postrelease. In the first year in the community, only 16% received any form of mental health treatment; by the end of year three, nearly 40% had been rearrested (Lovell, Gagliardi, & Peterson, 2002).

In this chapter, I will review the historical factors underlying incarceration of large numbers of seriously mentally ill individuals, explore a commonly held view that increased funding of routine civil outpatient services would lower incarceration rates, and summarize clinical, social, and legal factors that create barriers to effective outpatient treatment. In the last section, I examine emerging models for the provision of transitional and outpatient services to this population.

Historical Background

Deinstitutionalizaton

From the beginning, there has been a connection between institutionalization and incarceration. In 1825, the Reverend Louis Dwight, shocked by what he witnessed while delivering Bibles to inmates in jails, formed the Boston Prison Discipline Society to advocate for better treatment of the mentally ill (Grob, 1973). The attention that he brought to the degrading conditions in jails, and his insistence that the mentally ill belonged in hospitals, led the state legislature to create the State Lunatic Asylum in Worcester, the first state psychiatric hospital. When it opened in 1833, half of the newly admitted patients came from jails, houses of corrections, and almshouses.

Dorothea Dix picked up the crusade in 1841. At that time, she was a 39-year-old teacher who agreed to teach Sunday school at the East Cambridge Jail, outside of Boston. She was appalled at the conditions, particularly the way the mentally ill were treated, and began a systematic survey of the conditions in other jails and almshouses, ultimately visiting 300 county jails, 500 almshouses, and 18 prisons in several states (Grob, 1973). She became the leading advocate for the creation of state institutions and has been credited with the creation of 32 such institutions in 20 states.

In 1880, the government undertook a census of "insane persons" in the United States (Wine, 1888). At the time, when the U.S. population stood at approximately 50 million, 92,000 insane persons were identified. Of these, 41,000 were in the 75 newly created state institutions. Fewer than 400 mentally ill inmates were located in jails or prisons, which at that time housed more than 58,000 people. Thus, less than 1% of the incarcerated population was identified as mentally ill. Following this snapshot, the issue of the criminalization of the mentally ill disappeared for almost a century.

The era of institutionalization peaked in the mid-1950s, with a total institutionalized mentally ill population of about 560,000 (Appelbaum, 1994; Hoge, Appelbaum, & Geller, 1989). It is important to recognize that institutionalization reflected a societal preference for segregation, isolation, and control of the mentally ill. The mentally ill were afforded few rights with respect to involuntary confinement and treatment. Under prevailing laws, psychiatrists held broad discretionary powers to initiate commitment based on a vague "need for treatment" standard. Those subject to commitment were afforded few procedural safeguards. Committed individuals were regarded as being globally incompetent, either by law or by social practice. The status of being committed, therefore, rendered individuals unable to enter contracts (such as rental agreements), to get married, or to vote. These legal disabilities served to further isolate the mentally ill and to place them under the control of family and others.

The process of deinstitutionalization began with two developments in the field of psychiatry (Appelbaum, 1994; Hoge et al., 1989). The first development was the rise of the community psychiatry movement. This influential movement grew out of the experiences of psychiatrists in WWII, who found the most effective management of combat fatigue to be brief treatment and quick return to duty. This approach was applied domestically, as psychiatrists focused on the importance of maintaining patients' relationships in the community and promoting rapid reintegration of hospitalized patients back into preexisting family and social structures. The move to an outpatient-oriented mental health system received a substantial boost when President John Kennedy signed into law the Community Mental Health Centers Act of 1963 (Title II, Public Law 88–164) providing federal support for construction of local outpatient treatment facilities for the mentally ill and developmentally disabled. The second development was the introduction of chlorpromazine (Thorazine®) into clinical practice in 1954, the first effective antipsychotic medication. As a result, psychotic episodes could be treated rapidly and patients could be returned more quickly, and more safely, to their homes.

The pace of deinstitutionalization increased during the 1960s, with the introduction of federal health insurance programs that stimulated the rise of private sector psychiatric hospital units. In addition, state legislatures evinced growing reluctance to fund the rising costs of public sector institutional care. On the legal front, civil commitment laws were dramatically transformed between the late 1960s and the mid-1970s (Appelbaum, 1994; Hoge et al., 1989). This wave of libertarian reform replaced the old "need for treatment" standard with a requirement that "dangerousness" be demonstrated. More stringent procedural safeguards, including higher standards of proof, were put into place. During this era, there was significant expansion of patients' rights, including the legal presumption of competence for committed patients, that accelerated deinstitutionalization. The reform movement increasingly empowered the mentally ill to take control of their destiny.

At present, there are roughly 55,000 patients hospitalized in state and county facilities (Manderscheid et al., 2002). It is estimated that roughly 12,000 of these are confined in forensic psychiatric hospitals, pursuant to court-ordered pretrial evaluations or, alternatively, following criminal court adjudication as not guilty by reason of insanity.

Increasing Societal Reliance on Punishment and Incarceration

During the period of rapid deinstitutionalization, there were important developments in correctional policy that helped set the stage for criminalization of the mentally ill. Beginning in the early 1970s, the United States began to rely increasingly on incarceration as a solution to societal problems (Travis, 2002). This is reflected most dramatically in the rate of incarceration per 100,000 adults. For several decades, this rate held steady at about 100. In the 1970s, the rate rose to more than 500 per 100,000; if one includes parole and probation supervision, to more than 700 (U.S. Census Bureau, 2004). Within a decade, the United States became the global leader in the use of incarceration.

A full discussion of the factors underlying the sea change in correctional policy is beyond the scope of this chapter. However, a few developments are important to understanding incarceration of the mentally ill. First, the drug culture took root in the 1960s. By the 1970s, it was perceived that treatment-based approaches to the "war on drugs" had failed; federal and state policymakers began to turn to punishment. Indeed, much of the increase in the incarceration rate can be attributed to drug-related offenses (Travis, 2002). The widespread availability of drugs of abuse has proven to be particularly problematic for many of the mentally ill, who seem to be vulnerable to abuse and addiction, and who suffer destabilization as a result. Although hard evidence is not available, it is likely that the mentally ill were disproportionately affected by the implementation of a broader range of drug-related offenses.

A second important factor underlying the higher rate of incarceration has been the reduction of judicial discretion with respect to sentencing and release decisions. Previously, judges could exercise wide discretion in the imposition of sentences. Moreover, sentences were indeterminate in nature, allowing parole boards to release inmates when they saw fit. Responding to concerns about racial discrimination in the exercise of discretion and political pressures to get tough on crime, legislatures enacted sentencing guidelines, reducing judges' authority (Travis, 2002). And, "truth in sentencing" legislation has ensured that inmates serve longer periods incarcerated.

Deinstitutionalization, therefore, occurred during a period of important social and correctional change. The mentally ill were released into a culture in which drug use was becoming endemic—a development that would provide ongoing challenges to the young and vulnerable, especially those at risk for psychiatric illness. Ready to exercise their newly found freedom, the deinstitutionalized entered a crime-weary society ready to punish their misdeeds. Moreover, they faced a criminal justice system less inclined to reduce the burden of punishment on the basis of mitigating factors such as mental illness.

Incarceration of the Mentally Ill

It appears self-evident that as more people have been incarcerated, the mentally ill would be included. But what is the basis for the widely accepted conclusion that there has been an increase in the rate of incarceration of the mentally ill? The evidence is largely inferential in nature. The silence on incarceration of the mentally ill that had prevailed since the national census of "insane persons" in 1880 was broken in the early 1970s. In the wake of civil commitment reform and deinstitutionalization in California came reports that the mentally ill were appearing in increasing numbers in jails, and reports from prisons soon followed (Abramson, 1972; Stelovich, 1979; Swank & Winer, 1976; Whitmer, 1980).

Even today, it is difficult to determine with precision the prevalence of mental illness in correctional settings. In the 1980s, several groups of researchers applied modern diagnostic criteria to various incarcerated populations. Employing standardized assessment techniques, they reported rates of serious mental illness several times that of the nonincarcerated population. A study of male detainees at Cook County Jail found a lifetime prevalence of schizophrenia and bipolar disorder of 3.8 and 2.2%, respectively (Teplin, 1990). The Epidemiological Catchment Area (ECA) Study, a large-scale examination of the prevalence of mental disorders in the United States, reported 1-year prevalence rates for schizophrenia and bipolar disorder of

5% and 6%, respectively, in a sample of prison inmates (Robins & Regier, 1991). Steadman and coworkers, employing a somewhat broader definition of mental disorder, found 8% of New York State prisoners to be affected (Steadman, Fabisiak, Dvoskin, & Holohean, 1987).

In more recent years, the federal government has undertaken periodic surveys of inmates in jails, state prisons, and federal prisons, as well as those on probation. These surveys have constructed estimates of mental illness based on self-report of illness, treatment, or hospitalization. In a large sample—the 1997 Bureau of Justice Statistics (BJS) survey involved 30,000 individuals— an estimated 16.2% of state prisoners were found to have significant mental illness; 7.4% of federal prisoners; 16.3% of jail inmates; and 16.0% of those on probation (Ditton, 1999). The rate of mental disorders in subpopulations may be higher. For example, there is some evidence to suggest that incarcerated women have higher rates of mental illness than do incarcerated men (Teplin, Abram, & McClelland, 1996).

The estimates of mental illness in correctional settings have received support from collateral sources. For example, BJS surveys indicate that about 10% of state inmates are prescribed psychotropic medication (Beck & Maruschak, 2001). Based on these studies, as well as the experience of clinicians and administrators in the field, it is generally accepted that roughly 6 to 11% of jail and prison inmates have a serious mental illness (such as schizophrenia or bipolar disorder); approximately 10–15% have some form of mental disorder requiring treatment; and an even larger number may experience some symptoms during incarceration (James & Glaze, 2006). Of course, the rate of mental illness observed in a facility will depend on both the definition employed and the effectiveness of institutional procedures in identifying mentally disordered inmates and bringing them to clinical attention.

When one applies estimated percentages to the total population in corrections, the numbers are staggering. Based on the BJS estimates, there are more than 800,000 mentally ill individuals under the control of correctional authorities at any given time: 180,000 state prisoners, 8000 federal prisoners, 97,000 jail inmates, and 547,000 on probation. It is important to note that the jail population turns over rapidly, so that the annual intake is 10 to 20 times the average daily census. Thus, it is reasonable to estimate that a million or more mentally ill individuals are processed through our nation's jails every year.

Early Responses to Criminalization

As the mentally ill began to flood our jails and prisons, the first wave of responses from the psychiatric community focused on restrictive civil commitment laws as the chief culprit. In brief, these admittedly early analyses of the newly coined "criminalization" problem concluded that the incarcerated mentally ill were being jailed for nuisance offenses because civil commitment was no longer available to them and, moreover, that those being incarcerated were similar to long-term state hospital patients (Lamb, 1982; Lamb & Weinberger, 1998; Torrey, 1997). Thus, from the beginning, the problem of the criminalization of the mentally ill has been linked to the failures of deinstitutionalization. It is not surprising that commentators have seen a common solution for both problems: a marked increase in the provision of mental health services, particularly outpatient services. However, several studies offer evidence that simply providing access to psychiatric services would not significantly affect incarceration of the mentally ill.

The relationship between community mental health services and incarceration of the mentally ill was examined by Fisher and colleagues at the University of Massachusetts Medical Center (Fisher, Packer, Simon, & Smith, 2000). As a result of the settlement of a class action suit, for more than a decade prior to the study, western Massachusetts had received a substantially higher level of funding for outpatient adult mental health services than had central Massachusetts. In comparison with central Massachusetts, the western part of the state had nearly twice the resources per capita for a diverse range of outpatient services, including emergency services, case management, residential programs, clinical treatment, and support services. Comparing western and central Massachusetts, Fisher et al. found that the rate of hospitalization was 60% higher in central Massachusetts (396 days per 100,000 versus 247 days), presumably reflecting the lower intensity and availability of outpatient services. The research team examined jail admissions in western and central Massachusetts over a 6-month period. An overall rate of mental disorder of 9.7% was found (schizophrenia, 2.5%; major depression, 6.1%; bipolar disorder, 1.1%). No significant difference was found in the rate of mental illness in the two jurisdictions.

In another study, researchers compared the rates of prior psychiatric hospitalization in two groups of seriously mentally ill individuals: those who had been incarcerated and those who had not (Fisher et al., 2002). The rate of prior hospitalization in the incarcerated group was 52%, significantly higher than the comparison group. A recent review of aggressive community treatment and intensive case management found these treatment modalities had little or no effect on rates of arrest (Mueser, Bond, Drake, & Resnick, 1998). Thus, it appears that lack of access to the mental health system and to comprehensive outpatient services per se are not the critical factors in criminalization, at least for many individuals. These studies suggest that we must look deeper at the nature and quality of outpatient services. The failure of well-funded outpatient services to lower rates of incarceration of the mentally ill demands explanation and, ultimately, further empirical study.

The Mentally Ill in Corrections: Barriers to Outpatient Treatment

In this section, the characteristics of the mentally ill in correctional facilities are examined in order to better understand why outpatient treatment failure is so common. It is important to note at the outset that the incarcerated mentally ill bear a double burden of stigmatization. In characterizing this group, we should not lose sight of the fact that there is substantial diversity within the population, and varying problems and needs that require individualized approaches. Nonetheless, examination of group characteristics will help to explain why the incarcerated mentally ill are so challenging to treat and why outpatient treatment failure is so common. Are these "typical" patients who have been incarcerated in lieu of commitment?

Comorbidities

It has been consistently reported that correctional mentally ill populations have high rates of alcohol and substance abuse conditions comorbid with primary psychiatric disorders. Teplin (1994) examined comorbidity in her study of mental disorders in the Cook County Jail. Among male detainees with a severe mental disorder (here defined as schizophrenia, major depression, or bipolar disorder), 85% were found to have a comorbid alcohol abuse or dependence disorder; 58% were found to have a drug abuse or dependence disorder (nonexclusive). It should be noted that rates of primary substance abuse disorders in the incarcerated population as a whole are high. In the large ECA Study, described earlier, the rate of any substance abuse disorder was found to be 72% in the prison sample (56% alcohol related, 54% related to other drug use) (Robins & Regier, 1991). Based on its survey results, the BJS reported that mentally ill inmates when compared with non-mentally ill inmates had significantly higher rates of use of drugs and alcohol at the time of their offense and in the month prior to offense (Ditton, 1999).

Individuals with mental illness and substance abuse disorders, in general, have worse prognoses than those with uncomplicated mental illness. Comorbidity is associated with a higher degree of psychotic symptoms, depression and suicidality, violence, lower functioning, higher rates of noncompliance, treatment relapse and rehospitalization, and HIV infection (Osher & Drake, 1996). Inmates with comorbid mental illness and substance abuse disorders may be systematically excluded from treatment programs within correctional institutions (Hills, 2000). The availability of inpatient and outpatient programs equipped to address this population following release to the community is not sufficient to serve those in need. Moreover, many of the programs that do exist are unwilling to serve correctional populations or those recently released from incarceration. Finally, as previously noted, intoxication is a very common correlate of criminal behavior. Thus, recidivism is likely to be the outcome of relapses, which are a common feature of the course of substance abuse disorders. For example, a study in Massachusetts comparing mentally disordered offenders with and without a substance abuse diagnosis found higher rates of reincarceration in the dual diagnosis group (Hartwell, 2004).

A second important comorbid condition is antisocial personality disorder (APD). In a study of jail inmates, Abram and Teplin (1991) found rates of APD ranging from 68% in those with schizophrenia and major depression, to 82% in those with bipolar disorder. APD comorbidity also greatly complicates the treatment and management of mentally disordered offenders because it is associated with manipulative behavior and a predisposition to commit criminal acts (DSM-IV-TR, 2000).

Related Social Disabilities

Homelessness has been consistently found as a correlate of incarceration for the mentally ill. BJS statistics reveal that the mentally ill have roughly double the rates of homelessness as those without mental illness (state prisoners, 20% versus 9%; federal prisoners, 19% versus 3%; jail inmates, 30% versus 17%) (Ditton, 1999).

Homelessness among the mentally ill is associated with serious alienation from health systems and family, and treatment failure. Substance abuse disorders contribute to the problem. McGuire and Rosenheck (2004) reported relevant data from the Access to Community Care and Effective Services and Supports (ACCESS) demonstration project, which involved 18 sites in nine states. In this project, 5774 homeless individuals with severe mental illness were provided comprehensive, integrated services, including assertive community treatment and intensive case management. The sample was grouped into three roughly equal groups, based on incarceration history. A strong association was found between comorbidity with substance abuse and incarceration. The homeless mentally ill with no history of incarceration had rates of comorbid alcohol dependence (26%) or drug dependence (25%), significantly lower than those with a lifetime incarceration history of 6 months or less (alcohol dependence, 44%; substance dependence, 37%); and those with an incarceration history of more than 6 months (mean, 48.9 months; alcohol dependence, 57%; drug dependence, 51%). Those with long-term incarceration histories (greater than 6 months) also exhibited higher scores on psychiatric symptom measures. In a 1-year follow-up, those with longer incarceration histories spent more time in jail, and had lower service utilization, including outpatient treatment contacts, engagement in employment services, and substance abuse services. In addition, those with incarceration histories received lower public support payments.

Unemployment or reliance on federal or other public assistance is disproportionately found in the incarcerated mentally ill population. At the time of arrest or conviction, 39% of state prisoners, 38% of federal prisoners, and 47% of jailed mentally ill are unemployed (Ditton, 1999). These rates exceed those found in non-mentally ill prisoners.

Violent Behavior

The literature on the relationship of mental illness to violent or criminal behavior is voluminous. In the mentally ill, a strong relationship has been established between substance abuse comorbidity and violent behavior. In a carefully designed study, Steadman et al. (1998) followed more than 1000 patients who had been hospitalized for mental illness and compared their violent behavior with that of a comparison non-mentally ill group from the community. Data were collected from the mentally ill group for 1 year following discharge from the hospital. Based on patient and family reports, released patients with no comorbid substance abuse diagnoses were no more likely than the controls to commit a violent act. However, patients who were comorbid for substance abuse diagnoses were significantly more likely to be violent during the follow-up period (1-year prevalence rate of violence was 31%, compared to 18% in released patients without comorbidity). Swanson, Holzer, Ganju, and Jono (1990) reported similar findings in a reanalysis of ECA study data.

As discussed above, the mentally disordered correctional populations have high rates of risk-enhancing comorbid disorders. Therefore, it is not surprising to find violent behavior in incarcerated mentally ill people. The BJS data support this conclusion. Based on conviction offenses for prisoners and probationers, and charges faced for jail detainees, the BJS found higher rates of violent offenses in mentally ill inmates when compared with non-mentally ill inmates (state prisoners, 53% compared with 46% in non-mentally ill; federal prisoners, 33% and 13%; jail inmates, 30% and 26%; and probationers,

28% and 18%). The increased rate of violent offenses among the mentally ill extended to comparisons of inmates who were repeat offenders.

Mentally disordered offenders are a diverse group. While many are charged with or convicted of a violent offense, a substantial number are not. Indeed, as the BJS data summarized above indicate, most of the mentally ill in jail populations have been incarcerated for nonviolent offenses (Ditton, 1999). Nor is it necessarily correct to conclude that those facing violent offenses are best managed in the criminal justice system. Many may be safely diverted to treatment programs. On the other hand, from the standpoint of treatment providers and outpatient mental health systems, those who are violent, homeless, and suffering comorbidity will be difficult to engage successfully in treatment programs.

Treatment in Correctional Settings

The quality of care in correctional facilities has been the subject of scrutiny and litigation. This section summarizes the findings of recent studies with the purpose of highlighting aspects of correctional treatment that are problematic from the perspective of community providers.

Jails

As part of a National Institute of Justice-sponsored initiative, Steadman and Veysey (1997) surveyed 1053 jails of varying sizes regarding the mental health services provided; conducted more extensive telephone interviews with 100; and visited 10. They found that 84% of jails reported that less than one-tenth of inmates received any kind of mental health service. Based on the responses, Steadman and Veysey estimated that crisis intervention programs are available in only 43% of jails; psychiatric medications in 42%; inpatient care in 72%; special housing in 36%; and discharge planning in 21%. Smaller jails tended to provide no services beyond suicide screening and prevention. Case management or similar services designed to link detainees to treatment on release were seldom provided.

Prisons

Recent government reports provide some insight into the scope of mental health services in state prisons. The National Commission on Correctional Health Care, in a recent report to Congress (2002a), noted that "most jails and prisons do not conform to nationally accepted guidelines for mental health screening and treatment." Comparing federal surveys from 1988 and 2000, Manderscheid, Gravesande, and Goldstrom (2004) concluded that "the growth in prison facilities and the growth in prisoner populations are outstripping the more meager growth in mental health services," and warned that services are becoming less available. The inadequacy of services is illustrated by examining unmet treatment needs. Examining the status of mentally ill state prisoners due to be released within 12 months, Beck (2000) found that 43% had not received treatment. In addition, only about 20% of inmates with alcohol or substance abuse problems—not necessarily comorbid—had received treatment.

Many barriers to treatment exist in correctional settings, not least of which is inadequate funding. Other barriers that have been identified include inadequate training of correctional officers in identification and management of the mentally disordered, poorly trained mental health professionals, institutional bias toward characterizing the mentally ill as malingerers, and the use of segregation units to manage disruptive behavior caused by mental disorder (Center for Mental Health Services, 1995; National Commission on Correctional Health Care, 2002a,b; The Correctional Association of New York, 2004). In addition, in many institutions inadequate protection of privacy undermines treatment of the mentally ill: some inmates choose to forgo assessment and medications rather than risk being preyed on by inmates who target the impaired. And facilities often have no method to enforce treatment when psychotic inmates refuse medication.

The problem of inadequate treatment in correctional settings is not likely to be solved in the near future; providers of transitional services and outpatient care must take these treatment deficiencies and the resulting unmet needs into account when they develop care plans for their clients.

Reentry Problems

Facilitating successful return to the community and reintegration into family, work, and other social roles serves multiple purposes. Released inmates who are able to make a successful transition are less likely to recidivate or to place other burdens on societal resources. Moreover, assisting prisoners who have paid their debt to society seems fair. The problematic nature of prisoner reentry to society has received considerable attention over the last several years (Travis, 2002). There are many barriers to prisoner reentry that result from a variety of social policies, or that occur as a consequence of incarceration. The problems of transition to the community are frequently compounded in the mentally ill population.

Prisoners, particularly those being released after lengthy prison terms, are alienated from their families and communities. This is particularly true of the mentally ill, who have often become estranged from families as a result of their psychiatric disturbances. In addition, they face the pervasive societal stigmatization of mental illness, as well as that related to incarceration.

Social policies further impede the transition process. Mentally ill inmates are disproportionately reliant on public assistance and SSI or SSDI benefits in order to obtain needed treatment and to ensure continuity of care following release. However, these benefits are discontinued during incarceration and, following release, the process of reinstatement may take 45 to 90 days. This process is not automatic; negotiating the bureaucracy may be beyond the abilities of some of the serious mentally ill. In the absence of medical benefits, the prospects for receiving treatment or obtaining psychotropic medication are bleak. Barriers to transition extend to housing and general assistance. As previously discussed, the burden of homelessness falls disproportionately on the incarcerated mentally ill. For the homeless mentally ill leaving prison, some form of financial assistance and help negotiating the complex process of obtaining residential access is necessary. However, those who have served time for violent offenses may face exclusion from Section 8 housing and drug-related felons may face a lifetime ban from federal public assistance and food stamps. Generally, assistance negotiating the maze to find appropriate housing is not available.

Mentally ill individuals released from incarceration face significant barriers to receiving care. The public mental health system is increasingly resource-constrained and, in many jurisdictions, access to outpatient services is restricted or prioritized to patients released from civilian public hospitals. In other cases, services may simply not be made available to the incarcerated population. At the time of this writing, there is a pending class action lawsuit in New York City concerning the lack of programs for mentally ill individuals with substance abuse disorders who have been ordered into treatment as a result of parole violations. Because treatment programs are not available, they cannot be released (William G. and Walter W. v. Pataki). Many providers are reluctant to treat former inmates due to fear and concerns about liability.

Providing Transitional Services and Treatment

Discharge planning

Discharge planning is essential to ensuring continuity of care on release from incarceration. A recent survey of jail services (Steadman & Veysey, 1997) found that discharge planning was available to about 20% of discharged mentally ill inmates; smaller jails provided this service less often. There is no comparable study of discharge planning for those released from prisons. Given the longer period of incarceration and greater investment of resources at the point of release, there is greater opportunity for comprehensive discharge planning. However, anecdotally, it appears that transitional services in many prisons consists of supplying a few weeks worth of medication and a list of providers in the community. An important difference between discharge planning in jails and prisons arises because jails hold pretrial detainees as well as sentenced inmates. Detainees are often released within a few days. Therefore, discharge planning for detainees must, of necessity, occur in a context of incomplete information, ongoing mental health needs assessment, and uncertain release dates. Jail planning processes for detainees resemble crisis intervention programs (Hartwell & Orr, 2000).

Discharge planning for those released from jails has received increased national attention in the wake of a class action settlement requiring New York City to provide discharge planning services to inmates with mental illness released from Riker's Island, one of the largest jails in the country (Brad H. v. City of New York). The GAINS Center has published a best practices model for discharge planning (Osher, Steadman, & Barr, 2002). The APIC model is a pragmatic approach that is named for four steps: (1) assess the inmate's clinical and social needs, and public safety risks, (2) plan for the treatment and services required to address the inmate's needs, (3) identify required community and correctional programs responsible for postrelease services, and (4) coordinate the transition plan to ensure implementation and avoid gaps in care with community-based programs.

Program Elements

In recent years, a few specialized programs have emerged, designed to manage mentally ill inmates in the reentry process and in the postrelease period. These innovative programs, which have embraced the dual role of improving the treatment of this population and reducing rates of recidivism, have reported success, although in small or uncontrolled studies (Project Link, 1999; Ventura,

Cassel, Jacoby, & Huang, 1998; Lamberti et al., 2001; The Thresholds State, County Collaborative Jail Linkage Project, 2001). A survey of more than 300 county behavioral health directors resulted in the identification of 16 programs in nine states involving the management of the mentally ill on release from incarceration (Lamberti, Weisman, & Faden, 2004). Thirteen of the 16 programs addressed reentry and postrelease management of ordinary mentally ill jail inmates (the remaining three included two diversion programs and a specialized service to manage insanity acquittees).

In 1998 the state of California established the Mentally Ill Offender Crime Reduction Grant program (MIOCRG) that provided more than $80 M in grants to 30 programs in 26 counties to develop and evaluate projects to help mentally ill offenders avoid further involvement with the criminal justice system (California Board of Corrections, 2004). Grant recipients were free to design programs to meet local needs and to leverage existing resources. The programs that emerged varied in admission criteria and the precise composition of services. In some programs, participation was voluntary; others involved court mandates to participate as a condition of probation. Generally included in the enhanced program were the following services: assistance in securing disability entitlements, housing, vocational training, and employment; residential and outpatient mental health treatment; individual and group counseling; substance abuse education and counseling; life skills training; medication education, management, and support; transportation services; socialization training and support; advocacy; and crisis intervention.

In its final evaluation of MIOCRG, the California Board of Corrections identified assertive community treatment as the most common element, reported by 19 of the 30 programs. The second most common feature was the use of mental health courts (9 programs). Three major strategies were identified within the programs: the use of multidisciplinary teams, intensive case management, and flexible service delivery. In addition, medication management and having a clinic or center as bases of operations were found to be important program elements.

Grant recipients were required to randomize offenders into two groups: one receiving experimental, enhanced services and the other receiving treatment as usual; all to be followed for 2 years postrelease. Twenty programs provided data suitable for analysis, involving a total of more than 4700 inmates. Inmates receiving enhanced services had better criminal justice outcomes than those who received routine services. In the followup period, they were booked less often (53% versus 56%), convicted less often (35% versus 38%), were less likely to be jailed (54% versus 57%), and spent less time in jail (13.7 versus 15.2 days). More impressive differences were found in treatment outcomes. At the end of the follow up period, those receiving enhanced services were less likely to have a drug problem (45% versus 55%) or an alcohol problem (38% versus 49%). Functioning, as assessed by the Global Assessment of Functioning Scale, indicated that those receiving enhanced services were less likely to worsen (21% versus 32%). Similar differences were found in quality of life and social measures: those receiving enhanced services were less likely to be homeless (7% versus 12%) and to be economically insufficient throughout the followup period (30% versus 53%). All findings were statistically significant.

Qualitative evaluation of the various programs resulted in the identification of several factors related to success. These included interagency collaboration and multidisciplinary partnerships, comprehensive and flexible services, intensive case management, involvement of the court, mental health courts, assistance with benefits, use of flex funds, and residential assistance (California Board of Corrections, 2004).

Conclusion

Deinstitutionalization was a disruptive force in the provision of public sector psychiatric services. The shift to a community-based model has undoubtedly resulted in increased autonomy and a higher quality of life for many individuals who would have been institutionalized in an earlier era. However, the transition was not painless. In many communities, decades passed before community mental health care received minimally adequate funding, and fiscal constraints continue to limit the implementation of services throughout the country. In addition, the magnitude of the need for social support and outreach services for the severely mentally ill was not anticipated at the outset of deinstitutionalization. Nearly a generation passed before a conceptualization of aggressive community services was developed and began to serve as a model for care (Stein & Test, 1980). Finally, the early, widespread experience of revolving door readmissions for the seriously mentally ill appeared unsolvable, until the walls between hospital and outpatient providers were torn down, and they began to work collaboratively on discharge planning and transition to community management.

Public sector psychiatry has had limited success, however, with the incarcerated mentally ill population. Many of the most difficult patients are not being served, or are not served adequately, in existing outpatient treatment programs. It appears that this deficiency is not the result of shortfalls in funding outpatient services or failure to provide aggressive community treatment (Fisher et al., 2000; Mueser et al., 1998; McGuire & Rosenheck, 2004). Two potential explanatory factors emerge from this review.

First, the incarcerated mentally ill include disproportionate numbers of patients who are difficult to treat, and who are more resistant to being engaged in treatment. Second, correctional institutions, particularly our jails, have not embraced discharge and transition planning for the mentally ill.

The development of outpatient services for the correctional population will require treatment targeted for alcohol and substance abuse comorbidities. Beyond the specifics of treatment, the more daunting challenge will be engaging released inmates in treatment. As suggested by the evolution of public sector services, nominal discharge planning—for example, merely scheduling outpatient visits—is not likely to be successful. Correctional and outpatient providers need to work together to ensure individualized plans designed to provide continuity of care and to ensure compliance. The experience from the public sector is that investment in this process will result in substantial improvement in outpatient care for those who desire services, but have impairments that limit follow through.

At present, we do not know to what extent it will be possible to rely on strictly voluntary programs, or whether legal coercion will be necessary for some patients. The public sector outpatient system is based almost exclusively on voluntary service provision, and it has failed to address the needs of the correctional population adequately. However, this may be due to providers' reluctance to treat patients with a propensity for violence and/or manipulative behavior. The California Board of Corrections final report on the MIOCRG program identified one of the factors in success as involvement of the courts, suggesting some application of coercion was involved in ensuring compliance. However, half of the county programs relied exclusively on voluntary participation (California Board of Corrections, 2004). It is likely that staff dedication to the correctional population, a commitment to spanning the boundary between the criminal justice and treatment systems, and comfort with risk assessment and management of patients with a history of incarceration were important to success. Clearly, more research is necessary to understand the factors underlying treatment compliance and recidivism reduction.

Key Elements of Transition Planning (Based on the APIC model, Osher, Steadman, & Barr, 2002).

- Assess the inmate's clinical and social needs, and public safety risks. This assessment should identify unmet treatment needs, including treatment of alcohol- and drug-related problems. In addition, transition planners should review the inmate's past record of compliance and current level of interest in community-based treatment following release. Review of preincarceration treatment records and consultation with family members will be necessary in some cases. The inmate's plans and prospects for meeting housing and financial needs should be reviewed. The assessment of public safety risks should focus on past violent and criminal conduct. Efforts should be made to identify factors related to problematic behavior, particularly symptoms of mental illness, noncompliance with medication, and substance abuse.
- Plan for treatment and services required to address the inmate's needs. A comprehensive plan should be constructed that addresses the inmate's needs. The plan should identify and prioritize services necessary for a successful transition, including services needed to minimize the risk of recidivism. Inmates with serious mental disorders or significantly impaired decision-making capacities should be considered for long-term psychiatric treatment, guardianship, or, in some jurisdictions, outpatient civil commitment. Coercive measures should be strongly considered for inmates who have a pattern of noncompliance and symptoms of mental illness have been associated with violent behavior.
- Identify required community and correctional programs responsible for postrelease services. The availability of services will vary considerably from community to community. Transition planners should maintain lists of providers and programs willing to accept released inmates.
- Coordinate the plan to ensure implementation and avoid gaps in care with community-based programs. Special assistance should be given to the more serious mentally ill inmates who may have difficulty making and keeping appointments, negotiating transportation, or renewing SSI or SSDI benefits. Ideally, community-based providers will meet with their correctional counterparts and the inmate prior to release.

References

Abram, K.M., & Teplin, L.A. (1991). Co-occurring disorders among mentally ill jail detainees: Implications for public policy. *American Psychologist, 46*, 1036–1045.

Abramson, M.F. (1972). The criminalization of mentally disordered behavior: Possible side-effect of a new mental health law. *Hospital and Community Psychiatry, 23*, 101–106.

Appelbaum, P.S. (1994). *Almost a revolution: Mental health law and the limits of change*. New York: Oxford University Press.

Beck, A.J. (2000, April 13). *State and federal prisoners returning to the community: Findings from the Bureau of Justice Statistics*. Presented at the First Reentry Courts Initiative Cluster Meeting, Washington, DC.

Beck, A.J., & Maruschak, L.M. (2001). *Mental health treatment in state prisons, 2000*. Bureau of Justice Statistics Special Report, NCJ 188215. Washington, DC: U.S. DOJ.

California Board of Corrections. (2004). Mentally Ill Offender Crime Reduction Grant Program: Legislative Report.

Center for Mental Health Services. (1995). *Double jeopardy: Persons with mental illness in the criminal justice system. A report to Congress.*

Diagnostic and statistical manual of mental disorders, fourth edition, text revision (DSM-IV-TR). (2000). Washington DC: American Psychiatric Association.

Ditton, P.M. (1999). *Mental health and treatment of inmates and probationers*. Bureau of Justice Statistics Special Report, NCJ 174463. Washington, DC: U.S. DOJ.

Fisher, W.H., Packer, I.K., Banks, S.M., Smith, D., Simon, L.J., & Roy-Bujnowski, K. (2002). Self-reported psychiatric hospitalization histories of jail detainees with mental disorders: Comparison with a non-incarcerated national sample. *Journal of Behavioral Health Services and Research, 29,* 458–465.

Fisher, W.H., Packer, I.K., Simon, L.J., & Smith, D. (2000). Community mental health services and the prevalence of severe mental illness in local jails: Are they related? *Administration and Policy in Mental Health, 27,* 371–382.

Grob, G. N. (1973). *Mental institutions in America*. New York: Free Press.

Hartwell, S.W. (2004). Comparison of offenders with mental illness only and offenders with dual diagnoses. *Psychiatric Services, 55,* 145–150.

Hartwell, S.E., & Orr, K. (2000). Release planning. *American Jails,* Nov/Dec, 9–13

Hills, H.A. (2000). *Creating effective treatment programs for persons with co-occurring disorders in the justice system*. Delmar, NY: GAINS Center.

Hoge, S.K., Appelbaum, P.S., & Geller, J.G. (1989). Involuntary treatment. In A. Tasman, R.E. Hales, and A.J. Frances (Eds.), *American Psychiatric Press review of psychiatry: Volume 8* (pp. 432–450). Washington, DC: American Psychiatric Press.

James, D.J., & Glaze, L.E. (2006). *Mental health problems of prison and jail inmates*. Bureau of Justice Statistics Special Report, NCJ 213600. Washington, DC: U.S. DOJ.

Lamb, H.R. (1982). *Treating the long-term mentally ill*. San Francisco: Jossey–Bass.

Lamb, H.R,. & Weinberger, L.E. (1998). Persons with severe mental illness in jails and prisons: A review. *Psychiatric Services, 49,* 483–492.

Lamberti, J.S., Weisman, R.L., Schwarzkopf, S.B., Price, N., Ashton, R.M., & Trompeter, J. (2001). The mentally ill in jails and prisons: Towards an integrated model of prevention. *Psychiatric Quarterly, 71,* 62–77.

Lamberti, J.S., Weisman, R., & Faden, D.I. (2004). Forensic assertive community treatment: Preventing incarceration of adults with severe mental illness. *Psychiatric Services, 55,* 1285–1293.

Lovell, D., Gagliardi, G.J., & Peterson, P.D. (2002). Recidivism and use of services among persons with mental illness after release from prison. *Psychiatric Services, 53,* 1290–1298.

Manderscheid, R.W., Atay, J.E., Male, A., Blacklow, B., Forest, C., Ingram, L., Maedke, J., Sussman, J., & Ndikumwami, J. (2002). Highlights of organized mental health services in 2000 and major national and state trends. In R.W. Manderscheid & M.J. Henderson (Eds.), *Mental health, United States, 2002*. Rockville, MD: U.S. Department of Health and Human Services.

Manderscheid, R.W., Gravesande, A., & Goldstrom, I.D. (2004). Growth of mental health services in state adult correctional facilities, 1988 to 2000. *Psychiatric Services, 55,* 869–872.

McGuire, J.F., & Rosenheck, R.A. (2004). Criminal history as a prognostic indicator in the treatment of homeless people with severe mental illness. *Psychiatric Services, 55*, 42–48.

Mueser, K.T., Bond, G.R., Drake, R.E., & Resnick, S.G. (1998). Models of community care for severe mental illness: A review of research on case management. *Schizophrenia Bulletin, 24*, 37–74.

National Commission on Correctional Health Care. (2002a). *The health status of soon-to-be-released inmates: A report to Congress.* Volume 1.

National Commission on Correctional Health Care. (2002b). *The health status of soon-to-be-released inmates: A report to Congress.* Volume 2.

Osher, F.C., & Drake, R.E. (1996). Reversing a history of unmet needs: Approaches to care for persons with co-occurring addictive and mental disorders. *American Journal of Orthopsychiatry, 6*, 4–11.

Osher, F., Steadman, H.J., & Barr, H. (2002). *A best practice approach to community re-entry from jails for inmates with co-occurring disorders: The APIC model.* Delmar, NY: GAINS Center.

Project Link. (1999). Prevention of jail and hospital recidivism among persons with severe mental illness. *Psychiatric Services, 50*, 1477–1480.

Robins, L.H., & Regier, D.A. (1991). *Psychiatric disorders in America: The Epidemiological Catchment Area Study.* New York: Free Press.

Steadman, H.J., & Veysey, B.M. (1997). *Providing services for jail inmates with mental disorders.* NIJ Research in Brief.

Steadman, H.J., Fabisiak, S., Dvoskin, J., & Holohean, E.J. (1987). A survey of mental disability among state prison inmates. *Hospital and Community Psychiatry, 38*, 1086–1090.

Steadman, H.J., Mulvey, E.P., Monahan, J., Robbins, P.C., Appelbaum, P.S., Grisso, T., Roth, L.H., & Silver, E. (1998). Violence by people discharged from acute psychiatric inpatient facilities and by others in the same neighborhoods. *Archives of General Psychiatry, 55*, 393–401.

Stein, L.K., & Test, M.A. (1980). Alternative to mental hospital treatment: I. Conceptual model, treatment program, and clinical evaluation. *Archives of General Psychiatry, 37*, 392–397.

Stelovich, S. (1979). From the hospital to the prison: A step forward in deinstitutionalization? *Hospital and Community Psychiatry, 30*, 618–620.

Swank, G., & Winer, D. (1976). Occurrence of psychiatric disorders in a county jail population. *American Journal of Psychiatry, 133*, 1331–1333.

Swanson, J.W., Holzer, C.E., Ganju, V.K., & Jono, R.T. (1990). Violence and psychiatric disorder in the community: Evidence from the Epidemiologic Catchment Area surveys. *Hospital and Community Psychiatry, 41*, 761–770.

Teplin, L.A. (1990). The prevalence of severe mental disorder among male urban jail detainees: Comparison with the Epidemiologic Catchment Area Program. *American Journal of Public Health, 80*, 655–656.

Teplin, L.A. (1994). Psychiatric and substance abuse disorders among male urban jail detainees. *American Journal of Public Health, 84*, 290–293.

Teplin, L.A., Abram, K.M., & McClelland, G.M. (1996). Prevalence of psychiatric disorders among incarcerated women. I. Pretrial jail detainees. *Archives of General Psychiatry, 53*, 505–512.

The Correctional Association of New York. (2004). *Mental health in the house of corrections: A study of the mental health care in New York State prisons.* New York: Author.

The Thresholds State, County Collaborative Jail Linkage Project. (2001). Helping mentally ill people break the cycle of jail and homelessness. *Psychiatric Services, 52*, 1380–1382.

Torrey, E.F. (1997). *Out of the shadows: Confronting America's mental illness crisis.* New York: John Wiley & Sons.

Travis, J. (2002). *But they all come back: Facing the challenges of prisoner reentry.* Washington, DC: Urban Institute Press.

U.S. Census Bureau. (2004). Accessed July 11, 2006, at http://www.census.gov/compendia/statab/tables/06s0338.xls.

Ventura, L.A., Cassel, C.A., Jacoby, J.E., & Huang, B. (1998). *Psychiatric Services, 49,* 1330–1337.

Whitmer, G.E. (1980). From hospitals to jails: The fate of California's deinstitutionalized mentally ill. *American Journal of Orthopsychiatry, 50,* 65–75.

Wine, F. H. (1888). *Report on the defective, dependent and delinquent classes of the population of the United States.* Washington, DC: U.S. Government Printing Office.

Chapter 27

Sexual Predators: Diversion, Civil Commitment, Community Reintegration, Challenges, and Opportunities

Karen Terry

Introduction

Despite the intense public focus on predatory sexual offenders today, they are not a new threat. Sex offenders have always existed, and have been vilified as "monsters," "fiends," "psychopaths," and "predators" throughout this century (Jenkins, 1998). Several highly publicized cases of predatory sex offenders have saturated the media since the early 1990s, bringing forth an intense public, political, and academic interest. Many questions arise in regard to how to best manage this population: Should they be treated? Should they be chemically incapacitated? Can they be supervised effectively in the community? Do they have high levels of recidivism? Is it possible to predict who will reoffend?

The reality is that sex offenders constitute a heterogeneous population of individuals and there is neither a single theory to explain their behavior nor one universal system of managing them. Most sex offenders do not live in prisons or hospitals. Those who are convicted are often sentenced to probation; almost all of those who are incarcerated are eventually released to live in the community; and, most importantly, many will never come to the attention of authorities. Because of this, it is important to understand the best ways in which the public can be educated about this population of individuals, hypotheses about why some individuals begin to commit sexually deviant behavior, how to best treat that behavior, which offenders should be incapacitated, and how to manage offenders once they are released to the community.

Research on sexual offenses and offenders is generally discussed in the fields of criminal justice, law, sociology, and psychology, not in the arena of public health. However, as Gene Abel and his colleagues have noted (Abel, Lawry, Karlstrom, Osborn, & Gillespie, 1994; Abel & Osborn, 1992), sexual offenders, particularly those who abuse children, constitute a public health problem. They describe it as such because of the high rate of sexual victimization among adult males and females, and because of the high rate of victimization in organizations that supervise or are charged with working with children (e.g., schools, places of worship, youth organizations) (Abel et al., 1994). The effects of sexual victimization are often long-term and traumatic, and may put the victim at a higher risk of suicide, depression, and sexually transmitted diseases ("Perceptions," 1995).

In the last decade, a common reaction to sexual abuse, particularly child sexual abuse, has been to increase penalties for sexual offenders. While such measures may be appropriate responses to sexual abuse as a criminal problem, they do not necessarily reduce the public health problem. In order to reduce the rate of victimization and, thus, the public health problem, it is important to educate the public about the reality of sexual offending and focus on the most effective methods of treating and managing offenders living in the community. The purpose of this chapter is to further evaluate who is considered a sexual offender, the legislation that has been enacted for the incapacitation and management of offenders, and to explore the policy implications of this legislation from a public health perspective.

Sexual Offenses and Offenders

It is not easy to define "normal" or "deviant" sexual behavior, as definitions vary across time, cultures, and jurisdictions (Stermac, Segal, & Gillis, 1990). While some actions, such as forcible rape, are easily identified as deviant, the legally and socially acceptable boundaries of other sexual behaviors are not as clear. Sexual behaviors other than those for the purposes of procreation (e.g., homosexuality, incest, adultery, masturbation, bestiality, and sexual activity with children) have vacillated between social acceptance and criminalization (Terry, 2006, p. 5).

Throughout the United States, sexual offenses vary by type, degrees of severity, class of offense, and length of sanction. They can be comprised of acts that include contact (such as sexual assault and rape), acts that include noncontact behavior (such as exhibitionism), and acts involving the viewing, possession, or distribution of child pornography. Each state differs in regard to terminology, definition of who can be a victim or an offender (male and/or female), the class of felony or misdemeanor, the age of the victim (with those having younger victims being more serious offenders), and whether a consensual act can be considered an offense (e.g., sodomy, incest among adult family members). Generally, sexual offenses involve a lack of consent on the part of the victim and some level of intent to receive sexual gratification on the part of the offender.

Of the sex offenders who are known (namely, those in the criminal justice system), it is clear that they differ from other types of offenders in several ways: they tend to be older, better educated, of all racial and ethnic groups, and of all socioeconomic classes. Researchers studying the etiology of deviant sexual behavior identify many factors with this behavior, including:

physiological factors, a retarded psychosexual development, deviant sexual arousal, learned conditions, poor-quality attachments, loneliness and intimacy problems, poor social skills, low self-confidence and self-esteem, to name but a few. Additionally, many offenders exhibit paraphilic behavior, the features of which are recurrent, intense sexually arousing fantasies or urges involving either nonhuman objects, suffering or humiliation of oneself or one's partner, children or other nonconsenting persons (American Psychiatric Association, 2000). What is clear is that there is no single theory that can adequately explain the etiology or maintenance of deviant sexual behavior; they can simply provide a piece of the complex explanation for this behavior.

One of the reasons that sex offenders are scrutinized so carefully is because of the fear that they will reoffend. Despite the fact that there are no consistently reliable data about the levels of recidivism among sex offenders, a number of state legislatures have either explicitly or implicitly identified them as presenting a high risk for repeating their offenses. It is impossible to accurately assess the true extent of sexual offending and levels of recidivism, and studies present vastly different rates for numerous reasons. Sexual abuse is significantly underreported, and most studies of sex offenders analyze only those offenders known to the criminal justice system. According to the Bureau of Justice Statistics (2001), sex crimes have the lowest rates of reporting for all crimes, and the Sourcebook of Criminal Justice Statistics shows that 71.1% of victims of sex crimes did not report the crime to the police in 1999. Additionally, researchers define recidivism differently—from arrest for any further offense to conviction for another sexual offense—which has an effect on the rates of recidivism reported. Studies are consistent, however, in identifying the heterogeneity of this group of individuals and noting that they reoffend at different rates, depending on a number of static and dynamic characteristics.

Legislation

Despite the heterogeneity in types of sexual offenders, legislators have adopted several one-size-fits-all policies, such as Megan's Law and Sexually Violent Predator Legislation, in reaction to an increasingly public focus on sexual offenders. The laws have been challenged in state and federal courts of all levels in regard to their constitutionality and the fairness in their structure and application. Ultimately, the courts declared them constitutional, but their effectiveness in preventing cases of sexual abuse has yet to be measured.

Registration and Community Notification Laws ("Megan's Law")

In July 1994, 7-year-old Megan Kanka was raped and killed by a recidivist child molester who lived across the street from her in the New Jersey suburb of Hamilton Township. The assailant, Jesse Timmendequas, had been convicted of two previous sexual offenses against children. He was able to lure Megan into his house by inviting her to see his puppy, and, not aware of his history, she voluntarily followed him. Soon after her death, her parents began a campaign for more stringent laws about the identification of sexual offenders in the community. They claimed that if a convicted sex offender is living in the area, the community has a right to know so that parents can better protect their children. Their actions were pivotal to the development of federal and state laws regarding the collection and dissemination of information about sex offenders (Terry & Furlong, 2003).

Prior to Megan's death, only five states had laws that required sex offenders to register their personal information with a law enforcement agency. Megan's parents campaigned for both registration and notification of the sex offenders' whereabouts to the community in which they are living to become mandatory in all states. Many politicians, from local government to the President, supported the Kankas, believing that by notifying the communities about known sex offenders, it may be possible to protect the lives of children. As a result of Megan's murder and her parents' advocacy for new legislation, the federal government and all states enacted Registration and Community Notification Laws (RCNL), commonly referred to as "Megan's Law." The federal law, The Jacob Wetterling Crimes against Children and Sexually Violent Registration Program, required that states have a registry for sex offenders or lose 10% of federal funding for local and state law enforcement. All states implemented RCNL and none suffered a loss of funds; Massachusetts was the last state to enact the legislation, and did so on August 5, 1996.

The goal of Megan's Law is simple—to protect the community from known sex offenders—yet it consists of complicated guidelines and procedures that vary by state. Over the 10 years since their inception, RCNL statutes have evolved into a more uniform structure as a result of the thousands of cases heard in state and federal courts. In all states, RCNL requires sex offenders, on conviction or release from a correctional institution, to inform a law enforcement agency of their whereabouts within a specified time period. Offenders are required to provide the agency with, at a minimum, a photograph, fingerprints, name, address, and place of employment. The agency then stores this information in a registry and, for high-risk offenders, notifies the community. Offenders must verify their address annually or every 90 days, depending on the level of risk they pose. RCNL statutes still differ in the following ways, however (Terry and Furlong, 2003).

- Triggering offense. Most offenses that trigger registration are categorized as sexual offenses in the penal code. However, some states also include triggering offenses such as prostitution, child pornography, and kidnapping.
- Length of registration. Offenders must remain on the registry for a specified length of time, and that time varies by state and risk level of offender. Registration length varies from 10 years to life, and in some states offenders can apply for expungement from the registry after a certain amount of time.
- Registration of juveniles. Approximately two-thirds of the states require juvenile sex offenders to be included on the registry. However, the requirements differ by state, with some mandating only the registration of juveniles who are tried as adults, while others require registration for anyone convicted or adjudicated delinquent of a sexual offense. States also differ in regard to whether the community is notified about juvenile offenders and the length of registration.
- Time period in which to register/reregister. On conviction, release from an institution, change of residence, or, in some states, residence for a certain number of days in a different jurisdiction, offenders must register their address with the police. The time period that they have to register varies from 48 hours to 10 days. Additionally, they must check in and confirm their

address with the police annually or every 90 days, depending on the risk level of the offender.

- Risk assessment. States use differing methods of determining offenders' risk level, such as actuarial assessments or offense type. Higher-risk offenders will have to register for longer periods of time and are subject to higher levels of notification in most states.
- Method of notification. Although all states now have provisions for Internet notification of offenders, agencies in some jurisdictions also post flyers or send notices to homes in the immediate vicinity of the offenders, have 800 or 900 numbers to call to find out information about a particular individual, have a registry available for viewing in a police department, or send notices home with children from school.
- Information about offenders. Nearly half the states require DNA samples as part of the sex offender registration process, and some are beginning to track offenders through the use of Global Positioning Systems (GPS).
- Residency requirements. Many jurisdictions have created residency requirements for sex offenders, prohibiting them from living within a certain distance from schools, parks, recreational facilities, or any other places where children congregate. These residency restrictions can range from 500 feet to 2500 feet.

The variation in state procedures creates challenges for offenders and law enforcement. Although the past decade has seen a move toward more uniformity, many differences in statute and procedure still exist. In an effort to improve on the uniformity, the government has created a national database for registered sex offenders. While this will help overcome some problems that exist in a state system (e.g., law enforcement can search for suspects who may live in a different state), it still has flaws. In particular, it relies on information from states to send information to the national registry (Ashby, 2006).

Megan's Law has been challenged in the courts but is considered constitutional on all grounds. Because Megan's Law is civil and not criminal, it does not constitute punishment. As such, the U.S. Supreme Court has declared that RCNL does not violate due process, double jeopardy, equal protection, ex post facto, or bill of attainder clauses. The courts have more recently addressed issues of right to privacy, right to withdraw a guilty plea, challenges to the risk assessment process, criminalization of the lack of compliance (to the civil statute), and residency requirements.

Under RCNL, sex offenders must abide by particular regulations and are subject to varying degrees of supervision. However, the fact remains that they are living in the community. For the most serious sexual offenders who have completed their criminal sentences, some state legislatures decided that community supervision is not a sufficient means of management and control. Thus, they created laws to confine these "sexually violent predators."

Sexually Violent Predator Legislation

Registration and community notification laws were not the only type of legislation spawned after emotionally charged sex crimes in the 1990s. Several states enacted legislation allowing for "sexually violent predators" (SVPs) to be committed to a secure facility at the end of their criminal sentences (note: this is something of a misnomer, however, since most SVPs have not committed offenses traditionally viewed as "violent"). The purpose of this legislation is to incapacitate sexual offenders who are assessed as a risk to reoffend. This legislation assumes a relationship between mental disorder, risk, and sexual violence, and it relies on risk assessment tools to identify those who may pose a risk while living in the community.

SVP legislation is similar to Mentally Disordered Sex Offender laws, or "sexual psychopathy" laws, from the 1930s. Sexual psychopathy statutes were based on the underlying assumption that sexually deviant behavior results from a diagnosable disorder and is treatable. Sex offenders who were diagnosed as sexual psychopaths would be civilly committed to a mental institution instead of prison. Because of the subjective process for commitment and lack of standardized procedures for release, many psychiatric and mental health organizations suggested that these laws should be repealed. By the early 1990s, sexual psychopathy laws existed in only 13 states (American Psychiatric Association, 1999.) However, at this time several highly publicized cases of child sexual abuse and murder occurred and legislators re-created laws to incapacitate offenders identified as "sexual predators."

Washington was the first state to enact SVP legislation, and it did so through the Community Protection Act (CPA) in 1990. By January 2007, 20 states will have enacted some version of SVP legislation. An SVP is generally defined as any person who has been convicted of (or, in some states, charged with) a sexually violent offense and who suffers from a mental abnormality or personality disorder which makes the person likely to engage in predatory acts of sexual violence. According to the Kansas statute (which serves as a model for statutes in several other states since it was the first to be tested in the U.S. Supreme Court), SVP legislation was enacted specifically to target "a small but extremely dangerous group of SVPs who do not have a mental disease or defect that renders them appropriate for involuntary treatment…" (Kansas SVPA § 59-29a). The standard for commitment is more than a "mere predisposition" to violence, and there must be some indication of past sexually violent behavior and a present mental condition that is likely to cause similar violent behavior in the future. However, every state defines the level of risk necessary for commitment, and the standards vary from "highly probable" to "highly likely" to "more likely than not" to "likely" to reoffend (Doren, 2006).

SVP legislation is civil, not criminal, but the commitment process resembles a criminal adjudication process and sexual offenders have rights similar to those in a criminal trial. The first step is referral; sex offenders are referred to the court shortly before release from prison. The prosecuting attorney files the petition, and there is a hearing to determine if there is probable cause that the sex offender is an SVP. At the hearing, the sex offender has the right to notice of the hearing, an opportunity to be heard, right to counsel, right to present evidence, right to cross-examine witnesses, and the right to view and copy all petitions and documents in his or her file. If the court establishes that there is probable cause, the sex offender is then sent for evaluation by a psychiatrist. If the psychiatrist assesses the offender as dangerous, then a trial will be held within 45 days. At trial, the offender has a right to counsel, a jury trial, and an examination by an expert of his or her choice. In some states the prosecuting attorney must prove the case beyond a reasonable doubt; however, other states use a standard of only clear and convincing evidence since it is a civil trial. The verdict of the jury must be unanimous in order for commitment to ensure; if not, the court must declare a mistrial and set a retrial date within 45 days. If the jury determines that the offender is an SVP, he or she is transferred to the secure facility in that state. Each state must also provide for a way in which the SVP can move to a Less Restrictive Alternative (LRA) or can be conditionally or unconditionally released into the community. Despite the actions taken to ensure that SVPs can be released into the community, few are. As of May 2006, 2627 persons were civilly committed in the United States (with an additional 1019 civilly detained awaiting commitment), and 57 detainees have been released based on the recommendation of treatment staff (more have been released by order of the courts) (Deming, 2006).

Like Megan's Law, SVP legislation varies by state, though most follow the general guidelines for Washington and Kansas. All states must provide certain standards for the SVP process, including due process rights during the commitment process, availability of treatment while incapacitated, and LRA facilities. However, they differ in their definition of what constitutes a "sexually violent predator" (mental abnormality, mental disorder, or personality disorder that renders them dangerous); the likelihood for future deviant behavior (the likelihood of recidivating and the level of dangerousness—e.g., an "extremely high" rating of dangerousness, are "distinctively dangerous," etc.); the standards of proof for commitment (proof beyond a reasonable doubt, clear and convincing evidence, a preponderance of the evidence that a person is an SVP); length of commitment (indefinite, or there may be an evaluation every year or 2 years to determine if the SVP is rehabilitated); facility (the secure unit may be within a prison, a hospital, a special secure facility for SVPs, or, in Texas, an outpatient program); and cost (though cost is expensive everywhere, it varies depending on the facility, number of offenders incapacitated, types and amount of treatment, and legal issues).

The civil commitment process depends on the ability of clinicians to predict risk of reoffense. While risk assessment procedures have improved significantly over the past 20 years (e.g., see Hanson, 2005), there continues to be potential for high rates of false positives among the group of sex offenders as a whole. The risk assessment process differs by state, but most jurisdictions use actuarial-based instruments in conjunction with clinical assessments. Actuarial instruments attempt to predict future offending behavior based on offense history or personal (static) characteristics. If the offender displays characteristics similar to a class of offenders who have shown a high degree of recidivism, the risk is assessed as high since it is assumed that the offender will follow a similar pattern of reoffense. However, unless there is a high base rate and a high accuracy rate for a particular cohort, the likelihood of accurately predicting future risk is less than 50% (Janus & Meehl, 1997). Predictions of violence tend to be most accurate for certain types of cases, such as when there is a history of repeated violence (Litwack, 1993), there is evidence of psychopathy (Hemphill, Hare, & Wong, 1998; Quinsey, Lalumiere, Rice, & Harris, 1995), or there is a previous conviction for a sexual offense (McGrath, 1991). Risk assessment instruments are increasingly using multiple factors to assess risk. Instruments such as the Sex Offender Need Assessment Rating (SONAR) focus on dynamic factors and differentiate those that are stable (e.g., intimacy deficits) and acute (e.g., anger) (Hanson & Harris, 2001). However, the use of both dynamic (changeable) and static risk factors in assessment tools is still emerging, and, thus, more empirical work needs to be done to assess the combination of these factors in overall evaluations of offenders (Hanson, 2005).

Risk assessment is a feature of civil commitment at two points: prior to commitment and, once committed, during evaluations to determine whether the offender should be released. These are two very different situations; as difficult as future risk is to predict prior to commitment, it is even more difficult to assess whether an individual who is incapacitated is at a sufficiently low level of risk to be released. The reason for this is because so few sex offenders are released from civil commitment once incapacitated as SVPs, there is no accurate base rate for comparisons (Kemshall, 2001). Additionally, it is likely that if clinicians will err in their judgments, they will do so on the side of society (Alexander, 1993). If a psychologist approves an offender's release, he or she may be deemed responsible for any actions the offender takes once in the community.

Though controversial, SVP legislation has been tested in the courts and was ultimately found to be constitutional in the case of *Kansas v. Hendricks*, 521 U.S. 346 (1997). The concept of civil commitment is not new, and has long been an option for people with mental illnesses or serious mental disorders that give rise to a substantial threat of serious harm to oneself or others. Involuntary civil commitment statutes have continuously withstood constitutional challenges, despite the infraction on civil liberties to those confined. SVP legislation differs from regular civil commitment in two distinct ways: first, the requirement for commitment is a mental or personality disorder, not a mental illness (a lower threshold for commitment), and also because it involves the commitment of offenders after their criminal sentence has been completed. SVP legislation has been challenged on the grounds of ex post facto application, double jeopardy, due process, equal application, and vagueness of the statute.

The first case to test the constitutionality of SVP legislation was that of Terry Young in Washington State (*In re Young* 857 P2d 989 (Wash 1993)). The Court at that time declared the SVP clause of the CPA constitutional on the grounds that the legislation was civil and not criminal in nature and therefore did not constitute punishment. The first test of SVP legislation by the U.S. Supreme Court occurred in the case of *Hendricks* in 1997. Leroy Hendricks, a diagnosed pedophile, had a long history of sexual deviancy and had been convicted of molesting several young boys and girls beginning in 1955. He entered but never completed sex offender treatment programs, and admitted to harboring strong sexual desires for young children that he acted on when he got "stressed out." Hendricks challenged his civil commitment under the Kansas SVPA on substantive due process grounds, and claimed that the Act established criminal proceedings in violation of the ban on double jeopardy and ex post facto laws. The Court upheld Hendricks's commitment and declared SVP legislation constitutional on all grounds, stating that SVP legislation does not constitute punishment because the purpose of civil commitment is neither retribution nor deterrence. Interestingly, the Court also accepted the lack of treatment once incapacitated. Hendricks argued that treatment was not offered to him once he was detained, and the Court ruled that the SVPA is not punitive even if it fails to offer treatment for the mental abnormality. The Court called treatment an "incidental objective," and in his opinion, Justice Thomas claimed that preventive detention was an acceptable means of incapacitation for dangerous sexual predators.

Hundreds of other persons committed since Hendricks find themselves working within the confines of the Court's decision in his case, even though their own personal circumstances may vary significantly. As a result, they have little or no prospect for release in the foreseeable future (Purdy, 1997). For those who are released, they face the task of reintegration into the community under the auspices of Megan's Law.

In 2006, California passed "Proposition 83" (California, 2006), "Jessica's Law," which is currently being challenged in courts. Proposition 83:
Increases sentences and fines for sexual assault across the board.

- Expands and strengthens basic sexual assault punishment statutes, including those for "One-Strike" Sex Crimes, "Habitual Sex Offenders," and "Aggravated Sexual Assault of a Child."
- Increases the penalty to life imprisonment for kidnapping for the purpose of child molestation and for assault with the intent to commit sex crimes during a residential burglary.
- Expands the requirement for mandatory prison sentences and mandatory consecutive sentences for sex crimes.
- Requires registered sex offenders released on parole to wear a GPS tracking device for life.
- Requires offenders to pay for their own GPS equipment, if they are financially able.
- Prohibits registered sex offenders from living within 2000 feet of any school or park.
- Allows local governments to include additional sites they deem appropriate, such as a water park.
- Allows for the designation of predators as "sexually violent" after one offense, rather than waiting for a second strike.
- Allows for indefinite commitment to a state hospital until the SVP can prove to a court they no longer fit the criteria.
- Requires SVP's parole period to toll while in the state hospital so they still have to serve their parole time after discharge.
- Increases parole terms.
- Provides for parole terms of up to 10 years for the most heinous sex offenses (current law provides for parole terms from 3 to 5 years for various sex offenses).
- Keeps habitual sex offenders off the streets by denying the opportunity to reduce prison terms through the use of "good-time credits."
- Protects children from Internet luring: Allows law enforcement to act as decoys in order to engage and capture Internet predators.
- Increases penalties for possession of child pornography: Allows possession of child pornography to be prosecuted as a felony.
- Makes possession of child pornography a felony if the offender has a prior sex offense conviction.
- Imposes an additional 5-year prison term for persons who drug their victims in the commission of specified sexual crimes, such as rape.

Does Sex Offender Legislation Work?

To debate whether RCNL and SVP legislation is the best solution for how to deal with known sex offenders is moot. This legislation has been declared constitutional, is not likely to be repealed, and some states are even expanding their sex offender legislation to include acts such as mandatory chemical castration of recidivist sex offenders who live in the community and Community Supervision for Life (CSL). The question should now be how to make this legislation the most effective it can be for offenders, victims, and the community. In order to do that, it is important to understand the benefits and shortfalls of the legislation.

It is difficult to assess the effectiveness of RCNL, even a decade after its implementation. It is clear that RCNL can be used as an investigative tool after offenses occur, but no empirical studies provide evidence that RCNL prevents or reduces sexual abuse. Sexual abuse against children has been decreasing since the early 1990s, prior to the enactment of Megan's Law. It is possible that Megan's Law has played a role in the reduction of sexual abuse cases; however, this reduction may also be the result of more aggressive treatment, prosecution, and incarceration of offenders (Finkelhor & Jones, 2004).

The Kankas' argument for the creation of this legislation was a good one; RCNL may alert children to the presence of dangerous sex offenders within their neighborhood. However, a number of high-profile abductions in the summer of 2002 revealed a flaw in the premise of RCNL. Because it is imposed locally and only covers known offenders, it does not allow for the fact that many child killers (and many more nonviolent child molesters) are mobile and can abduct or abuse children out of the registration catchment area. RCNL will not prevent motivated offenders from abducting children from their homes (e.g., Elizabeth Smart) or in broad daylight (e.g., Samantha Runion), nor will it alert the community about individuals with no convictions for sexual offenses (e.g., Danielle van Dam). The rape and murder of Jessica Lunsford in 2005 revealed problems with risk assessment and compliance with the law, since alleged killer John Couey was assessed as being a moderate-risk sex offender and the community was therefore not notified about him and he was not living at the address that he registered with the police.

As RCNL regulations become stricter, it is not only possible but highly likely that sex offenders will move from one community to other less-restrictive ones, or they may abscond and choose not to register at all. In many jurisdictions, sex offenders have a low compliance rate with RCNL (e.g., officials in California could not verify the whereabouts of more than 33,000 sex offenders in 2002). With only the barest of resources devoted to this issue, the police in most jurisdictions are not able to verify compliance, resulting in a database that is incomplete and inaccurate. Threats of harm and acts of vigilantism also may inhibit offenders from registering their correct information with officials (e.g., the death of Joseph Gray and William Elliott, convicted sex offenders shot by Stephen Marshall in Maine after he saw their information on the state registry). When residency requirements become too strict, they can impede the efforts of community protection. An example of this can be seen in Iowa. Since legislators implemented residency requirements forcing sex offenders to live more than 2000 feet from anywhere that children may congregate, the number of unaccounted-for sex offenders has doubled; many offenders are homeless, living under bridges, at truck stops, etc.; many sex offenders are living together in the hotels that fit within the boundaries of the residency requirements; treatment providers focus only on compliance with the law, not with treatment for the offenders; and sex offenders with stable lives and jobs are forced to move and often lose their jobs (Barnhill & D'Amora, 2006).

In order to make RCNL as effective as possible at preventing sexual attacks, several things are necessary. First, sex offenders must abide by the terms of the legislation and provide accurate information to the police. Second, police departments must have the resources to investigate those offenders who abscond or provide false information. Third, community members must be able to access the information easily. The move toward Internet registries means that notification is more reactive than proactive, and most members of the community do not regularly search the public sex offender websites. Fourth, all websites that notify the community about sex offenders should also include information about sexual abuse and abusers. The public must be educated to understand that most sexual offenders are not known (because of the low levels of reporting of sexual offenses) and most acts of sexual abuse occur between individuals who are related to or otherwise know each other. This does not address the issues of vigilantism, how to increase reporting of offenses, or other problems with the legislation (e.g., how homeless offenders should register). However, without these factors occurring, RCNL is merely feel-good legislation with no basis for assisting the community.

Like RCNL, SVP legislation has several shortcomings. The aim of SVP legislation is to protect the community by incapacitating sex offenders and treating them. Incapacitating sex offenders will fulfill the utilitarian goal of community protection. So it is then important to consider whether the offenders are, in fact, being rehabilitated and reintegrated back into the community. To consider the question of rehabilitation, it is necessary to consider whether the medicalization of the sexual abuse problem is beneficial or harmful to the offenders and whether the treatment offered to offenders is appropriate for this population.

In order to assess the impact of civil commitment on sex offenders, it is possible to apply the principle of therapeutic jurisprudence. Therapeutic jurisprudence assesses how the law may act as a therapeutic agent by having a positive or negative effect on those going through the legislative process (La Fond, 1999; Wexler, 1990). SVP legislation seems to have a negative impact on the SVPs by discouraging them from taking responsibility for their conduct (La Fond, 1999). It forestalls any personal attributions of autonomy or responsibility for that condition and thus may be antitherapeutic. It takes the social (or public health) problem of sexual abuse and turns it into a medical one, thus diminishing the possibility that a person can be cured of that problem. The medicalization of sexually deviant behavior is not grounded in any articulated legal standard (Janus, 1997:350), and the hospital setting allows moral problems (such as sexual offending) to be recast (by the offenders and society) as medical problems. Thus, offenders do not take responsibility for their actions.

Additionally, medicalizing the sexual abuse problem and removing responsibility from the offender directly contrasts the goal of sex offender treatment, specifically the concept of relapse prevention. Relapse prevention is one part of cognitive–behavioral treatment programs that requires offenders to take control of their thoughts, fantasies, ideas, and actions (Pithers, Marques, Gibat, & Marlatt, 1983). It encourages them to take responsibility for and manage their behavior. Relapse prevention is considered to be the backbone of cognitive–behavioral treatment for sex offenders, and civil commitment contradicts the principles taught through it. If, however, SVPs do have mental disorders that render them in need of medical treatment, then it is unlikely that the treatment offered to them will be useful. Most secure facilities offer a standard cognitive–behavioral treatment program, which is generally considered to be the most effective type of treatment for sex offenders.

It is not clear whether cognitive–behavioral treatment methods are effective at rehabilitating SVPs, because not all of those committed actually participate in treatment. In May 2006, 1954 of the 3646 civilly committed and detained SVPs were participating in sex offender specific treatment programs (Deming, 2006). There are many reasons for the lack of participation, one of which is the paradox presented by their treatment disclosures. In order to be deemed "rehabilitated," SVPs must fully address their offending behavior in a treatment program. This includes acknowledging their cognitive distortions, fantasies, and lack of victim empathy, as well as offense histories and arousal patterns (13 states use polygraphs and 14 use the penile plethysmographs [PPG] for such assessments)(Deming, 2006). Disclosures of their deviant acts and fantasies during treatment may reduce their chances of release, as the treatment providers may view such factors as putting the offenders at a high risk of recidivating if back in the community.

Because so few SVPs are released, there is no research on the effectiveness of civil commitment. In order to be released, sex offenders must participate in treatment, must be "rehabilitated," and they must then be assessed as not being a high risk to recidivate again in the future. Because the SVPs are generally deemed high-risk offenders due to historical factors on risk assessment instruments (e.g., the violence used in their previous offenses), it is difficult for them to later be assessed as low-risk offenders. Once incapacitated, only the dynamic factors, such as acknowledgment of responsibility for their offenses, can be reassessed. When sex offenders are released, they face a daunting task: reintegration into a community that does not want them and, in some cases, actively keeps them out. RCNL requirements stipulate that the community be notified when an offender is released in the area. The SVPs must remain in the secure facility until their safety is assured and living conditions are secured. In many cases, this does not happen, and the offender is incapacitated well beyond the intended date of release (Carabello, 2006). This should not, and cannot, happen; unless we as a society want the current legislation to be deemed unconstitutional on the basis of cruel and unusual punishment and double jeopardy, we must make an effort to understand, treat, and effectively manage sexual offenders without violating their rights and creating a greater risk for them to reoffend.

Summary and Implications

Sex offender legislation is becoming increasingly punitive, with new policies and regulations being implemented regularly. Whether or not these policies are effective at reducing sexual victimization has yet to be empirically measured. In the meantime, policymakers can take some steps toward more effective management policies for this population.

- *Use empirical evidence when designing policy*. Many of the sex offender laws today are based on emotionally charged sex crimes against children. The crimes on which the legislation is based are rare, extreme cases, and do not represent the norm. The feel-good legislation that results is not necessarily in the best interest of the community, the victims, or the offenders. It is important to fully understand the risks and needs of this population before implementing legislation that is overly strict and ineffective at accomplishing the goal.

- *Education about the sex offender population.* It is imperative to educate both the public and those who manage and supervise sex offenders in the community. The key points to this education include: (1) sexual offenses are underreported, and it is impossible to fully understand this population without knowing the true population of abusers; (2) sexual abuse is significantly more likely to occur between family, friends, and acquaintances than strangers; and (3) ostracizing offenders from society will not help them to take responsibility for their offenses and, ultimately, reduce their chances of recidivating.

- *Sex offenders constitute a heterogeneous population.* Creating legislation that encompasses all sexual offenders will not allow for ideal or even effective management of this population. Sex offenders are not alike; they begin abusing for different reasons and there are different treatment and management strategies that will work for different types of offenders.

- *Risk assessment is faulty.* Though risk assessment procedures are improving, it is still impossible to accurately predict who will commit offenses in the future. As such, clinicians may over- or underpredict dangerousness, though they are most likely to err on the side of overprediction.

- *Reintegration is important.* Most sex offenders live in the community. It is important to integrate or reintegrate them into the community in order to reduce their chances of recidivating. Policies that are too strict do not work. This is now clear with the residency requirements that are being implemented. The problem of sex offenders in the community will not go away, and it is important for agencies to work together to determine the best system of management for offenders.

- *Focus resources on high-risk offenders.* By stretching treatment, management, and supervision resources across all sex offenders, those with the highest risks and most needs are not receiving enough attention. All sex offenders are not equal and do not pose an equal threat to the community, and targeted strategies are necessary in order to most effectively reduce the risk of reoffense. This can include a variety of management techniques (e.g., GPS tracking, treatment to intensive supervision).

- *Collaboration between agencies is necessary for effective management.* Multiple agencies are involved in the management of sex offenders in the community. The containment model of management, which focuses on the collaboration of multiple agencies, has shown to be most effective at supervising offenders in the community, particularly those who pose a high risk. This approach focuses on offender accountability, sex offender-specific treatment, intensive supervision, and surveillance, and is a victim-centered approach to sex offender management (Carabello, 2006).

References

Abel, G.G., Lawry, S.S., Karlstrom, E., Osborn, C.A., & Gillespie, C.F. (1994). Screening tests for pedophilia. *Criminal Justice and Behavior, 21*, 115–131.

Abel, G., & Osborn, C. (1992). Stopping sexual violence. *Psychiatric Annals, 22*, 301–306.

Alexander, R. (1993). The civil commitment of sex offenders in light of Foucha v. Louisiana. *Criminal Justice and Behavior, 20*, 371–387.

American Psychiatric Association. (1999). *Dangerous sex offenders: A task force report of the American Psychiatric Association*. Washington, DC: Author.

American Psychiatric Association.(2000). *Diagnostic and statistical manual of mental Disorders* (4th ed.). Washington, DC: Author.

Ashby, C.M. (2006). *National sex offender registry: New hires data has potential for updating addresses of convicted sex offenders*. Washington, DC: U.S. Government Accountability Office.

Barnhill, E., & D'Amora, D.A. (2006, September). *Extreme measures to control sex offenders: The ethics of silence in a politically charged climate*. Paper presented at the Association for the Treatment of Sexual Abusers Conference, Chicago.

Bureau of Justice Statistics (2001). *Sourcebook of Criminal Justice Statistics, 1999*. Washington, DC.; US Department of Justice.

California Proposition 83 Sex Offenders. Sexually Violent Predators. Punishment, Residence Restrictions and Monitoring. Initiative Statute, 2006.

Carabello, K. (2006, September). *Outpatient management of the sexually violent predator*. Paper presented at the Association for the Treatment of Sexual Abusers Conference, Chicago.

Deming, A.H. (2006, September). *Sex offender civil commitment program demographics and characteristics*. Paper presented at the Association for the Treatment of Sexual Abusers Conference, Chicago.

Doren, D.M. (2006, September). *Sexual offender civil commitment laws: Then and now*. Paper presented at the Association for the Treatment of Sexual Abusers Conference, Chicago.

Finkelhor, D., & Jones, L.M. (2004). *Explanations for the decline in child sexual abuse cases*. Washington, DC: Office of Juvenile Justice and Delinquency Protection.

Hanson, R.K. (2005). Twenty years of progress in violence risk assessment. *Journal of Interpersonal Violence, 20*, 212–217.

Hanson, R.K., & Harris, A. (2001). A structured approach to evaluating change among sexual offenders. *Sexual Abuse: A Journal of Research and Treatment, 13*, 105–122.

Hemphill, J.F., Hare, R.D., & Wong, S. (1998). Psychopathy and recidivism: A review. *Legal and Criminological Psychology, 3*, 139–170.

Janus, E.S. (1997). The use of social science and medicine in sex offender commitment. *New England Journal on Criminal and Civil Commitment, 23*, 347–386.

Janus, E.S., & Meehl, P.E. (1997). Assessing the legal standard for predictions of dangerousness in sex offender commitment proceedings. *Psychology, Public Policy, and Law, 3*, 33–64.

Jenkins, P. (1998). *Moral panic: Changing concepts of the child molester in modern america*. New Haven: Yale University Press.

Kemshall, H. (2001). *Risk assessment and management of known sexual and violent offenders: A review of current issues*. Police Research Series, Paper 140. London: Home Office.

La Fond, J.Q. (1999). Can therapeutic jurisprudence be normatively neutral? Sexual predator laws: Their impact on participants and policy. *Arizona Law Review, 41*, 375.

Litwack, T.R. (1993). On the ethics of dangerousness assessments. *Law and Human Behavior, 17*, 479–482.

McGrath, R.J. (1991). Sex offender risk assessment and disposition planning: A review of clinical and empirical findings. *International Journal of Offender Therapy and Comparative Criminology, 35*, 328–350.

Perceptions of child sexual abuse as a public health problem—Vermont, September 1995. (1997). *Morbidity and Mortality Weekly Report, 46*(34), 801–803.

Pithers, W.D., Marques, J.K., Gibat, C.C., & Marlatt, G.A. (1983). Relapse prevention with sexual aggressives: A self-control model of treatment and maintenance of change. In J.G. Greer & I.R. Stuart (Eds.), *The sexual aggressor: Current perspectives on treatment*. New York: Van Nostrand Reinhold.

Purdy, M. (1997, June 29). Wave of new laws seeks to confine sexual offenders. *New York Times* (Northeast ed.), p. A1, col. 1.

Quinsey, V.L., Lalumiere, M.T., Rice, M.E., & Harris, G.T. (1995). Predicting sexual offences. In J.C. Campbell (Ed.), *Assessing dangerousness: Violence by sexual offenders, batterers and child abusers*. Thousand Oaks, CA: Sage.

Stermac, L.E., Segal, Z.V., & Gillis, R. (1990). Social and cultural factors in sexual assault. In W.L. Marshall, D.R. Laws, & H.E. Barbaree (Eds.), *Handbook of sexual assault: Issues, theories and treatment of the offender*. New York: Plenum Press.

Terry, K.J. (2006). *Sexual offenses and offenders: Theory, practice and policy*. Belmont, CA: Wadsworth.

Terry, K.J., & Furlong, J.S. (2003). *Registration and community notification: A "Megan's Law" sourcebook* (2nd ed.). Kingston, NJ: Civic Research Institute.

Wexler, D.B. (1990). *Therapeutic jurisprudence: The law as a therapeutic agent*. Durham, NC: Carolina Academic Press.

Chapter 28

Electronic Health Records Systems and Continuity of Care

Ralph P. Woodward

Introduction: Making the Case for an Electronic Health Records Systems

The electronic health record system (EMR or EHR) has become a foundation principle in every modern solution offered as a method for improving health care. Despite encouragement from the federal government (Bush, 2004a,b, 2005), few state departments of corrections have implemented electronic medical records systems. This parallels the free world where paper medical records continue to predominate (Moore, 2006; Oliner, 2002). It is not clear why medical systems have been slow to adopt electronic medical records. Cost remains a substantial impediment for most correctional facilities but it cannot be expense alone. Hospitals possess elaborate computerized financial departments and correctional facilities commonly employ computerized booking and commissary programs, thus there is no objection to the use of computerized records in these settings. Indeed, hospital and clinic managers would see as foolhardy any attempt to run a health care business without a computerized financial system. The loss of a misplaced paper billing record would be seen as catastrophic, but surprisingly scant attention is given to the deplorable state of most paper medical records. When a paper chart cannot be recovered, we simply create another one—a process common enough that it is considered normal. This practice would be unacceptable in any other area of the medical business enterprise.

Most areas of technical service delivery have long since adopted electronic systems to contain errors and improve service—airline scheduling systems are electronic and there are no manual telephone switching systems in existence. Given the life and death scenario of medical services, it is unacceptable that error prone manual systems continue to be a major source of medical misadventure. On discharge from prison, inmates move through a series of unrelated health care providers accumulating diagnostic and medication errors as they move along. These errors are a substantial source of morbidity and medical expense. Were there a durable, portable electronic health record or some form of recoverable national medical record these errors could be reduced. There are no technical limitations to achieving these goals and they have been demonstrated in many local and European national projects.

Electronic health records are not new (Davis, Collen, Rubin, & Van Brunt, 1968; Korein, Goodgold, & Randt, 1966; Slack, Hicks, Reed, & Van Cura, 1966), and as systems are employed in real-world applications, sober assessments of what can or cannot be accomplished are becoming apparent (Sichel, 1997). There is now sufficient field experience to judge what impact electronic health records systems might have on correctional facilities and the ability of correctional facilities to interact with community health service providers. Can the purchase and installation of an electronic health records system improve the delivery of health services? Theory and current practice suggest yes—though success requires attention to detail and will come at some expense.

Professionally trained medical staffs have relatively little input into the design, budgeting, or purchasing of medical services within their correctional facilities. Thus, those who would best appreciate the benefits of an electronic health record are not in a position to advocate for its purchase. The benefits of an electronic health record may be unapparent to the nonmedical professional and it remains the task of the health services managers to convince administrators of the value in these systems. The excessive oversell of electronic medical records system and their purported benefits contributes to skepticism on the part of purchasers and undermines the credibility of the health services administrator. Electronic medical records are not a magic bullet solution to failing health care delivery systems. A well-managed health system with paper-based medical records can achieve the same good outcome as an electronic medical records system. A casually deployed and maintained electronic medical records system can result in the unrecoverable loss of confidential medical information.

Despite legitimate concerns associated with the use of electronic health records, all medical systems, including correctional medical departments, should anticipate that the purchase of an EMR is inevitable. In most cases this will require substantial investment in IT infrastructure, training, and institutional management practices. Early planning will be the best approach to a smooth transition.

Desirable features of electronic health records systems and how one might evaluate a system have been extensively reviewed (Bell et al., 2004) and tools are available to guide the purchaser (EMR Edge, 2006; Medical Strategic Planning, 2006) in making a choice. In making the argument for deploying an electronic medical record, health services managers should exercise caution in overstating traditional claims which represent generally unachievable results.

What Can Be Achieved Today?

The immediate benefit of an electronic medical record is that information is stored in digital format and therefore immediately recoverable and transportable over communications networks. This is an obligate first step if the medical record is to become part of a national health care database as envisioned by the National Institutes of Health (Committee on Data Standards for Patient Safety, 2003).

Electronic health records have a central location on a database server and can be accessed by multiple users at the same time. This immediately eliminates the problem of lost records especially when inmates are moved to new housing locations. In a well-designed system, multiuser access allows all chart contributors to write to a single centralized chart. This eliminates the possibility of multiple charts on a single inmate where each chart may contain different information. This reduces the possibility that different clinicians are pursuing different treatment goals unknown to the other and simultaneously reduces litigation exposure that results from multiple conflicting medical records on an individual.

Electronic medical records are transportable over existing networks and offer the possibility of a truly portable and possibly centralized health record. Digital storage media such as CD-ROMs are more durable than paper records and can be transported by inmates without any requirement for high-tech equipment beyond routinely available desktop computers. They are confidential and secure by nature, and the CD-ROM has no resale value on the street. The ability to connect correctional provider to community-based provider with a portable clinical record is a major goal of electronic health records.

Electronic health records hold great potential for reducing medical errors—primarily through containment of medication errors but also by eliminating illegible chart entries and providing physician prompts for various services. Current EMR offerings are able to detect simple errors such as medication dosing, adverse medication interactions and allergy alerts; but the potential exists to intercept cases where a treatment plan may be failing to achieve the desired endpoint.

Automated clinical decision making is theoretically possible but not common in commercially available EMRs. This kind of software has demonstrated its usefulness in ECG readings and could be extended to laboratory interpretation and possibly assist in choosing complex medication regimens. General diagnostic software, despite years of development, remains unreliable and controversial (Alexander, 2006; Coiera & Westbrook, 2006; Joch, 2006).

The ability to do sophisticated data analysis and mining on large datasets is already common in many industries. The EMR provides an exceptional opportunity to do CQI not on samples, but on entire datasets. It seems reasonable to assume that accrediting agencies will take advantage of this capability and future accreditation may require a level of reporting that can be achieved only with electronic medical records. Real-time and continuous analysis of a clinical database provides a rich source for trend analysis, productivity reporting, cost containment, and syndromic surveillance.

Ultimately the best argument for installing an electronic medical records system is that it may well be impossible to run a medical department without one. Billing services, responses to litigation, disease reporting to regulatory agencies, and performance reporting are likely to be the driving force in the purchase of an electronic health records system rather than purely clinical necessity.

What Cannot Be Routinely Achieved?

Traditional advantages ascribed to electronic health records system have for the most part not been borne out by actual practice—or come only at unreasonable expense. When these features are oversold by software retailers or Health Services Managers, disappointment in the performance of electronic records is the inevitable result. Compared to other software products, EMRs are not complicated pieces of engineering. Commercially available applications are passive systems that attempt to mimic the paper process in digital format. One could argue that there is little benefit in having a physician type the same progress note on a keyboard that could as easily be written on paper. Equally disabling is forcing staff to view a medical record on a small, congested display terminal when the record can more conveniently and accurately be reviewed on paper. These criticisms and others are valid largely because available software systems have failed to take full advantage of computational platforms. Benefits of electronic-based health records will be realized as the marketplace for electronic health records systems grows and as purchasers demand useful advanced features designed by medical professionals.

Eliminate Medical Records Departments and Reduce Medical Records Staffing

Health Services Managers are cautioned not to make this feature a primary argument in support of an electronic medical records system. Most facilities will not have the technical or financial ability to achieve a paperless system. Thus, there will be a need to maintain a traditional paper-based medical records system for outside documents that are not in electronic format. Primarily this will be hospital discharge summaries, consultant reports, radiology reports, and any document requiring an inmate's signature. Although not recommended, some correctional facilities may elect to print the electronic record and store a backup in paper. This will result in an even larger paper-based medical records system. Facilities that are successful in eliminating all paper will do so only with an IT (information technology) infrastructure that is many times more expensive than a traditional medical records department. The cost of going paperless is the cost of writing custom interfaces between various medical data providers who will have had no prior experience in exporting electronic medical information. An exception to this are laboratory vendors who have been moving data in HL7 (health level 7) format for many years.

While there are no technical impediments to encoding all medical data in HL7 (or other standard format), current systems adhere to few or no requirements and there is only weak consensus on what features or transmission protocols future systems should support.

Can Speed Up the Delivery of Health Services

Electronic health record systems are written by software retailers, not clinicians. Features are designed and marketed to business managers—the usual purchaser of the system. Software engineers design features that appeal to business managers and are usually marketed as time saving. Endless pull-down menus that attempt to list every eventuality and question can turn a simple patient encounter into a chore. It is not uncommon to watch medical staff do their work on paper and then to input their paper notes into the EMR at a later date. Medical staff are forced to alter their practices to suit the machinery—sometimes to the exclusion of the patient. The use of an EMR may seem alien to new users. Not because the computer is difficult to use, but because the medical process is usually adapted to suit the needs of the computer or more correctly the needs of the software engineer. Picking disease and symptom choices from a pull-down menu may give a clinician a false sense of security. Canned notes can create the illusion of a comprehensive medical plan where none exists. Paradoxically, electronic medical records can contain less information than paper records. Repetitive canned notes containing no novel information create databases where every patient appears to be a copy of the previous patient. This reduction in novel medical information reduces the usefulness of data mining algorithms—a vital medical management tool.

Expensive, with Reoccurring Licensure Costs

Unless you are using public domain software or an in-house developed application, expect to pay recurring "maintenance" costs. These costs amount to annual expenditures of 10–12% of total purchase cost and have little to do with actual product maintenance. You should also anticipate the need for regular upgrades as the manufacturer drops support for the previous version.

Records are HIPAA Compliant and More Secure Than Paper

Electronic record security can be very good and most systems are HIPAA compliant. To achieve full security requires intelligent assignment of access privileges and roles as well as good policies on system abuses. Access privileges and roles are used to carefully delineate who has access to privileged medical information. Adequate antivirus and possible firewall protection are a must. The simple act of allowing a laptop to travel home can compromise many confidential medical records. This was graphically demonstrated in May 2006 when a Veterans Affairs employee transferred 26 million military veteran's records to a CD and took them home to work on. The CD was subsequently lost during a burglary.

No Record Access When the System Goes Down

For those times when the system is unavailable, there must be an interim system. Large systems will rely on redundant servers; however, paper will be the interim system for small facilities. These temporary paper records must be transcribed into the EMR once the system is available. Casual backup and retrieval policies can lead to catastrophic loss of medical records.

What Kinds of Advanced Features are Possible with Today's Technology?

Retail stores take advantage of data-mining algorithms that look for associations between purchase transactions (Agrawal & Srikant, 1994) and are used to predict future purchase patterns for a specific shopper. This same algorithm could be applied to a large medical database to look for associative rules that would predict which inmates are at highest risk for suicide in a local facility and display that information in near real time. Network analysis is already a common computational tool used to predict the spread of contagious diseases. If applied to the closed system of a correctional facility, the analysis could direct administrators how to proceed with isolation and quarantine of inmates and staff to control the spread of in-house contagious diseases. These advanced features, while common in other software products, will have to wait for the next generation of corrections-specific electronic health records systems.

What Could Be Achieved If Correctional Physicians Took the Leadership

Two problems inhibit the wide-scale adoption of electronic health records systems in the field of corrections: (1) the high cost of installation, management, and maintenance and (2) the inability to move electronic medical information between dissimilar systems. Neither represents technical limitations. In countries with national medical policies, mandated data transfer protocols and government purchased or subsidized data infrastructures have resolved both issues (Anderson, Frogner, Johns, & Reinhardt, 2006). By contrast, in the United States, several hundred software retailers compete in a small medical market. No single EMR vendor has been able to predominate and thus lend support for one of the established data protocol standards. Standards groups such as HL7 have presented no compelling reason to software retailers to adopt published standards.

Surprisingly few HMOs have demanded that health care providers adopt electronic medical records capable of importing and exporting data in an ANSI standard format. Were large HMOs to require the use of a standard electronic health record, it would likely jump-start a disorganized health delivery system toward a national, portable health records system.

With more than 2 million persons behind bars (Department of Justice, Bureau of Justice Statistics, 2006), the correctional community should be seen as a major provider of medical and mental health services. The medical operational characteristics of jails and prisons are sufficiently similar across the country to be considered a single system. In fact, were correctional facilities to be viewed as a corporate HMO, it would rank in the top 10 for enrollment (Table 28.1). Hospitals that provide medical services to inmates

Table 28.1 Largest U.S. health maintenance organizations.

Plan name	Enrollment (12/31/03)
Kaiser Permanente of N. Calif.	3,229,531
Kaiser Permanente of S. Calif.	3,204,401
Blue Cross of Calif.	2,555,487
Health Net of Calif.	2,429,951
PacifiCare of Calif.	1,735,792

Source: Advanstar Communications, Inc. (Walker, 2004).

are major financial beneficiaries of the correctional establishment. It would not be unreasonable to expect them to participate in a dialog concerning the exchange of electronic medical documents.

Core functionality of electronic health records systems has recently taken a step toward uniformity when the Certification Commission for Healthcare Information Technology issued its first 22 certifications. However, those features do not address the basic needs of a correctional EMR and the unique way correctional medicine is practiced. Also, certification does not address the manner in which systems will exchange data.

Correctional accrediting bodies such as the National Commission on Correctional Health Care, the American Correctional Association, or leadership groups such as the Society of Correctional Physicians are in a position to define "correctional best practices" and data exchange standards. Hospitals that serve the correctional community should be expected to adopt these standards. Additionally, correctional leadership groups are in the best position to define core functionality and certify compliant systems. Failure to take the lead at this critical time will allow alien practices and inefficient processes to be forced on the correctional environment.

Although the correctional health care market is small, its impact on national health care is disproportionately large. Correctional professionals with the skill to write electronic database systems could realistically produce software that would streamline correctional health care practices, reduce errors, and yield useful management information.

Community Connections

What does it mean to transfer medical information electronically and how does this differ from moving a paper record? Consider that when we move a paper record, we first spawn a new record by copying the existing record. The sender of the record retains ownership of the original record and the receiver of the copied record incorporates the paper chart into a new data structure. That record structure is further modified over time and is passed on to the next provider. In this scenario the medical record is a collection of documents with multiple owners, in different formats, and spread over a large geographic area. Once a paper chart moves beyond its primary data owner (usually the medical office that initiated the chart), connecting the parts of the chart into a unified record is difficult. In most cases a physician will never see a complete medical record until plaintiff's attorney connects all the pieces in a malpractice case.

The mere presence of an electronic health record does nothing to repair this problem. Each electronic health record system has its own unique method of storing and retrieving data which is unknown to the next EMR. Thus, there are two problems to be solved: (1) produce an electronic health record that is universal in nature such that it can be accessed by any EMR software and (2) produce a transportable record that contains all entries by all providers regardless of the location or setting of health care. In theory, goal number (2) does not require an electronic record. One could envision a system where the patient retains physical ownership of a paper record and transports the record to the point of service delivery. However, the fragility of paper and the unreliability of the process make this implausible and unnecessary in a modern world. Before there can be electronic linkage between community providers and correctional providers, there must be a common platform for data exchange and a system that allows all parts of a medical record to be retrieved by legitimate users.

Toward a Common Platform for Data Exchange

Readers might be surprised to learn that ANSI-approved standards for the exchange of electronic medical data have been available for more than a decade. Equally surprising is that many commercial vendors of medical software are unaware of these protocols. Each vendor has adopted a style and method that is unique to its product, and to date any electronic connection between products has been through the design of custom interfaces. The most successful exchange protocols have been developed by large software houses and accepted by small vendors who have no choice if they wish to stay in business. In the medical industry and especially in the field of corrections, no software vendor has been able to market to more than a few clients and thus no *de facto* standards have emerged as they have in other industries. The current medical standards have been arrived at through painful and slow collaboration between many competing participants. In Europe, standards succeed through regulatory requirements. In other limited circumstances, standards have succeeded when they are given away for free as in open-source, public domain software. A major impediment to the adoption of standards and protocols is proprietary ownership of those standards. The American Medical Association owns the CPT codes, SNOMED (SNOMED, 2005) is owned by the American College of Pathologists, and DSM-4 codes are owned by the American Psychiatric Association. In each case, use of these established vocabularies requires payment to its owner (note: the National Library of Medicine has purchased a general use license for the use of SNOMED). We will discuss the various data exchange protocols later in this chapter.

Toward a Unified Medical Record

The challenge of a single source location for a patient's complete medical record is even more difficult than that of the portable medical record. This goal envisions some national data repository where all medical records would be written to or read from. While technically achievable, it would require changes to the legal structure to prevent antitrust suits and an upgrade in data bandwidth of existing transmission lines to support transfer of images and sound. Point-to-point fiber-optic connections would likely be required to avoid long transmission delays. Tradition has long held that the owner of the record and the primary provider are one and the same. In some cases owning the medical record is considered equivalent to owning the business exchange with the patient.

Introduction to Health Data Exchange Standards

Standards (e.g., specifications or protocols) are simply operating rules-of-the-road that have been agreed to by everyone. Common examples include: the QWERTY keyboard, the placement order of numbers on your telephone, driving on the right-hand side of the road, 120 volts from your electrical outlet, the amount of fat in regular milk, the size of a cord of wood, width of train tracks, height of truck trailers, and thousands more. Standards are neither good nor bad, and by agreeing to them we provide for the orderly running of society. Standards may arise through purposeful design (as will be the case here) or they may arise informally, usually because they are pushed by a dominant player in some industry.

Health Level 7 (HL7)

Health Level Seven (Health Level Seven, Inc., 2006) is an American National Standards Institute ANSI-accredited Standards Developing Organization (SDO), whose charter is to produce standards in the clinical and administrative data domain. This SDO was founded in 1987 and like other ANSI-accredited SDOs is a not-for-profit volunteer organization. Standards are developed by members who may include providers, vendors, payers, consultants, and government groups who have an interest in the development of clinical and administrative standards for health care. SDOs do not write software. Instead, SDOs like Health Level Seven develop specifications that are used by software architects to write electronic health records systems. In the case of HL7, the standards being written are messaging protocols that enable unrelated health care applications to exchange sets of clinical and administrative data.

Health Level Seven members, known as the Working Group, are organized into technical committees and special interest groups (SIGs). SIGs are responsible for looking at end-user needs in specific areas and bringing those needs to the attention of the HL7 Working Group. Currently there is a SIG involved in HL7 standards as they relate to community provision of mental health. There is no SIG specifically addressing community connections unique in the field of correctional medicine.

HL7 is a text-based encoding system that represents clinical data in a structured format that can be parsed by any EMR system that "speaks" HL7. The first version of the HL7 standard (V.2.x) was adopted 13 years ago and version 3.0 has recently been adopted. Although this standard is well established, it is unlikely that many health care clinicians will have heard of it and many electronic health records systems do not support it. The current primary clinical application of HL7 is the transmission of laboratory data to electronic medical records systems; beyond this application, little clinical data are exchanged between systems with HL7 coding. Purchasers of future systems should expect that all clinical data on their EMR can be encoded and transmitted in HL7.

HL7 is strictly text-based and while intended to be read by machine, is human-readable. Although the standard requires the message to be human-readable, it would be rare to encounter it in this form. Usually it is parsed and loaded in an EMR application for reading.

For Developers

There are several web sites that provide sample HL7 messages that can be used to test a system's ability to parse an HL7 message. HL7 version 2.x is a loosely defined protocol. Vendors are given freedom to omit fields and as a result messages vary significantly between vendors. Because it is not possible to predict in advance precisely what fields an HL7 message may consist of, there are many errors in parsing messages. Inevitably, importing HL7 messages successfully requires a semicustomized interface for each vendor your EMR system needs to connect to.

HL7 version 3.0 markedly reduces optionality of the message content and takes HL7 closer to a true plug and play data transfer protocol. Additionally, HL7 will utilize the widely accepted XML protocol to envelop HL7 message content which will further increase system interoperability. Unfortunately, the cost and complexity of upgrading existing systems from HL7 version 2.x to 3.0 will likely require purchasers to wait until new EMR applications are written.

Extensible Markup Language (XML)

XML (World Wide Web Consortium [W3C], 2005) has been selected as the data transfer protocol for version 3.0 of HL7. While HL7 messages will continue to appear as described above, they may be optionally enveloped in an XML structure. Because many applications and web browsers are already XML compliant, this change in HL7 version 3.0 will build on preexisting compatibility between systems. A complete XML document consists of three components: the data schema, a style sheet, and the document itself. The three elements may be physically separate or enclosed in a single XML transmission. The data schema provides information on how the data are to be interpreted (field names, data types, data constraints). This is required if the data are to be imported into some other application such as an EMR for processing, searching, or queries. The optional style sheet is used to instruct a browser or other application on how to display the document for reading.

The primary function of XML is not to encode the physical appearance of a document but to instruct the receiving system on how data are to be interpreted. The machine receiving data would know the names of fields, the type of data the field represented (text, number, dates, etc.), and any constraints on the data values that the fields could contain. Functionally it would be similar to e-mailing a friend an attachment containing a Microsoft Access™ database except that with XML the receiving machine would not have to be running Windows™, Access™, or other proprietary software. Neither the sending application nor the receiving application need have any knowledge about the other if both are XML-compliant applications. XML can contain tags that are customized for different purposes. Virtually every industry—music, geology, chemistry, architecture—has published defined XML tags specific to that industry. To date there are no correctional-specific tags, and health care tags specific to community-based providers are currently in development.

HL7 Clinical Document Architecture (CDA)

The brief discussions on HL7 and XML prepare us to review CDA, the protocol best suited to moving clinical data between community providers and correctional facilities (Dolan et al., 2006). For the purposes of this discussion we may consider CDA to be an amalgam of HL7 and XML. CDA uses the vocabulary and data types derived from the HL7 Reference Information Model (RIM version 3) but encodes them in XML rather than in HL7. CDA release two was accepted as an ANSI standard in May 2005, replacing the previous version approved in November 2000.

HL7 CDA is a text-based, markup standard that specifies the structure of a clinical document. These documents can be of any nature: patient encounters, discharge summaries, consultants, diagnostic reports as well as images and sounds included in those documents. Because they are fundamentally XML, a data schema (defined in the HL7 RIM) is used to parse the data and pass them to some other application. An optional style sheet provides instructions to a browser on how to view the document where no additional processing is to be done.

CDA is already widely used in EU nations whose near-term goal is to store patient health records in national information infrastructures. CDA will be the data-exchange protocol for the proposed U.S. national medical database and will be used by HIPAA for all data exchanges. Currently, the largest field application of CDA is at the Mayo Clinic.

With this in mind we can propose a scenario whereby a released inmate is provided with a copy of his or her medical records in CDA format burned onto an inexpensive CD ROM. Community providers, with access to nothing more sophisticated than a web browser, would be able to immediately view a complete medical record, with laboratory results, flow sheets, or radiographic images. If the provider had access to an HL7 CDA-compliant EMR, the record could be updated, queried, or in some other way processed by the EMR application.

Data exchange protocols are for the most part written by standards groups consisting of computer scientists and software vendors with relatively little input from the technical end-user—in this case clinicians. This is not as strange as it seems since it simply separates the message (clinical content) from the vehicle used to convey the message. Physicians who use a telephone to relay medical information are not expected to also design the switching circuits that transmit the message. The expectation of the HL7 CDA project is to deliver a completed set of standards to medical professionals who will in turn define best practices described in some standard vocabulary. Correctional professionals will play a role in defining those best practices and vocabularies for the specialized field of correctional medicine.

Continuity of Care Record

There are multiple and possibly competing standards being developed in parallel with HL7 CDA (Ferranti, Musser, Kawamoto, & Hammond, 2006).

The Continuity of Care Record (CCR) is a standard specification developed jointly by ASTM International, the Massachusetts Medical Society (MMS), the Health Information Management and Systems Society (HIMSS), and the American Academy of Family Physicians (AAFP).

The CCR is a core data set summarizing a patient's problems, medications, allergies, insurance, advance directives, and care plan. The data set is fixed and nonextensible thereby providing for reliability and predictability in data exchange. Like HL7 CDA, the CCR is encoded in XML and is human-readable. The message content can be wrapped in an HL7 message or CDA-compliant document.

Development of the CCR is proceeding in parallel with HL7 CDA but is likely to be a short-term solution. The CCR is in effect a comprehensive chart summary rather than the chart itself and is modeled after paper forms required in Massachusetts. Structure, codes, and message standards remain under design. This initiative has relatively weak support from other standards bodies and it seems reasonable that this effort will be absorbed into HL7 CDA. Nevertheless, the simplicity of the model will allow the CCR to operate in advance of EHR interoperability.

Simple Methods to Transfer Electronic Medical Data

It is common practice to transfer medical data electronically in the form of spreadsheets, word processor documents, e-mail attachments, or simple MS Access™ databases. One might argue that this is the predominant method for moving clinical data as this is how we currently receive our consultant reports, X-ray reports, hospital discharges, and transfer summaries. Most modern software applications allow documents to be saved in XML format. Several office applications (examples include Microsoft InfoPath™, Adobe Forms Designer) are specifically designed to store and forward data in structured XML format. Recently, Microsoft has demonstrated a project that constructs a medical record from a series of InfoPath™ XML forms. While such an application does not meet the Institute of Medicine's vision of a future national health care record, it does have the advantage of generating and storing documents that are already compatible with the HL7 CDA model. Documents generated in this fashion could be imported into some future HL7-compliant EMR with little difficulty.

Where Do We Go from Here?

Adequate standards exist for describing portable electronic documents thus permitting free exchange between correctional setting and community provider. Existing EMRs do not support these data exchange protocols in a usable way, indeed many software architects are unaware that these standards exist. Of the more than 200 manufacturers of electronic health records systems, none predominates in the market and there is inadequate incentive to have EMR systems compatible with one another. The HL7 CDA architecture as well as other transfer protocols envision that once the technical platform is in place, professional groups would provide the top layer functionality by defining best practices and standard professional vocabularies. Unfortunately, the end professional user is rarely invited at the design phase and the health industry is left with software that ultimately is a retail programmer's cartoon of how a layman might practice medicine.

Implementing an Electronic Medical Records System

☑ Assume that installation of an electronic health records system is inevitable. Budget makers should be introduced to the concept with sufficient lead time to prepare.

☑ Use on-line tools (www.emredge.com/emr_list.php) to broadly survey available products for cost and features. Correctional trade shows allow side-by-side comparisons of correctional oriented EMRs.

☑ Have a software health consultant review your needs and product choices. Your consultant will also calculate number of required terminals and minimum IT infrastructure necessary to run a system.

☑ Rely heavily on the experience of correctional systems that have successfully installed EMRs.

☑ Once a product is chosen, allow atleast 24 months to install and test the system.

☑ Budget for an adequate IT infrastructure.

☑ Meet with community providers and where possible adopt common platforms. If a particular clinic or hospital system predominates, consider adapting it to your correctional facility.

☑ Provide for regular staff training—usually in the form of a computer lab.

☑ Staff a help desk.

☑ If possible an IT staff member should be part of the medical team to assist in report writing, screen updates and custom interfaces.

Figure 28.1 Implementing an electronic medical records system.

Currently there are more than 2 million persons incarcerated in the United States. That population plus the prisons and jails that hold them constitute a large, continuous, well-defined health records environment that is well suited to its own set of standards. Those standards build on the existing HL7 CDA protocol that allows for movement of electronic health records between participating correctional facilities (as in the case of correctional interstate compacts) and with free world providers who provide cooperative services to correctional facilities. While a unified data exchange protocol is achievable now, there are multiple competing groups and there will always be local modifications to standards (Mattison, Dolin, & Laberge, 2004). Standardized vocabularies are available and already incorporated into many products (LOINC, 2005). Lastly there remains the tantalizing possibility that more ready acceptance of open source, public domain electronic health records systems may bring about wide-scale use of these applications in the correctional health setting (openEHR Foundation, 2004).

Organizations such as the National Commission for Correctional Health Care and the American Correctional Association are positioned for leadership roles in hosting meetings of IT and correctional professionals who would define data payloads, EMR core features, and best practices that would be encoded into standards that have meaning in the correctional environment. The volume of medical information stored and coded in these corrections-based standards would provide an incentive to software houses to design products compliant with these standards.

References

Agrawal, R., & Srikant, R. (1994). Fast algorithms for mining generalized association rules. *Proceedings of the 20th International Conference on Very Large Data Bases, Santiago, Chile*.

Alexander, G.L. (2006). Issues of trust and ethics in computerized clinical decision support systems. *Nurs Adm Q, 30*, 21–29.

Anderson, G.F., Frogner, B.K., Johns, R.A., & Reinhardt, U.E. (2006). Health care spending and use of information technology in OECD countries. *Health Affairs, 25*, 819–831.

Bell, D.S., Marken, R.S., Meili, R.C., Wang, C.J., Rosen, M., & Brook, R.H. (2004). Recommendations for comparing electronic prescribing systems: Results of an expert consensus process. *Health Affairs, Web Exclusive & Supplemental Exhibit*, May 25, W4305–W4317.

Bush, G.W. (2004a, January 20). State of the Union Address.

Bush, G.W. (2004b, April 26). Speech to the annual convention of the American Association of Community Colleges.

Bush, G. W. (2005, January 27). President Discusses Health Care Information Technology Benefits, Intercontinental Cleveland Clinic Suite Hotel, Cleveland, Ohio.

Certification Commission for Healthcare Information Technology. (2006). Retrieved October 15, 2006, from www.cchit.org/certified/2006/CCHIT+Certified+Products+by+Product.htm.

Coiera, E.W., & Westbrook, J.I. (2006). Should clinical software be regulated? *Med J Aust, 184*, 601–602.

Committee on Data Standards for Patient Safety. (2003). Key capabilities of an electronic health records system: Letter report (2003). Washington, DC: The National Academies Press.

Davis, L.S., Collen, M.F., Rubin, L., & Van Brunt, E.E. (1968). Computer-stored medical record. *Comput Biomed Res, 1*, 452–469.

Department of Justice, Bureau of Justice Statistics. (2006). *Prison and jail inmates at midyear 2005.* Retrieved October 14, 2006, from http://www.ojp.usdoj.gov/bjs/abstract/pjim05.htm.

Dolan, R.H., Alschuler, L., Boyer, S., Beebe, C., Behlen, F.M., Biron, P. V., & Shabo, A. (2006). HL7 clinical document architecture, release 2. *J Am Med Inform Assoc, 3*, 30–39.

EMR Edge. (2006). Electronic medical record review and rating. Retrieved October 14, 2006, from http://www.emredge.com/emr_list.php.

Ferranti, J.M., Musser, R.C., Kawamoto, K., & Hammond, W.E. (2006). The clinical document architecture and the continuity of care record: A critical analysis. *J Am Med Inform Assoc, 13*, 245–252.

Health Level Seven. HL7 Version 3 Development Framework (HDF). (2005). Ann Arbor, MI: Health Level Seven, Inc.

Health Level Seven. (2006). Retrieved October 15, 2006, from http://www.HL7.org.

International Organization for Standardization. (2006). Retrieved October 15, 2006, from http://www.iso.org. Last modified 2006-09-12.

Joch, A. (2006). Built to crash. *Hosp Health Netw, 80*(2), 34–36.

Korein, J., Goodgold, A.L., & Randt, C.T. (1966). Computer processing of medical data by variable-field-length format: II. Progress and application to narrative documents. *JAMA, 196*, 132–138.

Logical Observation Identifiers Names and Codes (LOINC). (2005). Available from http://www.loinc.org/. Accessed June 11, 2005.

Mattison, J.E., Dolin, R.H., & Laberge, D. (2004). Managing the tensions between national standardization vs. regional localization of clinical content and templates. *Medinfo, 11*, 1081–1085.

Medical Strategic Planning. (2006). EHR selector. Retrieved October 14, 2006, from http://www.ehrselector.com.

Moore, P.L. (2006). Taming the beast. *2006/2007 physicians practice technology guide. Physicians Practice* pp. 7–10.

Oliner, S.D. (2002). Information technology and productivity: Where are we now and where are we going? *Federal Reserve Bank of Atlanta Economic Review, 87*, 15–44.

openEHR Foundation (2004). Retrieved October 26, 2006, from http://www.openehr.org/.

Sichel, D.E. (1997). *The computer revolution: An economic perspective.* Washington, DC: The Brookings Institution.

Slack, W.V., Hicks, G.P., Reed, C.E., & Van Cura, L.J. (1966). A computer-based medical history system. *N Engl J Med, 274*, 194–198.

SNOMED Clinical Terms. College of American Pathologists. (2005). Available from http://www.snomed.org/. Accessed June 11, 2005.

Walker, T., Managed Healthcare Executive Online, July 1, 2004, retrieved at: http://www.managedhealthcareexecutive.com/mhe/article/articleDetail.jsp?id=108175.

World Wide Web Consortium (W3C). (2005). XML Schema Part 2: Data types. W3C working draft, May 6, 1999. Retrieved June 11, 2005, from http://www.w3.org/1999/05/06-xmlschema-2/.

Chapter 29

Community Health and Public Health Collaborations

Thomas Lincoln, John R. Miles, and Steve Scheibel

Since the majority of inmates are eventually released back to their communities, public health officials have begun to recognize the tremendous public health opportunity within corrections and the potential to benefit the community with reduced illness rates, financial savings, improved public safety, and better use of the existing health care system and resources (Travis, Solomon, & Waul, 2001) From a policy perspective, inmates' health care and their reintegration back into the community began to take on new importance with the increasing number of HIV/AIDS cases identified in correctional settings (Conklin, Lincoln, & Flanigan, 1998) Collaborations between corrections, community, and public health programs at both federal and state levels have increasingly been developed to take advantage of the incarceration episode to decrease the burden of illness on those incarcerated and the greater community (Klein, O'Connell, Devore, Wright, & Birkhead, 2002; Roberts, Kennedy, & Hammett, 2004).

While the costs of prisoner reintegration are great, the opportunities to enhance the health and safety of the community are gaining in importance. By the mid-1990s, public health workers working in communities with high rates of HIV and other sexually transmitted disease (STDs) began to recognize the strong relationship among diseases, drug use, and periods of incarceration in jails and prisons among those infected with HIV. The lack of comprehensive public health approaches and the organizational framework to support continuity of care were contributing to significant and preventable disease morbidity among individuals who were at high risk for HIV/AIDS, TB, STDs, hepatitis, and other health problems (Hammett, 1998; Kennedy, Roberts, & Hammett, 2001) The Health Resources and Service Administration (HRSA)'s Special Projects of National Significance (SPNS) targeting incarcerated populations during the mid-1990s found that this was a significant problem for recently released inmates with HIV disease where effective clinical management and ongoing treatment were essential to prevent further HIV transmission. SPNS found that program models that integrate correctional and community-based prevention, primary care, and other supportive services were more effective maintaining continuity of care and reducing risk behaviors (HRSA, 2002).

The costs and opportunities associated with reentry and long-term reintegration of ex-prisoners are important questions that need to be addressed.

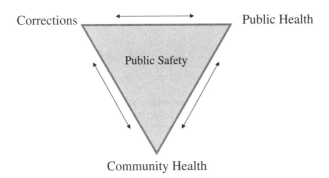

Figure 29.1 The Traid

How can corrections, public health, and communities work together to build a successful framework for reentry that addresses both the needs of the prisoner and those of the community to prepare for the return home (Freudenberg, 2004; Hammett, Roberts, & Kennedy, 2001; *Plan for Providing Medical Case Management and Support Services to Individuals with HIV Disease Being Released from Federal or State Prison—Report to Congress*, 2002)? And, most important, what types of policies can be realistically implemented to make a difference using current resources (Davis & Pacchiana, 2004; Hammett, 1998; Travis et al., 2001)?

Collaborations between public health and correctional agencies have evolved and are now an important venue of addressing the gaps in health care services for inmates. Public health departments have the mandate to prevent illness in the general population—particularly environmental and communicable diseases. Public health departments have the funds, staff, expertise, and other resources to help correctional facilities address the serious health needs of their inmates and thereby advance the cause of public health in their communities (Hammett, 1998; Klein et al., 2002) The same can be said for public health's interactions with community-based organizations (CBOs). Corrections and CBOs, in turn, need to collaborate as they share the same patients (though traditionally at different times) and families, and each have needed expertise and experience. Corrections, community health, and public health form a "triad" to maintain the health and safety of the entire community (see Figure 29.1).

Many types of collaborations exist between corrections and public health at a variety of levels (federal, state, local). State departments of corrections collaborate with public health at all levels but most often with state-level public health agencies. However, most collaborations are limited and focus only on the HIV-infected and/or mentally ill. While correctional, community, and public health systems value the collaborations, vast areas for improvement still remain, especially for the individual inmate on their release (Conklin, Lincoln, Wilson, & Gramarossa, 2002; *Corrections Agency Collaborations with Public Health: Special Issue in Corrections*, 2003).

The Public Health System

The Institute of Medicine Report, *The Future of the Public's Health in the 21st Century*, described government public health agencies as the backbone of the public health system. However, they stated that these agencies are clearly in

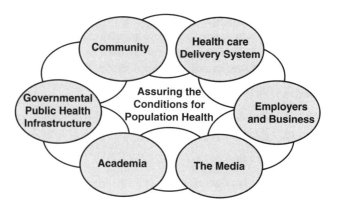

Figure 29.2 The Public Health System (Institute of Medicine 2002)

need of support and resources and that they cannot work alone. Public health agencies must build and maintain partnerships with other organizations and sectors of society, working closely with communities and community-based organizations, the health care delivery system, academia, business, and corrections. The health care delivery system plays a vital role in assuring the health of the public. Academic institutions train health and public health workers and conduct essential health-related research. Communities function as sites where health can either be supported or undermined. Through their various organizations and constituent entities, communities are major partners in the delivery of essential public health services that maintain health and safety (Institute of Medicine, 2002) Correctional settings play an essential role as public health "sentinels" (see Figure 29.2).

The nation's public health infrastructure covers the range of resources needed to deliver essential public health services to every community. This infrastructure is often described as a complex network of people, systems, and organizations working at the local, state, and national levels. The infrastructure includes all governmental and nongovernmental entities that provide any of these services. Environmental health, occupational health and safety, mental health, and substance abuse are integral components of the public health system. Service providers, such as managed care organizations, hospitals, nonprofit corporations, schools, faith-based organizations, correctional settings, and business, are also important parts of the public health infrastructure in many communities. ("Public Health Infrastructure, Healthy People 2010," 2004a)

The public health system is distinct from other parts of the health care system in two key respects: its primary emphasis on preventing disease and disability, and its focus on the health of entire populations, rather than individuals. Public health encompasses three core functions: assessment of information on the health of the community, comprehensive public health policy development, and assurance that public health services are provided to the community (Institute of Medicine, 2002) These functions have been further defined into 10 essential public health services.

Both the public and private sectors have key roles and responsibilities in public health. The nation is served by more than 3000 county and city health departments, more than 3000 local boards of health, 59 state and territorial health departments, tribal health departments, more than 160,000 public and

```
                    Exhibit 1:  Public Health in America

                Vision:  Healthy people in healthy communities
         Mission:  Promote physical and mental health and prevent disease, injury, and disability
Public health:
    ■   Prevents epidemics and the spread of disease
    ■   Protects against environmental hazards
    ■   Prevents injuries
    ■   Promotes and encourages healthy behaviors
    ■   Responds to disasters and assists communities in recovery
    ■   Assures the quality and accessibility of health services

Essential public health services:
    ■   Monitor health status to identify and solve community health problems
    ■   Diagnose and investigate health problems and health hazards in the community
    ■   Inform, educate, and empower people about health issues
    ■   Mobilize community partnerships and action to solve health problems
    ■   Develop policies and plans that support individual and community health efforts
    ■   Enforce laws and regulations that protect health and assure safety
    ■   Link people to needed personal health services and assure the provision of health care when otherwise unavailable
    ■   Assure a competent workforce – public health and personal care
    ■   Evaluate effectiveness, accessibility, and quality of personal and population-based health services
    ■   Research for new insights and innovative solutions to health problems.
                    http://www.health.gov/phfunctions/public.htm
```

Figure 29.3 Public Health in America (Public Health Functions Steering Committee, 1994)

private laboratories, and a series of federal health and environmental agencies that set national standards and provide funding, training, scientific guidance, and technical support. Their work is joined by a variety of managed care organizations, hospitals, numerous faith, civic, and volunteer groups, and key national associations. All must work together to ensure a healthy citizenry and a healthy environment. Unfortunately, this network of people, systems, and organizations is fragile and lacks adequate resources to address the complex issues found in communities today (Public Health Functions Steering Committee, 1994)

All public health services depend on the presence of basic infrastructure. Every categorical public health program—childhood immunizations, infectious disease monitoring, cancer and asthma prevention, drinking water quality, injury prevention, and many others—requires health professionals who are competent in cross-cutting and technical skills, public health agencies with the capacity to assess and respond to community health needs, and up-to-date information systems. Federal public health agencies rely on the presence of infrastructure systems at the local and state levels to support the implementation of their programs (Institute of Medicine, 2002).

In public health, a strong infrastructure provides the capacity to prepare for and respond to both acute and chronic threats to the nation's health, whether they are bioterrorism attacks, emerging infections, disparities in health status, or increases in chronic disease and injury rates. Such an infrastructure serves as the foundation for planning, delivering, and evaluating public health. The public health infrastructure comprises the workforce, data and information systems, and public health organizations. Research also is a key activity of public health infrastructure in identifying opportunities to improve health, strengthen information systems and organizations, and make more effective and efficient use of resources.

Health data and surveillance systems provide information on illness, disability, and death from acute and chronic conditions; injuries; personal, environmental, and occupational risk factors; preventive and treatment services;

and costs. To be most useful, public health data must be accessible, accurate, timely, and clearly stated and must adhere to strict confidentiality standards. The system must be linked with other data systems and must be linked with and integrated at the federal, state, and local levels. The systematic collection, analysis, interpretation, dissemination, and use of health data drive efforts to determine the health status of a population, plan prevention programs, and evaluate program effectiveness. If data are not available or are missing, problems can arise, especially for state and local health agencies. In particular, health problems may not be identified in high-risk populations, or the public intervention may not be timely enough. Information enables public health to direct preventive services and health promotion activities toward select populations such as corrections. The public health workforce must have up-to-date knowledge, skills, and abilities to deliver services effectively and carry out the core functions of assessment, policy development, and assurance of services. The importance of collaborating organizations in making the public health system effective often is overlooked.

The three components of the basic public health system are:

- *Workforce Capacity and Competency*: the expertise of the approximately 500,000 professionals who work in federal, state, and local public health agencies to protect the public's health.
- *Information and Data Systems*: up-to-date guidelines, recommendations, and health alerts and modern, standards-based information and communication systems that monitor disease and enable efficient communication among public and private health organizations, the media, and the public.
- *Organizational Capacity*: the consortium of local and state public health departments and laboratories, working side-by-side with private and community partners, to provide the essential services of public health.

Every health department fully prepared; every community better protected: These components are interrelated. Deficiencies in one area—or in one jurisdiction—have a ripple effect throughout the entire public health system. Therefore, the goal of strengthening public health's infrastructure is to achieve improvements in all three of these areas, in every part of the country. As with military preparedness, our public health system must be ready at all times to ward off threats and respond to crises. That same system can, through

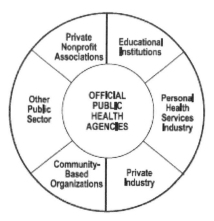

Figure 29.4 Public Health Workforce Framework (Kennedy and Moore, 2001)

community partnerships and efficacious interventions, elicit improvements in the health of its community residents. If the public health system is fully prepared to carry out the essential services, communities across the country will be better protected from both routine and acute health events (Institute of Medicine, 2002; Public Health Functions Steering Committee, 1994; "Public Health Infrastructure, Healthy People 2010," 2004b).

Public Health and Corrections Collaboration at Work

The missions of public health and corrections agencies can be complementary. Correctional facilities and inmate populations are part of the community, and public health is integral to public safety. While public health and correctional agencies are increasingly working together to improve the health of inmates and that of the community, there are many challenges and barriers that must be overcome. Correctional centers often do not recognize or accept a public health mission. Studies have found that most current collaborations are in disease surveillance, staff training, legislation and policy development, education/prevention programs, testing/screening/follow-up, and treatment services. There is little collaboration in diversion programs, quality assurance, clinical protocol development, discharge planning/transitional services, and laboratory services. To succeed, these arrangements require interaction and cooperation between the public health and correctional agencies and access to the inmate populations (Hammett et al., 1999).

The corrections system can also play an important role in the health of communities. Men and women confined in jails and prisons represent a public health opportunity. By reaching inmates, and the families and friends of those affected by the correctional system, health messages and interventions can be reinforced in the community. Devising new strategies to improve the health of those involved in the correctional system, and strengthening and developing new partnerships between corrections and public health are crucial activities for addressing the health objectives in *Healthy People 2010*.

Successful public health/corrections collaborations are much easier to develop and sustain when data are available to document the burden of disease within the inmate population. Limitations in the data from state prison systems and large city/county jails hinder our understanding of the true nature of the complex physical and behavioral conditions that must be addressed by correctional health providers. Moreover, this information is also needed by community public health providers to plan and prepare for their release back to the community. The NCCHC report, *The Health Status of Soon-to-Be-Released Inmates*, surveyed state prisons to collect data on the prevalence of chronic disease and mental illness among inmates. Only 19 of 41 states that responded indicated they collected data on the prevalence of asthma, diabetes, hypertension, and heart diseases in their systems. Jails had even less information due to the rapid turnover of inmates. Even basic demographic information was not always available. As a result, prevalence data from target diseases needed to be extrapolated from available data in civilian populations. Reporting of communicable disease was somewhat better, but only three conditions were tabulated with some consistency on a national basis: HIV/AIDS, TB, and selected STDs such as syphilis. Findings were similar for mental illness. Only

21 state systems indicated they had data on the number of inmates with mental disorders by diagnoses. Information was also sought on the number of inmates who had co-occurring alcohol dependency and other substance dependency disorders. Only a few systems could provide data and what was available was often facility specific. The wide variation in screening and discharge planning of soon-to-be-released inmates also limits public health and correctional care providers' knowledge of the degree of comorbidity in state prisons and large jails. This is especially true for soon-to-be-released inmates (Davis & Pacchiana, 2004; Hammett et al., 1999; Shuter, 2002).

Public Health's Role in Continuity of Care

Public health officials argue that the correctional setting provides access to high-risk populations and represents an important opportunity to do screening and to provide counseling and treatment to prevent further transmission of infectious disease, both during and after incarceration. However, there are significant implications for corrections. If prisons and jails improve the screening of inmates for certain conditions, then the correctional health care system has a duty to treat these individuals and to ensure that any medical treatment started during incarceration is continued on the inmate's release. From a public health perspective, this obligation is not just to the individual inmate, but also to the community at large in order to protect the public health. This is critical for those being released with communicable diseases such as HIV/AIDS or TB infection. For example, individuals with active TB put not only the correctional facility population at risk but also the entire community. Despite aggressive efforts by CDC and state and local health departments over the last two decades, TB infection remains a key public health problem, with state prison inmates identified as a high-risk population. (Davis & Pacchiana, 2004; Freudenberg, 2004; Varghese & Peterman, 2001).

State and local correctional health care systems have limited resources to provide services and the identification of additional medical needs will only place additional demand on an already overburdened system. On the other hand, public health departments have a role and should be proactive in disease surveillance among correctional populations. Improved information systems and better surveillance and collaboration between corrections and public health could produce a whole series of positive outcomes including:

• More resources for correctional health programs
• Better services
• A safer and healthier environment for inmates and staff
• Less disease returned to the community
• Improved community health

Surveillance data are important to establish health profiles of the populations housed in our nation's prisons and jails. It is essential that public health agencies assist correctional facilities in communicating data to state and local legislators about the burden of disease and the financial costs incurred by both correctional and public health providers.

Finally, prevention is a hard sell because it is difficult to demonstrate the cost-effectiveness of prevention programs. The payoff may be long term but for correctional systems it will be a challenge to justify the increased costs of enhanced screening and increased education and prevention activities when the benefits of cases averted are in the future. However, some recent examples of targeted screening and prevention programs in both jails and prisons demonstrate its effectiveness. During the 1990s almost one-third of Chicago's syphilis cases were identified as a result of intensified screening at the Cook County Jail. Florida identified over 17% of its early syphilis during a similar period from jail screening programs. In Rhode Island, Connecticut, New York, and New Jersey, during the late 1990s over 40% of all new HIV infections were identified in correctional settings. Data from the corrections demonstration project show that correctional facilities, especially jails, are important screening and treatment sites for STDs and HIV identification (HRSA, 2002). The outbreak and deaths associated with the multidrug-resistant tuberculosis outbreak in the mid-1990s in New York State resulted in the formation of tuberculosis task forces across the nation. Therefore, the benefits of effective public health intervention and prevention program in corrections will impact society at large, not just the jail or prison. Due to the cycle of incarceration, the benefits will also impact correctional systems as well. Who pays is the fundamental question. Prevention is easier to sell when corrections and public health are working together.

Understanding corrections and public health roles can be the foundation for better integration of services between corrections and the community. It can also serve to foster new approaches to address the health needs of inmates as they reenter the community at large (Davis & Pacchiana, 2004; Hammett, 1998).

Ethical and Legal Obligations

Since jails and prisons are part of the community at large, it is the responsibility of both corrections and public health officials to ensure that correctional facilities address relevant public health goals and objectives. Public health and corrections should establish liaisons at the local level with the jail or prison and public health that promote the health of inmates and the community at large (APHA Task Force on Correctional Health Care Standards, 2003).

The ethical obligation of health professionals practicing in the correctional settings should reflect the standards of care within the community. The legal obligations of correctional health care providers are the same as those who work in the community; they have, however, an additional obligation to adhere to local, state, and federal laws that govern the provision of services to prisoners as well as the Constitution, which states that the health system cannot be deliberately indifferent to prisoners' serious medical needs. Prisoners should only participate in biomedical research when they are treated as a protected class in accordance with federal regulations and community standards. Prisoners should have access to experimental treatments as long as protections are in place. Prison and jail health programs must also protect and promote the basic human rights of incarcerated individuals. No person should be tortured or be subjected to cruel, inhuman, or degrading treatment.

Finally, jails and prison health programs must have information systems and quality assurance procedures in place that allow them to monitor the performance of the health program, maintain epidemiologic information, and track access to care and services. Guidelines developed by ACA and NCCHC offer standards to ensure that these ethical and legal issues are addressed.

The Community/Public Health Model for Corrections

Over the past 13 years, the correctional health care program in Hampden County, Massachusetts, has been operating with goals and program structure designed to address the health of those currently incarcerated, as well as the health of the free public community from which they came and to which they will return. Key to this has been the integration with community health care. (The "porous walls" also permit collaboration with community partners in education, employment, and other programs besides health care.) At the conception of the program, the three disciplines at the table—the community health centers (CHCs), the public health department, and the Sheriff's department (the triad)—recognized that the incarcerated are temporarily displaced members of the community, with the same health and social issues whether in jail or the community (Conklin et al., 2002).

The health care model was designed to recognize and treat people in jail as community health center patients, support the community standard of care, foster local connections, promote neighborhood health care, and minimize transportation needs, but not overwhelm a particular community site with a disproportionate correctional health care load. In brief, at admission to the jail, patients are assigned to one of four health care teams based on their residential zip code proximity to the four CHCs participating in the program. For this facility of approximately 2000 prisoners, each of the four teams preferably comprises two physicians, a primary nurse, a nurse practitioner, and a case manager. The physicians and case managers are "dually based," with the majority of the physicians' time at the CHC and a half-day or two at the jail, and the majority of the case managers' time at the jail. The primary nurse and nurse practitioner are based only in the jail. Ongoing care is scheduled with the primary nurse, nurse practitioner, or physician. The primary nurse is the team care manager and coordinator, responsible for keeping track of team patients in the facility. The case managers focus much of their time on HIV case management and discharge planning, but also serve the same role for patients with other chronic medical conditions. A discharge planning nurse focuses on patients requiring hospitalization, long-term care, other complex medical discharge needs, or correctional classification issues, as well as standard medical reentry planning, and serves as a resource to the case managers.

As the program was developed, six important functions helped organize our thinking and were defined as the components of a public health model for correctional health care: early detection and assessment, comprehensive treatment, prevention and health promotion, education, continuity of care, and the use of data for programmatic and public health response (Conklin et al., 1998; Lincoln & Miles, 2006; Skolnick, 1998).

Early detection and assessment of health-related conditions, both for individuals and for groups, activates the care that follows. A good interview in the appropriate setting usually elicits much of the health and risk status information needed to guide the individual's care.

Appropriate screening for HIV, syphilis, chlamydia, gonorrhea, tuberculosis, diabetes, and hypertension was calculated to be cost effective in prisons and jails in general (National Commission on Correctional Health Care & National Institute of Justice, 2002). In Hampden County, rapid HIV testing and hepatitis C screening is voluntary, repeatedly offered and encouraged; syphilis testing is routine; chlamydia testing is routine but targeted by age (or risk factors in older patients); gonorrhea testing is done based on symptoms, on contact history, or if other tests show abnormalities; tuberculosis screening is routine for both active and latent disease; hypertension screening is routine; and some programs screen for diabetes. Alanine aminotransferase is included in the intake laboratory tests. Numerous other conditions need to be and are assessed for, particularly the highly prevalent problems in mental health, including substance abuse, and age- and sex-appropriate screening such as Pap smears, routine pelvic exams, and mammography.

Comprehensive treatment of the conditions identified through assessment is not isolated to the "purely medical" aspects but is necessarily biopsychosocial. It is often challenging in corrections to delineate what psychosocial goals have a reasonable chance of being successfully accomplished. In the community health model of the program, these difficult decisions and nuances are familiar to the health providers, as they are dealing with much of the same in community settings, and so have direct, practical knowledge of the community resources. In addition, they are aware of how the care behind the walls fits into the continuity of care.

Likewise, comprehensive treatment may not be limited to the patient. Important family needs can be identified and addressed with appropriate resources and collaboration. In addition to the usual community resources, a pilot program in part of our county entails referral of families with a member in jail to the neighborhood outreach workers (the North End Outreach Network Bridges Project). Each of these workers serves specific sections of a larger neighborhood region, rather than being tied to a particular funding agency's target group (elderly, substance abuse, etc.). Households with an incarcerated member are triggered to receive another assessment by the outreach worker. Difficulties at school for children with an incarcerated parent have been noted as a repeating theme, and can be identified and addressed.

Whether they are a household member or not, sexual or drug-injecting contacts of persons with sexually transmitted or bloodborne diseases are identified for counseling, testing, and treatment. Partner notification is provided as a service with provider referral by trained persons; this program is done in collaboration with the department of public health disease intervention specialist (DIS) who visits the jail on a frequent basis. These partner services are likely cost effective, as has been demonstrated for contacts of incarcerated males with chlamydia (Gift et al., 2006; Macke & Maher, 1999). Partner counseling and referral services can effectively identify sex and needle-sharing partners with previously undiagnosed HIV. HIV care workers can accomplish some of this effectively, but in other situations the DIS is better able to identify and engage contacts (as traditionally done for syphilis). Nationally this practice is underutilized (Centers for Disease Control and Prevention, 2003; Golden et al., 2003; Passin et al., 2006).

Specialty care is addressed through several approaches. The primary care practitioners in the jail have developed expertise for various conditions having a high prevalence (e.g., HIV, hepatitis C, gynecomastia, or chronic pain with addiction). This also benefits the community health center practices. Other specialty care may be managed by internal health providers outside the team structure, such as the tuberculosis prevention program, run by the infectious disease nurse and medical director in consultation with the CHC teams and state TB clinic. Specialty services with sufficient volume, such as optometry and orthopedics, are provided through on-site visits. When outside visits for specialty care are needed, patients are generally seen by the same specialists used by the corresponding CHC.

A prime example of *prevention and health promotion* is vaccination. While hepatitis A and B can be transmitted within correctional facilities (Macalino et al., 2004), most of the benefit of vaccination accrues to the longer period a person is back in the free community (Devasia et al., 2006; Gondles, 2005). Thus, the internal vaccination program efforts are largely supported by the public health department providing most of the vaccines. Other examples of prevention and health promotion include other vaccinations (influenza, pneumonia, varicella, and others), prenatal care for pregnant women, tobacco, drug, and alcohol relapse prevention, jail–community health and employment fairs, the diabetic/cardiovascular exercise program, and HIV and hepatitis counseling and testing. Economic modeling has demonstrated that there is at least as much cumulative prevention value for those testing negative as for those testing positive, primarily because of the far greater number of patients testing negative (Varghese et al., 2002; Varghese & Peterman, 2001).

While there has been substantial recognition of the immediate benefits and conversion to smoke-free facilities (May & Lambert, 1998), tobacco relapse prevention has received little attention in corrections (Chavez et al., 2004). While smoke-free facilities are healthier, the benefits are short term, as most inmates (98% at 6 months in our experience) resume tobacco use after release (Tuthill et al., 2002) Given that 75% or more of correctional populations are smokers, even small effects in relapse prevention represent a sizable population, many of whom are parents. Preliminary results of implementing a tobacco cessation education curriculum for correctional staff and inmates are encouraging but data on outcome following community reentry are lacking (Lincoln, Chavez, & Langmore-Avila, 2005) The tobacco-free status of the program was chosen for the benefit of both prisoners and staff, and as such completely prohibits staff from smoking on the entire grounds (as is often not the case in many "smoke-free" facilities)(Chavez et al., 2004).

A strong commitment to the health and well-being of staff members is an important part of the community health model. Wellness and fitness programs for staff are designed to promote health, enhance work morale, and support self-esteem, which in turn are seen doing the same for staff families and inmates.

Health education is such a major component of comprehensive treatment and prevention (as well as the other functional elements in the public health model) that it warranted separate consideration. For much of behavioral prevention work, education in the narrow sense is insufficient, and requires a broader definition. Effective education must be able to impact knowledge, attitudes, behavior, skills, and social norms. For instance, features of HIV risk behavior prevention programs that were found effective in meta-analysis were based on behavioral theory, and designed specifically to change HIV transmission risk behaviors. They were delivered to individuals by health care providers or counselors in an intensive manner, in settings where people with HIV receive routine services or medical care, and provided skills building, as well as addressing a myriad of issues related to mental health, medication adherence, and HIV risk behavior (Crepaz et al., 2006) Various educational methods are needed given the many different tasks, educational levels, and opportunities that exist in the correctional system. Our program addressed the needs of both staff and prisoners and included: written and video material; single and multiple sessions; individual and group sessions; instructor-led and peer-led sessions; voluntary (with incentives) and mandatory sessions; and formal and informal sessions. Often the measurable outcomes in education are incremental and cumulative, as formulated in the transtheoretical stages of behavioral change (Prochaska & Velicer, 1997). Repeat client-centered face-to-face education and counseling has been found to be effective and have high retention (Weinbaum, Lyerla, & Margolis, 2003). Though some settings, such as immediately following arrest "in lock-up," have not been found to be conducive to much health education, some relevant video and in-person presentations have resulted in greater acceptance of HIV testing (Fulton County, Chicago, Baltimore: H. R. Potter, PhD, & R. Voigt, MA, CDC, personal communication). In general, as educators working in both corrections and the free world will typically attest, enthusiasm for learning in corrections is high.

Peer-led education programs are very consistent with the community health paradigm. Because of the shorter length of stay, it has been more difficult for jails than prisons to provide peer-led programs—7% in jails as compared to 41% in prisons in a 1997 survey (Hammett et al., 1999). In this jail program that includes a sentenced population, it has been quite feasible. Peer education's important strengths include: credibility, effectiveness, cost-efficiency, benefit to educators in knowledge, allowance for informal learning moments throughout the week in housing settings, and the return of expertise to the community. These programs have proven inspirational and rejuvenating to the field (Boudin et al., 1999; Conklin et al., 1998; Hammett et al., 1999; Scott, Harzke, Mizwa, Pugh, & Ross, 2003). Randomized experimental evidence is limited, but much experience supports the approach, finding feasibility and positive changes in knowledge, attitudes, and beliefs (Scott et al., 2003; Shelton, 2001; St Lawrence et al., 1997; Vigilante et al., 1999). An innovative community-oriented peer-led program developed in a collaboration between the Center for AIDS Prevention Studies (UCSF), a community-based organization (Centerforce), and the staff and inmate peer educators inside a state prison "spans the fence" into the community with an education and prevention program not just for those incarcerated, but also one for the women who visit them (Grinstead, Zack, & Faigeles, 1999).

Continuity of care's importance is immediately obvious to most who work in health care and central to the design of the community health model. Of course, continuity of care depends on having an adequate level health care available in the community. A number of activities in this, as well as in other models, have been important in facilitating continuity of care (Hammett et al., 1999; Kennedy et al., 2001; Lincoln et al., 2006), including:

1. Attention first to needs that may be higher than health care in the *patient's priorities of daily living* hierarchy, such as food, housing, and/or transportation for themselves or their dependents. Transportation was the most common barrier to health care cited by our patients with chronic medical conditions after reentry (Lincoln et al., 2006). A study of reentry priorities of people leaving NYC jails found that only 30% of adults and almost no adolescents rated medical or health problems in their top three priorities.

Adult and adolescent males most often rate unemployment and educational needs among their top three needs while women regard substance abuse as a top priority. Both male and female adults rate housing as a high priority, while male adolescents do not. In most cases, caseworkers agreed with clients' self-assessment, though caseworkers were more likely to report that the male adolescents' substance use was a top problem than were the young men themselves (Freudenberg, 2006; Freudenberg, Daniels, Crum, Perkins, & Richie, 2005).

2. *Case management*, which addresses the aforementioned needs (Council of State Governments, 2004; Ehrmann, 2002; Freudenberg, 2004; "Michigan DOC: discharge planning starts early," 1999; Rich et al., 2001; Veysey, Steadman, Morrissey, & Johnsen, 1997). While various models exist, the case managers in the Hampden County jail program begin work with clients as soon as the need is identified, and follow them in the community as long as needed. Sometimes this is until the managers change jobs and move on from their position, highlighting the importance of the next item:

3. Development of a *personal connection* with the client before release. (J. J. Myers et al., 2003). In this population, which is familiar with the barriers to care including stigmatization and feeling judged, this (at least somewhat) familiar relationship can be a motivation and enhance the confidence to persist and follow-up with health care. This may be particularly important for women (Hammett, et al., 1999), and the many patients without established community health care providers.

4. *Dually based health care workers* (that is, HCWs who work with patients/clients both in the corrections program and in the community) not only promote a personal connection, but also bridge programs, bringing a community perspective into the correctional institution, and vice versa. This was judged a primary facilitator by patients after release (Lincoln et al., 2006). Besides providing continuity of care at reentry, this feature can provide continuity of care at incarceration (Council of State Governments, 2004).

5. Initiation of reentry planning in a *timely* manner, a significant aspect of which starts with admission. This is particularly important for jails, given the shorter stays and unexpected releases. With this model, it is even sometimes possible to begin reentry planning prior to the incarceration.

6. *Appointments scheduled* for follow-up health care in the community. This basic step was rated as very helpful by patients with chronic health conditions after they were released from the Hampden County jail. It may serve as a marker of a tangible discharge plan, and was found to be a leading predictor of follow-up (Hammett et al., 1999; Kennedy et al., 2003).

7. A *summary record* of important health conditions, medications, allergies, diagnostic studies, vaccinations, and other important treatments for each person released should be available to the community health provider at or prior to the time of the first visit. The use of electronic medical records (EMRs) facilitates this. Electronic transfer between compatible systems is the natural goal. Currently the health care staff at the Hampden County jail can access this information from several of the health centers' and hospital's electronic health records. Information from the jail is still sent to community providers by fax or paper, though even in this case, 24-hour access is available. Medical summaries are faxed on demand when patients present in the community and their record has not preceded them. This is quite

important for continuity. Of course, a summary record is just that and cannot replace firsthand familiarity with a patient. Likewise, firsthand familiarity does not guarantee total recall, and both the summary and more detailed medical record are needed in a timely manner when care shifts from jail to free world and vice versa.

8. Having necessary *medical benefits available promptly on release* is key, not just for medical care and medications, but for other requirements such as food, housing, and transportation. Initially, in Hampden County, fairly effective arrangements were made between local welfare offices and individual institutions—benefits were usually "denied" on application during incarceration but by maintaining the application within the system they could be activated on release. Currently, electronic application and communications facilitate work within the current Medicaid system; appropriate legislation, however, creates more widespread, dependable solutions to continuity of Medicaid benefits on release. In Hampden County, all the health centers and involved hospitals have free care programs that promote maintaining attendance at the health centers, but medications, medical equipment, and specialty care outside the health centers are difficult to obtain without income or coverage. Continuity of mental health care, in particular, is easier to maintain for those patients with Medicaid benefits (Morrissey et al., 2006)

9. *Geographic proximity*: the closer the correctional institution is to the neighborhoods and community organizations, the lower the barrier to dually based providers, on-site collaborations with the CBOs, HCWs coming from the primary neighborhoods of reentry, and other aspects of a community-integrated model. Jails can also serve as reentry sites for the prison system. In Hampden County, state prisoners planning to return to live in Hampden County may be transferred to serve the last 6 months or so of their sentence in the jail and have access to the local program and resources. The same practice exists in Virginia where partnerships with local jails and the state Department of Corrections allow selected prisoners to relocate from prison to a local jail in their community to receive transitioning services such as life skills workshops and assistance with housing and employment (Re-Entry Policy Council, 2004; Virginia Department of Corrections, 2003). When incarceration cannot occur in a facility with proximity and connections for reentry to the individual's planned locale, teleconferencing may be a consideration. The Threshold Prisons Project in Illinois arranges for incarcerated clients to have contact with social workers from their community for mental health care and other social services prior to reentry (Sadeanu, 2006).

Using Data for Program Improvement and Public Health Response

The data gathered for measuring quality reflects both what is feasible and how that quality is defined. In the model, those activities included in prevention, education, and continuity of care are tracked, as well as items of evaluation and treatment. So, for example, a basic quality assurance measurement tracked in the model is the rate at which patients attend their early appointments on reentry to the free community.

The Community-Oriented Model of Primary Care (COPC) and other quality improvement models require gathering information, in this case from the community, to formulate interventions, evaluating each intervention, and using that information to repeat the cycle. Community input in defining problems and setting priorities is important to COPC. Public health expands this process to a larger scale, and needs information from many sites. Jails have the ability to serve our public and our local communities by gathering this information, and as mentioned, jails can serve a sentinel early warning function as their structure can provide a window to a population with a particular profile of important risks that is otherwise hard to reach.

Collaborations

A multitude of collaborations are needed to support the community health model. In Hampden County, these are structured in various manners including through contracts, subcontracts, shared personnel, memoranda of agreement, volunteer arrangements, informal collaborations, and direct personal connections. Medicaid rates of payment are generally used, unless not feasible. As the health care landscape in the community changes, the correctional health program adapts. Some of the collaborations include:

- Community health centers
- Community mental health centers
- Community substance abuse programs
- State and City Departments of Public Health including the local tuberculosis and sexually transmitted disease clinics
- Hospitals, hospice, long-term care
- Laboratories
- Dental program
- Community care and case management programs
- Community outreach programs
- Internal security and other programs within the jail
- Community corrections programs, probation, and parole
- State prisons and juvenile programs
- State information technology department

The details of these would exceed this chapter's scope, but a few items not yet discussed bear comment.

Attention to the *training of community health care staff* regarding the special aspects of working in a correctional environment is very important. Most HCWs are unfamiliar with the environment, and even though their time within the jail may be limited, training, as with other new employees, is needed. Areas of emphasis include multiple boundary issues, regulations when friends or family are incarcerated, the role and structure of security, emergency procedures, and others. A guide for CBOs working with jails that includes advice on training is available from the New York State Department of Health ("How to Gain Access to County Jails for Delivery of HIV/AIDS Services: A Guide for Community-Based Organizations," 2004).

The same *laboratory* is used by the jail, three of the CHCs, and the largest hospital. Results are accessible via computers at all sites, and provide a seamless *information flow* through incarceration and reentry; for example, the basic ability to rapidly access prior chest radiology or hepatitis serology, can often save significant time, effort, cost, and concern.

The *community corrections* program, through which people complete sentences under electronic monitoring and live at home and participate in multiple programs, presents another opportunity for health issues to be addressed. Substance abuse treatment is contracted by the program through local resources that are able to continue providing care after completion of the individual's sentence. Health care is facilitated by a nurse on site at the day reporting facility who provides health care classes, counseling, and referral to the local community health centers. There are agreements in place with these health centers that streamline access. The community corrections program considers obtaining health care an aspect of self-care and recovery/rehabilitation. Medication continuity is supported and medications are supplied if necessary.

Outcomes from Hampden County

A number of quantitative and qualitative outcomes of this model of health care have been described, yet much better information is needed. With an interconnected, multifaceted program such as this, it is difficult to set up programmatic, randomized studies, to statistically isolate the key components or interventions, or find other means of comparison. One type of surrogate or process outcome could be a measure of the degree of correctional and community program integration, as proposed in the human services integration measure (Browne et al., 2004). As mentioned, follow-up appointments in the community are tracked for some conditions, and for HIV patients typically exceed 88%. A study of patients with a mix of chronic health conditions (most commonly hepatitis C, hypertension, and asthma) found that 65% of patients with scheduled appointments reported keeping their first appointment (Lincoln et al., 2006). A multivariate analysis with an instrumental variable approach designed to account for known or hidden bias, found that having the appointment scheduled ahead of time, correlated with increased primary care follow-up (Kennedy et al., 2003). The same group of patients reported improved overall health status, decreased health care visits, including emergency room visits, and fewer hospitalizations in the 6 months following jail, compared to their experiences prior to incarceration There was, however, no matched group or program available for comparison.

Costs of the health care program have been moderate. Though comparison metrics are limited, the 1999 NCCHC/NIC survey of 17 of the 30 largest U.S. jails found average health care costs of just under $8 per inmate-day (range $3.18 to $18.69), accounting for 15.3% of the jail operating budgets. Unfortunately, many of the jails' cost data did not include items such as mental health services or hospitalizations (Anno, 2001). In 1997, the Hampden County program, including all costs, was just under $6 per inmate-day and represented 8.5% of the jail operating budget (Conklin, et al., 1998), and in 2002 was just under $10 per inmate-day and 10% of operating budget.

Outcomes from Other Programs

In Rhode Island, the HIV program physicians and nurses care for patients in the correctional facility and continue their relationship into the community (Rich et al., 2001). The same program reported that women at high risk of HIV and reincarceration had lower recidivism rates than a historical control group (Vigilante et al., 1999). In four urban centers, continuity of medical care by a single health care provider was associated with decreased likelihood of female incarceration (Sheu et al., 2002). In a Cook County, IL, program that included some dually based HIV care providers, the follow-up rate was 60% for patients scheduled with the HIV Core Center program (Council of State Governments, 2004).

Several other correctional health case management programs have published relevant outcomes. For substance-abusing arrestees, case management was associated with more access to drug treatment and fewer crimes committed than for a control group who received only referrals or a single counseling session (Rhodes & Gross, 1997). Postrelease maternity case management was associated with decreased odds of low birth weight (Bell et al., 2004). Laboratory and pharmacy data from the Connecticut prison system with its transitional case management program found that the substantial improvement in HIV parameters gained in prison was subsequently lost in the 27% of HIV patients who were reincarcerated after an average of 4 months in the community (Springer et al., 2004). No results were reported on the other 73% in that study. The Centerforce Get Connected program provided HIV prevention case management to people leaving three California prisons and noted decreased HIV risk behaviors. It also suggested that health services may be important in the transition or reentry, and that longer term transitional case management (longer than 6 months) would avoid hand-offs that require restarting relationship building (J. Myers et al., 2005).

Two outcome trials are of particular importance as they included systematically matched comparison groups: Health Link and Project START. The Health Link program in New York City provides case management to incarcerated and formerly incarcerated individuals, assists community organizations that serve this population, and strengthens linkages between community organizations and city agencies to enhance postrelease services. Participants were randomly assigned to either a group that received full intensive discharge-planning and community case management services, or to one that received less-intensive discharge-planning services and no community-based services. The program produced modest beneficial impacts on some outcomes associated with greater service use. Males were more likely to attain a GED. Drug use may have decreased, although the patterns were mixed and inconsistent. Health Link had no impact on criminal justice system involvement or criminal activity; behaviors that cause the spread of HIV; overall use of health care or the likelihood of having health insurance; and employment rates or housing, social, and family situations (Freudenberg et al., 2005; Needels, James-Burdumy, & Burghardt, 2005; Richie, Freudenberg, & Page, 2001).

Project START is a multicentered study that compared a single HIV, hepatitis, and other sexually transmitted infections risk reduction session prior to release from prison with an enhanced program with an additional session before and four sessions after release that also addressed community reentry needs (e.g., housing, employment). The intervention spanning reentry demonstrated significant decrease in unprotected anal and vaginal sex (Wolitski & the Project Start Writing Group for The Project Start Study Group, 2006).

Another evaluation, important because of the analysis of difficulties encountered, comes from the Corrections Demonstration Project at the Fulton County Jail, Georgia (HRSA, 2002). They noted the lack of a clear project framework, staff roles and responsibilities, operational protocols, and political will to be formidable barriers throughout the project, leading to these recommendations for future projects:

Project Design:
- Establish theoretical, structural, and systematic integration of services prior to project implementation.
- Establish goals that are manageable and meaningful.
- "Buy in" from all affiliates and partners must be in place to maximize continuity of care.

Operational:
- Establish operational protocols and tools for service delivery and test these protocols prior to project implementation.
- Establish clear definitions of the deliverables.
- Establish formal Memorandum of Understanding and regular means for communication and dissemination of information with all partners and facilities.

The principles and approach described in the community health model are recommended in broader treatises on reentry (Council of State Governments, 2004; Travis, 2005), Likewise, it is consistent with other areas of public safety such as community policing, and other principles of reentry support.

Implementation of a Community Health Model for Corrections: A Case Study

There are many features of the community which must be taken into consideration when implementing a Community Health Model for correctional health care. In the ideal sense the jail would be considered another clinic in the network of clinics which provide health care to the underserved populations. The practitioners would divide their time between the jail and the community health clinics and the medical record information follows the patient without delay with the development of an integrated EMR. This provides for the possibility of a seamless transition between the jail and the surrounding community regarding health care including medical, dental, mental health, and substance abuse treatment. Another important aspect is that there is a mechanism for care for inmates postrelease once they have entered the jail, since they have in a sense enrolled into a community health care clinic and have generated medical information which can be shared with the surrounding community clinics and clinic appointments for medical care can be generated prior to release from the facility. Potentially there are many benefits to having this model implemented, but what are the considerations for utilizing this model?

One important consideration is the capacity of the community health clinic network to undertake the responsibility for health care of the inmates. There has to be a willingness and commitment from the clinic network to engage in correctional health care. From the community clinics' point of view they do not want to incur additional risk regarding financial loss from their involvement in the project and would not involve themselves in a competitive bidding process, typical of the privatization model. Also from the community clinics' point of view they would expect reasonable payment for the services provided for the inmates and these funds would support the community clinics in their needs as not-for-profit entities possibly to support ongoing and expand services. Thus, there are many types of contracts to consider ranging from full risk, shared risk, and little or no risk such as cost plus a percentage type arrangements. The possible advantage to the full-risk-type contract is that there is incentive to utilize on-site capabilities such as infirmaries or medical/mental health units, dental suites, telemedicine, and teleradiology to limit health care and correctional costs. These type contracts might be more appropriate for large jail facilities which deal with significant ongoing health care issues of the inmates and often are chronically short of correctional staff to move inmates between the community and the jail on an uninterrupted basis. These were some of the concerns when Unity Health Care contracted with Washington, DC DOC to provide medical care beginning October 1, 2006. Two months into this arrangement, the preliminary experience yielded a number of points to consider.

Conceptually, the community commits to the reality that the ex-offenders are part of their community and that it is probably better to take an active role in their lives regarding medical, mental health, and substance abuse than not. If the community views the inmates as an island, then this model is not for them. Thus, there needs to be a broad based consensus among the community politicians to provide support to the development of the complex relationship which needs to be developed between the community health clinics and the jail (medical record issues regarding electronic medical record which is the same as the clinics, legal issues, budgets, performance evaluations, contracts, and public health). A subcommittee was appointed by the mayor of Washington, DC to evaluate on an ongoing basis the health care of its inmates as well as the collaboration between the clinic network and the jail. The department of corrections is an essential element in the implementation of this novel paradigm. Leadership should be aware of the significant health care issues of the inmates and recognize the importance of excellent health care within the facility but also for the newly released inmate. Another important player in the initial consideration of the Community Health Model is the local Department of Health. There should be involvement at the beginning of consideration of implementation of this model to discuss the communities' public health issues including STDs, HIV, hepatitis C and B, tuberculosis, community-acquired MRSA, influenza, vaccination programs including HPV vaccine. Such discussions led to the recommendations for rapid HIV testing of all patients at booking as well as rapid chlamydia/gonorrhea testing. Public health initiatives or pilot projects can be discussed and included in the contract between the DOC and the clinic network. The Department of Corrections, Community Clinics, community/politicians, and the Department of Health should all be involved in the implementation of this model.

There are significant fiscal requirements for the consideration and implementation of the Community Health Model: monies for the evaluation of the facility to determine the state of medical diagnostic equipment and treatment units, crash carts, dispensing of medications systems, electronic medical records which interface with the jail system and speak to the surrounding community clinics regarding patient information, staff orientation, and education regarding new EMR and policies and procedures.

Thus, there may be additional up-front costs in implementing this model compared to bidding out the medical care to a private company, which may require activation energy in the form of a grant from a foundation or other source.

Program features of the Community Health Model in Washington, DC include continuity of provider between the jail and the community; quick access to medical information at inmate receiving or discharge (presumably without having to sign releases of information or other HIPAA restrictions); continuous quality improvement efforts within the jail but also comparing CQI of surrounding clinics; utilization management with practitioners who have admitting privileges at the referral hospitals and review by a trained registered nurse; adherence to policies and procedures that fulfill the requirements of the correctional accrediting associations; a close working relationship with the department of health; a strong postrelease case management program to ensure proper linkages are made to medical, mental health, pharmacy, substance abuse programs and social services as well as enrolling in various insurance programs such as Medicare, Medicaid, and ADAP. Referral services to medical subspecialties can be accessed via established relationships with the community clinics (e.g., Phoenix clinic for HIV and hepatitis C treatment). The Washington, DC jail is enrolling all inmates into the Unity clinic system and providing identifying health cards to the inmates on release regardless of whether or not they have an underlying chronic illness, an important distinction from the Hampden County model. Unity Health Care is a consortium of community Federally Qualified Health Centers (FQHC) providing health care for underserved persons in the Washington, DC area, and as such is entitled to (1) malpractice insurance and regulations that should discourage frivolous lawsuits and (2) group purchasing benefits regarding pharmaceuticals, laboratory services, and medical supplies.

Once embarking on the Community Health Model there are issues with staffing as well as implementation of procedures and protocols, critical to delivering health care in jails. The first issue with the staff is that there will be shared providers between the community clinics and the jail. On the one hand, there may not be the willingness of the clinic provider to work in the jail environment, and on the other hand the practitioner may be barred from practicing in the jail due to background issues. Thus, adequate staffing is always an issue for providers as well as nurses. The providers also have not had any orientation to correctional medicine, so resources must be allocated for training and orientation. The staffing matrix is negotiated between the clinics and the department of corrections. The Hampden County model uses predominately registered nurses, and nurse practitioners who are the inmate-patient providers. The Hampden County model does not have an infirmary and conducts nurse's sick call with standing orders for over-the-counter medications only. In contrast, the Washington, DC model uses an extensive infirmary and provides medical coverage with a variety of providers including medical doctors, nurse practitioners, and physician assistants. Nurse's sick call is guided by standard medical protocols with an EMR. The EMR will be linked to laboratory and the community clinic's EMR, allowing for on-site real-time comparisons of medical, mental health, and social services data and scheduling for postrelease appointments. Implementation of the EMR has been an ongoing process and is not functional at this time.

Table 29.1 Malpractice insurance and prescription benefits for satellites of Federally Qualified Health Centers: Washington. DC.

In 1992 the Federally Supported Health Centers Assistance Act (FSHCAA—PL 102–501, which amended Sec. 224 of the Public Health Services Act) created medical malpractice insurance for Federally Qualified Health Centers (FQHCs) through a program referred to as the FTCA medical malpractice program. In 1995 the FSHCAA was clarified and its sunset eliminated. Under these two provisions, many individuals connected with Section 330 health centers can be deemed federal employees for purposes of medical malpractice suits, thereby reducing or eliminating the need for their centers to purchase private medical malpractice insurance.

In Washington, DC, the jail site is listed on schedule b, providing malpractice coverage as a satellite under the umbrella of the FQHCs. One issue is that anyone who enters information onto the EMR or into the paper chart also be covered under FTCA. So, if there are agencies that perform HIV counseling and testing outside of the FQHC, this may jeopardize the covered status under FTCA. However, one can hire these individuals as employees of the CHC and this would take care of this issue. However, in the case of contractors the coverage is different. FTCA does cover contractors who are working full time (>32.5 hours per week) but not part time. However, FTCA does cover contractors if they work less than 32.5 hours per week if they provide services in family practice, OB-GYN, general internal medicine, or general pediatrics. Another instance would be hiring a full-time mental health practitioner to provide mental health care in jails rather than having a contractual relationship with a mental health group. However, if the mental health practitioner worked part time, they might not be covered under FTCA, unless they are hired as an employee of the FQHC.

There may also be prescription benefits associated with this which can be passed onto the jail such as 340(b) status. In Washington, DC, medications are purchased through an arrangement with St. Elizabeth's mental hospital (via a historical contract with the Department of War); thus, they do not use the 340(b) drug benefit. There is no legal precedence in using FTCA coverage for malpractice in the jail setting before Community Oriented Correctional Health Services (COCHS) started working with the DC jail.

The use of the EMR which is shared between the community clinics and the jail health center brings up some interesting HIPAA issues. One would think that corrections are exempt from HIPAA to allow access to medical information about the health status of an inmate. However, most community organizations do not recognize jails as HIPAA exempt and require signed releases to be generated with the resulting delay in the transfer of medical information. This delay in information flow may result in the delay of medical care and the issuance of critical medications to the inmate. This issue would be moot if there were interconnected EMRs between the clinics and the jail. Information technology departments of both corrections and the clinics must work in concert to develop such a system in conjunction with EMR vendors and consultants. An EMR approach to the medical record or limited EMR containing current medications, allergies, vaccinations, key results, and problem list could also be considered as a more expeditious method to transfer data as opposed to transferring the entire record.

There can be Department of Health initiatives which focus on correctional health care, and lend themselves to the Community Health Model. Most departments of health track the care and appropriate completion of treatment for active tuberculosis disease, but rarely track the treatment for latent tuberculosis infection. In the Community Health Model, clinics would follow the patients with latent tuberculosis infection during the course of their treatment. Chlamydia contacts are not routinely traced by the Department of Health in Washington, DC. Jails can actively screen for asymptomatic chlamydia/gonorrhea infection in both females as well as males with the urine tests. When implemented in San Francisco, the prevalence of chlamydia in young women was decreased by nearly one-half in a neighborhood with a high rate of incarceration at the local jail over the period from 1997 to 2004 (Barry, 2006). With linkages into the community-based clinic system, there exists the possibility to further trace STD contacts in the community when the diagnosis has been made of an index case at the jail. Thus, from a public health point of view, the Community Health Model of jail care with real-time communication with the EMR and continuity of providers assists in the diagnosis, treatment, and contact tracing of many contagious diseases, which are not routinely completed by the local Department of Health, often due to budgetary constraints. Other noteworthy examples of Department of Health initiatives which interface with jail health care include rapid HIV testing, hepatitis A and B vaccination programs, MRSA, and potentially HPV vaccination. Like the penal system caring for many of the mentally ill within a community, these facilities are taking on certain public health functions, not served by the local department of health, which improve the health of the community overall.

Monitoring the quality of health care in correctional facilities is a responsibility of both corrections as well as the medical care provider. Some expectations of quality can be written into the contract including the requirement for NCCHC or ACA accreditation. Often contracts will have specific sections relating to liquidated damages associated with lack of performance on a particular indicator (e.g., completed 14-day physical exams, Pap smears done, etc.). The fines are often determined by a representative of corrections, who works with the medical administration to determine what can be done to facilitate a corrective action plan. Other contracts do not specify liquidated damages for various performance indicators, but rather rely on accreditation efforts and a responsive grievance system to maintain or improve the level of health care provided. Likewise, it is important to have an outside monitor who reviews the health care of the facility in a comprehensive manner on a regular basis (reviews deaths, hospitalizations, infectious disease issues, chronic care clinics, women's health, and general medical care).

Measuring and evaluating outcomes in the Community Health Model may be an approachable topic. There is the benefit of having data on patient/inmates both within the community and in the jail health care center. With a strong case management system providing solid linkages to the community clinics as well as physically being within the community to follow up on released men and women, patients should stay in care and those with chronic medical/ mental illnesses should benefit. We can measure both process and outcomes. A process measure would be the percentage of HIV patients with appointments scheduled to see the clinic's HIV team in the community; an outcome measure would be the maintenance of an undetectable HIV viral load 90 days postrelease, after the patient had been placed on HIV medications and responded to this therapy while incarcerated (Springer & Altice, 2005) Other outcome measures are hemoglobin A1C in diabetes, emergency department visits/hospitalizations for asthmatics, emergency department utilization among clinic participants versus nonclinic patients, episodes of congestive health failure in patients on dialysis or with coronary artery disease, and so on. Outcomes data are very scarce when looking at medical care in the jail and seeing if the benefits continue once the inmate is released. More of this important information would be available with the Community Health Model because these data can be compared to the data generated within the clinic system and can be compared with the jail health care center. Ideally, the Community Health Model is a proactive system as opposed to a reactive system in that the emphasis is on uncovering illness and treating it early with case management and close follow-up with the same providers within the community. As there is no matched control group available for comparison, program evaluation will face the same challenges mentioned earlier in the section "The Community Public Health Model for Corrections"; nonetheless, the contract between Unity Health and the Washington, DC DOC represents a unique opportunity to evaluate both process and outcome measures of the quality of health care provided to the inmate-patients. Funding has been provided by the Robert Wood Johnson Foundation to evaluate health care at the Washington, DC Jail by the John Jay School of Criminal Justice in the next year.

References

Anno, B. J. (2001). *Correctional health care: Guidelines for the management of an adequate delivery system.* Washington, DC: National Institute of Corrections and National Commission on Correctional Health Care.

APHA Task Force on Correctional Health Care Standards. (Ed.). (2003). *Standards for health services in correctional institutions.* Washington, DC: American Public Health Association.

Barry, P. (2006, May 8–11). *Sexually transmitted infection screen in county jails is associated with a decrease in community prevalence of gonorrhea and chlamydia— San Francisco, 1977–2004.* Paper presented at the 2006 National STD Prevention Conference, Jacksonville, FL.

Bell, J. F., Zimmerman, F. J., Cawthon, M. L., Huebner, C. E., Ward, D. H., & Schroeder, C. A. (2004). Jail incarceration and birth outcomes. *J Urban Health, 81,* 630–644.

Boudin, K., Carrero, I., Clark, J., Flournoy, V., Loftin, K., Martindale, S., et al. (1999). ACE: A peer education and counseling program meets the needs of incarcerated women with HIV/AIDS issues. *J Assoc Nurses AIDS Care, 10*(6), 90–98.

Browne, G., Roberts, J., Gafni, A., Byrne, C., Kertyzia, J., & Loney, P. (2004). Conceptualizing and validating the human services integration measure. *Int J Integr Care, 4,* e03.

Centers for Disease Control and Prevention. (2003). Partner counseling and referral services to identify persons with undiagnosed HIV—North Carolina, 2001. *MMWR, 52*(48), 1181–1184.

Chavez, R. S., Oto-Kent, D. S., Porter, J., Brown, K., Quirk, L., & Lewis, S. (2004). *Tobacco policy, cessation, and education in correctional facilities.* West Sacramento, CA: National Commission on Correctional Health Care, National Network on Tobacco Prevention and Poverty, Health Education Council.

Conklin, T. J., Lincoln, T., & Flanigan, T. P. (1998). A public health model to connect correctional health care with communities. *Am J Public Health, 88,* 1249–1250.

Conklin, T. J., Lincoln, T., Wilson, R., & Gramarossa, G. (2002). *A public health manual for correctional health care.* Ludlow, MA: Hampden County Sheriff's Department.

Corrections agency collaborations with public health: Special issue in corrections. (2003). Longmont, CO: National Institute of Corrections Information Center, U.S. Department of Justice.

Council of State Governments. (2004). *Report of the Re-Entry Policy Council: Charting the safe and successful return of prisoners to the community.* New York: Re-Entry Policy Council.

Crepaz, N., Lyles, C. M., Wolitski, R. J., Passin, W. F., Rama, S. M., Herbst, J. H., et al. (2006). Do prevention interventions reduce HIV risk behaviors among people living with HIV? A meta-analytic review of controlled trials. *AIDS, 20,* 143–157.

Davis, L. M., & Pacchiana, S. (2004). Health profile of the state prison population and returning offenders: Public health challenges. *Journal of Correctional Health Care, 10,* 325–326.

Devasia, R. A., Jones, T. F., Kainer, M. A., Halford, S., Sheeler, L. L., Swift, J., et al. (2006). Two community hepatitis B outbreaks: An argument for vaccinating incarcerated persons. *Vaccine, 24,* 1354–1358.

Ehrmann, T. (2002). Community-based organizations and HIV prevention for incarcerated populations: Three HIV prevention program models. *AIDS Educ Prev, 14*(5 Suppl. B), 75–84.

Freudenberg, N. (2004). Community health services for returning jail and prison inmates. *Journal of Correctional Health Care, 10,* 369–397.

Freudenberg, N. (2006). Coming home from jail: A review of health and social problems facing US jail populations and of opportunities for reentry interventions citing Daniels J, Freudenberg N, Mosely J, Labriola M, Murrill C. Differing characteristics by age and gender of people leaving New York City jails. In preparation. Retrieved August 15, 2006, from http://www.urban.org/reentryroundtable/inmate_challenges.pdf

Freudenberg, N., Daniels, J., Crum, M., Perkins, T., & Richie, B. E. (2005). Coming home from jail: The social and health consequences of community reentry for women, male adolescents, and their families and communities. *Am J Public Health, 95,* 1725–1736.

Gift, T. L., Lincoln, T., Tuthill, R. W., Whelan, M., Briggs, L. P., Conklin, T. J., et al. (2006). A cost-effectiveness evaluation of a jail-based chlamydia screening program for men and its impact on their partners in the community. *Sex Transm Dis, 33,* S103–S110.

Golden, M. R., Hogben, M., Handsfield, H. H., St Lawrence, J. S., Potterat, J. J., & Holmes, K. K. (2003). Partner notification for HIV and STD in the United States: Low coverage for gonorrhea, chlamydial infection, and HIV. *Sex Transm Dis, 30,* 490–496.

Gondles, E. F. (2005). A call to immunize the correctional population for hepatitis A and B. *Am J Med, 118*(Suppl. 10A), 84S–89S.

Grinstead, O. A., Zack, B., & Faigeles, B. (1999). Collaborative research to prevent HIV among male prison inmates and their female partners. *Health Educ Behav, 26,* 225–238.

Hammett, T. M. (1998). *Public health/corrections collaborations: Prevention and treatment of HIV/AIDS, STDs and TB.* Washington, DC: U. S. Department of Justice, Office of Justice Programs, National Institute of Justice.

Hammett, T. M., Maruschak, L., & Harmon, P. (1999). *1996–1997 update: HIV/AIDS, STDs, and TB in correctional facilities* (NCJ publication No. 176344). Washington, DC: National Institute of Justice, Bureau of Justice Statistics, and Centers for Disease Control and Prevention.

Hammett, T. M., Roberts, C., & Kennedy, S. (2001). Health-related issues in prisoner reentry. *Crime Delinquency, 47,* 390–409.

How to gain access to county jails for delivery of HIV/AIDS services: A guide for community-based organizations. (2004). Retrieved March 1, 2005, from http://www.health.state.ny.us/diseases/aids/publications/cbo/docs/cojailguide.pdf.

HRSA. (2002). *Reports and studies: 2002 SPNS report to CARE Act grantees on thirteen SPNS initiatives.* Health Resources and Services Administration.

Institute of Medicine. (2002). *The future of the public's health in the 21st century.* Washington, DC: National Academy of Sciences.

Kennedy, S., Lincoln, T., Hammett, T. M., Roberts, C. A., Conklin, T. J., Tuthill, R. W., et al. (2003, November 19). *Effective linkage of jail inmates to community health care: Results from an evaluation of the public health model of correctional health care* [Oral presentation]. Paper presented at the 131st Annual Meeting of the American Public Health Association, San Francisco.

Kennedy, S., Roberts, C. A., & Hammett, T. (2001). *Discharge planning and continuity of care for HIV-infected inmates as they return to the community: A study of ten states.* Cambridge, MA: Prepared for Centers for Disease Control and Prevention by Abt Associates.

Kennedy, V.C. & Moore, F.I. (2001). A systems approach to public health workforce development. *Journal of Public Health Management and Practice 7*(4), 17–22.

Klein, S. J., O'Connell, D. A., Devore, B. S., Wright, L. N., & Birkhead, G. S. (2002). Building an HIV continuum for inmates: New York State's criminal justice initiative. *AIDS Educ Prev, 14*(5 Suppl. B), 114–123.

Lincoln, T., Chavez, R. S., & Langmore-Avila, E. (2005). US experience of smoke-free prisons. *BMJ, 331,* 1473.

Lincoln, T., Kennedy, S., Tuthill, R., Roberts, C., Conklin, T. J., & Hammett, T. M. (2006). Facilitators and barriers to continuing healthcare after jail: A community-integrated program. *J Ambul Care Manage, 29,* 2–16.

Lincoln, T., & Miles, J. R. (2006). Correctional, public and community health collaboration in the USA. In M. Puisis (Ed.), *Clinical practice in correctional medicine* (2nd ed.). St. Louis: Mosby.

Macalino, G. E., Vlahov, D., Sanford-Colby, S., Patel, S., Sabin, K., Salas, C., et al. (2004). Prevalence and incidence of HIV, hepatitis B virus, and hepatitis C virus infections among males in Rhode Island prisons. *Am J Public Health, 94,* 1218–1223.

Macke, B. A., & Maher, J. E. (1999). Partner notification in the United States: An evidence-based review. *Am J Prev Med, 17,* 230–242.

May, J. P., & Lambert, W. E. (1998). Preventive health issues for individuals in jails and prisons. In M. Puisis (Ed.), *Clinical practice in correctional medicine* (pp. 259–274). St. Louis: Mosby.

Michigan DOC: Discharge planning starts early. (1999). *AIDS Policy Law, 14*(22), 9.

Morrissey, J. P., Steadman, H. J., Dalton, K. M., Cuellar, A., Stiles, P., & Cuddeback, G. S. (2006). Medicaid enrollment and mental health service use following release of jail detainees with severe mental illness. *Psychiatr Serv, 57,* 809–815.

Myers, J., Zack, B., Kramer, K., Gardner, M., Rucobo, G., & Costa-Taylor, S. (2005). Get Connected: An HIV prevention case management program for men and women leaving California prisons. *Am J Public Health, 95,* 1682–1684.

Myers, J. J., Barker, T. A., Devore, B., Garner, J. E., Laufer, F. N., Porterfield, J., et al. (2003). CDC/HRSA HIV/AIDS intervention, prevention and continuity of care demonstration project for incarcerated individuals within correctional settings and the community: Part I , a description of corrections demonstration project activites. *Journal of Correctional Health Care, 9*(4), 453–486.

National Commission on Correctional Health Care & National Institute of Justice. (2002). *The health status of soon-to-be-released inmates: A report to Congress.* Washington, DC: U.S. Department of Justice.

Needels, K., James-Burdumy, S., & Burghardt, J. (2005). Community case management for former jail inmates: Its impacts on rearrest, drug use, and HIV risk. *J Urban Health, 82,* 420–433.

Passin, W. F., Kim, A. S., Hutchinson, A. B., Crepaz, N., Herbst, J. H., & Lyles, C. M. (2006). A systematic review of HIV partner counseling and referral services: Client and provider attitudes, preferences, practices, and experiences. *Sex Transm Dis, 33,* 320–328.

Plan for providing medical case management and support services to individuals with HIV disease being released from federal or state prison—Report to Congress.

(2002). Washington, DC: Health Resources and Services Administration, HIV-AIDS Bureau.

Prochaska, J. O., & Velicer, W. F. (1997). The transtheoretical model of health behavior change. *Am J Health Promot, 12*, 38–48.

Public Health Functions Steering Committee. (1994, December 14). Public health in America. Retrieved July 4, 2004, from http://web.health.gov/phfunctions/public.htm

Public Health Infrastructure, Healthy People 2010. (2004a). Retrieved July 4, 2006, from www.healthypeople.gov/document/html/volume2/23PHI.htm

Public Health Infrastructure, Healthy People 2010. (2004b). Retrieved October 6, 2004, from www.healthypeople.gov/Document/HTML/Volume2/23PHI.htm

Re-Entry Policy Council. (2004). *Report of the Re-Entry Policy Council: Charting the safe and successful return of prisoners to the community.* New York: Author.

Rhodes, W., & Gross, M. (1997). *Case management reduces drug use and criminality among drug-involved arrestees: An experimental study of an HIV prevention intervention.* Washington, DC: U.S. Department of Justice, National Institute of Justice.

Rich, J. D., Holmes, L., Salas, C., Macalino, G., Davis, D., Ryczek, J., et al. (2001). Successful linkage of medical care and community services for HIV-positive offenders being released from prison. *J Urban Health, 78*, 279–289.

Richie, B. E., Freudenberg, N., & Page, J. (2001). Reintegrating women leaving jail into urban communities: A description of a model program. *J Urban Health, 78*, 290–303.

Roberts, C. A., Kennedy, S., & Hammett, T. M. (2004). Linkages between in-prison and community-based health services. *Journal of Correctional Health Care, 10*, 333–368.

Sadeanu, A. (2006). Video-conferencing enhances reach of the Thresholds Prison Project. Retrieved August 24, 2006, from http://www.thresholds.org/newscontent.asp?ItemID=230&

Scott, D. P., Harzke, A. J., Mizwa, M. B., Pugh, M., & Ross, M. W. (2003). Evaluation of an HIV peer education program in Texas prisons. *Journal of Correctional Health Care, 10*, 151–173.

Shelton, D. (2001). AIDS and drug use prevention intervention for confined youthful offenders. *Issues Ment Health Nurs, 22*, 159–172.

Sheu, M., Hogan, J., Allsworth, J., Stein, M., Vlahov, D., Schoenbaum, E. E., et al. (2002). Continuity of medical care and risk of incarceration in HIV-positive and high-risk HIV-negative women. *J Womens Health (Larchmt), 11*, 743–750.

Shuter, J. (2002). Communicable diseases in inmates: Public health opportunities. In National Commission on Correctional Health Care (Ed.), *The health status of soon-to-be-released inmates: A report to Congress, Volume 2.* Washington, DC: U.S. Department of Justice.

Skolnick, A. A. (1998). Correctional and community health care collaborations. *JAMA, 279*, 98–99.

Springer, S. A., & Altice, F. L. (2005). Managing HIV/AIDS in correctional settings. *Curr HIV/AIDS Rep, 2*(4), 165–170.

Springer, S. A., Pesanti, E., Hodges, J., Macura, T., Doros, G., & Altice, F. L. (2004). Effectiveness of antiretroviral therapy among HIV-infected prisoners: Reincarceration and the lack of sustained benefit after release to the community. *Clin Infect Dis, 38*, 1754–1760.

St Lawrence, J., Eldridge, G. D., Shelby, M. C., Little, C. E., Brasfield, T. L., & O'Bannon, R. E., 3rd. (1997). HIV risk reduction for incarcerated women: A comparison of brief interventions based on two theoretical models. *J Consult Clin Psychol, 65*, 504–509.

Travis, J. (2005). *But they all come back: Facing the challenges of prisoner reentry.* Washington, DC: The Urban Institute Press.

Travis, J., Solomon, A. L., & Waul, M. (2001). *From prison to home: The dimensions and consequences of prisoner reentry.* Washington, DC: The Urban Institute Justice Policy Center.

Tuthill, R. W., Lincoln, T., Conklin, T. J., Kennedy, S., Hammett, T. M., & Roberts, C. A. (2002, October 21). *Does involuntary cigarette smoking abstinence among inmates during correctional incarceration result in continued abstinence post release?* [poster] Paper presented at the 26th National Conference on Correctional Health Care, Nashville, TN.

Varghese, B., Lincoln, T., Miller, A., Mugalla, C., Gift, T. L., Irwin, K. L., et al. (2002, October 21). *Economic evaluation of the HIV counseling and testing program at a county jail.* Paper presented at the 26th National Conference on Correctional Health Care, Nashville, TN.

Varghese, B., & Peterman, T. A. (2001). Cost-effectiveness of HIV counseling and testing in US prisons. *J Urban Health, 78,* 304–312.

Veysey, B. M., Steadman, H. J., Morrissey, J. P., & Johnsen, M. (1997). In search of the missing linkages: Continuity of care in U.S. jails. *Behav Sci Law, 15,* 383–397.

Vigilante, K. C., Flynn, M. M., Affleck, P. C., Stunkle, J. C., Merriman, N. A., Flanigan, T. P., et al. (1999). Reduction in recidivism of incarcerated women through primary care, peer counseling, and discharge planning. *J Womens Health, 8,* 409–415.

Virginia Department of Corrections. (2003). Pilot program offers reentry transition services to offenders. Retrieved October 18, 2004, from http://www.vadoc.state. va.us/offenders/institutions/programs/reentry.htm

Weinbaum, C., Lyerla, R., & Margolis, H. S. (2003). Prevention and control of infections with hepatitis viruses in correctional settings. Centers for Disease Control and Prevention. *MMWR Recomm Rep, 52*(RR-1), 1–36; quiz CE31–34.

Wolitski, R. J., & the Project Start Writing Group for The Project Start Study Group. (2006). Relative efficacy of a multisession sexual risk-reduction intervention for young men released from prisons in 4 states. *Am J Public Health, 96,* 1854–1861.

Chapter 30

Improving the Care for HIV-Infected Prisoners: An Integrated Prison-Release Health Model

Sandra A. Springer and Frederick L. Altice

Introduction

Highly active antiretroviral therapy (HAART) has remarkably transformed HIV disease into a chronic condition such that when patients completely suppress viral replication, they can expect to live a normal life expectancy. Unfortunately, many of those who might benefit most from HAART (e.g., illicit drug users, the mentally ill, and the socially and medically marginalized) are less likely to receive it, and when they do, less likely to adhere to treatment. Many of these individuals do not interface consistently with health care institutions in the community setting, yet when incarcerated, have an important opportunity not only to be identified as being HIV-infected, but also to initiate HAART if medically indicated.

The prevalence of HIV infection among prisoners is five to seven times greater among incarcerated persons compared to the general population (Crosland, Poshkus, & Rich, 2002; Spaulding et al., 2002). Prisons and jails house individuals with HIV who have not traditionally benefited from access to HIV care and antiretroviral therapy in community settings. Specifically, prisons are comprised of HIV-infected individuals with comorbid medical conditions such as substance use disorder and serious psychiatric illnesses and are socially marginalized through relapsing homelessness, poverty, and unstable living circumstances.

HIV care has resulted in impressive reductions in mortality in the New York prison system (CDC, 1999) and HIV/AIDS is no longer the leading cause of prison-related mortality nationally (Linder, Enders, Craig, Richardson, & Meyers, 2002). In nearby Connecticut where 98% of prescribed HAART regimens were within the Department of Health and Human Services guidelines, impressive increases in CD4 count and reductions in HIV-1 RNA levels were observed. Indeed, 59% of these prisoners achieved a viral load below the level of detection prior to release. Despite these successes, the one-quarter of subjects who were reincarcerated lost the viral load and CD4 benefits within 3 months after release to the community (Springer et al., 2004).

The revolving door of prison and jail results in one-quarter of all HIV-infected individuals in the United States becoming involved with the correctional system annually (Hammett, Harmon, & Rhodes, 2002). Owing to the sheer magnitude of the problem and the public health implications, developing effective linkages that result in sustained clinical benefit after release to the community is urgently needed. The challenge is finding a mechanism whereby HIV-infected prisoners receive necessary support, guidance, and structure as they transition from the highly structured environment of prison to the often-anticipated hopelessness, despair, unstable housing and social support relationships, and seemingly insurmountable obstacles on release (Thompson et al., 1998).

Many HIV-infected inmates are released to the community at an unprecedented pace (Beck, Karberg, & Harrison, 2002). One of the main goals in providing effective medical care to HIV-infected incarcerated persons is to hopefully maintain success of therapy on release into the community. This is not only important in maintaining the health and well-being of the released inmates, but also to decrease the transmission of HIV to members of the community after release. This is particularly true with the high prevalence of HIV risk behaviors reported by newly released HIV-infected inmates (Stephenson et al., 2005). A major risk behavior for newly diagnosed heterosexually acquired HIV infection among African-American women in the general population, who did not engage in high-risk behavior, was having sex with a partner who had a history of incarceration (Hammett et al., 2002). In the following sections, we will discuss the current state of knowledge on prison-release programs and provide some insight into future program development that might have implications for communities that struggle with continuity of care for people living with HIV/AIDS.

The challenge of providing continuity of care for released HIV-infected prisoners has been a formidable challenge, yet a number of programs have created successful forays to address this pervasive problem. Individual programs have responded to uniquely distinct challenges based on their specific population and geographical constraints. It seems clear that there are five distinct areas of focus for released HIV-infected prisoners. These include social stabilization that is often achieved through (1) adaptation of case management services for newly released prisoners, (2) continuity of antiretroviral therapy to preserve the benefit of treatment after the confines of incarceration, (3) continuity or initiation of substance abuse treatment, including the introduction of pharmacologically based opiate substitution or alcohol relapse prevention therapy prior to release, (4) linkages with appropriate treatment for mental illness, and (5) reducing HIV-risk taking behaviors as part of secondary prevention. These five important factors will be discussed in this chapter.

Adaptation of Case Management Services

Case management means that specific persons will coordinate medical and psychosocial care for individuals with complex medical needs such as HIV-infected soon-to-be-released prisoners. At present, case-management services are the mainstay of prisoner-release programs for HIV-infected inmates, with the intention to decrease recidivism, improve overall health, and decrease drug use. A few programs have demonstrated modest success in providing for unmet needs of HIV-infected released prisoners (housing, medical care, food) on release to the community; however, none of them have been able to demonstrate continued success with antiretroviral therapy (F. Altice & Khoshnood, 1997; Laufer, Arriola, & Dawson-Rose, 2002). Such projects have been implemented in Connecticut, Rhode Island, Massachusetts, and New York (Conklin, Lincoln, & Flanigan, 1998; Crosland et al., 2002; Flanigan et al., 1996). Table 30.1 provides summary details of release programs in the United States all of which are described in more detail below by geographic region.

California

A transitional program in the San Francisco jail called Homebase (Cloutier, 2002) provides direct linkage services between the local jail and community HIV providers. This program enrolls them in the AIDS Drug Assistance Program (ADAP) or MediCal insurance to help with overcoming barriers to antiretroviral therapy after release. It also directly delivers medications to clients and provides temporary housing, nursing care, case management, psychiatric services, and referral to drug treatment centers. As of June 30, 2002, 172 people have enrolled in the project and 94 have completed the study (Homebase, 2006). Unfortunately, there have not been any published data to support this program with regard to adherence to HIV medications and/or stabilization of biological outcomes.

Connecticut

Project TLC (F. Altice & Khoshnood, 1997) is a transitional case management program used to link inmates to care in Connecticut. It was the first such program for soon-to-be-released HIV-infected prisoners and began in

Table 30.1 Characteristics of prison-release programs.

State	CA[1]	CT[2]	NJ[3]	NY[4]	MA[5,3]	RI[6,7]	VA[8]
Prison (P) or Jail (J)	J	P	J	P	P	P	P
Worked with prisoner before release	Y	Y	Y	Y	Y	Y	Y
Services provided							
Case management and advocacy	Y	Y	Y	Y	Y	Y	N
Medical	Y	N	N	UN	N	Y	N
Nursing	Y	N	Y	UN	N	Y	N
Drug treatment	Y	N	N	Y	N	Y	N
Medication adherence	Y	N	Y	UN	N	UN	N
Housing	Y	N	N	UN	UN	UN	UN
Mental health	Y	N	N	UN	UN	UN	UN
Type of evaluation	O	O	D	O	D	O	D
Sample size	172	UN	UN	700	UN	97	UN
HIV clinical endpoints	N	N	N	UN	UN	N	UN

Y, yes; N, no; UN, unknown; NA, not applicable; O, observational; D descriptive.
[1] Cloutien (2002).
[2] F. Altice & Khoshnood (1997).
[3] Laufer et al. (2002).
[4] Richie et al. (2001).
[5] Conklin et al. (1998).
[6] Holmes et al. (2002).
[7] Rich et al. (2001).
[8] Kaplowitz et al. (2002).

1993. This program is operated by a community-based organization that has collaborated with the correctional system for years and works with the inmate to secure unmet needs during the 90 days prior to release and for 30 days in the community until the client can be transferred to a community-based case manager. Case managers meet the inmates at least twice prior to release to determine potential needs the inmate will require in the community on release. They schedule all appointments necessary on release and assist the client in obtaining such appointments including medical, mental health, and substance abuse treatment. ADAP approval is secured before release to the community. In an observational study of those who received the service compared to those who did not, the proportion who made it to their first medical appointment was 59% in the treatment group versus 15% in those not receiving the service. Retention in care was not measured. Recidivism to prison or jail did not differ for each group during the 1-year follow-up, but the mean time to reincarceration was shorter for Project TLC clients compared to the control group. Long-term clinical benefit such as continued antiretroviral benefit as measured by CD4 count and HIV-1 RNA viral load has not been measured, nor has relapse to illicit drug use been fully evaluated. More recently, this program has been successful in directly linking patients with a history of opioid dependence to methadone maintenance on the day of release.

New Jersey

The Visiting Nurses Association of New Jersey employs an HIV care coordinator and two outreach specialists assigned to the Monmouth County jail to provide HIV prevention, intervention, care, and discharge planning services to HIV-infected and high-risk uninfected inmates (Laufer et al., 2002). The outreach specialist provides all follow-up assessments to address adherence to prevention, care, and treatment regimens while the care coordinator provides prevention counseling and testing services. There is a reported network of services to offer inmates on release including mental health, substance use, medical care, housing, and other services. Once the inmate is released into the community, it is the care coordinator's responsibility to coordinate the service plan for each released inmate. No specific details regarding outcomes from this program have been reported.

New York

Health Link is a program that helps drug-using women released from New York City's Rose M. Singer Detention Center for Women at the Rikers Island Correctional Facility, improve their quality of life after release by working directly with the women throughout their jail term and on release to the community (Richie, Freudenberg, & Page, 2001). Such areas of attention included improving community organizations to serve ex-offenders and therefore to help decrease repeat arrests. From 1997 to May 2000, 700 women were enrolled in this program. Preliminary results from time period of 1994–1996 demonstrated that at 6 months, 46% of the enrolled women had been retained in the program, and at 12 months the retention rate was 35%. Women receiving comprehensive Health Link services had a reincarceration rate that was 21% lower than the usual jail services only group. This project does not specifically target HIV-infected individuals and would require careful assessment of those with HIV to determine if there is a benefit to this group. It is, however, one of the few jail-release programs that target an even more elusive group than released prisoners who have more time for planning for discharge.

A retrospective chart review of inmates who were paroled from New York correctional facilities (Hubbard, 2002) revealed that individuals who had experienced transitional planning were more likely to have undetectable viral loads postrelease (93% versus 77%) than those who did not receive transitional planning. This review shows that transitional programs alone are associated with the best clinical outcomes in this population and that structure for these individuals is paramount for improved health.

Massachusetts

One program from Hampden County Correctional Center in Ludlow, Massachusetts, links jail inmates to the community via a very systematic program which involves linking the inmates to a health care team headed by a physician from their neighborhood health center (Conklin et al., 1998). In this program, the physician who treats the inmate in jail will usually be that person's physician on release. Also, discharge planning begins while the inmate is still in jail. An assigned case manager links an inmate to appropriate social, psychiatric, and medical services in the inmate's geographical released area. Greater than 50% of the inmates discharged with HIV infection or other chronic illness received regular medical care in the community. Furthermore, the number of discharges receiving care in the community increased to greater than 80% when comprehensive discharge services were provided. Clinical outcome data, such as improvements in viral load or CD4 count, have not been reported.

Another program called the Transitional Intervention Program (TIP) (Laufer et al., 2002) provides linkages between the Department of Corrections and the community for HIV-infected inmates in Massachusetts. TIP serves all 13 county jails, 23 state prisons, and 61 Department of Youth Services Facilities in the state. TIP includes a team of providers whose responsibility is to link inmates to the community: a social worker within the incarceration facility coordinates transitional mental health care and substance use referrals; and a reintegration specialist, who is an ex-inmate, provides support for the released inmate. The inmates are discharged with appropriate links to primary, mental health care, substance use treatment, housing, benefits information, immigration services, family services, and education/employment training. The TIP team works with the person for up to 6 months postrelease. Data regarding clinical outcomes such as HIV-1 RNA viral load and CD4 T-cell count and return to drug abuse have not been reported.

Rhode Island

Project Bridge in Rhode Island links released incarcerated persons to primary care services via intensive case management (Holmes, Drainoni, & Rich, 2002; Rich et al., 2001). All prisoners in the sole combined jail and prison within Rhode Island have had mandatory HIV testing since 1989. All HIV-infected inmates are offered enrollment in Project Bridge within 30–90 days prior to release to the community. A social worker and case manager meet with the inmate who is then offered voluntary enrollment in the program which involves supportive services for a period of 18 months. Services include mental illness triage and referral, substance abuse assessment and treatment, appointments for HIV and other medical conditions, referral for housing and other entitlement assistance. Between January 1997 and June 2001, there were only 97 participants enrolled. Follow-up was successfully maintained for 98% for a 12-month period (patients were enrolled in a longitudinal study and paid for follow-up visits). Total enrollment at the end of study period was 58 (Crosland et al., 2002; Rich et al., 2001); HIV-1 RNA and CD4 count levels were not reported.

Virginia

A program from Virginia (Kaplowitz, Kaatz, & Weir-Wiggins, 2002) attempted to provide linkage with the inmate, parole officer, community provider, and department of corrections on inmate discharge. This service provided enrollment in the AIDS Drug Assistance Program (ADAP). They trained 425 probation and parole officers to be a link between HIV-infected parolees and community providers. Over 65% of the 150 HIV-infected inmates who returned for their parole visits kept their postdischarge medical appointments. The majority of released prisoners, however, did not keep their parole appointments.

These programs differ by issues of geography, whether or not the release facility was a prison or jail, and by specific features that are not likely replicable in other settings. Although these programs have provided benefit with regard to enhancing social support for soon-to-be-released HIV-infected prisoners, none have successfully demonstrated improved clinical benefit after release to the community. Some of the linkages to the community simply involve giving the soon-to-be-released prisoners a list of agencies that might help them apply for services, obtain health care, acquire a job, and apply for housing. Passive referrals have never been demonstrated to be effective for this population. Furthermore, many programs do not have a way to ensure that released prisoners will actually show up for appointments that are made prior to release or help them with adherence to HIV medications. Also, many released prisoners with histories of opiate dependency may not get adequate linkages to opiate substitution therapies such as methadone programs or see providers who can prescribe buprenorphine causing many to relapse to drug use which then leads to missed appointments and nonadherence to HIV medications.

For the most part, these variations in types of case management services for released prisoners alone have been unsuccessful in demonstrating overall improved HIV clinical outcomes such as decreased HIV-1 RNA viral load and improved CD4 T-cell count. Consistent case management services for homeless HIV-infected persons in the San Francisco area, however, not specifically developed for released prisoners, have been associated with improved CD4 count (Kushel et al., 2006). Such information suggests that continued intensive case management services after release, not just around the release time period, could be beneficial.

Transitioning to the community from prison is often chaotic and involves a complex array of health care linkages, housing and job searches, financial benefit application processes, psychosocial support, and effective drug rehabilitation treatment. Case management programs need to be modified to encompass the necessities such as housing, health care, drug treatment, employment, and insurance coverage for released prisoners. Furthermore, these services should have a continuity plan to allow for time for the released inmate to adjust to reintegrating into the community. Integration of such services will likely result in reductions in mortality and recidivism for released prisoners, as well as decrease HIV transmission to individuals in the community.

Directly Administered Antiretroviral Therapy (DAART)

AIDS mortality rate has substantially decreased in correctional facilities with the institution of highly active antiretroviral therapy (HAART) and chemoprophylaxis of opportunistic infections (OIs). The obstacles to continuing HAART after release to the community, however, include: substance abuse, mental illness, homelessness, unemployment, poverty, co-infection with other illnesses such as hepatitis B and C and tuberculosis, as well as adherence to complicated ART regimen (CDC, 2001; Glaser & Greifinger, 1993). It is important to determine more effective ways to address adherence to HAART for the recently released prisoner population so as to improve mortality as well as decrease transmission risk to the community.

Excellent adherence to HAART (e.g., taking medications >95% of the scheduled time) suppresses HIV viral load and increases CD4 cells, thereby keeping HIV-infected persons healthy and free from AIDS–associated opportunistic infections. Improvements in CD4 lymphocyte count and viral load have been described over a 5-year period in prisoners prescribed HAART in the Connecticut Department of Corrections. Overall, 59% of these 1844 patients achieved an undetectable viral load (Springer et al., 2004). However, this study failed to demonstrate continued success after these prisoners were released to the community with only transitional case management services. This is likely due to relapse to drug use and poor adherence to antiretroviral medications.

Directly administered antiretroviral therapy (DAART) provides a highly monitored setting where HAART can be offered. An outreach worker assists the person in taking medications on a daily or near-daily schedule with the goal of transitioning the person to taking medications on their own. The trained outreach worker can identify names of pills and explain side effects that the person can discuss with their physician as well as reinforce the need to take medications daily in order to avoid development of genotypic resistance and decrease the chance of acquiring AIDS-associated opportunistic infection. This method of medication administration may have particular appeal to recently released prisoners who do well in highly structured monitored settings. DAART can offer released prisoners encouragement to continue their excellent adherence to HAART therapy that they achieved while incarcerated. DAART has been demonstrated to be effective not only for prisoners (Babudieri, Aceti, D'Offizi, Carbonara, & Starnini, 2000; Fischl, Castro, & Monroig, 2001; Stephenson et al., 2005) but also for active IVDUs utilizing a mobile health care van (F. L. Altice, Smith-Rohrberg, Bruce, Springer, & Friedland, 2007; F. Altice et al., 2004) as discussed below.

Several studies have demonstrated improved clinical outcomes when DAART was employed in clinical settings. In a study of subjects enrolled in four clinical trials where prisoners received DAART and community participants received self-administered therapy (SAT), a significantly higher proportion of DAART patients in the prison had a nondetectable viral load after 80 weeks compared to the SAT group (95% versus 75%) (Fischl et al., 2001). Though impressive, the findings were obtained among highly motivated individuals who volunteered for a clinical trial. Patients in Italian prisons who received DAART were statistically more likely to achieve an HIV-1 RNA level below the limits of detection (62% versus 34%) and increase their CD4 count above 200 cells/ml (95% versus 68%) than those who self-administered their medications (Babudieri et al., 2000). In Connecticut, where female prisoners receive DAART, the reduction in viral load was 1.26 $\log_{10}$ compared to 0.86 $\log_{10}$ among men where DAART was not deployed (Springer et al., 2004).

In another study where DAART was not compared, SAT was found to produce increases in CD4 count similar to those described in clinical trials in a New York City jail (Shuter, 2002) and viral load and CD4 improvements were similar to those described in community settings for 170 Wisconsin prisoners (Sosman, Baker, & Catz, 2002). In contrast, in one small study of 34 prisoners in North Carolina where MEMS caps were used, DAART resulted in reduced adherence compared to SAT (Stephenson et al., 2005). Unfortunately, clinical outcomes were not compared and would have determined if medication administration recordkeeping resulted in the difference in adherence. The discrepancies of DAART outcomes in correctional settings are likely to reflect the way in which DAART is administered; for instance, in some settings, medication-taking is observed by a correctional officer. In such settings, it is surprising that any HIV-infected patient would take their medications.

More recently, two studies of DAART found differing results. In one study, 250 inner-city, low-income patients selected from screened patients were randomized to receive either DAART or intensive adherence case management or standard care for 6 months. Intention-to-treat analysis found no difference in adherence between the three groups; all were equally impressively highly adherent to their HAART regimens (Wohl et al., 2006). This study has been criticized, however, for its lack of demonstration that the DAART intervention itself had any likely benefit to patients, the choice of a study population without demonstrated problematic adherence, and analytical approaches that do not control for baseline characteristics (Smith-Rohrberg & Altice, 2006). A case–control study of 82 patients receiving DAART within Baltimore methadone clinics found the opposite results. Subjects who received DAART were compared to 809 patients who were receiving antiretroviral therapy as prescribed by their physicians as part of the Johns Hopkins HIV Cohort (Lucas et al., 2006). DAART subjects were significantly more likely to have an undetectable viral load and greater increase in CD4 cell count at 12 months than the comparison group of injection drug users (IDUs) who received methadone and self-administered their HAART.

A recent study of HIV-infected active drug users that used a randomized controlled design demonstrated that DAART was more effective at reducing HIV-1 RNA and increasing CD4 count than SAT (F. L. Altice et al., 2007). Further analyses demonstrated that the increased adherence by DAART subjects did not result in any increase in rate of development of genotypic resistance mutations(Smith-Rohrberg, Kozal, Springer, & Altice, submitted). DAART subjects were also more likely to have improved outcomes if they received enhanced services, such as increased access to health care and case management services(Smith-Rohrberg, Mezger, Walton, Bruce, & Altice, 2006).

The discrepancies in outcomes found in systems using DAART and self-administered therapy are likely explained by the variety of approaches used to define DAART. For instance, in some settings, correctional officers observe therapy. This will result in widespread nonadherence by HIV-infected individuals who do not want to disclose their HIV status. Other systems provide DAART only to those who are released from their housing units to pick up medications. Other programs insist on providing DAART at inconvenient hours (e.g., 4:00 a.m.), resulting in decreased attendance for many who work alternative shifts or for those on psychiatric medications that enhance sleep (Springer & Altice, 2005). Also, the studies which examine the usefulness of DAART can also be fraught with lack of generalizability as the recent Los Angeles study (Wohl et al., 2006) demonstrated. In this study, the majority of subjects did not have demonstrated problematic adherence and the DAART intervention had never been proven to be effective in pilot studies. For the remainder of subjects who were studied, there was a large percentage of highly motivated subjects as evidence by the high percentage of subjects achieving a nondetectable viral load(Smith-Rohrberg & Altice, 2006). Released prisoners, unlike the Los Angeles study subjects, have difficulty with adherence to medications. On release, in addition to the difficulty taking medications, they also face many competing demands, including: adequate and safe housing, access to medical and mental health care, making parole appointments, relapse to drug use, finding employment, as well as adjusting to the responsibilities of the family they were separated from during their incarceration period. The highly monitored setting of a DAART program can be beneficial for released prisoners by improving HIV care and developing less genotypic resistance (Daar, Cohen, Remien, Sherer, & Smith, 2003; Pollard, 2002), as well as offer motivation to decrease relapse to drug use, and decrease sexual risk behavior.

Substance Abuse Treatment

Over 75–80% of prisoners have a history of drug and alcohol problems prior to incarceration (Hammett et al., 2002). One of the most pressing needs facing released prisoners is relapse to illicit drug use and the start of the cycle that resulted in their prior incarceration.

Opiate Substitution Therapy

It is beyond the scope of this chapter to fully discuss how this might be accomplished. A recent review examines existing programs that utilize therapeutic communities and opiate substitution therapies such as methadone, LAAM, and buprenorphine (Smith-Rohrberg, Bruce, & Altice, 2004). For jail inmates whose stay within correctional settings is brief, induction and stabilization of opiate substitution therapy may be one way to serve as a bridge to treatment in the community. For prison inmates whose sentence is longer, initiation of substitution therapy prior to release can similarly assist with drug treatment needs. Below is a description of methadone and buprenorphine treatment, which are FDA-approved opiate substitution pharmacotherapies, used to effectively treat patients with DSM-IV criteria for opioid dependence. LAAM is not described as it is no longer available due to fatal cardiac toxicities associated with its use.

Methadone is a full opioid, mu-receptor agonist and has been shown in numerous studies to be effective in decreasing relapse to opiate use and improving retention rates in drug treatment programs. Furthermore, methadone treatment has many other benefits, including decreased criminal behavior and incarceration, improved social functioning, increased employment, and reduction in HIV risk behaviors. Several studies of methadone maintenance programs have been evaluated and have been successful in incarcerated settings in Canada (Sibbald, 2002), Australia (Dolan, Hall, & Wodak, 1996), and the United States (Tomasino, Swanson, Nolan, & Shuman, 2001). The best described program in the United States is within the jail setting in New York's Rikers Island. In Project KEEP (Key Extended Entry Program), inmates entering the prison already on methadone are maintained. The program also offers methadone initiation or supervised opiate withdrawal for opiate-dependent patients who are not receiving pharmacological treatment. Injection drug behaviors 6 months after release were reduced among Project KEEP participants who were maintained on methadone compared to those who were tapered off methadone (85% versus 37%). Retention in drug treatment 6 months after release, unfortunately, was modest with 27% of methadone maintained versus only 9% of those tapered off methadone remaining in treatment. The low retention was likely due to the suboptimal dose (~30 mg) of methadone provided to maintained patients (Magura, Rosenblum, Lewis, & Joseph, 1993). One limitation to use of methadone in the treatment of HIV has been the drug interactions between these two treatments (Bruce, Altice, Gourevitch, & Friedland, 2006; Khalsa, Genser, Vocci, Francis, & Bean, 2002) some of which may precipitate opiate withdrawal (F. L. Altice, Friedland, & Cooney, 1999).

Buprenorphine, a partial opioid, mu-receptor agonist, can be prescribed by community and correctional physicians who complete an 8-hour training program. This treatment for opiate dependence does not require the stringent regulations of a federally licensed methadone clinic. As a partial opiate-receptor agonist, buprenorphine does not produce serious adverse side effects such as respiratory depression that can result in lethal overdose. The potential for abuse exists, however, efforts in this regard have been thwarted through the co-formulation of buprenorphine with naloxone that when crushed and injected, results in marked opiate withdrawal symptoms. Buprenorphine has been shown to be equivalent to methadone with respect to relapse to drug use (Mattick, Ali, & White, 2002; Schottenfeld, Pakes, Oliveto, Ziedonis, & Kosten, 1997). Buprenorphine should not be co-administered in patients with benzodiazepine abuse, but may be safely prescribed when benzodiazepine prescription is not abused. Buprenorphine, with its safety profile and its relative lack of federally legislated constraints, opens up new possibilities for the supervised withdrawal and maintenance of prisoners with opiate dependence or abuse (Smith-Rohrberg et al., 2004) and has recently been adopted in jail settings in Connecticut and San Francisco.

While corrections-based buprenorphine programs have yet to be fully evaluated in the United States, the French have provided buprenorphine to opiate-dependent inmates since 1996 (Durand, 2001; Levasseur, Marzo, Ross, & Blatier, 2002). In a retrospective cohort study, 3600 medical files of French prisoners were analyzed to determine the comparative effectiveness of methadone, buprenorphine, and abstinence treatment following the legalization of prison-administered buprenorphine (Levasseur et al., 2002). Compared to abstinence-based treatment, both buprenorphine and methadone maintenance treatment within prison resulted in reduced recidivism rates after release. The early successes of the French experience with buprenorphine in corrections highlight the need to apply and evaluate buprenorphine within the U.S. correctional system as an effective treatment for opioid dependence and to reduce criminal activity and recidivism.

The use of buprenorphine and methadone as pharmacological treatment strategies to maintain an opiate-dependent person is evidence-based and the community standard of care. Such studies have shown decreases in relapse to drug use, decreases in recidivism rates, and improved adherence to antiretroviral therapy. Applying these models of treatment to correctional and prison-release programs should be carefully considered for those with HIV infection in order to reduce recidivism rates, reduce HIV risk behaviors, and enhance adherence to antiretroviral therapy. Buprenorphine is approved to be prescribed by primary care physicians and has been found to be as safe and effective as methadone at preventing relapse to opiate use, reduce recidivism rates as well as improve adherence to antiretroviral therapy and decrease morbidity (Durand, 2001; Levasseur et al., 2002; Schottenfeld et al., 1997)

Alcohol Treatment

In 2002, almost 50% of jail inmates reported symptoms of alcohol abuse or dependency prior to incarceration (Karberg & James, 2005) and in 1997 almost 60% of state and federal prisoners reported drinking alcohol at time of offense (Mumola, 1999). Heavy alcohol use has been associated with poor adherence to antiretroviral therapy for HIV-infected persons, as well as increased HIV-risk taking behaviors (Lucas, Gebo, Chaisson, & Moore, 2002; Theall, Clark, Powell, Smith, & Kissinger, 2006). Furthermore, active alcohol use has been found to have decreased likelihood of having suppressed HIV-1 viral load as compared to those who do not use alcohol (Palepu et al., 2003). Substance abuse treatment, defined as alcohol counseling, however, was not associated with improved adherence to antiretroviral medication or viral load suppression (Palepu, Horton, Tibbetts, Meli, & Samet, 2004). To date, alcohol pharmacotherapy simultaneously coupled with alcohol relapse prevention counseling for HIV-infected persons with problematic drinking or alcohol abuse/dependence has not been evaluated. Currently there are three FDA-approved medications for treatment of alcohol dependence: naltrexone, acamprosate, and disulfiram. Among HIV-infected patients, there are no studies of using combinations of these medications or when combined with effective alcohol counseling. This field is less evolved compared to similar studies among opioid-dependent patients receiving substitution therapy.

The following is a brief description of each of the approved treatments for alcohol dependence and problematic drinking.

Naltrexone is a full opioid receptor antagonist and is FDA-approved to prevent relapse to alcohol use in the treatment of alcohol dependence. It has been found in certain circumstances to prevent relapse to alcohol use in those who are alcohol dependent. Contraindications to its use are concurrent use of opiates or opioid substitution therapy (i.e. buprenorphine, methadone, LAAM) as it may precipitate withdrawal. Subjects who are currently receiving opiate substitution therapy or who are using prescription narcotics or heroin to control pain should be excluded from this treatment. Naltrexone is available in both oral and injectable formulations. It is dosed once a day and can be taken with daily antiretroviral therapy. Benefits of its use include less relapse to alcohol use and possibly improved adherence to antiretroviral regimens. Alcohol use has been associated with poor adherence to antiretroviral therapy and increased morbidity. Therefore, a once-daily medication that is FDA-approved for alcohol relapse prevention may be very helpful to decrease relapse to alcohol use and improve adherence to antiretroviral therapy. Injectable naltrexone has recently been approved, providing for once-monthly dosage that may further improve adherence to alcohol and HIV treatment. Poorly tolerated adverse events affect about 15% of patients treated with naltrexone and this principally includes minor side effects of nausea and headache. In certain persons a dose-dependent hepatotoxicity can occur with naltrexone and for this reason its use is contraindicated in patients who also have hepatic impairment due to cirrhosis. Therefore, those persons with elevated liver function tests three times normal and those with a past medical history of cirrhosis should be excluded from this treatment, as would be done in routine clinical care. Standard liver function tests should be monitored initially at 4 weeks and then at 8- to 12-week intervals (Kiefer & Mann, 2005; Mason, 2003; Roozen et al., 2006; Williams, 2005).

Acamprosate (Campral®), calcium homotaurinate, is believed to block glutaminergic *N*-methyl-D-aspartate receptors and activate gamma-aminobutyric acid type A receptors and was recently approved by the FDA for treatment of alcohol dependence. Acamprosate normalizes the deregulation of NMDA-mediated glutaminergic neurotransmission that occurs during chronic alcohol consumption and decreases the physiological mechanisms that may prompt relapse. Multiple studies have shown that this drug can reduce short- and long-term relapse rates in patients with alcohol dependence and can be used safely in those who are being treated with opiates or opiate substitution therapy. Furthermore, the safety profile of acamprosate is very favorable. The main adverse event reported across multiple trials is diarrhea, and in certain circumstances can precipitate renal insufficiency. The main downside to the use of this drug is that it must be administered three times a day, which may not be favorable for most persons. Diarrhea is avoided by gradually increasing the dose of acamprosate from one tablet of 333 mg by mouth three times a day to two tablets three times a day over 2 weeks. Renal insufficiency should be screened for prior to initiation of therapy and monitored at 4 weeks after initiation of therapy and then at 8- to 12-week intervals. Recent evaluations have found that the combination of acamprosate and naltrexone may be more effective combined than acamprosate alone (Kiefer & Mann, 2005; Mason, 2003; Williams, 2005).

Disulfiram (Antabuse®) inhibits acetaldehyde dehydrogenases. It has been used to treat alcohol dependence for more than 40 years and has very limited effectiveness. It has been shown to reduce frequency of drinking days; however, it has not been shown to improve relapse rates compared with placebo. Compliance with oral disulfiram is very low with dropout rates approaching 50%. This low compliance is due to the significant symptoms that can occur if one takes this medication after drinking alcohol. It should be taken at least 12 hours after abstaining from alcohol. If taken immediately after alcohol use, one can have symptoms of palpitations, flushing nausea, vomiting, and headache and in some cases one can develop myocardial infarction, respiratory depression, and death. It is prescribed at an initial dosage of 250 mg per day up to a maximum of 500 mg per day. Due to the significant problems with compliance and significant serious possibly fatal reactions, however, it is seldom recommended to be used in the primary care setting (Williams, 2005). Therefore, this would not be an ideal medication for use in released prisoners.

Injectable naltrexone has the most potential for released prisoners due to its effectiveness at preventing relapse to alcohol use and improved compliance. It cannot be used for those on opiate substitution therapy. Acamprosate has the advantage of being co-administered with opiate substitution therapy but has the disadvantage of possibly poor compliance due to its three times a day dosing intervals. All in all though, use of alcohol pharmacotherapy may provide improved adherence to antiretroviral therapy and improved clinical benefit with less relapse to alcohol use and lower recidivism rates and is worth studying in this population. Hence, it is worthwhile developing thoughtful prisoner-release programs that incorporate elements of DAART programs and pharmacological therapy that treats both opiate dependency and alcoholism. Integrating these components into prison-release programs may therefore have a stabilizing effect (addressing primary prevention needs of substance abuse) and provide the platform for other secondary needs such as adherence to HAART.

Mental Illness Treatment

Mental illness is highly prevalent in correctional institutions. The Bureau of Justice Statistics estimated that approximately one-third of state prisoners self-reported having some mental illness in the year 2000 (Feder, 1991). However, only 1.6% of all inmates or 10% of those identified as mentally ill were receiving any form of treatment for their psychiatric disorder. The majority of state prisons do not provide inpatient care for mental illness within the correctional facility and therefore mental illness is usually undiagnosed and untreated or improperly treatment during incarceration. For this reason, many prisoners are released to the community with improperly diagnosed or undiagnosed mental illness.

Mental illness, in particular major depressive disorder (MDD), is associated with poor adherence to medical care, including adherence to antiretroviral therapy (Bouhnick, 2002; Carrieri et al., 2003; Tucker, Burnam, Sherbourne, Kung, & Gifford, 2003; Turner et al., 2001). Untreated mental illness is also associated with increased risk of acquisition and transmission of HIV infection and potentially multidrug-resistant virus (F. L. Altice et al., 1998; Kozal et al., 2005; Stein, Solomon, Herman, Anderson, & Miller, 2003). Furthermore, recidivism rates are higher in released prisoners with comorbid untreated mental illnesses (Feder, 1991; Lovell, Gagliardi, & Peterson, 2002). Therefore, postrelease programs should also target linkage to community programs that also include treatment for mental illness.

Certain programs outside of and within the United States have recognized the significant unmet needs of released prisoners with mental illnesses and have tried to improve care on transition to the community. In the United Kingdom, a government–funded program has spent considerable time to determine appropriate needs of offenders with mental disorders especially targeting those who were repeat offenders to improve on linkages to the appropriate rehabilitation programs in the community (Badger, Vaughan, Woodward, & Williams, 1999).

Within the United States, an extensive proposed community reintegration program of male prisoners in the New Jersey Department of Corrections (NJ DOC) has described the costs associated with investing in actual linkages to mental health programs for those who are in need of continued treatment for mental illness after discharge to the community (Wolff, 2005). Approximately 16% of the inmates in New Jersey's prison system are classified as receiving "mental health treatment of some type" while in prison (a number which grossly underrepresents the true need). Approximately 67% of those inmates were identified as having a serious mental illness with the majority having major depression (41%), followed by schizophrenia (27%) and other Axis I disorders. This study describes considerable variation in what these prisoners actually "needed" for mental health care and their "placement characteristics" (e.g., nonviolent offenders; violent offenders). Patients were separated into two groups of need (not serious mental illness; serious mental illness) and two groups of "placement characteristics." Based on their cluster model, they estimated costs of investing into reentry planning and community-based treatment of these offenders.

This model is very interesting as it specifically targets the different treatment and coordination efforts needed for released offenders based on the degree of mental illness and degree of serious crime. Those with a higher degree of mental illness and more serious crime convictions require more comprehensive treatment and community services on transition to the community. Twenty percent of the NJ DOC released inmates have a special needs requirement each year. Planning community linkage and mental health treatment for released prisoners was proposed to be divided into two sections. The first step included four reentry planning tiers ranging from Tier 4 having the most extensive coordination for reentry into the community requiring 18 months of specialized coordination by a mental health professional beginning 6 months before release; to Tier 1 requiring the least amount of time with estimated 4 weeks of mental health professional experience only beginning 2 weeks prior to release to the community. Second, four community treatment alternatives were divided ranging from Tier 4, Assertive Community Treatment (ACT): where case management included one face-to-face meeting each week with a case manager, substance abuse counseling, and medication monitoring by a psychiatrist or nurse; to Tier 1 which was considered non-case managed care and involved the least amount of time for psychiatric treatment.

Estimates of costs suggest that the NJ DOC may not save money; however, the authors argue that such a four-tiered planning and treatment program would overall improve the public's investment by providing better allocated services and thereby reduce recidivism. At present there is no specific mental health needs-based community linkage program within the NJ DOC, but the authors provocatively suggest ways of improving treatment and transition to the community for released prisoners with comorbid mental illness.

Reducing Postrelease High-Risk Behavior

There is a significant degree of high-risk sexual behaviors and substance abuse among incarcerated persons prior to their incarceration, and in certain cases, albeit markedly reduced, during their incarceration (Stephenson et al., 2006). Most prisoners have a high degree of other sexually transmitted diseases besides HIV on entrance to correctional facilities including gonorrhea, syphilis, and chlamydia (Hammett et al., 2002). Studies have found that the prevalence of HIV and STDs are higher among female than male inmates. A quarter of all people living with HIV in 1999 were released from a prison or jail that same year in the southern United States (Hammett et al., 2002). Due to the high percentage of persons with HIV who are being released to the community from prison with significant high-risk sexual behaviors and high degree of comorbid STDs, it is likely that transmission of HIV and other STDs such as gonorrhea, chlamydia, and syphilis occurs on release to the community. A study of 932 male IDUs and 505 female IDUs, of which 26% of men and 35% of women were HIV–infected, found that female sex workers were more likely to have had incarceration in the previous 6 months, and more likely than non-sex workers to be HIV-infected (Tyndall et al., 2002). Furthermore, female sex workers were unlikely to use condoms with regular partners, used about 50% of the time with casual partners, and used about 80% of the time with paid customers. HIV seroconversion during the follow-up period of the study was documented in 10% of active female sex workers and 7% of other female IDUs who were not sex workers. Female drug users are more likely to sell sex to pay for their drug habit and are therefore more likely to put themselves at risk for HIV and other STD transmission.

In one recent study of 550 state prison inmates, 70% admitted to having multiple sex partners and 45% had unprotected sex with multiple partners prior to incarceration. Men who drank alcohol heavily in this cohort or had a risky partner were more likely to report unprotected sex with multiple partners (Margolis et al., 2006). Similarly, approximately 50% of a smaller cohort of 64 HIV-infected releasees from North Carolina prisons reported sexual activity after release, and a quarter of them reported engaging in unprotected sexual activity with their regular partners(Stephenson et al., 2006). More alarming, 33% of the released subjects reported having unprotected sex with partners they believed to be HIV-seronegative. Studies have also demonstrated that high–risk drug injection behavior occurs within prisons. One Spanish study also suggests that incarceration status does not itself lead to HIV risk reduction behaviors (Estebanez et al., 2002). There is therefore a significant opportunity for correctional facilities to offer prevention services to this high-risk population. Unfortunately, most of these prevention efforts have been limited to HIV counseling and testing but very few HIV prevention comprehensive programs have been evaluated.

Correctional facilities are an ideal area to test and integrate primary and secondary prevention-based programs to decrease high-risk sexual and drug use behavior prior to release to the community. Harm reduction programs such as needle exchange programs and condom provision have been used in the community and in prisons with good success (F. L. Altice, Springer, Buitrago, Hunt, & Friedland, 2003; Nelles & Harding, 1995). In fact, the World Health Organization (WHO) recommended in 1993 to increase availability of condoms for prisoners as well as include needle exchange programs (WHO, 1993). Linking prevention education with opiate substitution therapy can likely improve prevention of transmission of HIV further by limiting exposure to infected blood products (Longshore, Hsieh, & Anglin, 1994). Furthermore, other programs have studied intensive risk reduction education of prisoners and found this to reduce high risk-taking behavior after release to the community. One study in a men's prison in California provided eight consecutive 2-hour educational sessions on topics of HIV, including substance use and sexuality, to 97 men who were compared to 29 receiving standard care without an intensive health promotion intervention (Grinstead, Zack, & Faigeles, 2001). After release from prison, the intensive intervention group was less likely to have had sex since their release date and more likely to have used a condom after their release than the comparison group. Furthermore, the intervention group participants were less likely to have injected drugs or to have shared needles than the comparison group. This highly intensive educational initiative did appear to decrease HIV risk-taking behaviors in this incarcerated group of men suggesting its role for replication in other correctional facilities. Integration of prevention services along with substance abuse treatment and intensive case management would markedly reduce new HIV infections when these services are continued after release to the community. Programs should evaluate intensive case management services at time of release associated with continued prevention education regarding sexual and IDU risk-taking behaviors that are also linked with drug and alcohol treatment and mental health programs.

Conclusions

Released HIV-infected prisoners face many obstacles on reentry into the community. Such obstacles include access to medical care for their underlying HIV infection, mental health care, substance abuse treatment, as well as homelessness and unemployment. Intensive case management services can be effective if continued consistently after release, not just prior to release. The current case management programs in the United States designed for released prisoners have not demonstrated improved HIV clinical endpoints. DAART may be one effective way to improve adherence after release from prison. Many released prisoners were opiate dependent prior to incarceration and as such are likely to relapse to drug use. For those who meet criteria for opioid dependence, treatment with opiate substitution therapy either before or immediately on release is an essential ingredient to prevent relapse, overdose, and recidivism. Provocative programs that integrate DAART with opiate substitution therapy (and other services) will be part of the future landscape of prison-release programs. Furthermore, mental illness assessment and treatment should be offered with DAART and opiate substitution therapy, given the high degree of untreated comorbid mental illness that adversely affects adherence to antiretroviral therapy and increases risk of relapse to drug use. Future programs should be integrated with intensive educational programs about harm reduction that includes condom promotion and needle exchange within prisons to decrease transmission of HIV and other STDs within prison and after release to the community.

All in all, transition to the community for released HIV-infected prisoners is complicated but can be addressed simply by having a unified treatment program that offers access to HIV treatment, risk behavior education, substance abuse treatment, case management, and mental health care in one geographic localized area. This will provide the greatly needed structure for these persons and remove the confusion and chaos that often undermines the effective care they received while incarcerated.

References

Altice, F., & Khoshnood, K. (1997). *Transitional case management as a strategy for linking HIV-infected prisoners to community health and social services (Project TLC)*. Paper presented at the Connecticut Department of Public Heath.

Altice, F., Mezger, J. A., Hodges, J., Bruce, R. D., Marinovich, A., Walton, M., et al. (2004). Developing a directly administered antiretroviral therapy intervention for HIV-infected drug users: Implications for program replication. *Clin Infect Dis, 38*(Suppl. 5), S376–387.

Altice, F. L., Friedland, G. H., & Cooney, E. L. (1999). Nevirapine induced opiate withdrawal among injection drug users with HIV infection receiving methadone. *AIDS, 13*, 957–962.

Altice, F. L., Mostashari, F., Selwyn, P. A., Checko, P. J., Singh, R., Tanguay, S., et al. (1998). Predictors of HIV infection among newly sentenced male prisoners. *J Acquir Immune Defic Syndr Hum Retrovirol, 18*, 444–453.

Altice, F. L., Smith-Rohrberg, D., Bruce, R. D., Springer, S., & Friedland, G. (2007). Superiority of directly administered antiretroviral therapy compared to self-administered therapy among HIV-infected drug users enrolled in a six-month prospective, randomized controlled trial. *JAMA*, in press.

Altice, F. L., Springer, S., Buitrago, M., Hunt, D. P., & Friedland, G. H. (2003). Pilot study to enhance HIV care using needle exchange-based health services for out-of-treatment injecting drug users. *J Urban Health, 80*, 416–427.

Babudieri, S., Aceti, A., D'Offizi, G. P., Carbonara, S., & Starnini, G. (2000). Directly observed therapy to treat HIV infection in prisoners. *JAMA, 284*, 179–180.

Badger, D., Vaughan, P., Woodward, M., & Williams, P. (1999). Planning to meet the needs of offenders with mental disorders in the United Kingdom. *Psychiatr Serv, 50*, 1624–1627.

Beck, A., Karberg, J., & Harrison, P. (2002). *Prison and jail inmates at midyear 2001*. Retrieved from http://www.ojp.usdoj.gov/bjs/pub/pdf/pjim01.pdf

Bouhnik, A. D., Chesney M., Carrieri, P., Gallais, H. et al. (2002). Nonadherence among HIV-infected injecting drug users: the impact of social instability. JAIDS 31, Supp 3, S149–153. Retrieved from http://www.ojp.usdoj.gov/bjs/pub/pdf/satsfp97.pdf

Bruce, R. D., Altice, F. L., Gourevitch, M. N., & Friedland, G. H. (2006). Pharmacokinetic drug interactions between opioid agonist therapy and antiretroviral medications: Implications and management for clinical practice. *J Acquir Immune Defic Syndr, 41*, 563–572.

Carrieri, M. P., Chesney, M. A., Spire, B., Loundou, A., Sobel, A., Lepeu, G., et al. (2003). Failure to maintain adherence to HAART in a cohort of French HIV-positive injecting drug users. *Int J Behav Med, 10*, 1–14.

CDC. (1999). Decrease in AIDS-related mortality in a state correctional system— New York, 1995–1998. *MMWR, 47*(51–52), 1115–1117.

CDC. (2001). *Helping inmates return to the community*. Retrieved 2004 from www. cdc.gov/idu.

Cloutier, G. (2002, July 7–21). *Strategies to support treatment adherence in newly released HIV-positive prisoners*. Paper presented at the XIV International AIDS Conference, Barcelona, Spain.

Conklin, T. J., Lincoln, T., & Flanigan, T. P. (1998). A public health model to connect correctional health care with communities. *Am J Public Health, 88*, 1249–1250.

Crosland, C., Poshkus, M., & Rich, J. D. (2002). Treating prisoners with HIV/AIDS: The importance of early identification, effective treatment, and community follow-up. *AIDS Clin Care, 14*(8), 67–71, 76.

Daar, E. S., Cohen, C., Remien, R., Sherer, R., & Smith, K. (2003). Improving adherence to antiretroviral therapy. *AIDS Read, 13*(2), 81–82, 85–86, 88–90.

Dolan, K., Hall, W., & Wodak, A. (1996). Methadone maintenance reduces injecting in prison. *BMJ, 312*, 1162.

Durand, E. (2001). [Changes in high-dose buprenorphine maintenance therapy at the Fleury-Merogis (France) prison since 1996]. *Ann Med Interne (Paris), 152* (Suppl. 7), 9–14.

Estebanez, P., Zunzunegui, M. V., Aguilar, M. D., Russell, N., Cifuentes, I., & Hankins, C. (2002). The role of prisons in the HIV epidemic among female injecting drug users. *AIDS Care, 14*, 95–104.

Feder, L. (1991). A comparison of the community adjustment of mentally ill offenders with those from general population: An 18-month follow-up. *Law Hum Behav, 15*, 477–493.

Fischl, M., Castro, J., & Monroig, R. (2001). *Impact of directly observed therapy on long-term outcomes in HIV clinical trials*. Paper presented at the 8th Conference on Retroviruses and Opportunistic Infections, Alexandria, VA.

Flanigan, T. P., Kim, J. Y., Zierler, S., Rich, J., Vigilante, K., & Bury-Maynard, D. (1996). A prison release program for HIV-positive women: Linking them to health services and community follow-up. *Am J Public Health, 86*, 886–887.

Glaser, J. B., & Greifinger, R. B. (1993). Correctional health care: A public health opportunity. *Ann Intern Med, 118*, 139–145.

Grinstead, O., Zack, B., & Faigeles, B. (2001). Reducing postrelease risk behavior among HIV seropositive prison inmates: The health promotion program. *AIDS Educ Prev, 13*, 109–119.

Hammett, T. M., Harmon, M. P., & Rhodes, W. (2002). The burden of infectious disease among inmates of and releasees from US correctional facilities, 1997. *Am J Public Health, 92*, 1789–1794.

Holmes, L., Drainoni, M., & Rich, J. (2002, July). *Harm reduction focused case management for multiply diagnosed HIV-positive ex-offenders*. Paper presented at the XIV International AIDS Conference, Barcelona, Spain.

Homebase, P. (2006). Retrieved April 3, 2006, from www.sph.emory.edu/HIVCDP/california.htm.

Hubbard, M. (2002, July). *The effect of discharge planning on health outcomes for HIV-infected prison inmates*. Paper presented at the XIV International AIDS Conference, Barcelona, Spain.

Kaplowitz, L., Kaatz, J., & Weir-Wiggins, C. (2002, July). *Seamless transition of HIV+ inmates into community care in Virginia*. Paper presented at the XIV International AIDS Conference, Barcelona, Spain.

Karberg, J., & James, D. (2005). *Substance dependence, abuse, and treatment of jail inmates, 2002* (No. NCJ 209588). Washington , DC.

Khalsa, J., Genser, S., Vocci, F., Francis, H., & Bean, P. (2002). The challenging interactions between antiretroviral agents and addiction drugs. *Am Clin Lab, 21*(3), 10–13.

Kiefer, F., & Mann, K. (2005). New achievements and pharmacotherapeutic approaches in the treatment of alcohol dependence. *Eur J Pharmacol, 526*(1–3), 163–171.

Kozal, M. J., Amico, K. R., Chiarella, J., Cornman, D., Fisher, W., Fisher, J., et al. (2005). HIV drug resistance and HIV transmission risk behaviors among active injection drug users. *J Acquir Immune Defic Syndr, 40*, 106–109.

Kushel, M. B., Colfax, G., Ragland, K., Heineman, A., Palacio, H., & Bangsberg, D. R. (2006). Case management is associated with improved antiretroviral adherence and CD4+ cell counts in homeless and marginally housed individuals with HIV infection. *Clin Infect Dis, 43*, 234–242.

Laufer, F., Arriola, K., & Dawson-Rose, C. (2002). From jail to community: Innovative strategies to enhance continutity of HIV/AIDS care. *The Prison Journal, 82*, 84–100.

Levasseur, L., Marzo, J., Ross, N., & Blatier, C. (2002). Frequency of re-incarcerations in the same detention center: Role of substitution therapy. A preliminary retrospective analysis. *Ann Med Interne, 153*(3 Suppl.), 1S14–19.

Linder, J. F., Enders, S. R., Craig, E., Richardson, J., & Meyers, F. J. (2002). Hospice care for the incarcerated in the United States: An introduction. *J Palliat Med, 5*, 549–552.

Longshore, D., Hsieh, S. C., & Anglin, M. D. (1994). Reducing HIV risk behavior among injection drug users: Effect of methadone maintenance treatment on number of sex partners. *Int J Addict, 29*, 741–757.

Lovell, D., Gagliardi, G. J., & Peterson, P. D. (2002). Recidivism and use of services among persons with mental illness after release from prison. *Psychiatr Serv, 53*, 1290–1296.

Lucas, G. M., Gebo, K. A., Chaisson, R. E., & Moore, R. D. (2002). Longitudinal assessment of the effects of drug and alcohol abuse on HIV-1 treatment outcomes in an urban clinic. *AIDS, 16*, 767–774.

Lucas, G. M., Mullen, B. A., Weidle, P. J., Hader, S., McCaul, M. E., & Moore, R. D. (2006). Directly administered antiretroviral therapy in methadone clinics is associated with improved HIV treatment outcomes, compared with outcomes among concurrent comparison groups. *Clin Infect Dis, 42*, 1628–1635.

Magura, S., Rosenblum, A., Lewis, C., & Joseph, H. (1993). The effectiveness of in-jail methadone maintenance. *J Drug Issues, 23*, 75–99.

Margolis, A. D., MacGowan, R. J., Grinstead, O., Sosman, J., Kashif, I., & Flanigan, T. P. (2006). Unprotected sex with multiple partners: Implications for HIV prevention among young men with a history of incarceration. *Sex Transm Dis, 33*, 175–180.

Mason, B. J. (2003). Acamprosate and naltrexone treatment for alcohol dependence: An evidence-based risk-benefits assessment. *Eur Neuropsychopharmacol, 13*, 469–475.

Mattick, R., Ali, R., & White, J. (2002). Buprenorphine versus methadone maintenance therapy: A randomized double-blind trial with 405 opioid-dependent patients. *Addiction, 98*, 441–452.

Mumola, C. (1999). *Substance abuse and treatment, state and federal prisoners, 1997.* Retrieved from

Nelles, J., & Harding, T. (1995). Preventing HIV transmission in prison: A tale of medical disobedience and Swiss pragmatism. *Lancet, 346*, 1507–1508.

Palepu, A., Horton, N. J., Tibbetts, N., Meli, S., & Samet, J. H. (2004). Uptake and adherence to highly active antiretroviral therapy among HIV-infected people with alcohol and other substance use problems: The impact of substance abuse treatment. *Addiction, 99*, 361–368.

Palepu, A., Tyndall, M. W., Li, K., Yip, B., O'Shaughnessy, M. V., Schechter, M. T., et al. (2003). Alcohol use and incarceration adversely affect HIV-1 RNA suppression among injection drug users starting antiretroviral therapy. *J Urban Health, 80*, 667–675.

Pollard, R. B. (2002). Can HIV infection be treated successfully with a once-daily regimen? *AIDS Read, 12*(11), 489–490, 494–498, 500, 508.

Rich, J. D., Holmes, L., Salas, C., Macalino, G., Davis, D., Ryczek, J., et al. (2001). Successful linkage of medical care and community services for HIV-positive offenders being released from prison. *J Urban Health, 78,* 279–289.

Richie, B. E., Freudenberg, N., & Page, J. (2001). Reintegrating women leaving jail into urban communities: A description of a model program. *J Urban Health, 78,* 290–303.

Roozen, H. G., de Waart, R., van der Windt, D. A., van den Brink, W., de Jong, C. A., & Kerkhof, A. J. (2006). A systematic review of the effectiveness of naltrexone in the maintenance treatment of opioid and alcohol dependence. *Eur Neuropsychopharmacol, 16,* 311–323.

Schottenfeld, R. S., Pakes, J. R., Oliveto, A., Ziedonis, D., & Kosten, T. R. (1997). Buprenorphine vs methadone maintenance treatment for concurrent opioid dependence and cocaine abuse. *Arch Gen Psychiatry, 54,* 713–720.

Shuter, J. (2002). *Communicable diseases in inmates; public health opportunities.* Paper presented at the Health Status of Soon-to-be-Released Inmates.

Sibbald, B. (2002). Methadone maintenance expands inside federal prisons. *CMAJ, 167,* 1154.

Smith-Rohrberg, D., & Altice, F. L. (2006). Randomized, controlled trials of directly administered antiretroviral therapy for HIV-infected patients: Questions about study population and analytical approach. *Clin Infect Dis, 43,* 1221–1222; author reply 1222–1223.

Smith-Rohrberg, D., Bruce, R. D., & Altice, F. L. (2004). Review of corrections-based therapy for opiate-dependent patients: Implications for buprenorphine treatment among correctional populations. *J Drug Issues, 34,* 451–480.

Smith-Rohrberg, D., Kozal, M. J., Springer, S., & Altice, F. L. (submitted). Similar Rates of Genotypic Resistance Among HIV-Infected Drug Users Receiving Directly Administered Antiretroviral Therapy and Self-Administered Therapy: Results from a Six-Month Prospective, Randomized Controlled Trial. Unpublished Journal Article. Yale School of Medicine, Yale AIDS Program.

Smith-Rohrberg, D., Mezger, J., Walton, M., Bruce, R. D., & Altice, F. L. (2006). Impact of enhanced services on virologic outcomes in a directly administered antiretroviral therapy trial for HIV-infected drug users. *J Acquir Immune Defic Syndr Hum Retrovirol, 43*(Suppl. 1), S48–53.

Sosman, J., Baker, J., & Catz, S. (2002). *Clinical and immune recovery during antiretroviral therapy among HIV-infected prisoners.* Paper presented at the XIV International AIDS Conference, Barcelona, Spain.

Spaulding, A., Stephenson, B., Macalino, G., Ruby, W., Clarke, J. G., & Flanigan, T. P. (2002). Human immunodeficiency virus in correctional facilities: A review. *Clin Infect Dis, 35,* 305–312.

Springer, S. A., & Altice, F. L. (2005). Managing HIV/AIDS in correctional settings. *Curr HIV/AIDS Rep, 2,* 165–170.

Springer, S. A., Pesanti, E., Hodges, J., Macura, T., Doros, G., & Altice, F. L. (2004). Effectiveness of antiretroviral therapy among HIV-infected prisoners: Reincarceration and the lack of sustained benefit after release to the community. *Clin Infect Dis, 38,* 1754–1760.

Stein, M. D., Solomon, D. A., Herman, D. S., Anderson, B. J., & Miller, I. (2003). Depression severity and drug injection HIV risk behaviors. *Am J Psychiatry, 160,* 1659–1662.

Stephenson, B. L., Wohl, D. A., Golin, C. E., Tien, H. C., Stewart, P., & Kaplan, A. H. (2005). Effect of release from prison and re-incarceration on the viral loads of HIV-infected individuals. *Public Health Rep, 120,* 84–88.

Stephenson, B. L., Wohl, D. A., McKaig, R., Golin, C. E., Shain, L., Adamian, M., et al. (2006). Sexual behaviours of HIV-seropositive men and women following release from prison. *Int J STD AIDS, 17*, 103–108.

Theall, K., Clark, R., Powell, A., Smith, H., & Kissinger, P. (2006). Alcohol consumption, art usage and high-risk sex among women infected with HIV [Electronic Version]. *AIDS and Behavior*. Retrieved September 18, 2006.

Thompson, A. S., Blankenship, K. M., Selwyn, P. A., Khoshnood, K., Lopez, M., Balacos, K., et al. (1998). Evaluation of an innovative program to address the health and social service needs of drug-using women with or at risk for HIV infection. *J Community Health, 23*, 419–440.

Tomasino, V., Swanson, A. J., Nolan, J., & Shuman, H. I. (2001). The Key Extended Entry Program (KEEP): A methadone treatment program for opiate-dependent inmates. *Mt Sinai J Med, 68*, 14–20.

Tucker, J. S., Burnam, M. A., Sherbourne, C. D., Kung, F. Y., & Gifford, A. L. (2003). Substance use and mental health correlates of nonadherence to antiretroviral medications in a sample of patients with human immunodeficiency virus infection. *Am J Med, 114*, 573–580.

Turner, B. J., Fleishman, J. A., Wenger, N., London, A. S., Burnam, M. A., Shapiro, M. F., et al. (2001). Effects of drug abuse and mental disorders on use and type of antiretroviral therapy in HIV-infected persons. *J Gen Intern Med, 16*, 625–633.

Tyndall, M. W., Patrick, D., Spittal, P., Li, K., O'Shaughnessy, M. V., & Schechter, M. T. (2002). Risky sexual behaviours among injection drugs users with high HIV prevalence: Implications for STD control. *Sex Transm Infect, 78*(Suppl. 1), i170–175.

WHO. (1993). *World Health Organization guidelines on HIV infection and AIDS in prison*. Strasbourg: Council of Europe: Ministers of the State Members.

Williams, S. H. (2005). Medications for treating alcohol dependence. *Am Fam Physician, 72*, 1775–1780.

Wohl, A. R., Garland, W. H., Valencia, R., Squires, K., Witt, M. D., Kovacs, A., et al. (2006). A randomized trial of directly administered antiretroviral therapy and adherence case management intervention. *Clin Infect Dis, 42*, 1619–1627.

Wolff, N. (2005). Community reintegration of prisoners with mental illness: A social investment perspective. *Int J Law Psychiatry, 28*, 43–58.

Index

Printed in the United States of America.